DRUGS AND ANESTHESIA

Pharmacology for Anesthesiologists

Second Edition

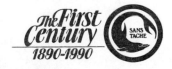

DRUGS AND ANESTHESIA
Pharmacology for Anesthesiologists

Second Edition
MARGARET WOOD, M.B. Ch.B., F.F.A.R.C.S.

Professor of Anesthesia
Associate Professor of Pharmacology
Departments of Anesthesiology and Pharmacology
Vanderbilt University School of Medicine
Nashville, Tennessee

ALASTAIR J. J. WOOD, M.B., Ch.B., F.R.C.P.

Professor of Medicine
Professor of Pharmacology
Departments of Medicine and Pharmacology
Vanderbilt University School of Medicine
Nashville, Tennessee

With nine contributors

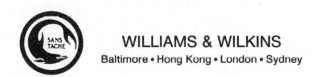

WILLIAMS & WILKINS
Baltimore • Hong Kong • London • Sydney

Editor: Timothy Grayson
Associate Editor: Carol Eckhart
Project Editors: Amy Walters Redmon, Susan Vaupel
Designer: JoAnne Janowiak
Illustration Planner: Ray Lowman
Production Coordinator: Anne Seitz

Copyright © 1990
Williams & Wilkins
428 East Preston Street
Baltimore, Maryland 21202, USA

Accurate indications, adverse reactions, and dosage schedules for drugs are provided in this book, but it is possible that they may change. The reader is urged to review the package information data of the manufacturers of the medications mentioned.

Printed in the United States of America

First Edition 1982

Library of Congress Cataloging in Publication Data

Drugs and anesthesia: pharmacology for anesthesiologists/[edited by] Margaret Wood,
Alastair J.J. Wood: with nine contributors.--2nd ed.
   p. cm.
  Includes bibliographies and index.
  ISBN 0-683-09253-7
  1. Anesthetics. 2. Pharmacology.   I. Wood, Margaret, 1946-
II. Wood, Alastair J. J.
[DNLM: 1. Anesthetics. 2. Pharmacology. QV 81 D794]
RD85.5D78 1990
615'.1'024617--dc 19
DNLM/DLC
for Library of Congress   89-5397
                                                      CIP

89 89 90 91 93
1 2 3 4 5 6 7 8 9 10

Dedicated to our children
ALASTAIR AND IAIN
without whose help this edition
would have been finished in half the time.

Preface to the Second Edition

Our goals remain the same: to apply a knowledge of the basic principles of pharmacology and pharmacokinetics to anesthesia and to illustrate the importance of these principles to the practicing anesthesiologist. Significant advances in therapeutics have been made since publication of the last edition, and new anesthetic drugs have been introduced into clinical practice. These changes have been incorporated into this new edition.

We have again chosen not to interpose references within the text to facilitate readability and the reader's ease of understanding; we have grouped the bibliographical references under subject headings so that the reader has more ready access to source material.

In spite of the trials of producing a second edition of this textbook, the combined authorship of an anesthesiologist and clinical pharmacologist has been maintained, and we hope this second edition will continue to be of value to both practicing anesthesiologists and those in training.

Margaret Wood
Alastair J. J. Wood

Preface to the First Edition _____

The purpose of this book is to fill a gap in the current anesthetic literature by providing a basic reference for the practicing anesthesiologist and also a textbook of pharmacology for the physician anesthetist in training, studying for board certification.

The underlying philosophy of our book is to apply a knowledge of the basic principles of pharmacology and pharmacokinetics to anesthesia, and to illustrate the importance of these principles to the practicing anesthesiologist.

Due to the complexity of therapeutic medical management today, the anesthetist must have not only a specialized knowledge of anesthetic agents, but also a knowledge of the wide spectrum of drugs that the patient may receive prior to surgery. The expanding role of anesthesiologists, particularly into the areas of intensive care and respiratory therapy, is increasing the number of drugs they use and the demands on their therapeutic and pharmacological knowledge. We have, therefore, included a detailed consideration of not only those drugs used principally by the anesthetist (such as neuromuscular relaxants and the volatile inhalational anesthetics) but also those drugs of importance used by other specialists, which the anesthesiologist will frequently encounter in daily clinical practice.

The book is divided into four parts. The first part includes general principles of pharmacology and pharmacokinetics; the second part of the book discusses the pharmacology and clinical use of the anesthetic agents themselves. The basic principles delineated in the first chapters are applied here to give a clearer understanding of the subject matter involved. The third part discusses cardiovascular pharmacology, an area particularly important to the anesthesiologist. The final part of the book deals in a systematic manner with the pharmacology of general therapeutic agents with a special relevance to anesthesia.

We hope that the combined editorship of a clinical pharmacologist and anesthesiologist will provide a textbook that is of use both to those anesthetists working for examinations, and also to the busy practicing anesthesiologist.

Contributors

Robert A. Branch, M.D., Ch.B., M.R.C.P.
Professor of Medicine
Professor of Pharmacology
Vanderbilt University School of Medicine
Nashville, Tennessee

Alan R. Brash, Ph.D.
Associate Professor of Pharmacology
Vanderbilt University School of Medicine
Nashville, Tennessee

Barry C. Corke, M.B., Ch.B., F.F.A.R.C.S.
Associate Professor of Anesthesiology
and Obstetrics and Gynecology
The University of North Carolina at
Chapel Hill
Chapel Hill, North Carolina

Michael H. Ebert, M.D.
Professor of Psychiatry and Pharmacology
Department of Psychiatry
Vanderbilt University School of Medicine
Nashville, Tennessee

John Feely, M.B., B.Ch., M.A., B.Sc., M.D.
F.R.C.P.(I)
Professor of Pharmacology and
Therapeutics
Trinity College
Dublin 2, Ireland

Russell G. McAllister, Jr., M.D.
Director, Department of Cardiopulmonary
Medicine
Glaxo, Inc.
Clinical Professor of Medicine
Duke University School of Medicine
Adjunct Professor of Pharmacology
University of North Carolina School of
Medicine
Research Triangle Park, North Carolina

Dan M. Roden, M.D.C.M., F.R.C.P.[C]
Professor of Medicine
Professor of Pharmacology
Vanderbilt University School of Medicine
Nashville, Tennessee

Richard C. Shelton, M.D.
Assistant Professor of Psychiatry
Department of Psychiatry
Vanderbilt University School of Medicine
Nashville, Tennessee

Raymond Woosley, M.D., Ph.D.
Chairman, Department of Pharmacology
Georgetown University School of
Medicine
Washington, D.C.

Contents

SECTION 4
GENERAL THERAPEUTICS

GENERAL PHARMACOLOGICAL PRINCIPLES

Drug Disposition and Pharmacokinetics

ALASTAIR J. J. WOOD

When physicians administer drugs to their patients, they do so in the expectation that the anticipated therapeutic effect will result. They are dismayed, therefore, when the patient either derives inadequate or no therapeutic benefit from the medication or, worse still, develops toxicity. It is often only at this stage in therapy that we examine the variables that ought to have been addressed prior to drug administration.

The aim of drug therapy is to deliver an effective concentration of drug to its site of action (target tissue) where it produces the desired therapeutic effect, while at the same time avoiding the delivery of drug concentrations that are high enough to produce toxicity. Individuals vary widely in their response to drugs. This variation is due to both differences in the concentration of drug available at the drug's site of action and differences in the individual's inherent sensitivity to the drug. An excessive drug concentration at the drug's site of action may result in toxicity, while inadequate concentrations will fail to produce a therapeutic effect. A dose response curve relating both the therapeutic response and adverse effects to drug concentration can be constructed (Fig. 1.1). The usual therapeutic concentrations within the so-called therapeutic window are those that produce therapeutic effects in a large proportion of patients while producing adverse effects in few. The ratio of plasma concentrations that produce therapeutic effects to those producing adverse effects is known as the *therapeutic ratio.* The higher the therapeutic ratio, the less likely is toxicity to occur at the usual therapeutic concentrations. An understanding of the factors determining drug concentrations within the body is crucial to rational drug use in patients and to achieving desirable plasma drug concentrations. Dost introduced the term "pharmacokinetics" in 1953 to describe the mathematical modeling of drug concentration activity relationships within the

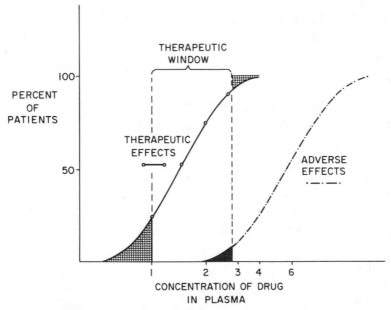

Figure 1.1.   Relationship between a drug's plasma concentration and its therapeutic and adverse effects.   The aim of pharmacokinetics is to achieve plasma drug concentrations within the "therapeutic window," i.e., concentrations that produce therapeutic effect in most patients while producing adverse effects in few. (With permission from Oates JA, Wilkinson GR: In *Harrison's Principles of Internal Medicine,* ed 12. New York, McGraw-Hill, 1989.)

body. Since that time, the term *pharmacokinetics* has come to be used to describe the study of drug disposition within the body, while the term *pharmacodynamics* has been used to describe the study of drug action.

PHARMACOKINETICS

The mathematical modeling of drug disposition requires a basic understanding of pharmacokinetic terms, which can easily be gained from consideration of the fate of a drug given intravenously. In the simplest case, in which a drug is administered intravenously and is distributed instantaneously, the body can be considered as a single container (compartment) to which the drug is added (Fig. 1.2). The concentration of drug in the container (C_{p0}) immediately following administration will then be

$$C_{p0} = \frac{\text{Dose}}{V_d} \qquad (1)$$

where V_d is the apparent volume in which the drug is distributed or the *volume of distribution* (the volume of the

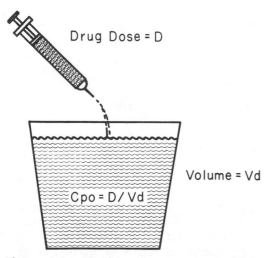

Figure 1.2. Single-compartment model in which, immediately following administration and assuming instantaneous distribution, the drug concentration in the container (C_{p0}) can be calculated from the dose (D) and the volume of the container (V_d) as D/V_d.

container in our example). It is important to note that this volume is *not* required to have any relationship to specific anatomical structures and that this situation can be generalized to any time following the drug's administration, when some drug elimination will have occurred, as

$$C_p = \frac{\text{Amount of drug in body}}{V_d} \qquad (2)$$

where C_p is the concentration of the drug at any time following the drug's administration. Thus the volume of distribution can be defined as

$$V_d = \frac{\textbf{Amount of drug in body}}{\textbf{Concentration in blood}} \qquad (3)$$

Following distribution, the drug is eliminated from the body by processes such as metabolism or renal excretion. Most drugs are eliminated by a *first-order* process, which implies that a *constant fraction* of the drug in the body is eliminated in any time period or that the rate of elimination is proportional to the amount of drug in the body at that time; i.e.,

Rate of elimination α amount of drug in body (Ab)   (4)

thus

Rate of elimination $= k_{el}Ab$ (5)

where k_{el} is the fractional elimination rate constant or the fraction of drug in the body eliminated in unit time and has units of time^{-1}. Of course, we do not usually know the amount of drug in the body at any time but can measure the plasma concentration (C_p).

Rate of elimination can then be expressed as

Rate of elimination $= Cl \times C_p$ (6)

where Cl or ***clearance*** **is the volume of plasma from which drug is completely removed in unit time.**

Combining Equations 5 and 6,

$$ClC_p = k_{el}Ab$$

but

$$Ab = C_pV_d \text{ (see Equation 2)}$$

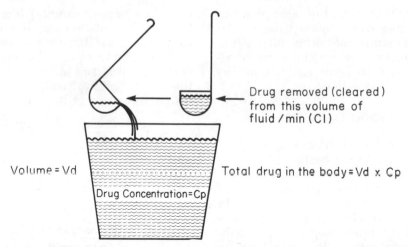

Figure 1.3. **Log plasma concentration versus time for a drug that, following intravenous administration, is instantly distributed (one compartment) and then is eliminated by a first-order process.** The slope of the line (k_{el}) is equal to $\dfrac{n\,C_{pl} - n\,C_{pl}/2}{t_{1/2}}$ (see text). In this example, the time taken for the plasma concentration to halve ($t_{1/2}$) is equal to 1 hour.

thus,

$$Cl = k_{el}V_d \qquad (7)$$

A characteristic of a first-order or exponential process is that equal fractions of the process occur in the same time. Thus, when plasma concentrations are plotted on a logarithmic scale against time, when elimination is first order, a linear plot will result (Fig. 1.3). (The exponential process can be expressed as $C_p = C_0 e^{-k_{el}t}$.) By definition, the slope of this line will be equal to $-k_{el}$ (because the slope of the line is the fraction eliminated in unit time or k_{el}).

The time taken for any plasma concentration to fall by one half is the *half-life* ($t_{1/2}$) and is the same at any concentration. For example, in Figure 1.3, the time taken to fall from C_{pl} to $\dfrac{C_{pl}}{2}$ equals the half-life if the slope is equal to k_{el} and ln C_{pl} is the natural logarithm of C_{pl}; i.e.,

$$k_{el} = \dfrac{\ln C_{pl} - \ln \dfrac{C_{pl}}{2}}{t_{1/2}}$$

but as

$$\ln C_{p1} - \ln \frac{C_{p1}}{2} = \ln \frac{C_{p1}}{\dfrac{C_{p1}}{2}} = \ln 2 = 0.693$$

Thus,

$$k_{el} = \frac{\ln 2}{t_{1/2}}$$

therefore,

$$k_{el} = \frac{0.693}{t_{1/2}} \qquad (8)$$

Substituting into Equation 7,

$$Cl = \frac{0.693V_d}{t_{1/2}} \qquad (9)$$

In theory, a first-order or exponential process will need infinite time to reach completion, but in practice, it is possible to calculate, in terms of half-lives, the amount of drug remaining in the body (Table 1.1; Fig. 1.3) and to show that after four half-lives the process is almost 94% complete. For example, it can be seen from Figure 1.3 that the drug concentration has fallen from 1000 ng/ml to 62.5

Table 1.1.
Relationship between Half-Life and
Amount of Drug Eliminated

No. of half-lives elapsed	Amount of drug remaining (%)	Amount of drug removed (%)
1	50	50
2	25	75
3	12.5	87.5
4	6.25	93.75
5	3.13	96.87

ng/ml after four half-lives have elapsed.

All of the principles of pharmacokinetics described previously can be visualized in terms of the ladle and container shown in Figure 1.4. The ladle (volume Cl) is dipped into the container (volume V_d) at a constant rate (say, once per minute). The drug contained in the ladle full of fluid or plasma is then removed from that fluid, and the drug-free fluid or plasma is returned to the container (Fig. 1.4). Thus, the amount of drug removed in unit time is the amount of drug in the ladle; i.e., $Cl \times C_p$. The fraction of the total drug removed in unit time (i.e., k_{el}) will be the volume of the ladle (Cl) divided by the volume of the container (V_d) (Fig. 1.4). Another extremely important principle is also demonstrated in this figure. If the volume of the container is increased, the fraction of drug removed in unit time (Cl/V_d) will be decreased, i.e., k_{el} will fall and the half-life or the time taken to remove 50% of the drug ($t_{1/2}$) (see below) will increase. No change will occur in the clearance (volume of the ladle), however, which is the primary determinant of drug concentration.

Thus, increasing the volume of distribution increases the elimination half-life

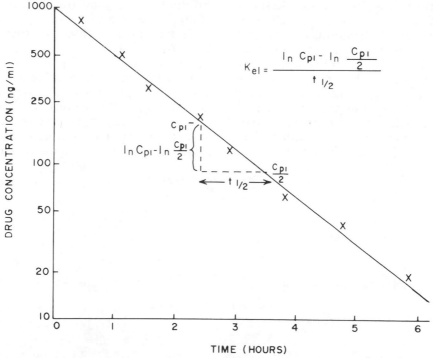

$$K_{el} = \frac{\ln C_{pl} - \ln \frac{C_{pl}}{2}}{t_{1/2}}$$

Figure 1.4. Conceptualization of pharmacokinetics. A ladle (volume = Cl) is dipped into a container (volume = V_d) of drug containing fluid (drug concentration = C_p) at regular intervals (say, once per minute). The drug is removed from the ladle, and now drug-free fluid is returned to the container. Thus, the volume of fluid *cleared* of drug in unit time is equal to the volume of the ladle (Cl). The fraction of drug removed in unit time is Cl/V_d, the rate constant of elimination (k_{el}).

but does not affect clearance. As clearance is independent of volume of distribution, clearance rather than half-life should be used as the preferred method of determining the efficiency of drug elimination.

Multicompartment Models

Up to this point we have assumed that following administration, a drug is instantly distributed in its volume of distribution. The situation is often not as simple as that, however, since distribution to all tissues does not occur equally fast. The more complex situation can be visualized in Figure 1.5, where the drug is rapidly distributed in the so-called central compartment and then slowly equilibrates with another (peripheral) compartment. The terms central and peripheral have no anatomical implication; rather, they imply differences in the rate at which drug distributes into them. During the period immediately following administration (distribution or α phase), a drug is moving from the central compartment to the peripheral compartment, resulting in a rapid fall in plasma levels until equilibrium is achieved between the drug in the tissues and in the blood. From that point, the tissue and blood concentrations fall in parallel due to drug elimination. This phase is known as the elimination of β phase. A two-compartment model such as this will result in a biexponential plot when plasma drug concentrations are plotted against time (Fig. 1.6). The biexponential has the form:

$$C_p = Ae^{-\alpha t} + Be^{-\beta t}$$

where C_p is the drug concentration at time t. A, α, B, and β are defined below.

The elimination (β) and distribution (α) processes are both first-order processes and therefore can be plotted separately as linear plots on a semilogarithmic scale. This can be done manually by "stripping away" the contribution that the β phase makes to the distribution curve. The β phase is extrapolated back to intercept the y axis. The intercept gives the value for $B(C_{p0})$ and the slope β. The values for the extrapolated β phase are subtracted from the measured values during the distribution phase, and the differences are plotted to give a line with a slope α and an intercept A, which represents the first-order distribution process. This is shown in Figure 1.6. The $t_{1/2\alpha}$ and $V_{d\alpha}$ can be determined from this line as outlined previously. It is, however, more usual to determine whether a one-, two-, or three-exponential curve describes the data best, by using a computer curve-fitting program to solve the appropriate equa-

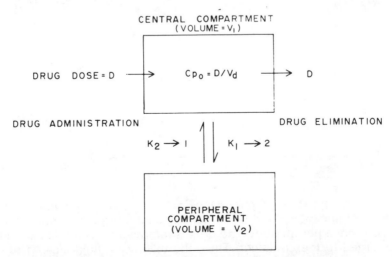

Figure 1.5.   Two-comparment model in which the drug is distributed instantaneously in the central compartment, but more slowly (with a rate constant of $K_{1 \to 2}$) to the peripheral compartment.

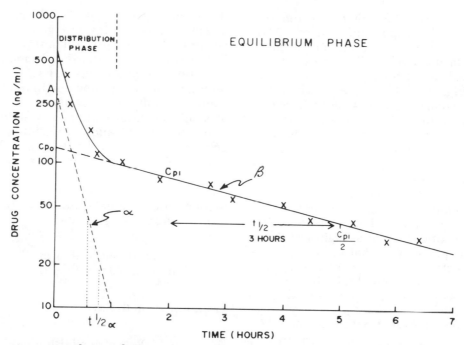

Figure 1.6. Log plasma drug concentration versus time for a drug that, following intravenous administration, is distributed rapidly into one compartment and more slowly into a second compartment (two compartment model).   There is a rapid fall in plasma levels following administration, which reflects distribution. Once equilibrium is achieved, the concentration falls exponentially due to elimination. The terminal or β phase has a *slope* β and can be extrapolated back to intercept the y axis at C_{p0}, which is the theoretical concentration that would have been achieved at zero time if the dose had been instantly distributed and that equals Dose/V_d. If the values of the back-extrapolated β phase are subtracted from the data during the distribution phase, the residuals can be plotted to give a straight line (---) with *slope* α and *intercept* A. The half-life of the α phase can be calculated and equals 0.2 hours in this case.

tions. The kinetics of the drug is then said to be described by a one-, two-, or three-compartment model.

Again, the half-life of elimination is the time taken for the concentration to fall by one-half during the elimination phase (3 hours in Fig. 1.6). Similarly, during the elimination phase, the other relationships derived previously for a one-compartment model are equally applicable.

Zero-Order Elimination

While most drugs are eliminated by first-order processes (constant proportion in unit time), some, such as alcohol, are eliminated by so-called *zero-order* processes *(constant amount in unit time)*. In

addition, and of particular importance, is the situation in which a first-order process changes to a zero-order process at high doses, so that whereas an increase in the dose of a drug eliminated by first-order kinetics will produce a proportional increase in plasma level, a similar increase in dose for a drug eliminated by zero-order kinetics will produce a much larger rise in plasma levels and a prolongation of the time needed to eliminate the drug. This can, therefore, be a very hazardous situation. Some drugs, such as phenytoin, salicylate, and theophylline, exhibit first-order elimination at low doses and zero-order elimination at higher doses because of saturation of the processes of elimination. This means that an increase in dose produces the expected and proportional increase in plasma levels until saturation is reached, when plasma levels will increase rapidly with very small further increases in the dose (Fig. 1.7). Conversely, when the plasma concentration is plotted against time, the rate of elimination increases as the plasma concentration falls (Fig. 1.8). Thiopental at doses required for induction of anesthesia (3.0 mg/kg) is eliminated by first-order kinetics. Thiopental at high dose (300 to 600 mg/kg), however, is eliminated by a zero-order process, resulting in unexpected prolongation of the recovery time following high-dose infusion compared with that following standard single doses. Figure 1.8 shows how the rate of thiopental elimination increases as plasma concentration falls.

Steady State Concentration

Up to this point we have considered only the disposition characteristics of a single intravenous injection. In practice, however, most drugs are given (a) by multiple doses or (b) by continuous infusion when it is important to maintain constant therapeutic effect, e.g., the continuous infusion of lidocaine in the treatment of ventricular arrhythmias. The plasma concentration at steady state (C_{ss}) achieved by continuous infusion can be determined from a knowledge of the clearance (Cl) and the rate of administration.

Because at steady state the rate of elimination must equal the rate of administration,

Rate of administration = Rate of elimination
Rate of administration = $Cl \times C_{ss}$

(from Equation 6) thus

$$C_{ss} = \frac{\text{Rate of administration}}{\text{Clearance}} \qquad (10)$$

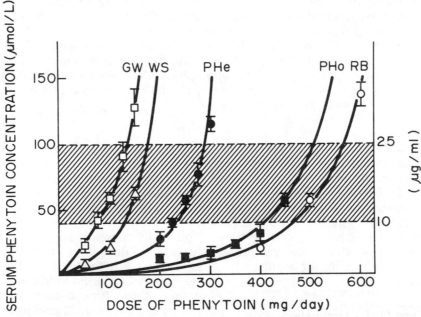

Figure 1.7.   Effect of increasing phenytoin doses on plasma phenytoin concentration.   At low doses, small increases in dosage produce proportional changes in plasma concentration. When higher doses are reached, however, a small increase in dose can produce a very large increase in plasma phenytoin concentration, resulting in toxicity. The therapeutic range is indicated by the *shaded area*. (With permission from Richens A, Dunlop A: Serum phenytoin levels in management of epilepsy. *Lancet* 2:247–248, 1975.)

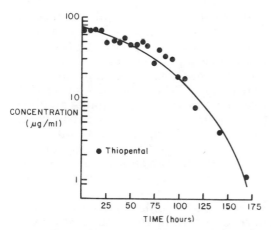

Figure 1.8. Plasma thiopental concentrations following high-dose thiopental infusion. The rate of elimination increases as the concentration decreases, demonstrating that at high doses thiopental is eliminated by a zero-order process. (Modified with permission from Stanski DR, Mihm FG, Rosenthal MH, Kalman SM: Pharmacokinetics of high-dose thiopental used in cerebral resuscitation. *Anesthesiology* 53:169–171, 1980.)

Similarly, when a drug that is eliminated by first-order kinetics is given intermittently, such that all of the drug has not been eliminated by the time the next dose is given, the drug will accumulate (Fig. 1.9). As this accumulation is a first-order process, it (like elimination, see Table 1.1) will be 94% complete after four elimination half-lives. Therefore, the time taken for a drug to achieve steady-state plasma concentration is about four half-lives. Thus, the longer the drug's elimination half-life, the longer it will take to accumulate to steady state. Obviously, with intermittent administration there will be considerable variability in the plasma drug concentration between doses (dosing interval). The average plasma concentration at steady state (C_{pav}) during intermittent dosing, however, can be calculated in a form analogous to Equation 10:

$$C_{pav} = \frac{\dfrac{Dose}{Dosing\ interval}}{Cl}$$
$$= \frac{Dose}{Dosing\ interval \times Cl} \qquad (11)$$

Loading Dose

When an effect is required immediately or, because of a drug's long half-life, it is impractical to wait until the drug has accumulated to steady state (four half-lives), a loading dose may be used to achieve the desired steady state therapeutic concentration (C_{ss}) rapidly. The loading dose required will be the total amount of drug that must be in the body to achieve the required plasma concentration (C_{ss}).

Thus from Figure 1.2 can be seen that

Loading dose required = Amount of drug required to be in body when plasma concentration is C_{ss}
= $C_{ss} \times V_d$ (from Equation 2)

But as V_d is often not readily available and the clinician may not know the desired plasma concentration, it is easier to

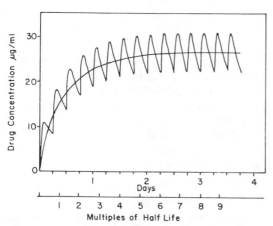

Figure 1.9. Drug accumulation to steady state following intermittent dosing (250 mg/every 6 hours) of a drug with a half-life of 9 hours. The *continuous line* joins the average drug concentration during the dosing interval. Accumulation is 94% complete after four half-lives (1.5 days). Time is shown in days and multiples of half-life.

express this in terms of the usual *maintenance* dosage regimen (e.g., 250 mg every 6 hours for the drug in Fig. 1.9).

As

$$C_{ss} = \frac{\text{Usual maintenance dose}}{\text{Dosing interval} \times Cl}$$
(from Equation 11)

substituting for C_{ss},

Loading dose required

$$= \frac{\text{Usual maintenance dose} \times V_d}{\text{Usual dosing interval} \times Cl}$$

but

$$\frac{V_d}{Cl} = \frac{1}{k_{el}} \text{ (from Equation 7)}$$

Loading dose required

$$= \frac{\text{Usual maintenance dose}}{\text{Usual dosing interval} \times k_{el}} \quad (12a)$$

or

$$= \frac{\text{Usual maintenance dose}}{\text{Fraction eliminated in dosing interval}}$$
(12b)

or

$$= \frac{\text{Usual maintenance dose}}{\text{Usual dosing interval}}$$

$$\times \frac{t_{1/2}}{0.693} \text{ (from Equation 8)} \quad (12c)$$

Depending on the information available to the clinician, any of these three equations (12a, 12b, or 12c) can be used to calculate the loading dose.

DRUG ABSORPTION

When a drug is taken by mouth, the speed of onset and the duration of its effect are partly determined by the rate and extent of its absorption from the gastrointestinal tract. Although theoretically absorption can occur anywhere within the gastrointestinal tract, the principal site of absorption is from the small intestine because of its enormous surface area. Thus, the rate at which drug leaves the stomach is a determinant of the speed of drug absorption. Narcotic analgesics markedly delay gastric emptying. General anesthesia and extradural anesthesia, on the other hand, do not affect gastric emptying. It is interesting that early labor does not affect gastric emptying, but late labor, i.e., 2 to 4 hours before delivery, does. Where rapidity of onset or bypassing of the drug-metabolizing systems of the liver is important to obtain therapeutic effect, however, sublingual or topical absorption may be utilized (e.g., with nitroglycerin). As absorption usually occurs by diffusion across lipoprotein cell membranes., the drug must be in a lipid-soluble form for absorption to occur. Accordingly, in the case of weak electrolytes that can exist in both ionized and unionized forms, depending on pH, absorption will be facilitated if the drug is in its unionized form. The effect of pH on the extent of ionization is determined by the drug's pKa (the pH at which it is 50% ionized). For a weak acid, an increase in the pH of one unit from the pKa will increase the degree of ionization to approximately 90% (see Table 1.4, page 23). This means that weak acids tend to undergo some absorption from the stomach where they are unionized, while bases do not. However, although theoretically under the alkaline conditions of the intestines an acid such as aspirin will be highly ionized (pKa = 3.4), resulting in poor conditions for absorption becaue of the large surface area of the small intestine and the prolonged contact that the drug has with the small intestine, this remains an important absorptive site.

The extent and rate at which drugs are distributed to tissues and the rate at which they enter the brain, and cross the placenta to reach the fetus, are dependent principally on:

1. The rate of delivery of the drug to the tissues, i.e., blood flow;
2. The extent of protein binding of the drug to the constituents of both blood and tissues;
3. The degree of lipid solubility and, hence, for weak acids and bases, their degree of ionization.

In addition to the use of such tradiional routes of administration as oral, intramuscular, and intravenous, the use of the transdermal route to achieve systemic effects has recently received attention. By using specially designed patches it is possible to overcome the fluctuation in plasma concentration usually produced by intermittent drug administration and to produce sustained drug concentrations for prolonged periods. Appropriately designed adhesive patches are now available that release a constant amount of drug to the skin surface for periods of as long as 1 week. In addition to providing sustained release, the transdermal delivery of drug also bypasses the first-pass hepatic metabolism to which drugs administered orally are subject. The transdermal approach has been used for a number of drugs, including clonidine, nitroglycerin, fentanyl, and hyoscine.

BLOOD FLOW

Not all of the organs and tissues of the body are perfused equally, so that in the few minutes immediately following a drug's intravenous administration, relatively more of the dose will reach those tissues that are highly perfused. Later, the drug will leave these tissues to move to the less well perfused tissues as equilibrium between drug in blood and drug in tissue becomes established there. Variation in tissue blood flow has an important influence on the disposition of thiopental, and clinical recovery from thiopental anesthesia is due to redistribution rather than elimination (see Chapter 8).

A particular case in which the anatomical distribution of blood flow is of great importance in drug disposition occurs in the case of drugs which are given orally and, following absorption, enter the portal venous system and pass to the liver. All of the drug must pass through the liver prior to entering the systemic circulation. Drugs such as lidocaine and propranolol are highly extracted by the liver, such that relatively little of the drug is able to pass through the liver and into the systemic circulation because most of the drug is metabolized and removed in its first passage through the

liver en route from the gut. This is known as *first-pass metabolism* and results in very poor systemic availability when the drug is given by mouth and considerable disparity between equieffective oral and intravenous doses (see Fig. 1.24, page 25). For example, an intravenous dose of propranolol of 0.055 mg/min (or approximately 80 mg/day) produces blood levels similar to those produced by oral administration of 240 mg/day. When drugs subject to extensive first-pass metabolism are given, it is necessary to keep this disparity between oral and intravenous doses in mind in determining how much of the drug to give systemically. First-pass metabolism is discussed in more detail later in this chapter.

PROTEIN BINDING

In plasma, drugs are bound to plasma proteins in a reversible fashion, i.e.,

$$\text{Drug} + \text{protein} \underset{K_2}{\overset{K_1}{\rightleftharpoons}} \text{Drug-protein complex}$$

so that drug exists in two forms in plasma—bound and free or unbound. The extent of protein binding is an important determinant not only of drug disposition but also of drug efficacy, since it is the free or unbound fraction of drug in plasma that is available for distribution outside the plasma space, for metabolism by drug metabolizing enzymes, for crossing biological membranes such as the placenta, and for binding to receptor sites and producing the drug's pharmacological effect. The extent to which a drug is protein bound is also important in facilitating its absorption. The free or unbound drug equilibrates across the cell membrane, so that in the plasma the proteins tend to reduce that free concentration, allowing more drug to cross the membrane faster and speeding absorption. The converse is also true for drugs leaving the plasma to enter the tissues where, disregarding other factors, the greater the degree of protein binding, the less drug will be available to leave the plasma space and, hence, the smaller will

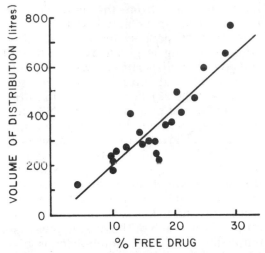

Figure 1.10. Relationship between the volume of distribution (V_d) of propranolol and the unbound fraction (% free drug) in a group of normal and diseased subjects. (Modified with permission from Branch RA, Jones J, Read AE: A study of factors influencing drug disposition in chronic liver disease using the model drug (+)-propranolol. *Br J Clin Pharmacol* 3:243–249, 1976.)

be the volume of distribution (Fig. 1.10). On the other hand, interactions such as displacement which increase the free fraction will also result in an increase in the volume of distribution. The extent of protein binding is important in determining relative concentrations of drug (total) in equilibrium across membranes. Because, once equilibrium is achieved, the free drug concentrations will be equal on either side of the membrane, the total concentrations depend on the extent of protein binding (Fig. 1.11). Thus, in the example shown in Figure 1.11, where the drug is 90% bound on one side of the membrane and the total concentration is 100 ng/ml., the free concentration will be 10 ng/ml. At equilibrium, this will equal the free concentration on the other side of the membrane, where the extent of protein binding is only 10% resulting in a total concentration of only 11 ng/ml and a total concentration ratio across the membrane of 9:1. Superficial examination might suggest that as the concentration on one side of the membrane is 9 times that on the other side, much greater pharmacological effects will be produced on the former side. The pharmacological effect, however, is also dependent on the free concentration, so that in spite of the total concentrations being 9-fold higher on one side of the membrane than on the other, it would be predicted that because the free concentrations are the same, the pharmacological effects will be similar on either side. This emphasizes the importance of taking protein binding into account when

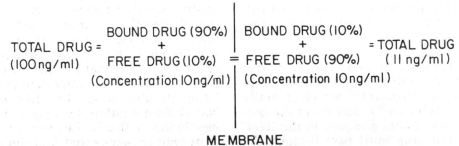

MEMBRANE

Figure 1.11. Disposition at equilibrium of a drug across a membrane when it is 90% bound in plasma on one side of the membrane and 10% bound in plasma on the other side of the membrane. Free concentrations on either side of the membrane will be equal. If, however, the drug is 90% bound on one side of membrane where its concentration is 100 ng/ml, the free concentration will equal 10 ng/ml. As this is the concentration that will equilibrate across the membrane, it will be equal on both sides of the membrane. On the other side of the membrane where the drug is only 10% bound, however, the total concentration will equal 11 ng/ml, giving a total concentration ratio of 9:1 across the membrane.

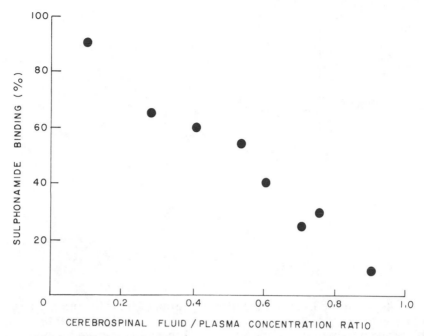

Figure 1.12. Relationship between the binding in plasma of a series of sulfonamides and their cerebrospinal fluid (CSF)/plasma concentration ratios. As the binding decreases and the free fraction increases, more drug can cross into the CSF, resulting in a higher CSF/plasma ratio. [Modified with permission from Smith SE, Rawlins M: *Variability in Human Drug Response.* London, Butterworths, 1973, p 47 (based on data from Garrod and O'Grady, In *Antibiotics and Chemotherapy,* ed 3. London, Churchill-Livingston, 1971).]

maternal/fetal ratios for drugs are compared (see Chapter 12 for a fuller discussion of this problem). The same considerations apply to the penetration of drugs across the blood-brain barrier and to their entry into the cerebrospinal fluid and brain tissues. Figure 1.12 shows the relationship between the extent to which a group of sulfonamides are bound to plasma protein and their ability to enter the cerebrospinal fluid. Distribution occurs even within the intravascular space with drug entering red cells according to the same principles, so that the ratio of drug concentration in blood to that in plasma (blood/plasma ratio) has also been shown to be proportional to the free fraction of drug in plasma (Figure 1.13).

Most drugs act by binding to receptor sites outside the intravascular space. It is the free fraction of the total drug in plasma that is available for leaving the intravascular space and binding to receptor sites, so that patients with a higher-than-normal unbound fraction of drug may show signs of pharmacological activity or toxicity at lower total drug levels. A good example of this is seen when the anticonvulsant phenytoin is used in patients with renal failure (see later in this chapter). In these patients, the free fraction is increased so that therapeutic effects occur at total drug concentrations below the usual therapeutic concentrations and toxicity occurs at total concentrations that would usually be considered to be within the therapeutic range, since in renal failure the free drug concentrations are higher than normal.

Disease states can exert a number of effects on the protein binding of drugs. For example, the concentration of albumin, to which many drugs are bound in plasma, may be reduced in patients with protein-losing renal disease, such as the nephrotic syndrome, and through failure to synthesize normal amounts of albumin, as in liver disease.

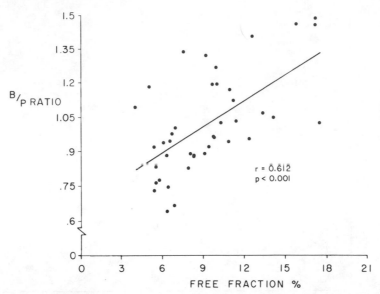

Figure 1.13.   Relationship between the blood/plasma (*B/P*) ratio and the free fraction of propranolol in plasma.   As the free fraction increases, more drug enters the red cells, causing the blood/plasma ratio to increase. (With permission from Wood M, Shand DG, Wood AJJ: Prapranolol binding in plasma during cardiopulmonary bypass. *Anesthesiology* 51:512–516, 1979.)

Table 1.2.
Drugs for Which α_1 Acid Glycoprotein (AAG) Is a Major Determinant of Plasma Binding

β-Adrenoceptor blockers	*Miscellaneous*
Alprenolol	Dipyridamole
Oxprenolol	Erythromycin
Pindolol	Metoclopramide
Propranolol	Prednisolone
Timolol	Progesterone
	Prazosin
Antiarrhythmics	*Opiates*
Aprindine	Methadone
Bupivacaine	Meperidine
Disopyramide	
Lignocaine	
Quinidine	
Calcium blockers	*Antidepressants and*
Verapamil	*psychoactive drugs*
Nicardipine	Amitriptyline
	Imipramine
	Nortriptyline
	Chlorpromazine
	Phencyclidine
	Triazolam

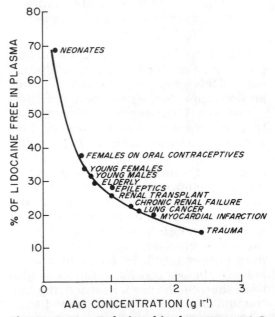

Figure 1.14.   Relationship between AAG concentration and unbound lidocaine (%) in plasma in various pathologic and physiologic states.   (Modified from Routledge PA: The plasma binding of basic drugs. *Br J Clin Pharmacol* 22:499–506, 1986.)

Table 1.3.
Pathophysiologic States Associated with Alterations in Plasma Proteins to Which Drugs Are Bound

Decreased albumin	Increased AAG	Decreased AAG
Burns	Burns	Neonates
Renal disease	Crohn's disease	Oral contraceptives
Hepatic disease	Renal transplantation	Pregnancy
Inflammatory disease	Infection	Estrogens
Nephrotic syndrome	Trauma	
Cardiac failure	Chronic pain	
Postoperative period	Myocardial infarction	
Malnutrition	Postoperative period	
Malignancy	Malignancy	
Neonates	Rheumatoid arthritis	
Elderly	Ulcerative colitis	
Pregnancy		

With permission from Wood M: Plasma drug binding implications for anesthesiologists. *Anesth Analg* 65:786–804, 1986.

Recently, it has been recognized that changes in α_1-acid glycoprotein (AAG) (an acute phase reactant protein) in certain disease states may be responsible for changes in the extent of protein binding in a number of basic drugs that are bound to this protein in plasma. Examples of drugs known to be bound to AAG are listed in Table 1.2. Chronic inflammatory diseases such as rheumatoid arthritis, inflammatory renal disease, and Crohn's disease (Table 1.3) are associated with a rise in AAG and, hence, an increase in the bound fraction of drugs such as chlorpromazine, lidocaine, and propranolol, which are highly bound to this protein (Fig. 1.14). In addition, certain acute inflammatory processes, e.g., following surgery, trauma, burns, or myocardial infarction, result in increased AAG concentrations and decreased drug binding (Table 1.3). The level of AAG is markedly reduced in the neonate, compared with that in the adult (Fig. 1.15), contributing to the reduction in the protein binding of a number of drugs in the neonate, including neuromuscular blocking agents *d*-tubocurarine and metocurine, propranolol, and lidocaine (see Fig. 1.34).

The contrasting effects on drug binding of changes in albumin and AAG are illustrated in burned patients in whom AAG

is elevated but albumin is reduced. This results in lowered binding of albumin bound drugs such as diazepam and increased binding of AAG bound drugs such as impramine (Fig. 1.16).

In addition to these quantitative differ-

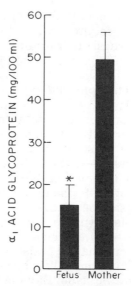

Figure 1.15. Concentrations in mothers and neonates. (With permission from Wood M, Wood AJJ: Changes in plasma drug binding and AAG in mother and newborn infant. *Clin Pharmacol Ther* 29:522–526, 1981.)

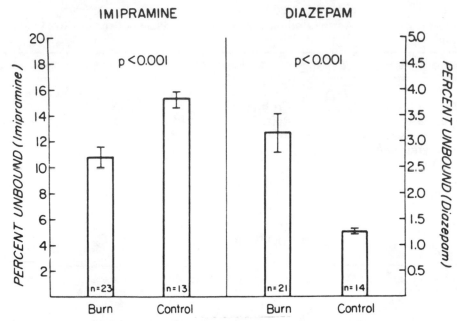

Figure 1.16.   Drug binding in burn patients.   The free fraction of imipramine is reduced, reflecting its increased binding and the elevated levels of AAG. Diazepam binding is reduced because of the lowered albumin concentration. (With permission from Martyn JAJ: Plasma protein binding of drugs after severe burn injury. *Clin Pharmacol Ther* 35:535–539, 1984.)

ences in the concentration of plasma proteins that cause alteration in the protein binding of drugs, other differences occur, such as those seen in renal failure where even in the face of normal plasma albumin concentrations the free fraction of phenytoin is increased. This may be due to either alteration in protein structure or the displacement of phenytoin from its binding sites by some metabolic product usually excreted by the kidneys. The result is that because of the higher free concentrations of phenytoin produced, the suppression of seizure activity occurs at lower total drug concentrations, and most importantly, toxicity occurs at total concentrations that, in patients with normal renal function, would be considered to be within the usual therapeutic range (Fig. 1.17). The defect in phenytoin's protein binding in uremia raises the free fraction from its usual value of around 7% to as high as 25%. The defect is not corrected by dialysis of the plasma but

can be corrected by exposure of the plasma to charcoal, suggesting the presence of a binding inhibitor. The half-life of phenytoin is reduced in uremia without any change in clearance, so that the usual total daily dose is required, but it should be given more frequently.

have been classified according to the substances shown to bind to them. On albumin, at least three separate drug-binding sites have been identified that bind diazepam, digitoxin, and warfarin. These drugs have been used as markers for these three binding sites. Compounds that share a common binding site may displace one another from that binding site. An example of such an interaction is seen when the anticonvulsants phenytoin and sodium valproate are coadministered (Fig. 1.18). Valproate binds to both the diazepam- and the warfarin-binding can be corrected by exposure of the plasma to charcoal, suggesting the pressite, while phenytoin binds to the warfa-

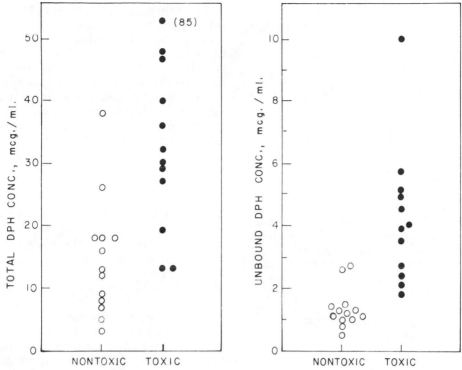

Figure 1.17.   Relationship of total and free phenytoin concentrations to toxicity. *Left hand panel* shows total phenytoin levels in patients who had signs of phenytoin toxicity and in those who did not. *Right hand panel* shows the concentrations of unbound or free phenytoin in the same patients. The use of free phenytoin concentrations greatly improves the discrimination between toxic and nontoxic patients. *DPH*, diphenylhydantoin. (With permission from Booker HE, Darcey B: Serum concentrations of free diphenylhydantoin and their relationship to clinical intoxication. *Epilepsia* 14:177–184, 1973.)

rin site. The plasma concentrations of valproate are much higher than those of phenytoin, so that the coadministration of valproate results in displacement of phenytoin from their shared binding site. Because of its lower concentration, phenytoin has minimal effects on valproate binding. By determining the binding site used by a drug it is possible to predict the likelihood of a displacement interaction occurring. For example, the penicillins, some hypoglycemics, and benzodiazepines displace diazepam from its binding site, whereas displacement of warfarin occurs with diuretics, phenytoin, sali-

cylic acid, and bilirubin which share the warfarin site.

Alterations in protein binding are usually only of importance for drugs that are highly protein bound, such as warfarin, propranolol, phenytoin, or diazepam. For example, for a drug that is usually 98% bound in plasma (2% free), reduction of the binding by only 2% will result in a doubling of the free fraction (Fig. 1.19, *drug A*), which may have profound pharmacological effects. For a drug that is only 70% bound in plasma (Fig. 1.19, *drug B*), however, a similar reduction in the bound fraction from 70% to 68% will

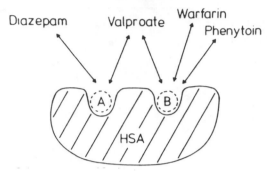

Figure 1.18. Binding of valproate and phenytoin to the diazepam- and the warfarin-binding site. Valproate binds to both the diazepam- and the warfarin-binding site. Because phenytoin also binds to the warfarin site, valproate can displace it from this site. (With permission from Kober A, Olsson Y, Sjoholm I: The binding of drugs to human serum. XIV. The theoretical basis for the interaction between phenytoin and valproate. *Mol Pharmacol* 18:237–242, 1980.)

cause a relatively small increase from 30% to 32% (a rise of only 7%) in the free fraction. Thus, this relatively small change in the free fraction would be unlikely to result in any clinically significant effects. In interpreting the therapeutic importance of reported changes in

drug binding, it is important to bear those relative changes in mind.

Drugs can be divided into two broad classes, depending on the avidity with which they are removed as they pass through the liver. This can be expressed as the fraction removed or extraction ratio. Drugs that are avidly removed from the blood by the liver, such as propranolol, are known as *high-extraction drugs*, but drugs that are poorly extracted, such as warfarin, are known as *low-extraction drugs* (see later). The extraction ratio of propranolol is around 78% after the first dose. As only 5% to 10% of the propranolol is unbound in plasma, the rate of removal is so high that the drug must be stripped from the plasma proteins to result in an extraction ratio that is much higher than the free fraction. For a drug such as warfarin or diazepam, however, this is not so. The extraction ratio is relatively low and is less than the free fraction. The significance of this is that for low-extraction drugs the extent of protein binding limits the rate of excretion or clearance, while for high-extraction drugs the clearance is independent of the extent of binding. The relationship between warfarin clearance and its free fraction is shown in Figure 1.20, and it can be seen that clearance increases as

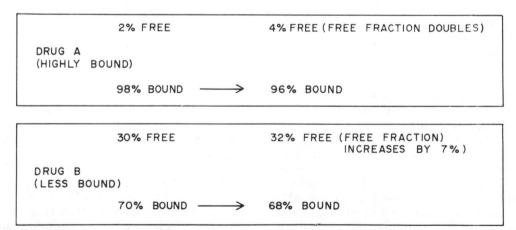

Figure 1.19. Contrasting effects of altered drug binding on a drug that is 98% (*A*) and 70% (*B*) bound in plasma. When the binding of *drug A* is reduced from 98% to 96%, the free fraction doubles (from 2% to 4%). When the binding of *drug B* is reduced by the same amount from 70% to 68%, however, the relative increase in free fraction is only 7% (from 30% to 32%).

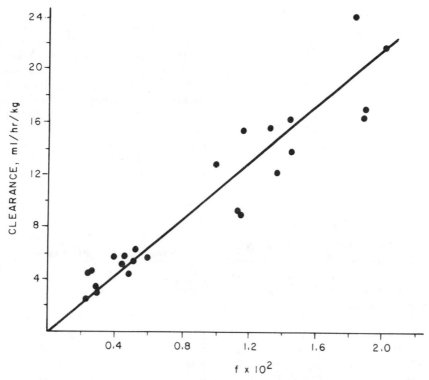

Figure 1.20. Relationship between the clearance of warfarin and the free fraction in plasma ($F \times 10^2$) in rats. As the free fraction increases for a low extraction drug such as warfarin, the clearance increases. (Modified with permission from Levy G: Clinical implications of interindividual differences in plasma protein binding of drugs and endogenous substances. In Benet LZ (ed): *The Effects of Disease States on Drug Pharmacokinetics.* Washington, DC, American Pharmaceutical Association, 1976, p 139.)

the free fraction increases. As the concentration of drug at steady state is dependent only on the dose and the drug's clearance; i.e.,

$$C_{ss} = \frac{\text{Rate of infusion}}{\text{Clearance}} \text{ (from Equation 10)}$$

the effects of altered protein binding on total steady-state drug concentrations will be different depending on the characteristics of the drug involved. The practical importance of these differences is shown in Figures 1.21 and 1.22. For a low-extraction drug (Fig. 1.21), if the free fraction is suddenly increased, for example, by a displacement interaction, the elevation in the free concentration will allow more of the drug to leave the intravascular space, resulting in a rise in the volume of distribution and a fall in the total drug concentration in plasma. With continued administration, however, the total concentration of drug would tend to recover, were it not for the clearance increasing, since, as described previously, for a low-extraction drug, the clearance is dependent on the free fraction. This increase in clearance will compensate for the rise in free fraction and will restore the free concentration to predisplacement levels, while the total drug concentration will be reduced. Thus after steady state has been reestablished, the free fraction will be higher and the total concentration will be reduced, resulting in an unchanged free concentration and, hence, no change in pharmacological effect.

For a high-extraction drug such as propranolol (Fig. 1.22), however, the rate of clearance is independent of the extent of

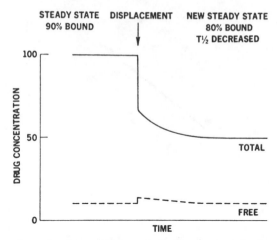

Figure 1.21. Effect of displacement from protein-binding sites on the total (———) and free (----) concentrations of a drug whose elimination is restricted by protein binding (low extraction). Following displacement, the free fraction of drug doubles, allowing more drug to be distributed outside the plasma space, causing the total concentration to fall. In contrast to Figure 1.22, however, with continued administration the higher free fraction results in an increased clearance (restrictive elimination), so that the total concentration falls and the free concentration is restored to predisplacement levels, although the total drug concentration has fallen to one half. (With permission from Shand DG, Mitchell JR, Oates JA: Pharmacokinetic drug interactions. In Gillette JR, Mitchell JR (eds): *Concepts in Biochemical Pharmacology. Handbook of Experimental Pharmacology 28/3.* New York, Springer-Verlag, 1975, p 295.)

protein binding (see previous paragraph). Thus, when the free fraction increases, there will be a similar fall in the total concentration because of the increase in the volume of distribution, but with continued administration in the face of an unchanged clearance, the total concentration will eventually be restored to its previous level. Because of the increase in the free fraction of propranolol, however, the free concentration will now be increased, resulting in an increase in pharmacological effect and possibly unex-

pected toxicity. An understanding of these predicted changes should assist in preventing adverse effects from the coadministration of drugs that displace one another at their protein-binding sites.

Although therapeutic drug monitoring usually only measures total drug levels, it has been shown that side effects of prednisone, phenytoin, and diazepam are more common in patients with low serum albumin, suggesting that measurement of the free concentration of such drugs might allow better prediction of toxicity. When free rather than total con-

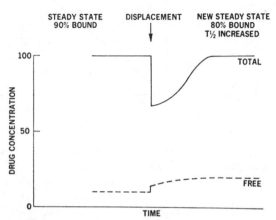

Figure 1.22. Effect of displacement from protein binding sites on the total (———) and free (----) concentrations of a drug whose elimination is not restricted by protein binding. Following displacement, the free fraction of the drug doubles, allowing more drug to be distributed outside the plasma space, causing the total concentration to fall. With continued administration, however, as the clearance is unaffected by protein binding (nonrestrictive elimination), the total concentration will return to predisplacement levels. This, coupled with the increased free fraction, results in an increase in the free concentration of drug. (With permission from Shand DG, Mitchell JR, Oates JA: Pharmacokinetic drug interactions. In Gillette JR, Mitchell JR (eds): *Concepts in Biochemical Pharmacology. Handbook of Experimental Pharmacology 28/3.* New York, Springer-Verlag, 1975, p 298.)

centration was used for monitoring phenytoin, an improvement in discrimination between toxic and nontoxic levels was found (Fig. 1.17).

Drug displacement interactions occur because many drugs and endogenous substances share common binding sites on plasma proteins. The clinical importance of the interaction will depend on the factors discussed previously, such as the extent of protein-binding, hepatic extraction ratio, and the therapeutic ratio.

DRUG IONIZATION AND PASSAGE ACROSS CELL MEMBRANES

The ease with which drugs cross cell membranes and the direction in which they move are partially dependent on the degree of ionization of the drug on either side of the membrane. The degree of ionization is dependent on the nature of the drug (acid or base), its pKa (negative logarithm of the acid dissociation constant), and the pH of its environment. Acids tend to be most highly ionized at high pH, while bases are most ionized at low pH. This is simply a function of the law of mass action. The ionized (H^+ and A^-) and unionized (HA) forms of an acid exist in equilibrium in solution as

$$H^+ + A^- \rightleftharpoons HA$$

The point at which this dissociation will establish equilibrium can be altered by the addition of hydrogen ions (i.e., lowering pH) that will shift the equilibrium to the right and, hence, reduce the degree of ionization. Thus, weak acids will tend to be relatively unionized at high concentration of hydrogen ions (low pH); the opposite is true for weak bases.

The Henderson-Hasselbalch equation relates the concentration of base [base] and acid [acid]:

$$pH = pKa + \log \frac{[base]}{[acid]}$$

Taking antilogarithms of both sides and rearranging,

$$\frac{[Base]}{[Acid]} = \text{antilog (pH} - \text{pKa)}$$

That is,

$$\frac{[Base]}{[Acid]} = 10^{(pH-pKa)}$$

For a weak acid it is the acid moiety that is unionized, while for a weak base it is the base that is unionized. Thus for an **acid,** this can be rewritten as

$$\frac{\text{Ionized}}{\text{Unionized}} = 10^{(pH-pKa)}$$

And for a **base,** as

$$\frac{\text{Unionized}}{\text{Ionized}} = 10^{(pH-pKa)}$$

For a weak acid a fall in pH of 1 unit from the pK will give

$$\frac{\text{Ionized}}{\text{Unionized}} = 10^{-1}$$

Thus a fall in pH of 1 unit will change the degree of ionization from 50% to approximately 10% (Table 1.4). Similar calculations can be made for weak bases.

For some membranes, such as in the stomach or placenta, the pH on either side of the membrane is different. Thus, the degree of ionization of a drug will be different on both sides of the membrane. In the gastrointestinal tract, this has implications for drug absorption, while entry of drugs into the fetus may be affected by the different pH on the maternal and fetal sides of the placenta, since equilibrium will be established for the nonionized portion of the drug. Figure 1.23 illustrates the situation for a weakly

Table 1.4.
Effect on Altered pH on Degree of Ionization of a Weakly Acidic Drug

	pH	% Ionized
Acidic	pK -2	1
	pK -1	10
	pK $-\frac{1}{2}$	24
	pK	50
	pK $+\frac{1}{2}$	76
	pK $+1$	90
Alkaline	pK $+2$	99

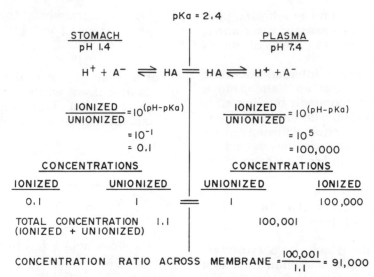

Figure 1.23.   Mechanism of "ion trapping."   A concentration gradient of 91,000 is established across the stomach for a weakly acidic drug with a pKa of 2.4, when the pH is 1.4 for the stomach contents and 7.4 for the plasma. The concentrations of unionized drug on either side of the membrane are equal and are arbitrarily given a value = 1.

acidic drug with a pKa of 2.4 in solution in the stomach, where the pH is 1.4. The drug can move from the stomach to the plasma (pH 7.4) until a total concentration ratio of 91,000 (actually 90,910) is established. Thus, weak acids are readily absorbed from the stomach, while bases are better absorbed from the more alkaline environment of the ileum and jejunum. In fact, because of the huge surface area and good blood supply, the small intestine is also an important site for absorption of weak acids in spite of the higher pH. Although Figure 1.23 represents the situation as static, in reality as drug is absorbed from the gastrointestinal tract it is continuously being removed by blood flow for distribution to the rest of the body and excretion. This helps to maintain the concentration gradient and facilitates absorption. On the other hand, when weak bases are administered systemically, they will tend to accumulate in the stomach because a concentration gradient opposite to that shown in Figure 1.23 for a weak acid will develop.

Similar effects are seen in the transfer of drugs across the placenta from mother to fetus, where the fetal pH is lower than

the maternal pH (see Chapter 12). This effect is known as ion trapping. The change in the degree of ionization with change in pH for a weakly acidic drug has been calculated and is shown in Table 1.4. It can be seen that a fall in pH of 1 pH unit from the pKa results in the degree of ionization decreasing from 50% to 10%. Similarly an increase in pH of the same magnitude from the pKa increases the degree of ionization from 50% to 90%.

DETERMINANTS OF HEPATIC DRUG CLEARANCE

The factors determining drug elimination vary depending on the characteristics of the drug in question. Elimination is best defined in terms of a clearance measurement that is the volume of blood from which drug is totally removed in unit time. Drug can be eliminated solely by renal excretion, by metabolism in the liver and/or in other organs, or by a combination of a number of these routes. For some drugs, the sole route of elimination is by metabolism in the liver. For such drugs, clearly the rate at which they are eliminated is dependent on both the liver's inherent ability to metabolize the drug and the amount of drug presented to the liver for metabolism. Drug reaches the liver via the portal circulation and by the hepatic artery. All drugs absorbed from the gut must, following absorption and passage through the portal venous system, pass through the liver prior to entering the systemic circulation. An appreciable proportion of drugs that are highly metabolized by the liver will, therefore, be removed from the blood prior to entering the systemic circulation. This phenomenon is known as *first pass metabolism* or first pass elimination (also called presystemic elimination) and results in a much smaller fraction of the dose entering the systemic circulation following oral administration than following intravenous administration (Figure 1.24). This results in a low systemic availability following oral administration and means that to obtain the same drug concentrations after oral administration as are obtained after intravenous administration a much larger dose must be administered.

Because of this central role performed by the liver in drug elimination, it is important to evaluate the effects on drug elimination of alteration in both the intrinsic ability of the liver to metabolize drugs and in the rate at which drugs are delivered to the liver through alteration in liver blood flow. The rate of removal

of drug from the body by the liver can be established by the hepatic clearance (Cl_H). By definition,

$$Cl_H = Q\left(\frac{Ca - Cv}{Ca}\right) \qquad (13)$$

where Cl_H is the hepatic clearance of the drug, Q is the hepatic blood flow, and Ca and Cv are the concentrations in the blood flow to the liver (mixed portal venous and hepatic arterial) and the effluent from the liver (hepatic venous), respectively. ($Ca - Cv$) is, therefore, the concentration gradient across the liver, and

$$\frac{(Ca - Cv)}{Ca} = E$$

where E is the extraction ratio. Therefore,

$$Cl_H = QE$$

Thus, **hepatic clearance (Cl_H)** depends on both liver blood flow and the liver's ability to remove the drug from blood as it passes through the liver, which in turn must depend on activity of the liver's drug-metabolizing enzyme systems. The intrinsic ability of the liver's drug-metabolizing enzyme systems can also be expressed as a clearance term ($Cl_{intrinsic}$). *In-trinsic clearance (Cl_{int})* **reflects the maximal ability of the liver to irrevers-**

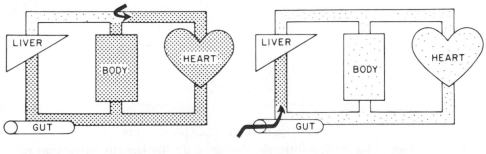

INTRAVENOUS   ORAL

Figure 1.24. Effect of presystemic elimination on the bioavailability of a drug. Following oral administration, all of the absorbed drug has to pass through the liver prior to entering the systemic circulation, so that for a drug that is highly extracted by the liver, relatively little will reach the systemic circulation, resulting in low bioavailability due to a high "first pass" effect. When the drug is administered intravenously, however, all of the drug enters the systemic circulation.

ibly remove the drug by all pathways and is independent of liver blood flow. It has been shown that

$$Cl_{H} = QE = Q \left[\frac{Cl_{int}}{Q + Cl_{int}} \right]$$

Thus, by rearrangement,

$$Cl_{int} = \frac{QE}{(1 - E)} \qquad (14)$$

Therefore, the *hepatic clearance* (Cl_H) of a drug is controlled by the two independent variables—hepatic blood flow and the intrinsic ability of the liver to metabolize drugs, i.e., Cl_{int}. Therefore, an increase in intrinsic clearance produced, for example, by enzyme induction will result in an increase of the extraction ratio (E). Because of the complex relationship between Cl_H, Q, and Cl_{int}, however, the magnitude of the change in E

depends on the initial Cl_{int} (Fig. 1.25). For drugs with a low Cl_{int}, a rise in intrinsic clearance due to an increase in enzyme activity will produce an almost proportional increase in the extraction efficiency (Fig. 1.25 *inset*) and hepatic clearance. However, for drugs with a high initial intrinsic clearance, increasing the intrinsic clearance has almost no effect on either the extraction ratio or hepatic clearance.

Change in the rate of drug delivery to the liver, i.e., liver blood flow, also affects liver clearance and extraction ratio but in opposite directions. Thus an increase in liver blood flow results in a fall in the extraction ratio (Fig. 1.26). For a drug with a high initial extraction ratio or intrinsic clearance, this fall in extraction ratio is relatively small and is almost linear, but for a drug with a low intrinsic clearance and extraction ratio, the in-

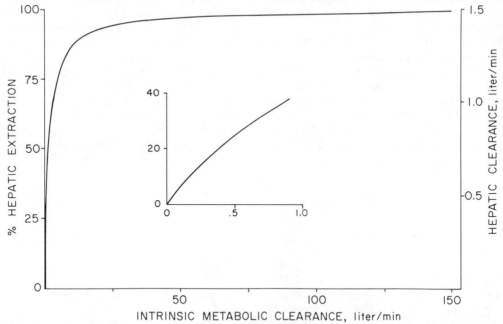

Figure 1.25.   Effect of increasing intrinsic clearance on the hepatic extraction ratio and hepatic clearance when liver blood flow (Q) equals 1.5 L/min.   For a drug that is totally metabolized in the liver, hepatic clearance equals the systemic or intravenous clearance. The *inset* shows an expanded scale for low values of Cl_{int}. For drugs with a high intrinsic metabolic clearance (>15 L/min), further increases in intrinsic clearance produce very little change in hepatic extraction ratios or systemic clearance. (With permission from Wilkinson GR, Shand DG: A physiological approach to hepatic drug clearance. *Clin Pharmacol Ther* 18:377–390, 1975.)

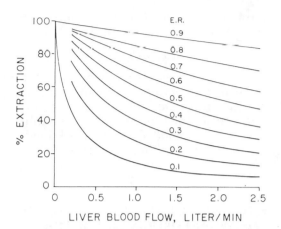

Figure 1.26. Effect of increasing liver blood flow on extraction ratio for drugs with different extraction ratios. Each *curve* represents a drug whose extraction ratio (*E.R.*) at 1.5 L/min is shown above that point. For drugs with a high extraction ratio, there is an almost linear fall in hepatic extraction ratio with increasing liver blood flow in the physiological range (0.5 to 2.5 L/min). For drugs with a low extraction ratio, however, there is little change in hepatic extraction ratio with increases in the liver blood flow over the same physiological range. (With permission from Wilkinson GR, Shand DG: A physiological approach to hepatic drug clearance. *Clin Pharmacol Ther* 18:377–390, 1975.)

crease in liver blood flow produces a large fall in extraction ratio, which to some extent compensates for the increase in blood flow. These changes in extraction ratio mean that for drugs with a high initial extraction ratio and intrinsic clearance, changes in liver blood flow produce an almost proportional change in hepatic clearance. For drugs with a low intrinsic clearance, however, changes in liver blood flow *over the physiological range* (0.5 to 2.5 L/min) produce little change in hepatic clearance (Fig. 1.27).

Drugs can, therefore, be classified according to their extraction ratios as high- or low-extraction compounds. The effects of changes in intrinsic clearance (Cl_{int}) or liver blood flow (Q) will be quite different in these two groups.

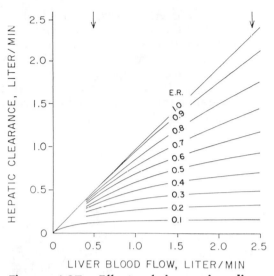

Figure 1.27. Effect of increasing liver blood flow on the hepatic clearance of drugs with varying extraction ratios. Each *curve* represents a drug whose extraction ratio (*E.R.*) at 1.5 L/min is shown above that flow. For drugs with a low extraction ratio, increase in liver blood flow within the physiological range (indicated by *arrows*) produces very little change in hepatic clearance. For a drug with a high extraction ratio, however, increases in liver blood flow produce an almost proportional increase in hepatic clearance, which for drugs that are totally metabolized by the liver is identical to the systemic or intravenous clearance. (With permission from Wilkinson GR, Shand DG: A physiological approach to hepatic drug clearance. *Clin Pharmacol Ther* 18:377–390, 1975.)

Clearance can be calculated as

$$\frac{D}{AUC}$$

where D is the dose administered and AUC is the area under the concentration/time curve (e.g., the area under the concentration/time curve shown in Fig. 1.6). Thus systemic clearance or the clearance following intravenous administration (Cl_s) will be defined as

$$Cl_s = \frac{D_{iv}}{AUC_{iv}}$$

where D_{iv} and AUC_{iv} are, respectively, the dose and the area under the concentration/time curve following intravenous administration. For a drug that is eliminated only by hepatic metabolism, Cl_s must equal the heptic clearance (Cl_H). The clearance following oral administration (Cl_o) can be calculated as

$$Cl_o = \frac{D_o}{AUC_o}$$

where D_o and AUC_o are, respectively, the dose administered orally and the area under the concentration curve following oral administration. Following oral administration and assuming complete absorption, only a fraction of the dose (F) enters the systemic circulation (see Fig. 1.24). This fraction, which enters the systemic circulation, will be handled identically to that which is administered intravenously, so that the practical effect is to reduce the apparent dose (see Fig. 1.24). Thus,

$$Cl_s = \frac{FD_o}{AUC_o}$$

$$\frac{Cl_s}{F} = \frac{D_o}{AUC_o}$$

But the fraction (F) of the oral dose that escapes metabolism as it passes through the liver on its "first pass" is equal to $(1 - E)$, where E is the extraction ratio. Thus, from the previous equations,

$$\frac{Cl_s}{F} = \frac{D_o}{AUC_o} = Cl_o$$

Therefore,

$$\frac{Cl_s}{1 - E} = \frac{D_o}{AUC_o}$$

and as

$$Cl_s = QE$$

$$Cl_o = \frac{D_o}{AUC_o} = \frac{Cl_s}{1 - E} = \frac{QE}{(1 - E)}$$

Therefore,

$$Cl_o = \frac{QE}{(1 - E)}$$

But Cl_{int} also equals $QE/(1 - E)$ (see Equation 14), so that for a drug that is completely absorbed and is completely metabolized only by the liver,

$$Cl_o = Cl_{int}$$

This is operationally extremely useful, in that it is, therefore, possible to calculate the intrinsic clearance, systemic clearance, extraction ratio, bioavailability and liver blood flow from a knowledge of the disposition characteristics of the drug when it is administered both orally and intravenously.

EFFECTS OF CHANGES IN LIVER BLOOD FLOW AND DRUG-METABOLIZING ACTIVITY ON DRUG DISPOSITION

As indicated previously, drugs can be classified as high- and low-extraction compounds according to their intrinsic clearance. From Figures 1.26 and 1.27, it will be recalled that the effects of altering liver blood flow on hepatic clearance depends on the drug's intrinsic clearance (or extraction ratio). It is possible, therefore, to predict the effects of alteration in hepatic blood flow and changes in intrinsic clearance on the disposition characteristics of the drug from a knowledge of its initial intrinsic clearance.

The effect of increasing intrinsic clearance, for example, due to increased enzyme activity produced by enzyme induction on the plasma drug concentrations following both oral and intravenous administration of a high- and low-extraction drug is shown in Figure 1.28. For a low-extraction drug $(E = 0.10)$ (Fig. 1.28, *left hand panel*), doubling the intrinsic clearance from 0.167 to 0.334 L/min results in an almost proportional increase from 0.10 to 0.18 in the extraction ratio. Half-life decreases to about one half of its previous value, and the clearance following both oral and intravenous administration is increased to almost the same degree.

On the other hand, doubling the intrinsic clearance of a high-extraction drug $(E = 0.90)$ (Fig. 1.28, *right hand panel*) only increases the extraction ratio from 0.90 to 0.95 and has almost no effect on the drug's half-life. The most striking difference, however, is the disparate effects on

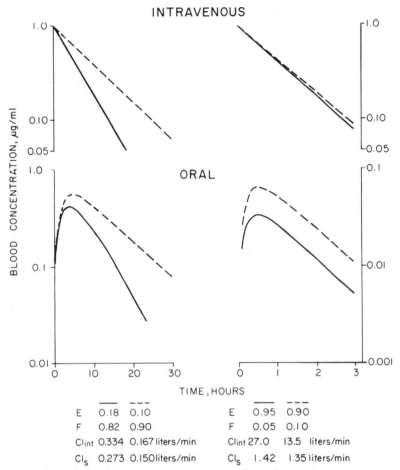

Figure 1.28. **Effect of doubling intrinsic clearance (Cl_{int}) on the concentrations in blood following the intravenous *(upper panels)* and oral administration *(lower panels)* of equal doses of two completely metabolized drugs.** The *left hand panels* show a low-extraction drug (E = 0.10) and the *right hand panels* show a high-extraction drug (E = 0.90) at a liver blood flow of 1.5 L/min. Doubling of the Cl_{int} of a low-extraction drug *(left hand panel)* results in an almost proportional increase in Cl_s and E. Doubling of the Cl_{int} of a high-extraction drug *(right hand panel)*, however, causes almost no change in Cl_s, so that the bioavailability (1 − E) is halved. (With permission from Wilkinson GR, Shand DG: A physiological approach to hepatic drug clearance. *Clin Pharmacol Ther* 18:377–390, 1975.)

the clearance following oral (Cl_o) and intravenous (Cl_s) administration. The clearance and the area under the concentration/time curve following intravenous administration are virtually unaffected, while following oral administration the clearance doubles, the drug concentrations in blood are reduced, and the area under the concentration/time curve halves. As the bioavailability (F) is equal to Cl_s/Cl_o and as Cl_o increases much more

than Cl_s for a high-extraction drug when the intrinsic clearance doubles, the bioavailability will be almost halved. Thus, for a low-extraction compound, when the intrinsic clearance or drug-metabolizing ability is increased, the clearance following oral or intravenous administration will be increased by approximately the same extent. For a high-extraction compound, however, increasing intrinsic clearance will significantly increase only

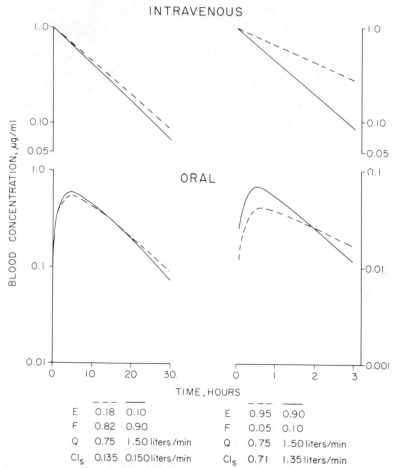

Figure 1.29. Effect of doubling hepatic blood flow *(Q)* on the concentration in blood of a low-extraction drug *(E = 0.10) (left hand panels)* and a high-extraction *(E = 0.90) (right hand panels)* drug following intravenous *(upper panels)* and oral *(lower panels)* administration. Doubling liver blood flow has little effect on the intravenous (Cl_s) or oral clearance (Cl_o) of a low-extraction drug, whereas it doubles the intravenous but does not affect the oral clearance of a high-extraction drug. (With permission from Wilkinson GR, Shand DG: A physiological approach to hepatic drug clearance. *Clin Pharmacol Ther* 18:377–390, 1975.)

oral clearance, there being little change in systemic or intravenous clearance.

The effects of doubling hepatic blood flow are shown in Figure 1.29 for a low- and a high-extraction drug. For a low-extraction drug (Fig. 1.29, *left hand panel*), doubling hepatic blood flow has no appreciable effect on the oral or systemic clearance or half-life. For a high-extraction drug, on the other hand, doubling hepatic blood flow (Fig. 1.29, *right hand panel*) reduces the half-life and increases

the systemic (intravenous) clearance. Oral clearance, however, will be unaffected, so that bioavailability (F) will increase.

In summary, an increase in drug-metabolizing ability (Cl_{int}) increases the extraction ratio and both oral and systemic clearance for a low-extraction drug. For a high extraction drug, however, increasing intrinsic clearance increases only oral clearance and, hence, reduces bioavailability. Increasing blood flow, on the

Table 1.5.
Effect of Increased Hepatic Blood Flow and Enzyme Activity on the Disposition of High and Low Extraction Compounds (No Change Implies No Pharmacologically Significant Change)

	Low extraction drug (E < 30%)	High extraction drug (E > 70%)
Effect of increased hepatic blood flow on		
Systemic clearance (Cl_s)	No change	Increased
Oral clearance (Cl_o)	No change	No change
Bioavailability (F)	No change	Increased
Half-life ($t_{1/2}$)	No change	Decreased
Effect of increased enzyme activity on		
Systemic clearance (Cl_s)	Increased	No change
Oral clearance (Cl_o)	Increased	Increased
Bioavailability (F)	No change	Decresased
Half-life ($t_{1/2}$)	Reduced	No change

other hand, does not affect the oral or the systemic (intravenous) clearance of a low-extraction drug but does increase the systemic (intravenous) clearance of a high-extraction drug. Thus, low-extraction drugs can be visualized as having enzyme-dependent kinetics, while the kinetics of high-extraction drugs are blood flow dependent. The kinetics of drugs with intermediate extraction ratios will be partially dependent on both liver blood flow and drug-metabolizing ability. The effects of changes in drug-metabolizing ability and hepatic blood flow on the disposition of low- and high-extraction drugs are summarized in Table 1.5, and examples of both types of compounds are given in Table 1.6.

EFFECTS OF AGE AND DISEASE ON DRUG DISPOSITION

Age

Frequently, the pharmacokinetics of drugs are defined in groups of healthy, normal, young male volunteers. The patients to whom the drugs are subsequently administered therapeutically, however, are often elderly with perhaps multiple disease processes. It is, therefore, important to evaluate the effects of both age and disease states on drug disposition.

As age advances, renal function deteriorates, resulting in impaired elimination of drugs such as digoxin, cimetidine, or pancuronium, which are excreted to a significant extent by the kidneys (Fig. 1.30). The degree of impairment in the excretion of such drugs parallels the fall in creatinine clearance. The disposition of drugs that are metabolized may also be affected by aging. For example, it has been shown that the blood concentrations of propranolol are twice as high in people over 35 than in those under that age (Fig. 1.31). Age is not the only factor causing this elevation in propranolol concentrations, however. When the effects of smoking were examined, it was found that the concentrations of propranolol in blood were 2 times as high in nonsmokers as in smokers (Fig. 1.32). In fact, smoking and aging appear to interact, so that only in smokers did the propranolol clearance fall with age, suggesting that perhaps as people age they become resistant to the known, enzyme-inducing effects of cigarette smoke.

Other dispositional changes found in the elderly include an increase in the volume of distribution of diazepam with a consequent prolongation of diazepam's half-life but with no change in the clearance. In addition to changes in the drug-metabolizing ability, it has also been shown that liver blood flow falls with age

Table 1.6.
Examples of Drugs That Are Thought to Have Either Low or Intermediate-to-High Extraction Ratios in Humans

Low extraction drugs
Amobarbital
Antipyrine
Mepivacaine
Warfarin
Tolbutamide
Phenytoin

Intermediate-to-high Extraction Drugs
Analgesics
  Acetylsalicyclic acid
  Meperidine
  Morphine
  Nalorphine
  Naloxone
  Pentazocine
  Propoxyphene
Psychoactive Agents
  Imipramine
  Nortriptyline
  Protriptyline
  Perphenazine
β-Receptor agonists and antagonists
  Alprenolol
  Metoprolol
  Propranolol
  Oxprenolol
  Salbutamol
  Isoproterenol
Others
  Lidocaine
  Indocyanine green

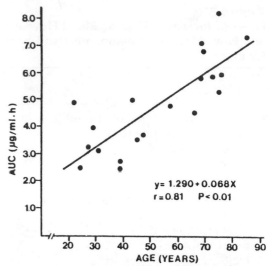

$$y = 1.290 + 0.068X$$
$$r = 0.81 \quad P < 0.01$$

Figure 1.30.   Effect of age on blood cimetidine concentrations. Cimetidine concentrations increase with advancing age due to decreased renal function. Seventy to 80% of cimetidine is excreted renally. (With permission from Redolfi A, Borgogelli E, Lodola E: Blood level of cimetidine in relation to age. *Eur J Clin Pharmacol* 15:257–261, 1979.)

(Fig. 1.33), suggesting that the elimination of drugs whose rate of removal is dependent on liver blood flow will be impaired in elderly patients.

Recently, it has become clear that there are pharmacokinetic differences at the other extreme of age. A number of physiological processes in neonates differ from those in adults and even from those in older infants and children. For example, both acetylcholinesterase and pseudocholinesterase levels are reduced in the blood of premature and full-term newborns. Adult levels are not reached until 1 year of age. In spite of the reduced pseudocholinesterase levels, however, newborns are more resistant to succinylcholine than are adults.

Plasma protein binding of a number of drugs is reduced in the newborn because of qualitative and quantitative differences in plasma protein, reduced blood pH, and the presence of elevated levels of endogenous substances that compete for binding sites. Recently, it has been shown that AAG levels are substantially reduced in newborn infants (Fig. 1.15). This contributes to the reduced binding of a number of drugs in the neonate, while the lower albumin concentrations in mothers at term account for the reduced binding of albumin-bound drugs, such as diazepam, in the mother (Fig. 1.34). This reduced protein binding results in increased volume of distribution for a number of drugs in the neonate.

The liver's ability to metabolize drugs in the neonate also seems to differ from

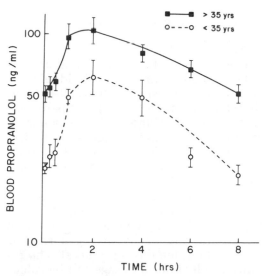

Figure 1.31. Effect of age on blood propranolol concentrations. The concentrations in the subjects over 35 years of age are more than twice as high as those under 35 years of age. (With permission from Vestal RE, Wood AJJ, Branch RA, Shand DG, Wilkinson GR: Effects of age and cigarette smoking on propranolol disposition. *Clin Pharmacol Ther* 26:8–15, 1979.)

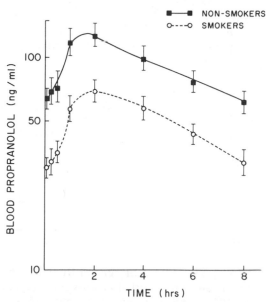

Figure 1.32. Effect of smoking on blood propranolol concentrations. The concentrations in smokers are less than half those in nonsmokers. (With permission from Vestal RE, Wood AJJ, Branch RA, Shand DG, Wilkinson GR: Effects of age and cigarette smoking on propranolol disposition. *Clin Pharmacol Ther* 26:8–15, 1979.)

that in the adult. All metabolic processes are not affected equally, however. For example, in the newborn the hydroxylation of diazepam and mepivacaine is reduced much more substantially than is demethylation of these compounds. Glucuronidation is impaired in newborns and premature infants due to reduced glucuronyl transferase activity resulting in accumulation of drugs such as chloramphenicol for which this is their major route of metabolism. The high concentrations of chloramphenicol in infants have resulted in toxicity (gray baby syndrome) which may be fatal. The impaired ability of the liver to eliminate a number of drugs results in a prolongation of the half-life in newborns compared with that in adults or older children (Table 1.7).

The elimination of renally excreted drugs is also reduced substantially in both premature and full-term newborns because of their poor renal function for the first 6 to 12 months of extrauterine

life. This means that drugs such as the aminoglycoside antibiotics and the penicillins whose elimination is dependent upon adequate renal function require careful adjustment of dosage regimen and, ideally, regular monitoring of plasma drug concentrations to prevent excessive accumulation and toxicity.

The use of digoxin in neonates and infants remains a controversial subject; however, it appears that infants aged 1 month to 2 years require higher doses (corrected for body weight) than do neonates or older children. It has been suggested that the half-life of digoxin is shorter in children aged 1 month to 2 years than in others and that the volume of distribution is higher in children, neonates, and infants. Suggestions that the myocardial sensitivity to digoxin alters with age have been made, but this remains an area of controversy. Never-

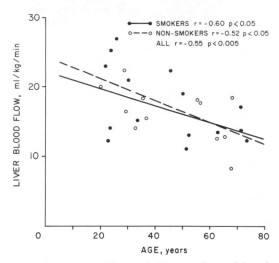

Figure 1.33. Effect of age on liver blood flow in smokers and nonsmokers. Liver blood flow fell with age independently of smoking habits. (With permission from Vestal RE, Wood AJJ, Branch RA, Shand DG, Wilkinson GR: Effects of age and cigarette smoking on propranolol disposition. *Clin Pharmacol Ther* 26:8–15, 1979.)

theless, clearly the dosage requirements for digoxin are far different in infants and children than in adults, and both plasma digoxin concentration and therapeutic effect should be monitored carefully. A suggested dosage scheme is given in Table 1.8.

Table 1.7.
Plasma Half-Lives of Drugs in Newborns and Adults

	Half-life (hr)	
	Newborns	Adults
Acetaminophen	3.5	1.9–2.2
Bupivacaine	25	1.3
Diazepam	25–100	15–25
Digoxin	60–107	30–60
Meperidine	22	3–4
Mepivacaine	8.7	3.2
Oxazepam	21.9	6.5
Theophyline	24–36	3–9

Effect of Disease

RENAL DISEASE

The presence of disease is another variable that adds to the interindividual variability in drug response. It is self-evident that for drugs that are principally excreted by the kidneys the presence of severe renal disease will significantly impair excretion. Fortunately, it is relatively easy to quantitate the extent of a patient's renal impairment from the creatinine clearance. Because of the reduced excretion, the drug dosage must be modified either by giving the usual dose less frequently or by giving a smaller dose at the same dosing interval. The required reduction in dosage can be calculated from a knowledge of the normal renal clearance (Cl_R) and nonrenal clearance (Cl_{NR}) of the drug. The dosage required in any patient can then be calculated as

Dose required in patient with renal insufficiency

$$= \text{Usual dose} \times \frac{\text{Patient's drug clearance}}{\text{Normal drug clearance}}$$

The patient's drug clearance is calculated as follows:

$$\text{Total clearance} = \text{Renal clearance } (Cl_R)$$
$$+ \text{ Nonrenal clearance } (Cl_{NR})$$

The patient's renal clearance can be calculated by comparing the patient's creatinine clearance (Cl_{CR}) to a normal clearance of 100.

$$\text{Patient's } Cl_R = \text{Normal } Cl_R$$
$$\times \frac{\text{Patient's } Cl_{CR}}{100}$$

Thus, the patient's total drug clearance

$$\text{Normal } Cl_R \times \frac{\text{Patient's } Cl_{CR}}{100}$$
$$+ Cl_{NR}$$

The effects of renal impairment on individual drugs are discussed in the appropriate chapters.

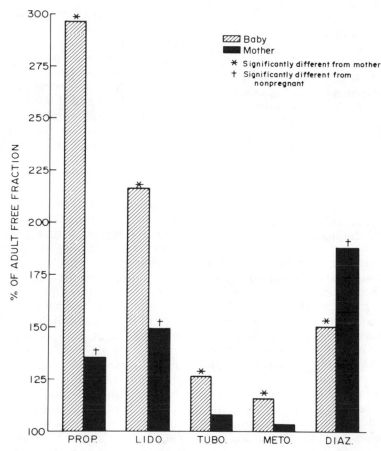

Figure 1.34.   Free fraction of propranolol *(Prop.)*, lidocaine *(Lido.)*, tubocurarine *(Tubo.)*, metocurine *(Meto.)*, and diazepam *(Diaz.)* in the neonate and mother expressed as a percentage of the nonpregnant adult value.   (Data are taken with permission from Wood M, Wood AJJ: Changes in plasma drug binding and α_1 acid glycoprotein in mother and newborn infant. *Clin Pharmacol Ther* 29:522–526, 1981.)

Table 1.8.
Oral Digoxin Doses (μg/kg) for Infants and Children

	Premature and low birth weight infants	Term neonates	Infants (1–12 mos)	Children	Adolescents
Total digitalizing dose*	20–30	30	35	40	15–20
Daily maintenance dose*	5–10	10	15–20	10	3.6–4.5

With permission from Gorodischer R: Cardiac drugs. In Yaffe S J (ed): *Pediatric Pharmacology. Therapeutic Principles in Practice.* New York, Grune & Stratton, 1980.
*Total digitalizing dose should be divided into three doses over 24 hours. Maintenance dose should be divided into 2 doses.

LIVER DISEASE

Liver disease will affect the excretion of drugs that are predominantly metabolized. Unfortunately, there is no liver function test that can quantitate the degree of liver impairment in the same way as the creatinine clearance can for renal disease. Clearly, in chronic liver disease, however, elimination of a number of drugs is impaired. Three factors should be considered in evaluating the alteration in drug disposition in liver disease:

1. Altered protein binding;
2. Altered drug-metabolizing ability; and
3. Portasystemic shunting.

Chronic liver disease produces changes in both the drug-metabolizing ability of the liver (intrinsic clearance) and the hepatic circulation. Total liver blood flow may be reduced; in addition, portasystemic shunting causes some of the portal blood flow to enter the systemic circulation directly, bypassing the liver's drug-metabolizing systems. The reduction in liver drug-metabolizing ability and altered hepatic hemodynamics reduces the clearance and increases the systemic availability (amount of drug entering the systemic circulation following an oral dose) of a number of normally highly extracted drugs (high clearance drugs), such as propranolol, meperidine, and pentazocine. In the case of propranolol, the clearance following oral administration is halved and the systemic availability is increased from 38% in normals to 54% in cirrhotics, resulting in higher concentrations and a longer half-life (Fig. 1.35).

The elimination of low-extraction drugs whose clearance is controlled principally by liver drug-metabolizing ability may also be altered in liver disease. For example, theophylline clearance is reduced in cirrhosis, resulting in an increased risk of toxicity. The effects of liver disease on the elimination of low-extraction drugs, however, depend on the metabolic pathways normally responsible for the drug's elimination, as it appears that all pathways are not affected equally by liver disease. For example, the clearance of both diazepam and chlordiazepoxide, which are oxidized by the microsomal mixed-function oxidase system, is reduced in liver disease. Drugs such as oxazepam and lorazepam, however, which are eliminated through con-

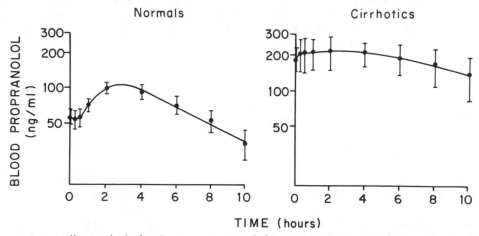

Figure 1.35. Effect of cirrhosis on propranolol concentrations. The concentration of propranolol after oral administration. The peak concentrations in the cirrhotic patients *(right hand panel)* are twice those in the normal patients. (With permission from Wood AJJ, Kornhauser DM, Wilkinson GR, Shand DG, Branch RA: The influence of cirrhosis on steady-state blood concentrations of unbound propranolol after oral administration. *Clin Pharmacokinet* 3:478–487, 1978.)

Table 1.9.
Effects of Route of Metabolism on Clearance of Benzodiazepines in Liver Disease

	Initial route of metabolism	Cirrhosis	Hepatitis
Diazepam	Oxidation	Decrease	Decrease
Chlordiazepoxide	Oxidation	Decrease	Decrease
Lorazepam	Glucuronidation	No change	No change
Oxazepam	Glucuronidation	No change	No change

With permission from Wilkinson GR, Branch RA: Effects of hepatic disease on clinical pharmacokinetics. In Benet LZ, et al (eds): *Pharmacokinetic Basis for Drug Treatment.* New York, Raven Press, 1984.

jugation pathways such as glucuronidation, are eliminated normally in both cirrhosis and viral hepatitis (Table 1.9). Oxazepam and lorazepam would, therefore, appear to be better choices for administration to patients with liver disease than is diazepam or chlordiazepoxide. In addition to the toxicity caused by elevated drug concentrations due to slowing of drug elimination, patients with chronic liver disease also exhibit increased sensitivity to a number of drugs.

CARDIAC FAILURE

Lidocaine is a drug that is highly metabolized by the liver, making its clearance, following intravenous administration, flow dependent. It is not unexpected, therefore, that the reduction in hepatic blood flow in cardiac failure would result in reduced lidocaine clearance. Thus, when lidocaine is used to suppress ventricular arrhythmias in patients with cardiac failure, a lower-than-normal rate of infusion should be used. In addition, because the volume of distribution is lower in such patients, a reduction should be made in the loading dose. Lidocaine is metabolized to two active and potentially toxic metabolites (see Chapter 11), monoethylglycinexylidide (MEGX) and glycinexylidide (GX). These metabolites are normally eliminated by both the kidney and by metabolism, so they too may accumulate excessively in cardiac failure. The excretion of digoxin and theophylline has also been reported to be impaired in patients with cardiac failure.

**THERAPEUTIC PLASMA
CONCENTRATION MONITORING**

From the previous discussions, the difficulties in predicting the plasma drug concentrations that a given dose will produce should be clear. Because of the large interindividual variability, measurement of plasma drug concentration can be used to assure that drug concentrations within the "therapeutic window" are achieved. Drug concentration measurements are most helpful when there is a relatively wide interindividual variability in steady-state plasma drug concentration, when the therapeutic ratio is low, and when it is hard to define underdosage or overdosage clinically. Certain patient groups, such as those with renal or hepatic disease and those receiving multiple drugs when drug interactions may occur (see Chapter 4), are clearly at special risk of developing excessive drug concentrations. Certain characteristics of the drug itself are also important in determining the usefulness of measuring plasma drug concentrations. There must be a reasonably constant relationship between plasma drug concentration and effect, preferably both therapeutic and toxic. The drug and not a metabolite, unless the metabolite is measured, should be responsible for producing these effects. Lastly, the effects of the drug should be reversible. A further practical point is that an assay for the drug must be available. There are now a number of drugs for which plasma measurements are widely available, and the therapeutic and toxic concentrations of some are shown in Table 1.10.

Table 1.10.
Therapeutic Drug Concentrations

Drug	Therapeutic range*
Carbamazepine	3–10 μg/ml
Digitoxin	10–20 ng/ml
Digoxin	0.5–2 ng/ml
Ethosuximide	60–100 μg/ml
Lidocaine	4–6 μg/ml
Phenobarbital	10–25 μg/ml
Phenytoin	10–25 μg/ml
Primidone	<10 μg/ml
Procainamide	4–8 μg/ml
Propranolol	50–100 ng/ml
Quinidine	2–5 μg/ml
Theophylline	10–20 μg/ml
Thiocyanate†	<100 μg/ml†

*Therapeutic range: therapeutic effects are seen in most patients with this range while few patients develop toxicity until concentrations are above this range.
†Thiocyanate levels during nitroprusside therapy above 100 μg/ml are frequently assoicated with toxicity.

PHARMACOKINETICS IN THE PERIOPERATIVE PERIOD

Little attention has been devoted to the study of pharmacokinetics in the perioperative period, so that very few data are available. Most of the research in this area has been performed in laboratory animals, and definitive studies in humans are limited. On average, patients receive 10 different drugs while in hospital, so the potential for drug interactions to occur during the perioperative period is great.

Absorption

Gastric and intestinal motility is reduced in the early postoperative period, suggesting that absorption of drugs administered orally may be impaired. In addition, it has been shown that administration of narcotic analgesics causes impaired absorption of acetaminophen used as a model compound. The use of anticholinergics such as atropine as a premedicant also delays drug absorption.

Drug Binding and Distribution

During the catabolic phase after surgery and trauma, there is increased nitrogen loss with increased albumin breakdown; albumin levels fall, whereas globulin concentrations may increase with resultant decrease in the albumin/globulin ration. Plasma α_1-acid glycoprotein concentrations increase after surgery and trauma.

Because of the postoperative fall in plasma albumin, the binding of phenytoin is reduced postoperatively, which as expected is associated with an increase in volume of distribution. It is important to note, however, that for a drug such as phenytoin, whose clearance is low and is dependent on drug binding, the fall in total phenytoin concentrations with continued phenytoin administration will restore the free concentration of phenytoin to normal, in spite of the elevated free fraction, For other drugs, such as quini-

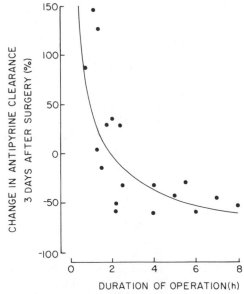

Figure 1.36.   Relationship between duration of surgery and change in antipyrine clearance 3 days postoperatively compared to 1 day prior to surgery. (With permission from Pessayre D, Allemand, H, Benoist C, Afifi F, Francois M, Benhamou JP: Effects of surgery under general anesthesia on antipyrine clearance. *Br J Clin Pharmacol* 6:505–513, 1978.)

dine, binding increases after surgery, probably because of the rise in the concentration of α_1-acid glycoprotein to which a number of drugs, such as propranolol, chlorpromazine, and lidocaine, are also bound (see page 17). Cardiopulmonary bypass for patients with ischemic heart disease is associated with no change in lidocaine clearance on the first postoperative day, but 3 days after surgery, α_1-acid glycoprotein concentrations are doubled, and free fraction is decreased, resulting in a 40% decrease in volume of distribution. Lidocaine clearance was also decreased (42%) 3 days after surgery.

Thus changes in the plasma binding of drugs in the perioperative period may cause changes in the volume of distribution and, possibly, changes in drug uptake. In addition, the changes in the distribution and amount of blood flow to various organs that occurs during anes-

thesia may also affect drug uptake and distribution.

Metabolism

Antipyrine elimination has been studied in patients preoperatively and 3 days postoperatively, and its clearance, which reflects drug-metabolizing ability, was increased in patients whose surgery lasted 2 hours or less but was decreased in those whose surgery lasted longer (Fig. 1.36). This suggests that the effects of surgery and anesthesia on drug metabolism may be dependent on both the duration and, also probably, the nature of the surgery and/or anesthesia undertaken. Halothane has been shown to inhibit drug metabolism in laboratory animals. Other volatile anesthetics may also inhibit drug metabolism (Fig. 1.37). The clearance of fentanyl and lidocaine is reduced during halothane anesthesia in

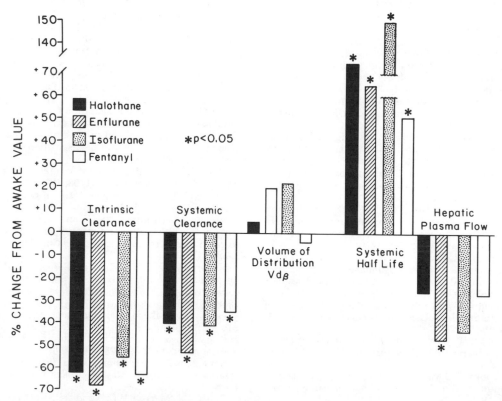

Figure 1.37.   Effects of administration of halothane, isoflurane, enflurane, and fentanyl on propranolol disposition in the dog.   (Data are from a series of studies by M. Wood.)

humans, and after cardiopulmonary bypass the clearance of digoxin and fentanyl is reduced.

Altered Liver Blood Flow

The rise in liver blood flow following
surgery might also be expected to alter
bioavailability and the clearance of drugs
whose hepatic extraction is flow dependent (see page 32). In the perioperative
period, however, the effects of altered
liver blood flow are relatively unex-
plored. In contrast, the fall in hepatic
blood flow that commonly occurs during
general anesthesia (Fig. 1.37) may be reflected in decreased drug clearance and
increased blood concentrations for
highly extracted drugs administered intravenously in the perioperative period.
Thus, many of the physiological changes
that occur in the perioperative period are
likely to affect drug elimination; the
pharmacokinetic significance of many of
these changes, however, remains to be
determined in humans.

BIBLIOGRAPHY

Bennett WM, Aronoff GR, Morrison G, Golper
TA, Pulliam J, Wolfson M, Singer I: Drug prescrib-
ing in renal failure: dosing guidelines for adults. *Am
J Kidney Dis* 3:155–193, 1983.

Benowitz NL, Meister W: Pharmacokinetics in
patients with cardiac failure. *Clin Pharmacokinet*
1:389–405, 1976.

Bjornsson TD: Nomogram for drug dosage adjustment in patients with renal failure. *Clin Pharmacokinet* 11:164–170, 1983.

Booker HE, Darcey B: Serum concentrations of
free diphenylhydantoin and their relationship to
clinical intoxication. *Epilepsia* 14:177–184, 1973.

Branch RA, James J, Read AE: A study of factors
influencing drug disposition in chronic liver disease, using the model drug (+)-propranolol. *Br J
Clin Pharmacol* 3:243–249, 1976.

Chelly, JE, Hysing ES, Abernethy DR, Doursout
MF, Merin RG: Effects of inhalational anesthetics
on verapamil pharmacokinetics in dogs. *Anesthesiology* 65:266–271, 1986.

Chennavasin P, Brater DC: Nomograms for drug
use in renal disease. *Clin. Pharmacokinet* 6:193–
214, 1981.

Cockcroft DW, Gault MH: Prediction of creatinine clearance from serum creatinine. *Nephron*
16:31–41, 1976.

Crooks J, O'Malley K, Stevenson IH: Pharmacokinetics in the elderly. *Clin Pharmacokinet,* 1:280–
296, 1976.

Elfström J: Drug pharmacokinetics in the postoperative period. *Clin Pharmacokinet* 4:16–22, 1979.

Fremstad D, Bergerud K, Haffner JFW, Lunde
PKN: Increased plasma binding of quinidine after
surgery: a preliminary report. *Eur J Clin Pharmacol*
10:441–444, 1976.

Gibaldi M, Levy G: Pharmacokinetics in clinical practice. 1. Concepts. *JAMA* 235:1864–1867,
1976.

Gibaldi M, Levy G: Pharmacokinetics in clinical
practice. 2. Applications. *JAMA* 235:1987–1992,
1976.

Gorodisher R: Cardiac drugs. In Yaffe SJ (ed): *Pediatric Pharmacology. Therapeutic Principles in
Practice.* New York, Grune & Stratton, 1980.

Holley FO, Ponganis KV, Stanski DR: Effects of
cardiac surgery with cardiopulmonary bypass on lidocaine disposition. *Clin Pharmacol Ther* 35:617–
626, 1984.

Hug CC: Pharmacokinetics of drugs administered
intravenously. *Anesth Analg.* 57:704–723, 1978.

Hull CJ: Pharmacokinetics and pharmacodynamics. *Br J Anaesth* 51:579–594, 1979.

Klotz U: Pathophysiological and disease-induced
changes in drug distribution volume: pharmacokinetic implications. *Clin Pharmacokinet* 1:204–218,
1976.

Klotz U, Avant GR, Hoyumpa A, Schenker S, Wilkinson GR: The effects of age and liver disease on
the disposition and elimination of diazepam in
adult man. *J Clin Invest* 55:347–359, 1975.

Koch-Weser J: Serum drug concentrations as
therapeutic guides. *N Engl J Med* 287:227–231, 1972.

Krauss JW, Desmond DV, Marshall JF, Johnson
RF, Schenker S, Wilkinson GR: The effects of aging
and liver disease on the disposition of lorazepam in
man. *Clin Pharmacol Ther* 24:411–419, 1978.

Martyn JAJ, Abernethy DR, Greenblatt DJ:
Plasma protein binding of drugs after severe burn
injury. *Clin Pharmacol Ther* 35:535–539, 1984.

Mather LE, Runciman WB, Illsley AH, Carapetis
RJ, Upton RN: A sheep preparation for studying interactions between blood flow and drug disposition:
V: the effects of general and subarachnoid anaesthesia on blood flow and pethidine disposition. *Br J Anaesth* 58:888–896, 1986.

Morselli PL: Clinical pharmacokinetics in neonates. *Clin Pharmacokinet* 1:81–98, 1976.

Nimmo WS: Effect of anaesthesia on gastric motility and emptying. *Br J Anaesth* 56:29–36, 1984.

Nimmo WS, Heading RC, Wilson J, Tothill J, Prescott LF: Inhibition of gastric emptying and drug absorption by narcotic analgesics. *Br J Clin Pharmacol*
2:509–513, 1975.

Nyberg L, Wettrell G: Digoxin dosage schedules
for neonates and infants based on pharmacokinetic
considerations. *Clin Pharmacokinet* 3:453–461,
1978.

Pessayre D, Allemand H, Benoist C, Afifi F, Francois M, Benhamou JP: Effects of surgery under general anesthesia on antipyrine clearance. *Br J Clin
Pharmacol* 6:505–513, 1978.

Rane A, Wilson JT: Clinical pharmacokinetics in
infants and children. *Clin Pharmacokinet* 1:2–24,
1976.

Reilly CS, Merrell WJ, Wood AJJ, Koshakji RP,
Wood M: Comparison of the effects of isoflurane
and fentanyl-nitrous oxide-atracurium anesthesia

on propranolol disposition in dogs. *Br J Anaesth* 60:791–796, 1988.

Reilly CS, Wood AJJ, Koshakji RP, Wood M: The effect of halothane on drug disposition: contribution of changes in intrinsic drug metabolizing capacity and hepatic blood flow. *Anesthesiology* 63:70–76, 1985.

Reilly CS, Wood AJJ, Koshakji RP, Wood M: Effect of enflurane anaesthesia on drug disposition in the dog. *Br J Anaesth* 58:802P, 1986.

Richens A, Dunlop A: Serum phenytoin levels in management of epilepsy. *Lancet* 2:247–248, 1975.

Richey DP, Bender AD: Pharmacokinetic consequences of aging. *Ann Rev Pharmacol Toxicol* 17:49–65, 1977.

Roberts RJ: Drug therapy in infants. In *Pharmacologic Principles and Clinical Experiences.* Philadelphia, WB Saunders, 1984.

Routledge PA: The plasma protein binding of basic drugs. *Br J Clin Pharmacol* 22:499–506, 1986.

Shand DG, Mitchell JR, Oates JA: Pharmacokinetic drug interactions. In Gillette JR, Mitchell JR (eds): *Concepts in Biochemical Pharmacology. Handbook of Experimental Pharmacology 28/3.* New York, Springer-Verlag, 1975.

Sheiner LB, Stanski DR, Vozeh S, Miller RD, Ham J: Simultaneous modeling of pharmacokinetics and pharmacodynamics: application to d-tubocurarine. *Clin Pharmacol Ther* 25:358–371, 1979.

Smith SE, Rawlins M: *Variability in Human Drug Response.* London, Butterworths, 1973.

Stanski DR, Mihm FG, Rosenthal MH, Kalman SM: Pharmacokinetics of high-dose thiopental used in cerebral resuscitation. *Anesthesiology* 53:169–171, 1980.

Vestal RE, Wood AJJ, Branch RA, Shand DG, Wilkinson GR: Effect of age and cigarette smoking on propranolol disposition. *Clin Pharmacol Ther* 26:8–15, 1979.

Wettrell G, Andersson KE: Clinical pharmacokinetics of digoxin in infants. *Clin Pharmacokinet* 2:17–31, 1977.

Wiklund L: Postoperative hepatic blood flow and its relation to systemic circulation and blood gases during splanchnic blockade and fentanyl analgesia. *Acta Anesth Scand* 19 (Suppl 58):5–28, 1975.

Wilkinson GR: The effects of liver disease and aging on the disposition of diazepam, chlordiazepoxide, oxazepam and lorazepam in man. *Acta Psychiat Scand Suppl* 274:56–74, 1978.

Wilkinson GR, Shand DG: A physiological approach to hepatic drug clearance. *Clin Pharmacol Ther* 18:377–390, 1975.

Wood AJJ, Kornhauser DM, Wilkinson GR, Shand DG, Branch RA: The influence of cirrhosis on steady state blood concentrations of unbound propranolol after oral administration. *Clin Pharmacokinet* 3:478–487, 1978.

Wood AJJ, Vestal RE, Spannuth CL, Stone WJ, Wilkinson GR, Shand DG: Propranolol disposition in renal failure. *Br J Clin Pharmacol* 10:561–566, 1980.

Wood AJJ, Vestal RE, Wilkinson GR, Branch RA, Shand DG: Effect of aging and cigarette smoking on antipyrine and indocyanine green elimination. *Clin Pharmacol Ther* 26:16–20, 1979.

Wood M: Plasma drug binding: implications for anesthesiologists. *Anesth Analg* 65:786–804, 1986.

Wood M, O'Malley K, Stevenson IH: Drug metabolizing ability in operating theatre personnel. *Br J Anaesth* 46:726–728, 1974.

Wood M, Shand DG, Wood AJJ: Propranolol binding in plasma during cardiopulmonary bypass. *Anesthesiology* 51:512–516, 1979.

Wood M, Wood AJJ: Changes in plasma drug binding and α, acid glycoprotein in mother and newborn infant. *Clin Pharmacol Ther* 29:522–526, 1981.

Yaffe SJ (ed): *Pediatric Pharmacology. Therapeutic Principles in Practice.* New York, Grune & Stratton, 1980.

Yeh TF: *Drug Therapy in the Neonate and Small Infant.* Chicago, Year Book, 1985.

2

Drug Metabolism

ALASTAIR J. J. WOOD

Many drugs are metabolized prior to elimination from the body. Usually these drugs, which are themselves relatively nonpolar lipid-soluble compounds, are metabolized to more polar less lipid-soluble metabolites which are excreted more readily. The lipid-soluble parent drug is excreted relatively slowly because of the ease with which back diffusion occurs from the urine in the renal tubules. It has been shown that, were it not for metabolism, a highly lipid-soluble agent such as thiopental would have a half-life of approximately 100 years. However, metabolism to more polar less lipid-soluble compounds reduces the reabsorption from the renal tubules and, therefore, speeds elimination. Usually these metabolites have less pharmacological activity than the parent compound, but this is by no means always so. For example, the acetylated metabolite of procainamide, N-acetyl-procainamide, has antiarrhythmic activity and in fact is now available as an antiarrhythmic in its own right. Also, the metabolites of the local anesthetic lidocaine (see Chapter 11) are pharmacologically active. The pharmacological effects of some drugs are due almost entirely to their metabolites. For example, the antineoplastic effects of cyclophosphamide are due to the production of an active metabolite within the body. A large number of examples of pharmacologically active metabolites are now recognized. The production of metabolites may be associated with toxicity not seen with the parent compound. The significance and production of such toxic metabolites are discussed in detail in Chapter 4. Although the term *detoxification* has sometimes been used synonymously with drug metabolism, the fact that metabolites may occasionally be toxic or active makes its usage inappropriate.

PATHWAYS OF DRUG METABOLISM

There are four basic reactions which drugs may undergo in the body:

$$
\left.\begin{array}{l}
\text{oxidation} \\
\text{reduction} \\
\text{hydrolysis}
\end{array}\right\} \text{—Phase I}
$$
$$\text{conjugation —Phase II}$$

$$\text{Drug} \xrightarrow[\text{Enzymes}]{\overset{\text{Phase I}}{\text{Oxidation}}} \overset{\text{Phase II}}{\underset{\text{Enzymes}}{\text{Reduction}}} \xrightarrow{} \overset{}{\underset{}{\text{Conjugated}}} \text{Metabolites}$$

The reactions can be further subdivided into Phase I and Phase II reactions. Phase I reactions include oxidation, reduction, and hydrolysis, while Phase II reactions are synthetic in nature. Examples of Phase II reactions include the production of glucuronides, sulfates, and acetylated and methylated derivatives of drugs and their metabolites. The end result of almost all Phase I and Phase II reactions is the production of more polar and more water-soluble metabolites whose excretion is more rapid than that of the parent compound.

Phase I Reactions

DRUG OXIDATION

Drug oxidation is carried out by a series of enzymes located in the smooth endoplasmic reticulum of the liver, kidney, and other tissues. The largest amount of these enzymes is found in the liver which is, therefore, the principal site of metabolism for a large number of drugs. When the cells are homogenized, the endoplasmic reticulum is disrupted, and fragments of endoplasmic reticulum can be concentrated by centrifugation in what is known as the *microsomal fraction*. This is prepared by centrifuging the liver homogenate slowly (1200 $\times$ g) for 30 minutes, removing the supernatant, and centrifuging again (100,000 $\times$ g) to obtain the pellet of microsomes. This contains an iron-containing hemoprotein called *cytochrome P-450*, so called because of its absorption peak at 450 nm when it combines with carbon monoxide. Cytochrome P-450 or a family of closely related cytochromes are central to the oxidation of a large number of drugs, other exogenously administered compounds, and endogenous substrates within the body. The cytochrome P-450 system is also known as the mixed-function oxidase system because it involves both reduction and oxidation steps as outlined in Figure 2.1. It requires the presence of nicotinamide adenine dinucleotide phosphate (NADPH) and molecular oxygen (O_2). The molecule of oxygen is split with one atom of oxygen going to oxidize each molecule of drug and the other oxygen atom being incorporated into a molecule of water.

Drug combines with the oxidized form of P-450 (Fe^{3+}) to which an electron is transferred from the oxidation of NADPH to $NADP^+$ by the flavoprotein, NADPH-cytochrome c reductase, resulting in reduced drug-P-450 complex (Fe^{2+}). The reduced drug-P-450 complex then binds a molecule of oxygen (O_2) to form a drug-P-450 oxygen complex which, when it receives an additional electron, forms oxidized P-450, oxidized drug, and water. The reader should bear in mind when following these reactions that a gain of electrons is reduction, while electron loss results in oxidation. It is now clear that the rate of this reaction is determined more by the activity of the enzyme NADPH-cytochrome c reductase than by the activity of P-450 itself.

The enzyme system described previously is present not only in the liver but also in other tissues including the kidney, intestinal mucosa, and adrenal cortex where it is responsible for the hydroxylation of steroids, and, in fact, it

was in the adrenal that some of the earliest studies on the cytochrome P-450 mixed-function oxidase system were performed.

It is customary to think of enzymes as being relatively substrate specific. The fact that so many compounds may be metabolized by the cytochrome P-450 system might therefore appear surprising. It is likely, however, that there are really a large number of different forms or isozymes of P-450. A suggestion that at least two forms of P-450 exist comes from the differences in the absorption spectra produced when different substrates combine with P-450. When the light from a spectrophotometer beam passes through a solution containing P-450 and carbon monoxide, the absorption peak occurs at 450 nm; however, when drug is added to the solution, the absorption peak changes. These changes can be plotted as a difference spectrum (Fig. 2.2). Practically this is done by having light of known wavelengths shine through two cuvettes in a dual beam spectrophotometer and plotting the difference between the absorption in the drug-free P-450 solution in one cuvette and that in the other cuvette to which drug substrate has been added to the P-450 solution. Substrates can then be classified according to the difference spectra produced. Type I drugs have a maximum difference of absorption in the range of 385 to 390 nm, while for type II substrates, it is in the range of 425 to 435

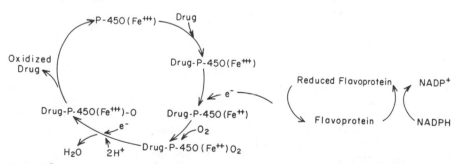

Figure 2.1. Electron transfer by the cytochrome P-450 (mixed-function oxidase system). NADPH is oxidized to $NADP^+$ by the flavoprotein, NADPH-cytochrome c reductase, resulting in an electron transfer to the oxidized form of P-450, P-450 (Fe^{3+}), and its reduction to P-450 (Fe^{2+}). A complex is then formed with oxygen. The addition of another electron results in the production of water and oxidized drug.

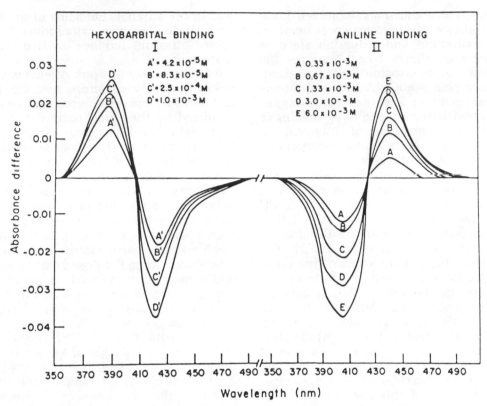

Figure 2.2. Difference spectra for drugs binding to P-450. (With permission from Mannering GJ: Microsomal enzyme systems which catalyze drug metabolism. In LaDu BN, Mandel HG, Way EL (eds): *Fundamentals of Drug Metabolism and Drug Disposition*. Baltimore, Williams & Wilkins, 1971, pp 206–252.

nm. An increasing concentration of substrates increases the difference in absorption as shown in Figure 2.2. Drugs such as hexobarbital, aminopyrine, ethylmorphine, and the volatile anesthetics have a type I difference spectrum, while, for example, aniline and acetanilide produce type II difference spectra. Type I substrates can accelerate the rate of reduction of P-450 by NADPH while type II substrates usually slow this reduction.

Although the number of drugs which undergo oxidation by the mixed-function oxidase system and the number of pathways involved may appear to be unmanageably large, confusion can be avoided by recognizing that all of these reactions can be regraded as oxidations or hydroxylations.

The metabolism of thiopental illustrates how apparently diverse metabolic pathways actually involve the identical step of oxidation to achieve the end result of decreased lipid solubility, increased polarity, and ease of excretion.

ALIPHATIC OXIDATION

Oxidation of the side chain (aliphatic oxidation) of thiopental by the P-450 system converts the highly lipid-soluble thiopental to the more polar, more water-soluble thiopental carboxylic acid which, following conjugation with glucuronic acid, is readily excreted in the urine.

DESULFURATION

Thiopental is also desulfurated to pentobarbital again by an oxidative step.

DEHALOGENATION

Although dehalogenation may appear to be different from the oxidations discussed so far, in fact, it too involves oxidation of a carbon-hydrogen bond to form an intermediate which is unstable and spontaneously loses H-x (where x is a halogen atom). The dehalogenation step involved in the metabolism of halothane is performed by the oxidation of the carbon atom bearing the two halogens which results in halogen loss. It is important to note that the presence of three halogens (in this case, fluorine) on a terminal carbon makes that carbon relatively resistant to dehalogenation. Dehalogenation of methoxyflurane with liberation of fluorine is associated with the production of polyuric renal insufficiency.

There are a number of other pathways of metabolism such as N-dealkylation (responsible for the demethylation of morphine to normorphine), o-dealkylation, etc., which are well reviewed in the bibliography at the conclusion of this chapter.

The *reductive* pathway deserves further attention, both because of its importance in the metabolism and toxicity of halothane and because of the apparent contradiction that it too involves the mixed-function oxidase or cytochrome P-450 system. Under conditions of low oxygen tension, halothane can be reduced by the P-450 system. The low oxygen tension allows the P-450 system to transfer electrons not to oxygen, as it usually does, but directly to the substrate, in this case halothane, allowing direct reduction of halothane (electron gain). This only occurs under conditions of reduced oxygen tension when insufficient oxygen is present to compete for the electrons and is thought to have implications for halothane toxicity. This pathway is discussed in more detail in Chapter 9.

HYDROLYSIS

Only esters and amides are metabolized by hydrolysis. The enzymes responsible (esterases and amidases) are found both in plasma and tissues including the liver. However, the enzymes are present, not in the microsomal fraction, but in the soluble fraction and do not involve cytochrome P-450. Hydrolysis is an important pathway for the degradation of the local anesthetic procaine. Hydrolysis of succinylcholine by plasma cholinesterase is responsible for the rapid termination of this drug's effect. An inherited defect in the ability of plasma cholinesterase to hydrolyze succinylcholine is responsible for prolonged paralysis in some patients (see Chapters 5 and 10).

Esmolol (see Chapter 14) is a β-adrenergic blocking agent with a very short half-life (approximately 9 minutes) in humans. It is metabolized by an esterase contained in the cytosol of red cells but not by plasma esterase. Thus, in contrast to succinylcholine, esmolol's metabolism does not demonstrate genetic polymorphism.

Phase II Reactions

Phase II reactions, in contrast to those of phase I, are synthetic in nature when the drug, or more commonly its metabolite, reacts with an endogenous substrate to form a conjugate. The conjugates are usually more water soluble and, hence, more easily excreted than the parent compound. Conjugation reactions can occur when the drug contains a reactive group, such as carboxyl ($-COOH$), primary amine ($-NH_2$), sulfhydryl ($-SH$), or hydroxyl ($-OH$), which is capable of acting as a substrate for the enzymes of conjugation. If the drug itself does not contain such groups, then it will require metabolism and insertion of such a group by phase I enzyme systems before conjugation can occur. The endogenous substrates used for conjugation by the body come from the compounds used in the metabolism of carbohydrates (glucuronic acid) and amino acids (glutathione and methionine). These conjugating agents do not, however, interact directly with the drug or its metabolites, but do so through an activated form.

GLUCURONIC ACID CONJUGATION

Glucuronic acid conjugation is a major route of drug metabolism with a large portion of the metabolites in urine or bile being in this form. The glucuronic acid is derived from readily available glucose and has to be activated through the synthesis of uridine diphosphate glucuronic acid (UDPGA). The enzyme glucuronyl transferase is then responsible for the transfer of glucuronic acid from UDPGA to the drug or its metabolite to produce the glucuronide of the drug.

UDP-glucuronic acid

$$+ \text{ drug (or metabolite)} \xrightarrow[\text{transferase}]{\text{glucuronyl}}$$

$$\text{drug-glucuronic acid} + \text{UDP}$$

The conjugation with the large hydrophilic glucuronic acid moiety renders the drug or metabolite more water soluble, less lipid soluble, and more highly ionized at physiologic pH, so that reabsorption from the renal tubules is less. The glucuronide conjugate is eliminated by excretion in the urine and/or bile, the biliary route being more important for the high-molecular-weight (over 400) compounds. Sometimes, if the glucuronide is readily hydrolyzed, reabsorption of the parent compound may occur from the gut resulting in an enterohepatic circulation.

ABNORMALITIES OF GLUCURONIDE FORMATION

The rate of glucuronidation is an important determinant of the rate of excretion of bilirubin. In normal newborn infants, the activity of glucuronyl transferase is markedly reduced, so that in situations such as hemolytic disease of the newborn where the bilirubin load is increased, the ability to conjugate the relatively fat-soluble bilirubin to its less lipid-soluble and more easily excreted glucuronide is inadequate. This causes accumulation of bilirubin and deposition in the brain which results in kernicterus. This is worsened if drugs such as novobiocin, which reduce glucuronidation, are administered to such infants. Phenobarbital increases the rate of formation of glucuronyl transferase and, for that reason, it has been given to mothers prior to delivery or to newborn infants following delivery to increase their rate of glucuronidation of bilirubin. Because of their

inability to glucuronidate and excrete it normally, chloramphenicol accumulates to toxic concentrations in newborn infants, resulting in the "gray baby" syndrome characterized by cardiovascular collapse, cyanosis, and death. Glucuronidation is also reduced in pregnancy, probably because of elevated levels of progesterone and pregnanediol.

ACETYLATION

For some compounds such as procainamide, hydralazine, and isoniazid, acet-

Table 2.1.
Ethnic Distribution of Acetylator Phenotype

Ethnic group	Rapid acetylators (%)
Asiatic origin	
Canadian Eskimo	95–100
Korean	89
Japanese	88–90
Alaskan Eskimo	79
American Indians	79
Chinese	78–85
Filipino	72
Canadian Indians	63
African origin	
American Negro	49–58
Africans	43–51
European origin	
Latin Americans	67
Italian	51
USA whites	43–48
German	43
USA Greek	40
Swiss	39
British	38–40
USA Italian	36
USA Scandinavian	32–49
Swedes	32–49
Canadians	30–41
Mediterranean origin	
USA Askenazi	45
Israeli Askenazi	33
Israeli Non-Askenazi	31
Israeli Baghdad Jews	25
Egyptians	18

With permission from McQueen EG: Pharmacological basis of adverse drug reactions. In Avery GS (ed): *Drug Treatment.* New York, Adis Press, 1980.

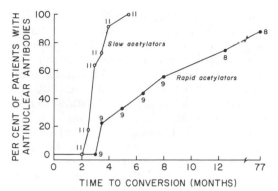

Figure 2.3.   Positive antinuclear antibodies (ANA) in patients receiving procainamide therapy.   Slow acetylators develop positive ANA faster than do rapid acetylators. (With permission from Woosley RL, Drayer DE, Reidenberg MM, Nies AS, Carr K, Oates JA: Effect of acetylator phenotype on the rate at which procainamide induces antinuclear antibodies and the lupus syndrome. *N Engl J Med* 298:1157–1159, 1978.)

ylation is an important pathway of metabolism. In humans the rate at which acetylation occurs is bimodally distributed; i.e., the population falls into two groups, slow acetylators and fast acetylators. The proportion of fast and slow acetylators in the population is genetically determined and varies between races with Caucasians having about 50% fast acetylators, while as many as 88 to 90% Japanese are fast acetylators (see Table 2.1). The rate of acetylation has implications for toxicity, with slow acetylators developing positive antinuclear antibodies following procainamide therapy at a faster rate than fast acetylators (Fig. 2.3).

MERCAPTURIC ACID SYNTHESIS

Although only a small fraction of a drug is usually excreted as a mercapturic acid conjugate, it is now recognized that this can reflect a very important pathway of detoxification. Mercapturic acid conjugates are formed after the drug or, more usually, its metabolite has combined with the sulfhydryl (-SH) groups of glutathione. This appears to be an important

pathway in the "mopping up" of toxic and highly reactive intermediates which are sometimes produced during drug metabolism. An example of this is seen with overdosage of acetaminophen (Tylenol). This drug is metabolized to a toxic metabolite which covalently binds to liver proteins and produces hepatic necrosis. This only occurs when an overdose is taken because at normal doses any toxic metabolites produced can react with glutathione and go on to form mercapturic

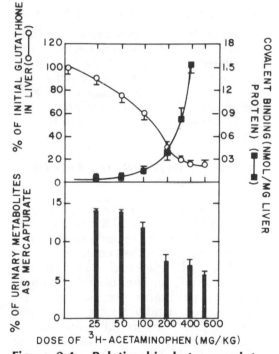

Figure 2.4.   Relationship between glutathione depletion, covalent binding, and mercapturate formation following increasing doses of acetaminophen administered to hamsters.   As the dose is increased, glutathione is depleted until covalent binding of acetaminophen metabolites occurs to liver proteins (*upper panel*). Because of depletion of glutathione, less is available for conjugation and, hence, the fraction of drug excreted as the mercapturate is reduced. (With permission from Jollow DJ, Thorgeirsson SS, Potter WZ, Hashimoto M, Mitchell JR: Acetaminophen-induced hepatic necrosis. VI. Metabolic disposition of toxic and nontoxic doses of acetaminophen. *Pharmacology* 12:251–271, 1974.)

acid conjugates. However, when an overdose is taken, the glutathione in the liver is used up, allowing the toxic metabolites to bind covalently to liver proteins. In Figure 2.4, the relationship between glutathione depletion and covalent binding to liver macromolecules is shown. As glutathione is depleted, covalent binding increases, and the proportion of the drug excreted as the mercapturate in the urine decreases, reflecting the loss of the ability to conjugate toxic metabolites to mercapturates through glutathione.

OTHER PATHWAYS OF CONJUGATION

Other pathways of conjugation include the formation of sulfates, amides, and methylated derivatives of the drug or its metabolites. As always, the usual result of such reactions is to reduce the degree of lipid solubility, reduce the pharmacological activity, and speed the rate of excretion.

FACTORS AFFECTING THE RATE OF DRUG METABOLISM

It is now clear that numerous factors can affect the rate at which drugs are metabolized. These can include such apparently diverse factors as genetic composition, alcohol, cigarette consumption, concomitant drug administration, environmental pollutants, occupation, nutritional status, and various hormones. Some of these factors alter the rate of drug metabolism through changes in the activity of the drug-metabolizing enzymes. Drugs which increase the activity of the drug-metabolizing enzymes are known as enzyme-inducing agents. This normally occurs through an increased rate of synthesis of the microsomal drug-metabolizing enzyme systems.

Enzyme Induction

The classic compounds used to increase the rate of drug metabolism in animal studies have been phenobarbital and the polycyclic hydrocarbons, such as 3-methylcholanthrene (3-MC). It is clear that the polycyclic hydrocarbons act differently to increase the rate of drug me-

tabolism. For example, phenobarbital increases the rate of metabolism of a much larger number of drugs than does 3-methylcholanthrene administration. In addition, administration of the polycyclic hydrocarbons results in the production of a modified form of cytochrome P-450, which has an absorption peak when bound to carbon monoxide, not at 450 nm as in untreated animals, but at 448 nm. This has been called cytochrome P-448.

In humans, the effects of enzyme-inducing agents are usually studied by demonstrating that the interacting compound or environmental factor changes the clearance of a marker drug. Antipyrine has been widely used as a marker of drug metabolism in humans because it is entirely metabolized by the liver, is relatively poorly protein bound, and is distributed only in body water. Thus, changes in its clearance reflect changes in its rate of metabolism. An example of the utility of this technique is shown in Figure 2.5. The clearance of antipyrine was shown to be higher in a group of op-

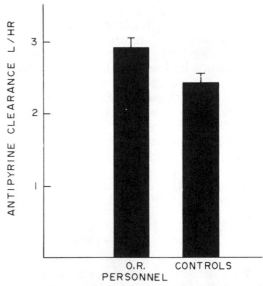

Figure 2.5. Increased clearance of antipyrine in operating room personnel. (With permission from Wood M, O'Malley K, Stevenson H: Drug metabolizing ability in operating theatre personnel. *Br J Anaesth* 46:726–728, 1974.)

Table 2.2.
Inducers of Drug Metabolism in Humans

Drugs
  Phenobarbital
  Other barbiturates
  Phenytoin
  Rifampin
  Glutethimide
  Carbamazepine
  Phenylbutazone
  Spironolactone
Other factors
  Cigarette smoking
  Charcoal broiled beef
  Dietary protein/carbohydrate ratio

Table 2.3.
Inhibitors of Drug Metabolism in Humans

Chloramphenicol
Sulfaphenazole
Phenylbutazone[a]
Cimetidine
Monoamine oxidase inhibitors
Disulfiram
Allopurinol
Ketoconazole

[a]Reduces clearance of *S*-warfarin and accelerates clearance of *R*-warfarin.

erating room personnel than in a group of other hospital personnel, suggesting that the drug-metabolizing ability is increased in those who work in the operating room. Other drugs can be used as markers of drug-metabolizing ability. For example, smoking increases the clearance of propranolol and results in lower concentrations in smokers in contrast to nonsmokers (Figure 1.32). The implications of such drug interactions are reviewed in Chapter 4. Examples of drugs which have been shown to increase drug metabolism in humans are listed in Table 2.2.

Enzyme Inhibition

Although studied both in vitro and in animals, clinical implications of enzyme inhibition have only recently been addressed. It will be clear that enzyme inhibition is potentially of more clinical importance because inhibition of the drug-metabolizing enzymes will result in reduction in drug clearance and elevation in drug concentration, contributing to either toxicity or excessive pharmacological effect. Some of the drugs which have been shown to inhibit drug metabolism in humans are listed in Table 2.3. Again the clinical implications are discussed in Chapter 4.

In addition to the use of marker drugs to define the activity of the drug-metabolizing enzymes in humans, changes in the disposition of endogenous compounds have been monitored as an index of drug metabolism; changes in the plasma concentrations of γ-glutamyl transpeptidase, the excretion of D-glucaric acid, and urinary 6β-hydroxycortisol have all been utilized.

Pharmacogenetics

The well-recognized polymorphism for the pathways of acetylation and hydrolysis is described earlier in the chapter; however, only a small number of drugs are metabolized by either of these pathways. Most drugs are metabolized through oxidative pathways, and genetic polymorphism for the oxidative pathways has now been recognized.

DEBRISOQUINE POLYMORPHISM

Genetically determined defects in the metabolism of sparteine and debrisoquine were the first oxidation defects to be identified. Subsequently these were shown to reflect alterations in the activity of the same cytochrome P-450 isozyme. Debrisoquine, an adrenergic-neuron blocking agent used in the treatment of hypertension in Europe, is metabolized principally by oxidation to 4-hydroxy debrisoquine. The ability to metabolize debrisoquine by this pathway is impaired in 8 to 10% of the United States and United Kingdom populations resulting in two distinct populations (*polymorphism*): a poor metabolizer group and an extensive metabolizer group. This polymorphism has been shown to be geneti-

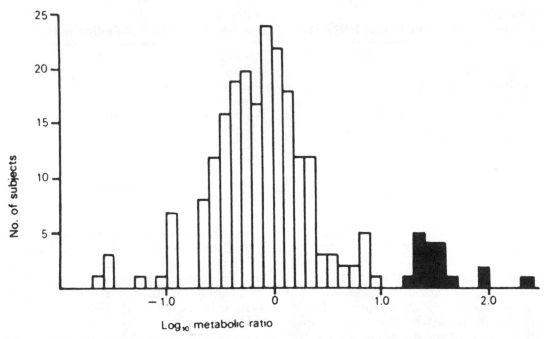

Figure 2.6.   Genetic polymorphism of debrisoquine metabolism. The distribution of the debrisoquine metabolic ratio (ratio of unchanged debrisoquine to 4-hydroxy debrisoquine in the urine) shows there to be two populations. Ninety percent of the population *(open bars)* are extensive metabolizers with a metabolic ratio <12 ($\log_{10}$, 1.1), and 10% of the population *(solid bars)* are poor metabolizers with a metabolic ratio > 12. (With permission from Woolhouse NM, Andoh B, Mahgoub A, Sloan TP, Idle JR, Smith RL: Debrisoquine hydroxylation polymorphism among Ghanaians and Caucasians. *Clin Pharmacol Ther* 26:584–591, 1979.)

cally determined *(genetic polymorphism).* An individual's ability to metabolize debrisoquine can be assessed by determining the *metabolic ratio* which is defined as the ratio of the amount of drug excreted unchanged in the urine to that of the metabolite (Fig. 2.6). Multiple isozymes of cytochrome P-450 which are genetically determined exist, each of which is responsible for the metabolism of certain drugs. The poor metabolizer phenotype is due to inheritance of a homozygous recessive genotype and is presumed to be due to either the complete absence or the presence of a functionally inadequate cytochrome P-450 isozyme.

The clinical importance of this genetically determined impairment of debrisoquine metabolism stems from the wide spectrum of drugs whose metabolism is also impaired in poor metabolizers of de-

brisoquine (Table 2.4). The consequences of the impaired drug metabolism in poor metabolizers depend on the contribution that the impaired pathway makes to the drug's overall clearance and also whether the metabolite whose production is impaired is pharmacodynamically active. If the impaired metabolic pathway makes a large contribution to the drug's overall clearance, then high and potentially toxic plasma drug concentrations may occur in poor metabolizers given usual therapeutic doses. Conversely, the inability to produce an active metabolite may reduce the drug's therapeutic effects.

The antiarrhythmic effects of encainide are due to both encainide itself and the production of active metabolites (see Chapter 16). The ability to produce these metabolites is impaired in patients who

Table 2.4.
Examples of Drugs Whose Metabolism Is Impaired in Poor Metabolizers of Debrisoquine

---

β-Adrenergic blockers
  Alprenolol
  Bufuralol
  Metoprolol
  Propranolol
  Timolol
Antihypertensives
  Guanoxan
Antiarrhythmics
  Encainide
  Propafenone
  Sparteine
Psychotropic agents
  Amitriptyline
  Desiprimine
  Nortriptyline
  Dextromethorphan
Others
  Perhexiline
  Phenformin

---

are poor metabolizers. This means that, because of their reduced ability to metabolize encainide, very high encainide concentrations and low metabolite concentrations are achieved in poor metabolizers, and thus they depend on encainide itself to produce therapeutic effects. In contrast, extensive metabolizers rapidly metabolize encainide to active metabolites, which are then responsible for the antiarrythmic effects of encainide.

OTHER OXIDATIVE POLYMORPHISMS

Since the identification of the debrisoquine/sparteine polymorphism, other oxidative polymorphisms have been identified, e.g., mephenytoin and tolbutamide. The ability to metabolize the two stereoisomers of the anticonvulsant mephenytoin exhibits genetic polymorphism. The frequency of poor metabolizers of mephenytoin depends on the population studied and ranges from 3% in a Caucasian to 18% in a Japanese population. Because of the multiplicity of P-

450 isozymes which exists, it is likely that other examples of genetic polymorphism of oxidized drugs will be recognized in the future.

BIBLIOGRAPHY

Alyares AP, Kappas A, Eiseman JL, Anderson KE, Pantuck CB, Pantuck EJ, Hsiao KC, Garland WA, Conney AH: Intraindividual variation in drug disposition. *Clin Pharmacol Ther* 26:407–419, 1979.

Brown BR: Drug biotransformation and anesthesia. In *Current Problems in Anesthesia and Critical Care Medicine*. Chicago, Year Book, 1978, pp 1–29.

Clark DWJ: Genetically determined variability in acetylation and oxidation: therapeutic implications. *Drugs* 29:342–375, 1985.

Cohen EN, VanDyke RA., Trudell JR: *Metabolism of Volatile Anesthetics. Implications for Toxicity.* Reading, MA, Addison-Wesley, 1977.

Conney AH: Pharmacological implications of microsomal enzyme induction. *Pharmacol Rev* 19:317–366, 1967.

Conney AH: Environmental factors influencing drug metabolism. In LaDu BN, Mandel HG, Way EL (eds): *Fundamentals of Drug Metabolism and Drug Disposition*. Baltimore, Williams & Wilkins, 1971.

Conney AH, Welch R, Kuntzman R, Chang R, Jacobson M, Munro-Faure AD, Peck AW, Bye A, Poland A, Poppers PJ, Finster M, Wolff JA: Effects of environmental chemicals on the metabolism of drugs, carcinogens, and normal body constituents in man. *Ann NY Acad Sci* 179:155–172, 1971.

Coon MJ: Drug metabolism by cytochrome P-450: progress and perspectives. *Drug Metab Dispos* 9:1–4, 1981.

Daly J: Enzymatic oxidation at carbon. In Brodie BB, Gillette JR (eds): *Concepts in Biochemical Pharmacology. Handbook of Experimental Pharmacology 28/2*. New York, Springer-Verlag, 1971, pp 285–311.

Eichelbaum M: Defective oxidation of drugs: pharmacokinetic and therapeutic implications. *Clin Pharmacokinet* 7:1–22 1982.

Eichelbaum M: Polymorphic drug oxidation in humans. *Fed Proc* 43:2298–2302, 1984.

Estabrook RW: Cytochrome P-450, its function in the oxidative metabolism of drugs. In Brodie BB, Gillette JR (eds): *Concepts in Biochemical Pharmacology. Handbook of Experimental Pharmacology 28/2*. New York, Springer-Verlag, 1971, pp 264–284.

Gelboin HV: Mechanisms of induction of drug metabolism enzymes. In LaDu BN, Mandel HG, Way EL (eds): *Fundamentals of Drug Metabolism and Drug Disposition*. Baltimore, Williams & Wilkins, 1971.

Gelehrter TD: Enzyme induction. *N Engl J Med* 294:522–526, 589–595, 646–651, 1976.

Goldstein A, Aronow L, Kalman SM: Drug metabolism. In *Principles of Drug Action: The Basis of Pharmacology*. New York, John Wiley & Sons. 1974, pp 227–300.

Jacqz E, Hall SD, Branch RA: Genetically determined polymorphisms in drug oxidation. *Hepatology* 6:1020–1032, 1986.

Jollow DJ, Thorgeirsson SS, Potter WZ, Hashimoto M, Mitchell JR: Acetaminophen-induced hepatic necrosis. VI. Metabolic disposition of toxic and nontoxic doses of acetaminophen. *Pharmacology* 12:251–271, 1974.

Kalow W: Ethnic differences in drug metabolism. *Clin Pharmacokinet* 7:373–400, 1982.

LaDu BN: Genetic factors modifying drug metabolism and drug response. In LaDu BN, Mandel HG, Way EL (eds): *Fundamentals of Drug Metabolism and Drug Disposition*. Baltimore, Williams & Wilkins, 1971.

Mandel HG: Pathways of drug biotransformation: biochemical conjugations. In LaDu BN, Mandel HG, Way EL (eds): *Fundamentals of Drug Metabolism and Drug Disposition* Baltimore, Williams & Wilkins, 1971.

Mannering GJ: Microsomal enzyme systems which catalyze drug metabolism. In LaDu BN, Mandel HG, Way EL (eds): *Fundamentals of Drug Metabolism and Drug Disposition* Baltimore, Williams & Wilkins, 1971, pp 206–252.

Mehta MU, Venkataramanan R, Burckart GJ, Ptachcinski RJ, Yang SL, Gray JA, Van Thiel DH, Starzl TE: Antipyrine kinetics in liver disease and liver transplantation. *Clin Pharmacol Ther* 39:372–377, 1986.

O'Malley K, Crooks J, Duke E, Stevenson IH: Effect of age and sex on human drug metabolism. *Br Med J* 3:607–609, 1971.

Park BK, Breckenridge AM: Clinical implications of enzyme induction and enzyme inhibition. *Clin Pharmacokinet* 6:1–24, 1981.

Raghuram TC, Koshakji RP, Wilkinson GR, Wood AJJ: Polymorphic ability to metabolize propranolol alters 4-hydroxypropranolol levels but not beta blockade. *Clin Pharmacol Ther* 36:51–56, 1984.

Smith SE, Rawlins MD: *Variability in Human Drug Response*. London, Butterworths, 1973.

Smuckler, EA: Metabolism of halogenated compounds. In Brodie BB, Gillette JR (eds): *Concepts in Biochemical Pharmacology. Handbook of Experimental Pharmacology 28/2*. New York, Springer-Verlag, 1971, pp 367–377.

Spoelstra P, Teunissen MWE, Janssens AR, Weeda B, Van Duijn W, Koch CW, Breimer DD: Antipyrine clearance and metabolite formation: the influence of liver volume and smoking. *Eur J Clin Invest* 16:321–327, 1986.

Uetrecht JP, Woosley RL: Acetylator phenotype and lupus erythematosus. *Clin Pharmacokinet* 6:118–134, 1981.

Vessell ES: Polygenic factors controlling drug response. Individualization of drug therapy. *Med Clin North Am* 58:951–963, 1974.

Vesell ES, Penno MB: A new polymorphism of hepatic drug oxidation in humans: family studies of antipyrine metabolites. *Fed Proc* 43:2342–2347, 1984.

Vestal RE, Wood, AJJ: Influence of age and smoking on drug kinetics in man. Studies using model compounds. *Clin Pharmacokinet* 5:309–319, 1980.

Vestal RE, Wood AJJ, Branch RA, Shand DG, Wilkinson GR: The effects of age and cigarette smoking on propranolol disposition. *Clin Pharmacol Ther* 26:8–15, 1979.

Wang T, Roden DM, Wolfenden HT, Woosley RL, Wood AJJ, Wilkinson GR: Influence of genetic polymorphism on the metabolism and disposition of encainide in man. *J Pharmacol Exp Ther* 228:605–611, 1984.

Wedlund PJ, Aslanian WS, McAllister CB, Wilkinson GR, Branch RA: Mephenytoin hydroxylation deficiency in Caucasians: frequency of a new oxidative drug metabolism polymorphism. *Clin Pharmacol Ther* 36:773–780, 1984.

Williams RT: Pathways of drug metabolism. In Brodie BB, Gillette JR (eds): *Concepts in Biochemical Pharmacology. Handbook of Experimental Pharmacology 28/2*. New York, Springer-Verlag, 1971, pp 226–242.

Wood AJJ, Vestal RE, Shand DG, Wilkinson GR, Branch RA: The effects of aging and cigarette smoking on antipyrine and indocyanine green elimination. *Clin Pharmacol Ther* 26:16–20, 1979.

Wood M., O'Malley K, Stevenson IH: Drug metabolizing ability in operating theatre personnel. *Br J Anaesth* 46:726–728, 1974.

Woolhouse NM, Andoh B, Mahgoub A, Sloan TP, Idle JR, Smith RL: Debrisoquine hydroxylation polymorphism among Ghanaians and Caucasians. *Clin Pharmacol Ther* 26:584–591, 1979.

3

Drug Receptor Interactions

ALASTAIR J. J. WOOD

DRUG RECEPTOR INTERACTIONS

In Chapter 1, the factors influencing the delivery of a therapeutic drug concentration to its site of action are discussed. The variables of patient compliance with the therapeutic regimen, dosage, absorption, volume of distribution, protein binding, and rate of elimination are all of importance in determining the concentration of drug finally available at its site of action. In addition, variability also exists in patients' intrinsic sensitivity to a given drug concentration, so that in a group of patients in whom it is possible to achieve similar plasma drug concentrations, some patients may show an adequate therapeutic effect, some may show no effect, while still others may show evidence of toxicity. Recently, a number of the factors that determine these differences in sensitivity or pharmacodynamics have been identified.

Many drugs initiate a series of events leading to their effect by binding to some specific macromolecule which can be conceptualized as a "receptor." The concept that drugs might act by binding to receptors was first suggested by Langley in 1905, when he postulated that the actions of nicotine and curare at the myoneural junction might be mediated by a specific "receptive substance." Ehrlich in 1913 also made use of the same concepts to account for the actions of certain chemotherapeutic agents.

Until recently, the receptor concept remained just that—a useful theoretical concept on which it was possible to visualize and model the relationship between drug concentration and effect.

However, it is now possible to directly label and isolate receptors from tissue and to study their functional and structural characteristics. It is now recognized, for example, that alteration in receptors can modulate drug effects. The purpose of a receptor may be visualized as 2-fold.

1. **Recognition.** The receptor must be able to recognize the specific hormone, neurotransmitter, drug, etc., to which it responds.
2. **Transmission.** The receptor must have the ability to relay the signal that a molecule of agonist has bound to it so that the appropriate response may follow.

Binding of the ligand to the receptor usually produces some conformational change in the receptor, which in some way conveys the signal that binding has occurred. Receptors for neurotransmitters and hormones have been studied in detail and appear to fall into three types:

1. Receptors for the polypeptide hormones and catecholamines, which are situated on the external surface of the plasma membrane of responsive cells;
2. Receptors for the steroid hormones which are found in the cytoplasm of cells;
3. Receptors for thyroid hormones which are found in the chromatin of the target cells.

In general, there are a number of steps (Fig. 3.1) between the recognition by the receptor of a drug and the production of its effect. These will be examined in detail in relation to the β-adrenergic receptor, although many of the principles also apply to other receptor systems.

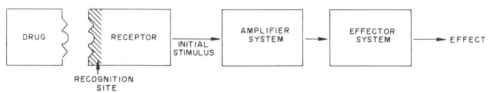

Figure 3.1.   Steps in the production of a pharmacodynamic effect following binding of drug to the receptor.

STRUCTURE AND FUNCTION OF THE β-ADRENERGIC RECEPTOR

The receptor adenylate cyclase system contains three separate components (Fig. 3.2):

1. The receptor recognition site itself whose structure is shown in Figure 3.3;
2. The guanine nucleotide regulatory protein;

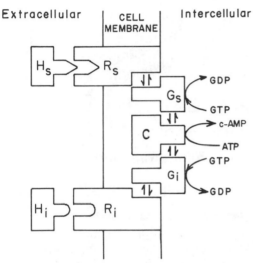

Figure 3.2. Model of adenylate cyclase activation or inhibition by a hormone. The binding of hormone (H_s or H_i) to the receptor results in either stimulation, if it is a stimulatory receptor (R_s) (see Table 3.1), or inhibition, if it is an inhibitory receptor (R_i). The binding of hormone to the receptor enhances the association of guanosine triphosphate *(GTP)* to a guanyl nucleotide regulatory protein. The GTP-regulatory protein complex then activates adenylate cyclase (C). After its activation, the enzyme converts adenosine triphosphate *(ATP)*, in an ATP-Mg^{2+} complex, to cyclic adenosine monophosphate *(cAMP)*, which activates protein kinase to phosphorylate proteins such as intracellular enzymes. (With permission from Lefkowitz RJ, Caron MG, Stiles GL: Mechanisms of membrane-receptor regulation: biochemical, physiological, and clinical insights derived from studies of the adrenergic receptors. *N Engl J Med* 310:1570–1579, 1984.)

3. The catalytic moiety ultimately responsible for the synthesis of cyclic AMP.

The $β_1$- and $β_2$-adrenergic receptors are single chain glycoproteins organized in a characteristic fashion as shown in Figure 3.3. There are seven membrane spanning domains. Part of the molecule is outside the cell for recognition and binding of ligands.

Binding of a hormone to a receptor linked to the adenylate cyclase system ultimately either stimulates or inhibits the catalytic component. For example, binding of β-receptor agonists to β-adrenergic receptors stimulates, whereas binding to $α_2$-adrenergic receptors inhibits cyclic AMP production (Table 3.1).

Two types of guanine nucleotide regulatory proteins (G proteins), G_s and G_i, interact with the stimulatory and inhibitory receptors, respectively. Both G proteins are trimers composed of 3 subunits: $α_s$, $β$, and $γ$ in the case of G_s; and $α_i$, $β$, and $γ$ in the case of G_i. Thus, $α_s$ and $α_i$, respectively, distinguish stimulatory from inhibitory G proteins (Fig. 3.4) and are also the site of binding of guanyl nucleotides (GDP and GTP).

Following binding of an agonist to a stimulatory receptor, the agonist-receptor complex interacts with the appropriate G protein (Fig. 3.2) (G_s). This interaction facilitates the replacement of GDP

Table 3.1.
Examples of Receptors Stimulating or Inhibiting Adenylate Cyclase

Stimulatory receptors (R_s)	Inhibitory receptors (R_i)
$β_1$ + $β_2$-Adrenergic	$α_2$-Adrenergic
Adenosine (A$_2$)	Adenosine (A$_1$)
ACTH[a]	Acetylcholine
Vasopressin	(muscarinic)
Glucagon	Opiates
Prostaglandin E$_1$	Somatostatin
hCG[a]	
Vasointestinal	
peptide (VIP)	

[a]ACTH, adrenocorticotropic hormone; hCG, human chorionic gonadotropin.

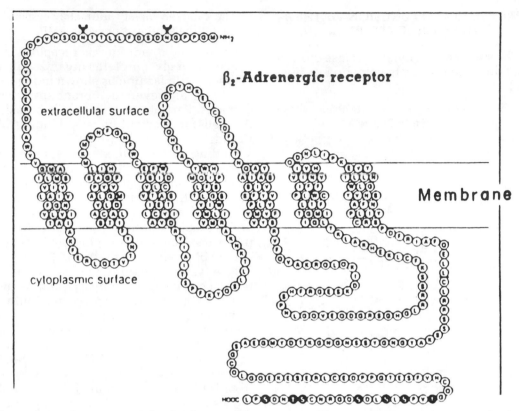

Figure 3.3.   Structure of the β-adrenergic receptor.   The receptor contains seven hydrophobic regions which span the lipid membrane. The extracellular recognition site is also shown along with the intracellular part of the receptor which is subject to phosphorylation. (With permission from Lefkowitz RJ, Benovic JL, Kobilka B, Caron MG: β-Adrenergic receptors and rhodopsin: shedding new light on an old subject. *Trends Pharmacol Sci* 7:444–448, 1986.)

by GTP which results in activation of the G protein and by the production of conformational change in the adenylate cyclase enzyme, activation of the enzyme to convert ATP to adenosine 3′,5′-monophosphate (cyclic AMP). Cyclic AMP then acts as a "second messenger" by activating various protein kinases which phosphorylate intracellular proteins. As these intracellular proteins are frequently enzymes, phosphorylation will result in a change in the enzyme activity.

For example, binding of epinephrine to the β-receptor of cells involved in glycogen synthesis results in cyclic AMP generation and phosphorylation of the enzyme glycogen synthetase with a resultant decrease in its activity and inhibition of glycogen synthesis from glu-

cose. On the other hand, glycogen breakdown to glucose is increased.

The way in which the receptor-hormone interaction is linked to effect through the amplifier system of cyclic AMP generation has important implications; for example, when adenylate cyclase is stimulated, it may generate more cyclic AMP than is required to saturate the next step so that a maximal effect may be produced by a drug or hormone stimulating only a fraction of the total receptors, meaning that a proportion of the receptors are so-called "spare receptors." Therefore, stimulation of all receptors may not be required to generate a maximal effect. In addition to direct stimulation of receptors by agonist binding, it is possible to raise cyclic AMP levels in

Stimulation   Inhibition

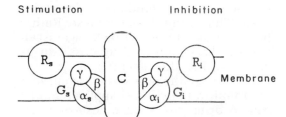

Membrane

Figure 3.4.   Structure of G protein.   The receptor (*R*) communicates with the adenylate cyclase or catalytic component (*C*) through the appropriate G protein (G_i or G_s). The G proteins are trimers composed of α, β, and γ subunits. The G_s and G_i proteins differ in their α subunits (α_s and α_i, respectively). (With permission from Helmreich EJM, Pfeuffer T: Regulation of signal by β-adrenergic hormone receptors. *Trends Pharmacol Sci* 6:438–443, 1985.)

other ways. For example, because cyclic AMP is converted to the inactive 5'-AMP by the enzyme, phosphodiesterase inhibition of this enzyme by the methylxanthines, such as theophylline, raises cyclic AMP levels and mimics many of the effects of β-adrenergic receptor stimulation, e.g., bronchodilation, increased cardiac output, etc.

Although the actions of a large number of hormones appear to be mediated by stimulation or inhibition of intracellular cyclic AMP (Table 3.1), it should not be assumed that all hormones act through a cyclic AMP-mediated system. For example, steroid hormones appear to act in a quite different way. Steroids, which are more lipid soluble than the polypeptides and catecholamines, pass through the cell membrane and enter the cell where they bind to receptors situated in the cell cytoplasm. The receptor-steroid complex which is now activated, perhaps by changing the conformation of the receptor so that a nuclear binding site is exposed, binds to chromatin situated in the cell nucleus. The receptor-steroid-chromatin combination in some way regulates the concentrations of specific messenger RNA. As the rate of synthesis of proteins is dictated by the levels of messenger RNA, alteration in protein synthe-

sis occurs. For example in the liver, binding of steroids to receptors in hepatic cells results in an increase in certain amino transferases and results in increased gluconeogenesis. Thus, the effects of the steroids are produced through messenger RNA-mediated alterations in protein and enzyme synthesis.

DOSE-RESPONSE RELATIONSHIPS

It is axiomatic in clinical medicine that there is a relationship between drug dosage, or concentration at the site of action, and response, whether that response is the desired therapeutic effect or some undesired toxic effect. The desire to relate drug dosage to effect requires an examination of drug dose response relationships.

It is the experience of every clinician that increasing the dose of a drug will in many cases increase the intensity of that drug's effect until a maximum effect is achieved. Further increases in dose at that point will produce no further increase in effect, but may be associated with toxicity. This may be expressed graphically as a hyperbolic dose-response curve (Fig. 3.5). Practically this curve may appear to have an intercept on

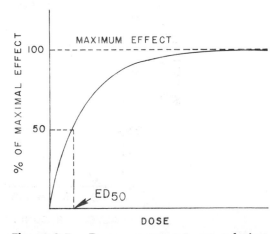

Figure 3.5.   Dose-response curve relating dose to the intensity of effect.   When the maximal effect is achieved, no further increase in effect is seen with further increase in dose. The dose producing 50% of maximal response is the ED_{50}.

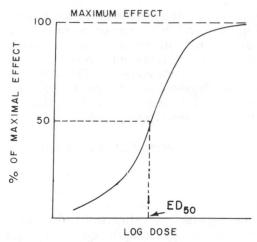

Figure 3.6. Log dose-response curve. Note the "linear" portion of the log dose-response curve during which small increases in dose will produce a relatively large increase in effect.

the dose axis because there will be doses which, when administered, produce effects which are too small to detect. Eventually with increasing dose, a dose will be reached which produces a detectable effect. This is the *threshold dose.* Rather than plotting drug dose directly against effect, the logarithm of drug dose can be plotted against the effect (Fig. 3.6).

The slope of the dose-response curve is important in the clinical application of a drug. A drug with a steep dose-response curve will show marked increase in effect for small increases in dose, while those with a shallow dose-response curve will require relatively large increases in dose to produce a similar increase in effect.

For some drugs, the effect is of an "all or none" type and, therefore, a dose-response curve has to be plotted as the percentage of patients who respond to any given dose. The drug concentration at which half the population responds is called the ED_{50}.

Examples of ED_{50} are common in anesthesia. In 1946, Robbins defined anesthetic ED_{50} as the concentration of anesthetic at which 50% of mice failed to right themselves for 15 seconds when placed in a rotating bottle with a known

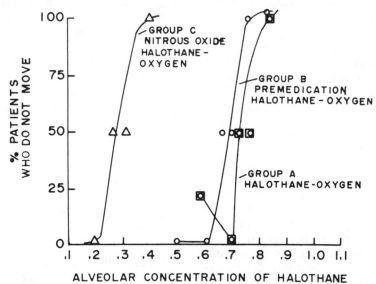

Figure 3.7.   Dose-response curve to halothane and oxygen (□); premedication, halothane and oxygen (○); and when nitrous oxide is added (△).   The percentage of patients who do *not* move in response to a surgical incision is plotted against the end-tidal halothane concentration. (Data taken with permission from Saidman LJ, Eger EI: Effect of nitrous oxide and of narcotic premedication on the alveolar concentration of halothane required for anesthesia. *Anesthesiology* 25:302–306, 1964.)

concentration of anesthetic. An example of anesthetic ED_{50} in humans is the concept of MAC, which is defined as the minimum anesthetic concentration in the alveolus at which 50% of patients moved in response to a surgical incision. Thus, the determination of MAC requires the measurement of end-tidal anesthetic concentration and the patient's response to skin incision. A dose-response curve can then be plotted as the percentage of patients who show an anesthetic response, i.e., do not move during the incision at different doses (alveolar concentration of anesthetic) as shown in Figure 3.7.

MODELS OF DRUG RESPONSE

In order to predict drug effects, it is useful to be able to model the relationship between drug concentration and effect.

The Log Linear Pharmacodynamic Model

The magnitude of response is frequently plotted against the logarithm of drug concentration (Fig. 3.6). This has the advantage of providing a linear portion of the curve in the range of 20 to 80% of the maximal response that can be analyzed using relatively simple techniques. However, use of this model has some limitations. (*a*) Analysis of the linear portion of the curve does not allow prediction of the maximal effect (E_{max}) nor does it predict that no drug effect will be produced when no drug is present (drug concentration is zero).

The E_{max} Model

This model more accurately represents the situation depicted in Figure 3.5. It calculates the effect (E) at any drug concentration (C) as:

$$E = \frac{E_{max} \cdot C}{EC_{50} + C}$$

where E_{max} is the maximal response, and EC_{50} is the drug concentration producing 50% of the maximal response. In contrast

to analysis of the linear portion of the log linear concentration response curve, use of this equation will allow determination of E_{max} and also predicts that, in the absence of drug, no effect will be produced, i.e., when $C = 0$, E will also equal 0.

The Sigmoid E_{max} Model

The simple hyperbolic function represented by the E_{max} model may be inadequate to represent the concentration effect relationship for some drugs. The addition of an extra parameter (N) may improve the fit of the data. Using this model:

$$\text{Effect} = \frac{E_{max}\, C^N}{EC_{50N} + C^N}$$

The value given to N will influence the slope of the curve. Changing the value of N will alter the shape of the dose-response curve (Fig. 3.8). This model has been used to model drug effect for some of the intravenous anesthetic agents (see Chapter 8, Fig. 8.7).

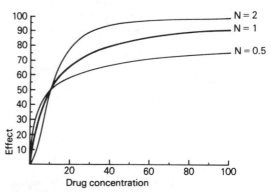

Figure 3.8. The relationship between drug concentration and effect predicted by the simple E_{max} model ($n = 1$) and by the more complex sigmoid E_{max} model. Note when *n* is greater than 1 the central portion of the curve steepens, but at values of *n* less than 1, the curve is steeper initially but shallower at high concentrations. (Modified from Holford NHG, Sheiner LB: *Clin Pharmacokinet* 6:429–453, 1981.)

RELATIONSHIP BETWEEN DRUG RECEPTOR BINDING AND RESPONSE: DISSOCIATION CONSTANT

When drugs or hormones combine with receptors, a reversible reaction takes place that can be represented as:

$$D + R \overset{\kappa_1}{\rightleftharpoons} DR$$

where D is the drug, R is the receptor, DR is the drug-receptor complex, and k_1 is the forward rate constant. The rate of drug receptor association is dependent on the drug $[D]$ and unoccupied receptor $[R]$ concentration, i.e,

Rate of association α $[D][R]$

Therefore,

Rate of association $= k_1 [D][R]$

However, this reaction is reversible:

$$DR \overset{\kappa_2}{\rightleftharpoons} D + R$$

and the dissociation of drug receptor complex depends only on the concentration of drug receptor complex $[DR]$, i.e.,

Rate of dissociation $= k_2[DR]$

where k_2 is the rate constant. Now at equilibrium, the rate of dissociation must equal the rate of association. Therefore,

$$k_1[D][R] = k_2[DR]$$

or

$$\frac{[D][R]}{[DR]} = \frac{k_2}{k_1} = K_d$$

The ratio of k_2/k_1 is the equilibrium *dissociation* constant (K_d) $(k_1/k_2$ is the equilibrium *association* constant, $K_a)$.

When half the receptors are occupied by drug, then the concentration of unoccupied receptors must equal the concentration of occupied receptors, i.e. $[DR] = [R]$. Thus, $[R]$ and $[DR]$ cancel out in the previous equation, so that at 50% receptor occupancy:

$$K_d = [D]$$

That is, the free drug concentration required to half saturate receptors is equal to the dissociation constant K_d. There-

fore, the lower the drug concentration which half saturates the receptors (K_d), the greater is the drug's affinity for the receptor.

A. J. Clark's theories of drug action which were developed in the 1920s assumed that the intensity of effect produced by drug binding to receptor was dependent on the fraction of receptors occupied by the drug and that maximal drug effect occurred when all of the receptors were occupied. While this is a useful model of drug-receptor relationships, it is clearly not applicable to all such interactions, and some of the problems with such assumptions will be discussed later. However, if it is assumed that

$$D + R \rightarrow DR \rightarrow \text{Effect}$$

and that effect is proportional to the fraction of receptors occupied, then the equations applied previously to drug receptor interactions are equally applicable to drug effects. Thus, saturation of receptors would produce maximal effects, and half-maximal effect would be produced at half-maximal receptor occupancy which occurs at a drug concentration equal to K_d. This is analogous to E_{max} and EC_{50} discussed in the previous section.

Thus, the greater the drug's affinity for the receptor, the lower the drug concentration required to produce half-maximal effect. This is often described loosely as potency. So that drugs A and B in Figure 3.9 both produce the same maximal effect and have parallel dose-response curves, but drug B required 10 times higher drug concentration to produce the same effect. Thus, a drug's affinity for its receptor is an important characteristic of the drug which determines its relative potency. For example, in Figure 3.9 drug A could be said to be 10 times more potent than drug B.

INTRINSIC ACTIVITY

It will be recognized by any clinician that, though two drugs may have a similar effect, the maximal effect achieved by one may be different from that produced by another. For example, though mor-

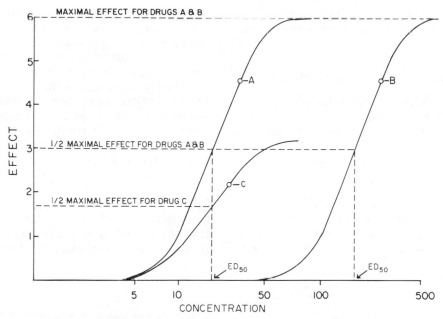

Figure 3.9.   Log dose-response curves for three drugs.   Drugs A and B produce the same maximal effect, but B requires concentrations 10-fold higher than A. The ED_{50} for A is 17 while for B it is 170. Drug C has the same ED_{50} as A; i.e., free concentrations which produce half-maximal effect are the same, but C produces a smaller maximal effect. Thus, A and B differ only in their affinity for the receptor and are both full agonists with A being 10 times more potent than B. However, C is only a partial agonist, but its affinity (K_d) for the receptor is the same as A. Curve C could also represent the dose-response curve to an agonist in the presence of a noncompetitive blocker which, in the absence of the blocker, produced dose-response *curve A.*

phine and codeine are both analgesics, it is clear that morphine has a much greater analgesic effect than even maximal doses of codeine. This raises the concept of *intrinsic activity*. It could be said that the intrinsic analgesic activity of morphine is greater than that of codeine. When such situations are found with drugs which bind to the same receptor, drugs with high, intermediate, and zero activity may all exist. Those with high activity being full agonists; with intermediate, partial agonists; and those with no activity, antagonists. An example of the response to a partial agonist is shown by drug C in Figure 3.9. The maximal effect produced by drug C is only approximately one-half that produced by either A or B. However, the drug concentration required to produce half of C's maximal effect (K_d) is identical to that of drug A. Thus, although drug C has a lower maximal effect than either A or B, its affinity for the receptor is similar to A and greater than B. Thus, two independent and important properties of drugs defining the characteristics of their dose-response curves are *intrinsic activity* (also sometimes called efficacy), which determines the maximal response produced, and *affinity*, which determines the position of the dose-response curve and, hence, relative potency. Increased affinity (reduction in K_d) moves the dose-response curve to the left.

Clearly it is not possible to explain differences in intrinsic activity in terms of Clark's receptor occupancy theory, which related activity to the fraction of receptors occupied, as both partial agonists and antagonists in sufficient concentration can occupy all of the receptors without producing either maximal response, or in the case of antagonists, any response.

Occupation Activation Model

A modification to the original model assumes that receptors can exist in two states, activated and nonactivated, and that response is proportional to the fraction of receptors in the activated state. Therefore, when an agonist binds to a receptor, it converts the receptor from the nonactivated to the activated state. Full agonists are able to convert most of the receptors which they occupy to the activated state, while competitive antago-

nists convert none and partial agonists convert only a fraction of the receptors which they occupy to the activated state.

More recently, these concepts have been extended with the recognition that the ability to stimulate the β-receptor by full and partial agonists may reflect their ability to cause coupling of receptor to G protein (G_s) (see "Structure and Function of the β-Adrenergic Receptor").

The effects of a partial and full agonist at β-receptors are shown in Figure 3.10.

When a partial agonist is administered in the presence of a full agonist, the effects will depend on the relative concentrations of full and partial agonists, so that at concentrations of the full agonist

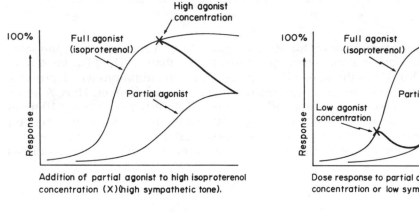

Addition of partial agonist to high isoproterenol concentration (X)(high sympathetic tone).

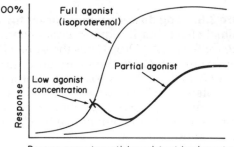

Dose response to partial agonists at low isoproterenol concentration or low sympathetic tone.

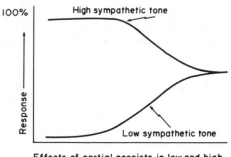

Effects of partial agonists in low and high sympathetic tone.

Figure 3.10.   Dose-response curves to full and partial agonists.   Isoproterenol stimulation of β-adrenoceptors is shown as an example of the effects of a full agonist. A full agonist causes a maximal response which is greater than that of a partial agonist. When increasing concentrations of a partial agonist are added to a full agonist, the effect of the full agonist is reduced to the maximal effect of the partial agonist *(upper left)*. At lower concentrations of a full agonist *(upper right),* the partial agonist will increase the effect of the low concentration of full agonist to the maximum effect of the partial agonist. The effect of partial agonist in the setting of low and high sympathetic tone or low and high concentrations of a full agonist is shown *(bottom)*.

which produce maximal effect, increasing doses of the partial agonist will competitively antagonize the effect of the full agonist. This will result in reduction of the effect to the level of the maximal effect produced by the partial agonist (Figure 3.10). On the other hand, at low concentrations of the full agonist which are below that which would produce the maximal effect of the partial agonist, addition of the partial agonist will increase the effect but only to the maximal effect of the partial agonist. As all of the receptors become occupied by the partial agonist, the dose-response curves will converge toward that of the maximal effect of the partial agonist (Figure 3.10).

Spare Receptors

Spare receptors exist when occupancy of only a few receptors by a full agonist results in a maximal response. As the rate of formation of drug-receptor complexes [DR] is proportional to the concentration of both drug [D] and receptor [R]

$$[DR] \propto [D][R]$$

the presence of so-called spare receptors, i.e., more receptors than are needed to elicit a maximal response, confers a biological advantage by increasing the rate of formation of drug-receptor complexes and increasing the sensitivity to low agonist concentrations. Spare receptors can be quantitated as the fraction of receptors which can be irreversibly blocked without reduction of the maximal response.

Many receptor-effector systems are coupled to enzymes. For example, in the cyclic AMP system described previously, activation of the receptor can stimulate adenylate cyclase to produce more cyclic AMP than is required to saturate the next step in the pathway. This means that a maximal response distal to cyclic AMP generation can be produced from the system when only a fraction of the receptors is activated.

At the neuromuscular junction, many more acetylcholine receptors exist than are required to elicit a muscle action potential so that a large proportion of the re-

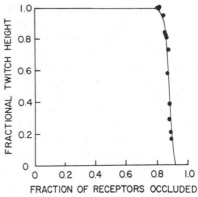

Figure 3.11. Demonstration of the effect of "spare receptors" on the margin of safety of neuromuscular transmission. The fractional twitch height following stimulation is shown at increasing concentrations of tubocurarine which result in an increasing proportion of receptors being occupied by tubocurarine. No change is produced until around 80% are occupied. (With permission from Waud BE: Neuromuscular blocking agents. In *Current Problems in Anesthesia and Critical Care Medicine*. Chicago, Year Book, 1977.)

ceptors can be blocked by a competitive antagonist, such as curare, before neuromuscular transmission fails. In fact, if fractional twitch height is plotted against the fraction of the receptors blocked (occupied by the antagonist) (Fig. 3.11), no change occurs in the twitch height produced until around 80% of the receptors are occupied by antagonist, and by the time 90 to 95% of the receptors are occupied by the antagonist, no response occurs. This has been described as the margin of safety for neuromuscular transmission.

Antagonists

Antagonists are drugs which, though they bind to receptors and prevent an agonist from binding, do not themselves initiate an effect. Competitive antagonists bind reversibly to the receptor so that if the antagonist is present in relatively high concentrations, the agonist will not gain access to the receptor. On the other hand, if the agonist is present in sufficient concentration, it will still be able to occupy the receptors and to exert the same effect as in the absence of the antagonist; however, higher concentrations of agonist will be required. The dose-response curves A and B in Figure 3.9 (page 63) could be produced by an agonist in the absence (A) and presence (B) of a competitive antagonist. It is important to note that a competitive antagonist has the effect of shifting the dose-response curve to the right without affecting either its shape or the maximal effect produced. It should also be clear that for competitive antagonists such as the β-adrenergic blockers there can be no such thing as "complete β blockade" as at any concentration of β blocker, the effect can be overcome provided sufficient agonist is administered (see Chapter 14).

The ratio of the dose of agonist required to produce the same response in the presence of antagonist to that required in the absence of antagonist is the dose ratio (DR) or concentration ratio (CR) if concentrations are used. It will be clear that the greater the degree of competitive blockade the greater will be the dose ratio. This is illustrated for curare in Figure 3.12 where increasing concentrations of tubocurarine shift the dose-response curve to carbachol to the right in a parallel fashion. In the presence of 10^{-7} M tubocurarine, 12μM carbachol is required to produce the same degree of depolarization as is produced by 6.4 μM carbachol when no tubocurarine is present giving a concentration ratio (CR) of 12 : 6.4 or 1.9.

Schild demonstrated that:

$$(CR - 1) = B/K_B$$

where CR is the concentration ratio defined previously, B is the concentration of antagonist, and K_B is the antagonist's equilibrium dissociation constant. From the Schild equation above, it follows that when the concentration or dose ratio equals 2:

$$B = K_B$$

and, in addition, that the concentration ratio will be linearly related to the antagonist concentration with a slope of $1/K_B$.

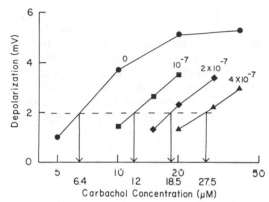

Figure 3.12.   Effect of increasing concentrations of tubocurarine on carbachol-induced depolarization. Increasing concentrations of tubocurarine move the dose-response curves to the right in a parallel fashion. The dose of carbachol required in the presence of 10^{-7} tubocurarine to produce a depolarization of 2 mV is 12 μM, while in the absence of tubocurarine, a 6.4 μM concentration is required, giving a dose ratio of 12:6.4 or 1.9. (With permission from Waud BE: Neuromuscular blocking agents. In *Current Problems in Anesthesia and Critical Care Medicine.* Chicago, Year Book, 1977.)

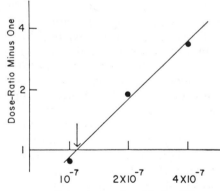

Figure 3.13.   Schild plot relating log (DR−1) to log tubocurarine concentration. (Note both *axes* are plotted on log scales.) Data are from Figure 3.12. The *intercept* gives the K_B, and the *line* has a slope of 1 for a competitive antagonist. (With permission from Waud BE: Neuromuscular blocking agents. *Current Problems in Anesthesia and Critical Care Medicine.* Chicago, Year Book, 1977.)

It is more usual, however, to plot the log(dose ratio − 1) against the logarithm of the antagonist concentration (Fig. 3.13). For a competitive antagonist such as tubocurarine, this should be linear and have a slope of 1. The equilibrium dissociation constant (K_B) can be determined as the antagonist concentration when $(DR − 1)$ equals 1 (or the dose ratio equals 2 as in the previous paragraph),

which can be determined from the intercept on the Schild plot (Fig. 3.13).

Noncompetitive antagonists act by binding irreversibly to receptors or by reducing the responsiveness of the effector system. Therefore, by reducing the number of receptor-effector units available to respond, they reduce the maximal effect produced by agonists, if no spare receptors are present, without altering the af-

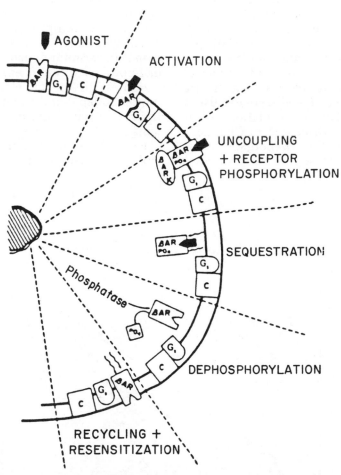

Figure 3.14. Mechanisms of desensitization. Following stimulation of receptor by agonist and receptor G protein coupling, a cytosolic enzyme, BARK, phosphorylates the receptor causing dissociation of the receptor from the G protein (uncoupling). Subsequently the phosphorylated receptor is sequestered away from the cell membrane so that it is no longer available for binding to agonists. Dephosphorylation then occurs, and eventually the receptor cycles back to the cell surface causing resensitization. More prolonged exposure to agonists causes a loss of receptors from the total population (including externalized and internalized receptors). (Modified from Lefkowitz RJ, Benovic JL, Kobilka B, Caron MG: β-Adrenergic receptors and rhodopsin: shedding new light on an old subject. *Trends Pharmacol Sci* 7:444–448, 1986.)

finity of the agonist for these receptors which are not blocked. An example of such antagonism is shown in Figure 3.9 (page 63). The dose-response curve in the presence (C) and absence (A) of a noncompetitive blocker is shown. It can be seen that the concentration of agonist (K_d) required to produce half-maximal effect is unaltered, but the maximal effect is reduced.

Some competitive antagonists used clinically are really partial agonists but, when available in concentrations sufficient to occupy most of the receptors, prevent their occupation by the full agonist and, therefore, reduce their effect to the maximal effect produced by a partial agonist. Examples of this effect are shown in Figure 3.10 and were discussed above. Partial agonists in relation to opiate receptors are discussed in Chapter 7 and in relation to the adrenergic nervous system in Chapter 14.

Receptor Regulation

Chronic exposure to agonists frequently results in an attenuation over time of the response produced even when the agonist concentration is kept constant. This phenomenon has been called desensitization, tachyphylaxis, or tolerance. Desensitization may involve actual reduction of receptor number (receptor down-regulation) or impairment of communication between the receptor and the adenylate cyclase enzyme itself (receptor coupling). Conversely, receptor sensitivity may be increased by an increase in receptor density (up-regulation) or improved receptor enzyme communication. With the development of techniques to label and isolate receptors and improve understanding of the mechanisms involved in receptor adenylate cyclase communication, the factors responsible for receptor desensitization have

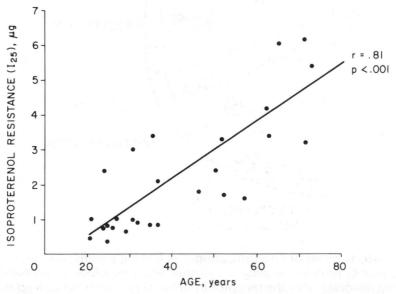

Figure 3.15.   Effect of age on the resistance to isoproterenol-induced rise in heart rate.   As age increases, the dose of isoproterenol required to raise the heart rate by 25 beats per minute (I_{25}) increases so that the elderly require 4 to 5 times more isoproterenol to raise their heart rate than the young. (With permission from Vestal RE, Wood AJJ, and Shand DG: Reduced β-receptor sensitivity in the elderly. *Clin Pharmacol Ther,* 26:181–186, 1979.)

been defined. Desensitization can be of two types, homologous or heterologous.

When responsiveness is lost only to agonists of the same class as the desensitizing agonist, this is *homologous desensitization*, whereas the loss of responsiveness to a wide range of stimulants has been termed *heterologous desensitization*. Understanding receptor desensitization requires familiarity with the details of receptor adenylate cyclase coupling outlined earlier in this chapter.

The steps involved in receptor agonist binding and subsequent desensitization are outlined in Figure 3.14.

When agonist binds to the β-adrenergic receptor, the formation of the receptor-G protein complex is promoted (receptor coupling). The conformational change produced in the G protein by this association initiates the steps which stimulate the production of cyclic AMP. In addition, in the receptor itself a conformational change makes the receptor susceptible to phosphorylation by the enzyme β-adrenergic receptor kinase (BARK) (Fig. 3.14). BARK has the distinction of only phosphorylating the receptor when it is occupied by agonist. The phosphorylated receptor dissociates from the G protein causing "uncoupling." Subsequently, the phosphorylated receptor is

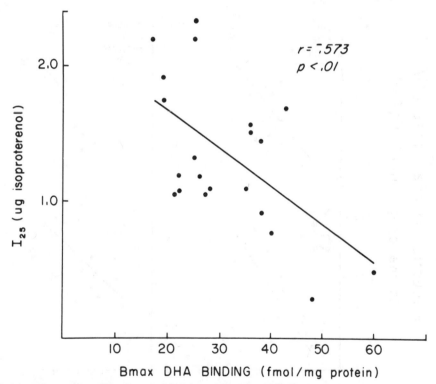

Figure 3.16. Receptor density and isoproterenol responsiveness. Relationship between the cardiac resistance to isoproterenol measured as the dose of isoproterenol required to produce a 25-beat/min (BPM) rise in heart rate (I_{25}) and the number of receptors on leukocyte membranes (B_{max}). The higher the number of β-receptors, the more sensitive the individuals were to isoproterenol, i.e., the lower the dose of isoproterenol required to produce a 25 BPM rise in heart rate. (With permission from Fraser J, Nadeau J, Robertson D, Wood AJJ: Regulation of human leukocyte beta receptors by endogenous catecholamines: relationship of leukocyte to beta receptor density to the cardiac sensitivity to isoproterenol. *J Clin Invest* 67:1777–1784, 1981.)

sequestered away from the cell surface, resulting in the receptor being inaccessible to agonist which cannot cross the lipid cell membrane (Fig. 3.14). Dephosphorylation of the receptor within the cell occurs, and eventually the receptor is recycled back to the cell surface, resulting in resensitization. More prolonged exposure to agonist results in loss of receptors, so that the total number of receptors including both those on the cell surface and internalized is reduced. Therefore, a number of steps appear to be involved in receptor desensitization (Fig. 3.14):

1. Receptor phosphorylation;
2. Receptor G protein uncoupling;

3. Receptor internalization;
4. Loss of receptors.

Many of these steps can be measured directly by *ex vivo* techniques, e.g., receptors coupled to G protein exhibit high affinity for agonists (i.e., bind agonists more avidly), whereas those uncoupled from G protein have a lower affinity for agonists.

In contrast to homologous desensitization which involves the specific enzyme BARK in *heterologous desensitization*, phosphorylation of the receptor is produced by cyclic AMP-dependent protein kinase.

Insulin receptor regulation may be important in the pathogenesis of diabetes,

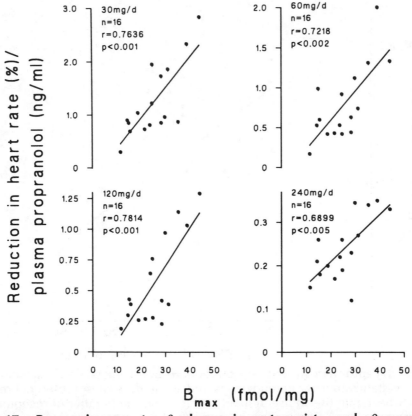

Figure 3.17. Responsiveness to β-adrenergic antagonists and β-receptor function. Relationship between the cardiac sensitivity to the β-blocker propranolol (reduction in heart rate during exercise/plasma propranolol) and β-receptor density following 30, 60, 120, and 240 mg of propranolol per day. (With permission from Zhou HH, Silberstein DJ, Koshakji RP, Wood AJJ: Interindividual differences in beta receptor density contribute to variability in response to beta receptor antagonists. *Clin Pharmacol Ther,* 45:587–592, 1989 .)

where carboyhdrate intake, by stimulating insulin release, may produce down-
regulation of insulin receptors and,
hence, a fall in the sensitivity to insulin.
If the ability of the pancreas to compensate for the reduced sensitivity by producing more insulin is impaired, then diabetes will result.

In addition to mediating desensitization or tachyphylaxis, alterations in receptor function appear to be important
determinants in interindividual responsiveness to both agonists and antagonists.
In the case of the β-adrenergic receptor,
alterations in many of the steps illustrated in Figure 3.14 have been demonstrated and may be associated
with changes in β-receptor sensitivity *in
vivo*.

A number of disease states may have
an abnormality in receptor regulation as
their basis. For example, it has been
shown that antibodies to β-receptors
exist in some asthmatics and that this
may explain the bronchospasm seen in
such patients. Antibodies have been
demonstrated to acetylcholine receptors
in a high proportion of patients with myasthenia gravis. Other factors have been
shown to influence receptor responsiveness in humans. For example, it has been
shown that the elderly are more resistant
to the isoproterenol-induced rise in heart
rate, so that to produce the same rise in
heart rate (25 beats/min) requires 4 to 5
times as much isoproterenol in the elderly compared to the young (Fig. 3.15).

In addition, the elderly exhibit impaired coupling of the receptor to G protein so that a smaller proportion of their
receptors are in the *high affinity* state.
This alteration may contribute to their
reduced sensitivity to β-receptor agonists.

Alterations in receptor number have
also been demonstrated following
chronic exposure to sympathetic agonists, such as bronchodilators, which resulted in a reduction in the number of β-
receptors. The number of β-receptors is
an important determinant of response to
both β-receptor agonists and antagonists
(Figures 3.16 and 3.17) so that the greater
the number of β-receptors, the greater

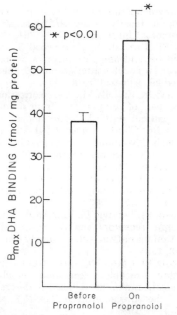

**Figure 3.18. Effect of three weeks of
treatment with propranolol on β-receptor
density on polymorphonuclear cells in
man.** Receptor density is increased because of blockade of down-regulation by
circulating catecholamines. (Data taken
with permission from Fraser J, Nadeau J,
Robertson D, Wood AJJ: Regulation of
human leukocyte beta receptors by endogenous catecholamines: relationship of leukocyte beta-receptor density to the cardiac
sensitivity of isoproterenol. *J Clin Invest*
67:1777–1784, 1981.)

the individual's sensitivity to both β-re-
ceptor agonists and antagonists.

Exposure to endogenous levels of catecholamines also results in decrease in
receptor number. Conversely, chronic β
blockade, by releasing the receptors from
their chronic down-regulated state,
causes an increase in receptor number
(Fig. 3.18).

Thus, receptor regulation and receptor
responsiveness are yet other variables
which have to be considered in evaluating a patient's response to drugs.

BIBLIOGRAPHY

Receptors

   Fraser J, Nadeau J, Robertson D, Wood AJJ: Regulation of human leukocyte beta receptors by en-

dogenous catecholamines: relationship of leukocyte beta-receptor density to the cardiac sensitivity to isoproterenol. *J Clin Invest* 67:1777–1784, 1981.

Galant SP, Duriseta L, Underwood S, Insel PA: Decreased beta-adrenergic receptors on polymorphonuclear leukocytes after adrenergic therapy. *N Engl J Med* 299:933–936, 1978.

Greenacre JK, Conolly ME: Desensitization of the β-adrenoceptor of lymphocytes from normal subjects and patients with phaeochromocytoma: studies in vivo. *Br J Clin Pharmacol* 5:191–197, 1978.

Helmreich EJM, Pfeuffer T: Regulation of signal by β-adrenergic hormone receptors. *Trends Pharmacol Sci* 6:438–443, 1985.

Huganir RL, Greengard P: Regulation of receptor function by protein phosphorylation. *Trends Pharmacol Sci* 8:472–486, 1987.

Lefkowitz RJ, Benovic JL, Kobilka B, Caron MG: β-Adrenergic receptors and rhodopsin: shedding new light on an old subject. *Trends Pharmacol Sci* 7:444–448, 1986.

Lefkowitz RJ, Caron MG, Stiles GL: Mechanisms of membrane-receptor regulation: biochemical, physiological, and clinical insights derived from studies of the adrenergic receptors. *N Engl J Med* 310:1570–1579, 1984.

Levitzki A: Regulation of hormone sensitive adenylate cyclase. *Trends Pharmacol Sci* 8:299–303, 1987.

Maze M: Clinical implications of membrane receptor function in anesthesia. *Anesthesiology* 55:160–171, 1981.

Norman J: Drug-receptor reactions. *Br J Anaesth* 51:595–601, 1979.

Sibley DR, Lefkowitz RJ: Molecular mechanisms of receptor desensitization using the β-adrenergic receptor-coupled adenylate cyclase system as a model. *Nature* 317:124–129, 1985.

Swillens S, Dumont JE: A unifying model of current concepts and data on adenylate cyclase activation by β-adrenergic agonists. *Life Sci* 27:1013–1028, 1980.

Vestal RE, Wood AJJ, Shand DG: Reduced beta-adrenoceptor sensitivity in the elderly. *Clin Pharmacol Ther* 26:181–186, 1979.

Zhou HH, Silberstein DJ, Koshakji RP, Wood AJJ: Interindividual differences in beta receptor density contribute to variability in response to beta receptor antagonists. *Clin Pharmacol Ther*, 45:587–592, 1989.

Dose Response Relationships

Quasha AL, Eger EI, Tinker JH: Determination and applications of MAC. *Anesthesiology* 53:315–334, 1980.

Tallarida RJ, Jacob LS: *The Dose-Response Relation in Pharmacology.* New York, Springer-Verlag, 1979.

*E*max *Model*

Holford NHG, Sheiner LB: Understanding the dose-effect relationship: clinical application of pharmacokinetic-pharmacodynamic models. *Clin Pharmacokinet* 6:429–453, 1981.

Swerdlow BN, Holley FO: Intravenous anaesthetic agents: pharmacokinetic-pharmacodynamic relationships. *Clin Pharmacokinet* 12:79–110, 1987.

4

Drug Interactions and Adverse Drug Reactions

ALASTAIR J. J. WOOD

ADVERSE REACTIONS TO DRUGS
    Mechanisms
    Exaggeration of the Intended Pharmacological Effect
    Toxicity Unrelated to a Drug's Primary Pharmacological Activity

DRUG INTERACTIONS
    Pharmacokinetic Interactions
    Pharmacodynamic Interactions

ADVERSE REACTIONS TO DRUGS

It is now recognized that every drug can produce untoward consequences, even when used according to standard or recommended methods of administration. When used incorrectly, the drug's effectiveness may be reduced, or adverse reactions can be expected to occur more frequently. The administration of several drugs during the same period of time may also result in adverse interactions among drugs.

Patients receive on the average 10 different drugs while hospitalized. The sicker the patient, the more drugs are given, and as expected, there is a corresponding increase in the likelihood of adverse drug reactions. When fewer than six different drugs are given to hospitalized patients, the probability of an adverse reaction is about 5%, but when more than 15 drugs are given, the probability is over 40%. A small group of widely used drugs accounts for a disproportionate number of reactions. A number of studies have shown that aspirin, digoxin, anticoagulants, diuretics, antimicrobials, steroids, and hypoglycemic agents accounts for as many as 90% of all reactions.

Most adverse reactions to drugs may be classified into two groups. The most frequent are those that result from the exaggerated but predicted pharmacological action of the drug (type A). Other adverse reactions ensue from toxic effects on cells that result from mechanisms unrelated to the intended pharmacological actions (type B). These, therefore, are often unpredictable, are frequently severe, and result from a number of recognized as well as undiscovered mechanisms. Some of the mechanisms of extrapharmacological toxicity include direct cytotoxicity, the initiation of abnormal immune responses, and the perturbation of metabolic processes in individuals rendered susceptible by genetic enzymatic defects.

Exaggeration of the Intended Pharmacological Effect

By prior consideration of the known factors that modify drug action, these adverse reactions are often preventable.

ABNORMALLY HIGH DRUG CONCENTRATION AT THE RECEPTOR SITE

Increased concentration at the site of action due to pharmacokinetic variability is the usual cause of exaggerated pharmacological effect. For example, reduction in the volume of distribution, in the rate of metabolism, or in the rate of excretion all will result in a higher-than-expected concentration of the drug at the receptor site with a consequent increase in pharmacological effect. An increase in the dose of a drug which exhibits nonlinear kinetics, such as phenytoin, may produce a proportionately greater increase in the blood level, resulting in toxicity. (See Chapter 1 for a detailed discussion of these variables.)

Genetic variability in drug metabolism may also result in abnormally high drug concentrations. For example, approximately 10% of the Caucasian population of the United States or the United Kingdom are poor oxidizers of the antihypertensive debrisoquine. A large number of other drugs (Table 2.4) are also poorly metabolized in this 10% segment of the population, so that they will be at particular risk of elevated drug concentrations and concentration-mediated toxicity.

ALTERATION IN THE DOSE-RESPONSE CURVE

An altered dose-response curve due to increased receptor sensitivity will result in an increase in drug effect at the same concentration (see Chapter 3). An example of this is seen in the excessive response to the anticoagulant warfarin at normal and lower-than-normal blood levels in the elderly.

THE SHAPE OF THE DOSE-RESPONSE CURVE

The shape of the dose-response curve also determines the likelihood of the development of adverse drug reactions. These drugs with a steep dose-response curve are more likely to be associated with dose-related toxicity because of the small increase in dose required to produce a large change in pharmacological effect. (See Chapter 3 for a detailed discussion.)

CONCOMITANT DRUG THERAPY

Concomitant drug therapy may affect the pharmacokinetics or pharmacodynamics of other drugs. Pharmacokinetics may be affected by alterations in bioavailability, protein binding, or the rate of metabolism or excretion. Pharmacodynamics may be altered by competition for receptor sites, by prevention of the drug's access to its site of action, or by antagonism or enhancement of the drug's pharmacological effect. These subjects have been discussed in detail in the preceding chapters.

Toxicity Unrelated to a Drug's Primary Pharmacological Activity

CYTOTOXIC REACTIONS

Our understanding of these so-called "idiosyncratic" reactions has greatly improved recently as it has become clear that many of these reactions are due to irreversible binding of drug or metabolites to tissue macromolecules by shared electron (covalent) bonds. Some chemical carcinogens such as the alkylating agents combine directly with DNA. However, it is more commonly only after metabolic activation to chemically reactive metabolites that covalent binding occurs. This metabolic activation usually occurs in the microsomal mixed-function oxidase system, the hepatic enzyme system which is responsible for the metabolism of many drugs (see Chapter 2). During the course of drug metabolism by these pathways, reactive metabolites of some drugs may be produced which covalently bind to tissue macromolecules, causing tissue damage. Because of the highly reactive nature of these metabolites, covalent binding often occurs close to the site of production, such as the liver, but the mixed-function oxidase system is found in other tissues as well.

Although the relevance to humans remains to be determined, it is interesting to note that such a mechanism has been described for the production of hepatotoxicity with halothane in rats. When rats are exposed to halothane under hypoxic conditions and following stimulation of the drug-metabolizing enzymes with phenobarbital or other enzyme-inducing agents, hepatic necrosis results. This necrosis appears to be associated with the production of reactive intermediates which bind covalently (see Chapters 2 and 9).

No drug is completely without side effects, and it is important to remember that a side effect in one patient may be the desired pharmacological effect in another. Recent improvements in drug regulation allow physicians to prescribe drugs with considerable confidence as to their purity, bioavailability, and effectiveness. However, while regulatory bodies try to ensure that drugs with serious toxic potential are not marketed, physicians have to constantly weigh the potential toxicity against the possible benefits.

DRUG INTERACTIONS

Patients frequently receive two or more drugs simultaneously. In addition, many patients presenting for anesthesia are receiving medications other than those immediately associated with their surgery. In any situation in which more than one drug is administered, the potential for a drug interaction exists. These interactions fall into two types:

Pharmacokinetic interactions in which the administration of one drug alters the disposition of another and, hence, alters the concentration of drug at the receptor site; and

Pharmacodynamic interactions in which one drug alters the response to another.

Pharmacokinetic Interactions

Pharmacokinetic interactions produce changes in the drug concentration at the receptor site by altering absorption, elimination, or distribution.

PHARMACEUTICAL INCOMPATIBILITY

Pharmaceutical incompatibility occurs because one drug reacts chemically or physically with another, usually when they are added to infusion fluids or mixed in the same syringe. Thiopental is precipitated by many drugs and should not be mixed with succinylcholine or ketamine. Trichloroethylene should not be used in a circuit containing soda lime as trichloroethylene is decomposed to form, among other substances, the neurotoxic product dichloroacetylene. Single or multiple addition of drugs to infusion fluids may result in interaction. Cephaloridine, isoproterenol, insulin, calcium, and hydrocortisone should not be added to sodium bicarbonate infusions. Mannitol solutions and blood are incompatible.

ALTERATION IN ABSORPTION

Reduction in the absorption of tetracyclines occurs when aluminum-containing antacids are administered simultaneously. Ion exchange resins, such as cholestyramine, result in decreased bioavailability and lower concentrations of

thyroxine, digoxin, and warfarin when they are coadministered.

The administration of narcotic analgesics during labor has been shown to slow gastric emptying and result in delayed absorption of acetaminophen. It is likely that the absorption of other drugs would also be delayed by narcotics administered during labor. Alteration in absorption may also occur from sites other than the gut. For example, the absorption of local anesthetic is slowed when it is mixed with epinephrine, thus reducing the peak plasma concentrations and lessening the likelihood of systemic reactions. Absorption interactions may also occur in the lungs, an example being the second gas effect where rapid uptake of nitrous oxide concentrates other anesthetic agents, such as halothane or en-

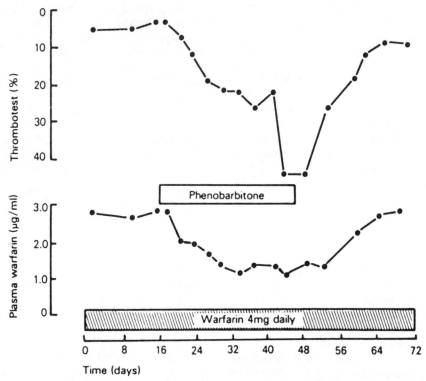

Figure 4.1.   Change in steady-state warfarin concentration following phenobarbitone administration.   Phenobarbitone reduces plasma warfarin concentration, which results in a reduction in the degree of anticoagulation (rise in thrombotest). (With permission from Park BK, Breckenridge AM: Clinical implications of enzyme induction and enzyme inhibition. *Clin Pharmacokinet* 6:1–24, 1981.)

flurane, resulting in higher alveolar concentrations (see Chapter 9).

ALTERATION IN DRUG-METABOLIZING ENZYMES

Many drugs are eliminated by metabolism by the mixed-function oxidase systems in the liver (see Chapter 2). The activity of these enzymes can be increased by enzyme-inducing agents, such as the barbiturates or the antibiotic rifampin. Increased drug-metabolizing enzyme activity results in more rapid metabolism and excretion of durgs which are metabolized by these enzyme systems, resulting in lower drug concentrations. An example of this effect is shown in Figure 4.1, where phenobarbitone was administered to a patient already stabilized on the anticoagulant warfarin. The increased rate of warfarin metabolism and fall in warfarin plasma concentrations resulted in a shortening of the prothrombin time (reflected by a rise in the thrombotest) and loss of anticoagulant control. Potentially more serious is the rise in warfarin concentrations and increase in the degree of anticoagulation after discontinuation of the inducing agent. This can result in excessive anticoagulation and hemorrhage when the patient has been stabilized on the anticoagulant in the presence of the inducing agent.

Inhibition of drug metabolism will result in increased drug concentrations and excessive pharmacological effect. Cimetidine is a potent inhibitor of drug metabolism and has been shown to impair the elimination of warfarin, diazepam, antipyrine, and propranolol. In addition, cimetidine reduces the clearance of lidocaine.

Anesthetic agents themselves also affect drug disposition (see Chapter 1, page 38). The volatile anesthetics inhibit the metabolism of oxidized drugs, but glucuronidation may be relatively unaffected by anesthesia. In addition to the direct effect of anesthetic agents on drug metabolism, anesthetics may also alter drug disposition through their hemodynamic effects on organ blood flow and, hence, drug delivery to the organs of

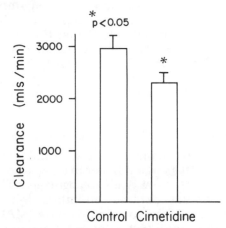

Propranolol
Oral Clearance

Figure 4.2. **Effect of cimetidine on propranolol clearance.** (With permission from Feely J, Wilkinson GR, Wood AJJ: Reduction of liver blood flow and propranolol metabolism by cimetidine. *N Engl J Med* 304:692–695, 1981.)

drug excretion, such as the liver and kidney. The effects of anesthesia on drug disposition have been discussed in Chapter 1.

Allopurinol, which inhibits the enzyme xanthine oxidase and hence the conversion of xanthine to uric acid, also inhibits the metabolism of synthetic xanthine derivatives, such as 6-mercaptopurine, resulting in elevated plasma concentrations and an increase in toxicity when allopurinol is added to 6-mercaptopurine treatment.

Drugs that produce inhibition of plasma cholinesterase prolong the action of succinylcholine (see Chapter 10). Drugs that induce drug-metabolizing enzymes can alter the metabolism of methoxyflurane, possibly resulting in the release of nephrotoxic levels of fluoride ion (see Chapter 9).

ALTERATION IN PROTEIN BINDING

Alteration in drug concentrations at the receptor site may occur through changes in the protein binding of one drug produced by the coadministration of another. This may result in displacement of one drug from its protein binding sites so that a higher free drug concentration will exist transiently. The long-term consequences of these displacement interactions depend on whether the drug's clearance is increased by the increased free fraction (see Figs. 1.21 and 1.22). Protein-binding interactions are only of importance for drugs who protein binding is high (>90%).

MONAMINE OXIDASE INHIBITORS

The interaction of these antidepressants with a large number of sympathomimetics is now well recognized. The monoamine oxidase inhibitors inhibit the enzyme monoamine oxidase (MAO) which is responsible for the metabolism of a number of endogenous and exogenous sympathomimetics. This results in an increased store of catecholamines accumulating within the synaptic nerve endings.

The administration of drugs which cause catecholamine release to patients receiving MAO inhibitors may result in a hypertensive crisis because of the greater-than-normal amounts of catecholamines released. Thus, amphetamines, ephedrine, and metaraminol may all produce excessive peripheral release of catecholamines resulting in hypertension. In addition to drugs, monoamines in food such as tyramine, which is present in large quantities in cheese and other foods, reach the systemic circulation because they are not destroyed by the MAO in the liver as they enter from the gut via the portal circulation. Tyramine acts as an indirect-acting sympathomimetic, causing release of the catecholamines from the adrenal medulla and nerve endings where they are present in abnormally high concentrations, so that their release causes a hypertensive crisis. Other foods containing high concentrations of tyramine include wine, chocolate, and yeast-containing foods or drinks. The hypertensive crisis produced by such compounds can be life threatening and may result in an intracerebral hemorrhage.

MAO inhibitors have also been shown to enhance the effects of general anesthetic agents and, when meperidine is given in conjunction with MAO inhibitors, a syndrome of excitation, rigidity, coma, and hyperpyrexia has been described.

REDUCTION IN RENAL CLEARANCE

A recently recognized interaction is that involving digoxin and quinidine. When quinidine is added to digoxin therapy, an increase in the serum digoxin concentration results. On average, there is a doubling of the serum digoxin level, but there is considerable interindividual variability with the increase ranging up to 5-fold. Quinidine causes displacement of digoxin from both myocardial and peripheral tissue stores with a consequent reduction in the volume of distribution. In addition, the renal clearance of digoxin is reduced by 25 to 30%, while the glomerular filtration rate or creatinine clearance is unchanged. It has been postulated that the fall in renal excretion is due to a reduction in the renal tubular secretion of digoxin. The importance of this interaction is seen in the high frequency with which signs of digoxin toxicity have been reported. It is, therefore, recommended that caution be exercised when quinidine is added to digoxin therapy, that the dose of digoxin be reduced, and that serum digoxin concentrations be monitored carefully. Interestingly, quinidine does not appear to affect the elimination or volume of distribution of digitoxin.

ALTERED EXCRETION THROUGH THE LUNGS

Drugs that depress ventilation, such as narcotics, may delay pulmonary excretion of inhalational anesthetics.

LIMITATION OF DRUG ACCESS TO ITS SITE OF ACTION

Preventing a drug from reaching its site of action will reduce the drug's pharmacological effect. An example of this action is seen with the adrenergic neuron blockers, such as guanethidine, guanadrel, debrisoquine, and bethanidine, which are taken up by the norepinephrine pump into adrenergic nerve endings. Inhibitors of norepinephrine uptake, such as the tricyclic antidepressants and chlorpromazine, also inhibit the uptake of guanethidine and so, by preventing its entry into the adrenergic neurons, block guanethidine's antihypertensive effect. Amphetamine also antagonizes guanethidine's antihypertensive effect, but by a different mechanism. These interactions are discussed more fully in Chapter 15.

Pharmacodynamic Interactions

Pharmacodynamic interactions are often less well recognized because of the difficulty in quantitating drug effect accurately enough to demonstrate the change. However, well-described interactions can occur at the neuromuscular junction causing the aminoglycoside and polymyxin antibiotics such as streptomycin, neomycin, or gentamicin to enhance the effects of curare and other neuromuscular blocking agents resulting in prolonged neuromuscular blockade. These are discussed in Chapter 10.

The more common pharmacodynamic interactions involve drugs with similar actions producing additive effects. For example, the coadministration of two drugs with sedative activity will result in greater sedation than was produced by either drug alone.

Drugs acting at the same receptor site will also interact in a predictable way. For example, the administration of a β blocker will antagonize the effects of a β-receptor stimulant administered as a bronchodilator. Similarly, atropine will antagonize the effects of simultaneously administered cholinergic agents.

The inhalational agents enhance the dysrhythmic effects of endogenous and exogenous catecholamines, and epinephrine dosage should be limited under these circumstances (see Chapter 13). Antihypertensive drugs, which deplete catecholamine stores (e.g. reserpine),

may render the patient liable to hypotensive episodes during anesthesia. Thiazide therapy may cause hypokalemia, increasing the toxicity of digitalis and altering the action of nondepolarizing muscle relaxants. β-Adrenergic receptor blocking drugs may potentiate the cardiovascular depressant effects of inhalational anesthetic agents and reduce the sympathetic response to stress and hypovolemia; however, there is good evidence to indicate the β-adrenergic receptor blocking agents should be continued up to the time of surgery. Volatile anesthetics may also potentiate cardiovascular depression in patients receiving calcium channel-blocking agents; bradycardia, hypotension, and heart block may occur (see Chapter 18).

Lidocaine interacts with muscle relaxants (Chapter 10) and lowers MAC for halothane and nitrous oxide. The interaction of levodopa (see Chapter 6) with inhalational anesthetic agents is of concern to anesthesiologists because significant blood pressure instability may occur if the patient is anesthetized with halothane. Patients receiving tricyclic antidepressants may develop arrhythmias and cardiovascular instability during anesthesia. In addition, a dangerous pressor response may occur if such patients are given epinephrine, norepinephrine, and some sympathomimetic amines.

The interactions reviewed in this chapter should not be taken as an exhaustive list, but rather are included only as examples of the various mechanisms by which one drug can interfere with the pharmacological effect of another. Only by limiting the number of drugs prescribed and by remaining alert to the potential for drug interactions will it be possible to reduce the actual frequency with which such interactions occur in practice.

BIBLIOGRAPHY

Brown DD, Spector R, Juhl RP: Drug interactions with digoxin. *Drugs* 20:198–206, 1980.

Bruce DL: Alcoholism and anesthesia. *Anesth Analg* 62:84–96, 1983.

Chung F: Cancer, chemotherapy, and anesthesia. *Can Anaesth Soc J* 29:364–371, 1982.

Cooke JE: Drug interactions in anesthesia. *Clin Plast Surg* 12:83–89, 1985.

Davies DM (ed): *Textbook of Adverse Drug Reactions*, ed 3. New York, Oxford University Press, 1985.

Dodson ME: Adverse reactions and anaesthesia. *Adverse Drug React Bull* 96:352–355, 1982.

Doering W: Quinidine-digoxin interaction. Pharmacokinetics, underlying mechanism, and clinical implications. *N Engl J Med* 301:400–404, 1979.

Edwards R: Anaesthesia and alcohol. *Br Med J* 291:423–424, 1985.

Feely J, Wilkinson GR, Wood AJJ: Reduction of liver blood flow and propranolol metabolism by cimetidine. *N Engl J Med* 304:692–695, 1981.

Gallagher JD, Lieberman RW, Meranze J, Spielman SR, Ellison N: Amiodarone-induced complications during coronary artery surgery. *Anesthesiology* 55:186–188, 1981.

Grogono AW, Seltzer JL: A guide to drug interactions in anaesthetic practice. *Drugs* 19:279–291, 1980.

Hager WD, Fenster P, Mayersohn M, Perrier D, Graves P, Marcus FI, Goldman S: Digoxin quinidine interaction: pharmacokinetic evaluation. *N Engl J Med* 300:1238–1241, 1979.

Halsey MJ: Drug interactions in anaesthesia. *Br J Anaesth* 59:112–123, 1987.

Liberman BA, Teasdale SJ: Anaesthesia and amiodarone. *Can Anaesth Soc J* 32:629–638, 1985.

Mitchell JR, Cavanaugh JH, Arias L, Oates JA: Guanethidine and related agents. III. Antagonism by drugs which inhibit the norepinephrine pump in man. *J Clin Invest* 49:1596–1604, 1970.

Mitchell JR, Potter WZ, Hinson JA, Snodgrass WR, Timbrell JA, Gillette JR: Toxic drug reactions. In Gillette JR, Mitchell JR (eds): *Concepts in Biochemical Pharmacology. Handbook of Experimental Pharmacology 28/3.* New York, Springer-Verlag, 1975.

Ochs RH, Pabst J, Greenblatt DJ, Dengler HJ: Noninteraction of digitoxin and quinidine. *N Engl J Med* 303:672–674, 1980.

O'Malley K, Stevenson IH, Ward CA, Wood AJJ, Crooks J: Determinants of anticoagulant control in patients receiving warfarin. *Br J Clin Pharmacol* 4:309–314, 1977.

Park BK, Breckenridge AM: Clinical implications of enzyme induction and enzyme inhibition. *Clin Pharmacokinet* 6:1–24, 1981.

Rawlins MD: Drug interactions and anaesthesia. *Br J Anaesth* 50:689–693, 1978.

Selvin BL: Cancer chemotherapy: implications for the anesthesiologist. *Anesth Analg* 60:425–434, 1981.

Smith TN, Corbascio AN (eds): *Drug Interactions in Anesthesia*, ed 2. Philadelphia, Lee & Febiger, 1986.

Wood AJJ, Oates JA: Adverse reactions to drugs. In Braunwald E, Isselbacher KJ, Petersdorf RG, Wilson JD, Martin JB, Fauci AS (eds): *Harrison's Principles of Internal Medicine*, ed 11. New York, McGraw-Hill, 1987.

Wood M: Complications of prior drug therapy. In Orkin FK, Cooperman LH (eds): *Complications in Anesthesiology*, ed 2. Philadelphia, JB Lippincott, 1989.

DRUGS AND ANESTHESIA

5

Cholinergic and Parasympathomimetic Drugs. Cholinesterases and Anticholinesterases

MARGARET WOOD

Acetylcholine (ACh) is the neurotransmitter or chemical mediator at a large number of sites in the peripheral and central nervous systems of many vertebrates, including man. It is traditional to refer to nerves that release acetylcholine from their terminals as cholinergic nerves.

Cholinergic or cholinomimetic drugs act at sites in the body where acetylcholine is the chemical transmitter of the nerve impulse. They may be divided into three groups:

1. **Choline esters:** (carbachol, methacholine);
2. **Alkaloids:** (pilocarpine, muscarine, arecoline);
3. **Anticholinesterases:** cholinesterase inhibitors, by preventing the destruction of acetylcholine, produce intensified cholinergic effects (physostigmine, neostigmine, pyridostigmine, edrophonium).

PHYSIOLOGY OF THE PARASYMPATHETIC NERVOUS SYSTEM

The autonomic nervous system is divided into two divisions—sympathetic and parasympathetic. The preganglionic fibers of the sympathetic nervous system arise from the thoracolumbar segments of the spinal cord, while the corresponding preganglionic fibers of the parasympathetic nervous system have a craniosacral origin. These preganglionic fibers synapse in autonomic ganglia from which arise postganglionic fibers that then innervate either adrenergic or cholinergic receptors situated throughout the body (Fig. 5.1). The autonomic or involuntary nervous system innervates the heart, blood vessels, glands, viscera, and smooth muscle and, therefore, controls and integrates the autonomic functions of the body. Nerve impulses are transmitted across the synapses and neuroef-

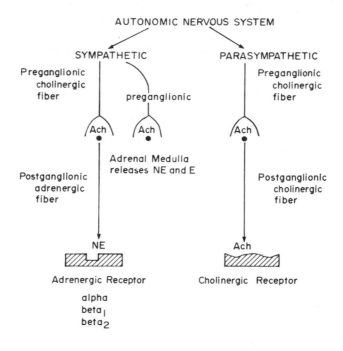

Figure 5.1. Diagram of the autonomic nervous system.

fector junctions of the autonomic nervous system by means of specific chemical agents called neurotransmitters. The neurotransmitter for the adrenergic receptor is norepinephrine and that for the cholinergic receptor is acetylcholine. The neurotransmitter of all preganglionic autonomic nerve fibers, all postganglionic parasympathetic fibers, and a few postganglionic sympathetic fibers (e.g., sweat glands) is acetylcholine. Acetylcholine is also the transmitter at the motor neuromuscular junction.

Acetylcholine and cholinergic drugs thus act at the following sites:

1. **Parasympathetic Nervous System**
   autonomic ganglia
   postganglionic nerve terminals
2. **Sympathetic Nervous System**
   autonomic ganglia
   some postganglionic nerve endings, e.g., sweat glands
3. **Neuromuscular Junction**
4. **Central Nervous System**
5. **Blood Vessels**

Acetylcholine has a direct vasodilator action on arterioles. The physiological responses of the effector organs to cholinergic stimulation are summarized in Table 5.1. Knowledge of these effects allows one to predict the actions of cholinergic and anticholinergic drugs at the cholinergic receptor.

SYNTHESIS, STORAGE, AND RELEASE OF ACETYLCHOLINE

Acetylcholine is synthesized from acetylcoenzyme A and choline within the nerve terminal under the control of the enzyme, choline acetyltransferase (formerly known as choline acetylase). Choline acetyltransferase catalyzes the final step in the synthesis of acetylcholine—the acetylation of choline with an acetyl group from acetylcoenzyme A. The choline required is taken up from the extracellular fluid into the nerve terminal by the process of active transport, and the final step, the acetylation of choline, takes place in the axonal cytoplasm. Acetylcholine is then stored in synaptic

vesicles at the nerve terminals in constant amounts or "quanta." The storage and release of acetylcholine have been the subject of intensive investigation and are best understood at the neuromuscular junction. In the absence of motor nerve stimulation, a succession of these storage vesicles undergoes spontaneous rupture or discharge and releases packets or quanta of acetylcholine, producing small areas of depolarization (miniature end plate potentials), none of which is great enough to generate a propagated muscle contraction. When a strong impulse arrives at the motor nerve terminal, a large number of vesicles rupture, and sufficient acetylcholine is released to produce depolarization of the motor end place and contraction of the muscle results. The simultaneous rupture of a large number of synaptic vesicles appears to depend on the presence of calcium ions.

In close association with acetylcholine is the enzyme acetylcholinesterase (AChE) which is responsible for the rapid destruction and hydrolysis of acetylcholine to choline and acetic acid. There is another enzyme in the tissues and the plasma that is also capable of hydrolyzing acetylcholine and other choline esters, called pseudocholinesterase or plasma cholinesterase. However, diffusion and hydrolysis by plasma cholinesterase play only a minor role in the termination of the action of acetylcholine.

CHOLINERGIC RECEPTORS—NICOTINIC AND MUSCARINIC RECEPTORS

Cholinergic receptors have been divided into two types, "muscarinic" and "nicotinic," because muscarine and nicotine were found to stimulate them selectively (Fig. 5.2). The peripheral actions of acetylcholine are 2-fold: the effects of its release at parasympathetic postganglionic fibers are mimicked by the action of muscarine and blocked by atropine and are, therefore, called muscarinic effects. Nicotinic effects of the neurotransmitter are seen at the skeletal neuromuscular junction and autonomic ganglia (includ-

Table 5.1.
Physiological Responses of Effector Tissues to Cholinergic Nerve Transmission

Tissue	Response
Eye	
Sphincter muscle (iris)	Contraction—miosis
Ciliary muscle	Contraction—for near vision as part of the convergence-accommodation reflex
Heart	
S-A node	Decrease in heart rate (vagus)
Atria	Decrease in contractility
A-V node	Decrease in conduction velocity; A-V block
Ventricle	Possible slight decrease in contractility
Lung	
Bronchial smooth muscle	Stimulation—bronchoconstriction
Bronchial glands	Stimulation—increased secretions
Stomach	
Motility and tone	Increase
Sphincters	Relaxation
Secretions	Stimulation
Intestine	
Motility and tone	Increase
Sphincters	Relaxation
Secretions	Stimulation
Bladder	
Detrusor	Contraction
Trigone and internal sphincter	Relaxation
Sex organs	Erection (male)
Sweat glands	Increased secretion
Adrenal medulla	Secretion of norepinephrine and epinephrine
Exocrine glands	
Pancreas	Increased secretion
Salivary	Increased secretion
Lacrimal	Increased secretion
Pharyngeal	Increased secretion

ing the adrenal medulla) and are mimicked by nicotine and blocked by the neuromuscular blocking agents and the ganglionic blocking agents, respectively. It is now known that nicotine in low doses stimulates and at high doses blocks autonomic ganglia. The same has also been shown to be true for nicotine at the neuromuscular junction. It should also be noted that muscarinic receptors may exist in the absence of cholinergic innervation, e.g., in blood vessels and the placenta.

The muscarinic receptors have recently been classified into subtypes based on their affinity for agonist and antagonist compounds; it is thought that at least two exist (M_1 and M_2). A new selective muscarinic competitive antagonist, pirenzepine, e.g., has a high affinity for

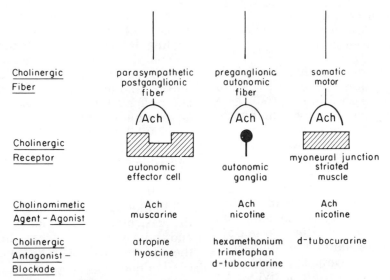

Cholinergic Fiber	parasympathetic postganglionic fiber	preganglionic autonomic fiber	somatic motor
Cholinergic Receptor	autonomic effector cell	autonomic ganglia	myoneural junction striated muscle
Cholinomimetic Agent – Agonist	Ach muscarine	Ach nicotine	Ach nicotine
Cholinergic Antagonist – Blockade	atropine hyoscine	hexamethonium trimetaphan d-tubocurarine	d-tubocurarine

Figure 5.2.   Nicotinic and muscarinic receptors.   *Ach,* acetylcholine. The cholinergic receptors have been divided into nicotinic and muscarinic; the peripheral actions of acetylcholine at the postganglionic parasympathetic nerve terminals are mimicked by muscarine and blocked by atropine, and can be demonstrated on the heart, smooth muscle, and exocrine glands. The nicotinic actions of acetylcholine, seen at the skeletal neuromuscular junction and autonomic ganglia, are mimicked by nicotine and blocked by the neuromuscular blocking agents and the ganglionic blocking agents, respectively.

one but not the other of the two most widely recognized subtypes. Receptor subtypes with a high affinity for pirenzepine predominate in autonomic ganglia, while those with low affinity are found in the myocardium and smooth muscle. Thus, pirenzepine specifically inhibits the M_1 subtype but not the M_2 receptor, has a high affinity for muscarinic receptors in the parietal cell, and therefore inhibits gastric secretion without associated side effects on the central nervous system, heart, eye, and bladder.

CHOLINE ESTERS

STRUCTURE-ACTIVITY RELATIONSHIPS

Acetylcholine, the acetyl ester of choline, is a quaternary ammonium compound that possesses a cationic (positively charged) head joined by a chain of two carbon atoms to an ester grouping. The chemical structures of acetylcholine and the other important choline esters are given in Figure 5.3. These compounds may differ from acetylcholine in three ways (Table 5.2):

Table 5.2.
Comparative Pharmacology of the Choline Esters

Choline ester	Susceptibility to hydrolysis	Muscarinic actions				Nicotinic actions
		CVS	Gut	Bladder	Eye	
Acetylcholine	+++	++	++	++	+	++
Methacholine	+	+++	++	++	+	+
Carbachol	−	+	+++	+++	++	+++
Bethanechol	−	±	+++	+++	++	−

1. relative muscarinic activity;
2. relative nicotinic activity;
3. resistance to enzymatic hydrolysis.

The degree of muscarinic activity falls if the acetyl group is replaced, but in some instances, substitution produces a compound that resists enzymatic hydrolysis. For example, carbachol (where the acetyl group is replaced by carbamyl) possesses both muscarinic and nicotinic actions, but is almost totally resistant to hydrolysis by either acetylcholinesterase or plasma cholinesterase (pseudocholinesterase). Bethanechol, which possesses mainly muscarinic and little nicotinic activity, is also resistant to the cholinesterases. Although both carbachol and bethanechol possess muscarinic activity, the cardiovascular effects are not marked, and gastronintestinal and urinary effects predominate. Due to β-methyl substitution, acetyl-β-methylcholine, or methacholine, is a poor nicotinic agonist and, therefore, has predominantly muscarinic activity which is most evident on the cardiovascular system. In addition, its duration of action is more prolonged than acetylcholine because it is hydrolyzed by acetylcholinesterase at only a third the rate of acetylcholine and is almost totally resistant to hydrolysis by plasma cholinesterase.

CARDIOVASCULAR EFFECTS

Acetylcholine has a negative chronotropic and inotropic effect on the heart. A small dose of acetylcholine (1 to 5 μg/kg) given by intravenous injection to the anesthetized cat causes a fall in blood pressure due to vasodilation and, in addition, a reflex tachycardia mediated through the aortic and carotid baroreceptors. Larger doses result in bradycardia due to the direct action of acetylcholine on the heart. Because of the rapidity of the enzymatic hydrolysis of acetylcholine, the fall in blood pressure is short lived. The hypotension and bradycardia are muscarinic effects and are prevented by the administration of atropine. Very large doses (500 to 1000 times the dose required to elicit the muscarinic effect) of acetylcholine when given with atropine cause a large rise in blood pressure. The atropine blocks the muscarinic effects revealing the nicotinic effects of sympathoadrenal discharge and stimulation of the autonomic ganglia, with resultant hypertension and tachycardia. The neuromuscular effects when seen consist of fibrillary twitchings of muscle followed by a transient loss of power. The actions of acetylcholine alone are too short lived and widespread to be of clinical use.

GASTROINTESTINAL EFFECT

Stimulation of the smooth muscle of the gastrointestinal tract, gall bladder, and biliary ducts occurs. In addition, there is enhanced secretory activity. Defecation may result.

GENITOURINARY EFFECTS

Stimulation of the smooth muscle of the urinary tract occurs, with relaxation of the internal sphincter which may cause micturition.

Other Choline Esters

Methacholine, carbachol, and bethanechol are little used today.

METHACHOLINE (ACETYL-β-METHYLCHOLINE)

Methacholine is destroyed by cholinesterase less readily than acetylcholine and is potentiated by anticholinesterase drugs. It has predominant cardiovascular muscarinic effects and has been used in the treatment of supraventricular tachycardia. Side effects include profound hypotension, syncope, bradycardia and heart block, nausea and vomiting, precipitation of bronchospasm, defecation, micturition, sweating, lacrimation and salivation, etc.

CARBACHOL (CARBAMYLCHOLINE)

Carbachol is a very potent and relatively nonselective cholinergic agonist, possessing both muscarinic and nicotinic activity. It has been used in the past for its stimulatory effect on the bladder and gastrointestinal tract. It has a fairly long duration of action of about 2 hours because the carbamate substitution protects it from hydrolysis by either true or pseudocholinesterase, and its actions are therefore not potentiated by anticholinesterases. Its side effects are predictable and include cardiovascular effects, salivation, lacrimation, urination, defecation, and abdominal cramping.

BETHANECHOL (CARBAMYLMETHYLCHOLINE)

Bethanechol has a long duration of action because it is also resistant to cholinesterases and its actions are predominantly muscarinic. If a cholinergic agent is to be used to stimulate the smooth muscle of the gastrointestinal tract and urinary bladder then bethanechol is the preferred drug due to its lack of nicotinic activity and relatively mild cardiovascular effects. It has been used in the treatment of gastric retention following bilateral vagotomy, congential megacolon, and urinary retention.

CHOLINE ALKALOIDS

Pilocarpine, muscarine, and arecoline are the three major naturally occurring cholinomimetic alkaloids.

PILOCARPINE

Pilocarpine is the chief alkaloid obtained from the leaves of *Pilocarpus*, a genus of trees and shrubs found in South America. Pilocarpine has a direct muscarinic effect and very little nicotinic effect. Its chief use today is as a topical miotic agent in ophthalmological practice, where it is used in the treatment of glaucoma to reduce intraocular pressure and to reverse the mydriasis produced by atropine.

METOCLOPRAMIDE

Metoclopramide is a procainamide derivative that has powerful peripheral cholinergic effects and centrally antagonizes cerebral dopamine receptors. Metoclopramide increases gastric peristalsis, causes dilation of the pylorus, and thus increases gastric emptying. These effects on the proximal gut have been termed "gastrokinetic" and are abolished by nar-

cotic analgesics and atropine, but not by vagotomy. The antiemetic effects of metoclopramide result from its antagonism of dopamine receptors in the central nervous system. Therapeutic uses include the management of nausea and vomiting; increasing peristalsis in diagnostic radiography and gastrointestinal intubation, gastroesophageal reflux, and esophagitis; and reducing gastric volume prior to emergency and obstetric anesthesia.

Metoclopramide is rapidly absorbed from the gut, and oral bioavailability varies between 30 and 100%. The plasma elimination half-life is about 4 hours and is prolonged by renal impairment. The most common side effects are nervousness, somnolence, and dystonic reactions.

The suggested dose is 10 to 20 mg administered slowly intravenously or 5 to 15 mg, orally. Metoclopramide has been used by anesthesiologists to accelerate gastric emptying prior to anesthesia and to reduce perioperative nausea and vomiting. When 10 mg of metoclopramide is administered intravenously followed later by 50 mg of meperidine, gastric emptying is accelerated, but when a higher dose (150 mg) of meperidine is administered simultaneously with a 10-mg intramuscular dose of metoclopramide, the ability of metoclopramide to accelerate gastric emptying appears to be lost. Thus, when atropine and metoclopramide or opioids and metaclopramide are administered together, the effects are cancelled out. The use of metoclopramide as part of an anesthetic regimen to reduce gastric volume and acidity is further discussed in Chapter 23.

Cisapride is another gastrointestinal prokinetic drug; it increases lower esophageal pressure and increases the rate of gastric emptying. It has been shown to reverse morphine-induced delay in gastric emptying in patients about to undergo anesthesia induction. However, it has no antidopaminergic properties, and extrapyramidal side effects (associated with metoclopramide) have not been reported. Cisapride acts by enhancing the release of acetylcholine in the myenteric plexus of the gastrointestinal tract. The future role of cisapride in anesthetic practice remains to be fully evaluated.

CHOLINESTERASES

There are two enzymes present in humans capable of hydrolyzing esters of choline.

1. **Acetylcholinesterase** (AChE), also known as specific or true cholinesterase, is found in the region of cholinergic nerve fibers and in red cells. It is not found in plasma. It is responsible for the hydrolysis and inactivation of acetylcholine released during cholinergic transmission at cholinoceptive sites, such as the neuromuscular junction.
2. **Butyrocholinesterase** (BuChE), also known as nonspecific cholinesterase, plasma cholinesterase, or pseudocholinesterase is synthesized in the liver and is found in the liver, plasma, kidney, and intestine. Its physiological function is not known, but it is responsible for the hydrolysis of the depolarizing neuromuscular relaxant succinylcholine and the ester-type local anesthetic agents. Pseudocholinesterase will be considered in more detail later in this chapter.

Acetylcholinesterase

Acetylcholine possesses a positively charged quaternary ammonium group, being the acetyl ester of choline (Fig 5.3) and is hydrolyzed by the enzyme acetylcholinesterase. Acetylcholinesterase has two active sites—an anionic site and an esteratic site. The exact structure of the active sites of acetylcholinesterase is a controversial subject, but it is thought that the quarternary nitrogen group of acetylcholine is attracted to negative phosphate groups at the anionic site of the enzyme and that the carbon atom of the carbonyl group is attracted to a positively charged nucleophilic group at the esteratic active site, possibly consisting of histidine and serine. The anionic or negatively charged site binds acetylcholine and orients it correctly as the substrate for hydrolysis. There is evidence that it is the esteratic site that is primarily concerned with hydrolysis or cleavage of the ester bond of aceylcholine. The esteratic site contains an electronegative

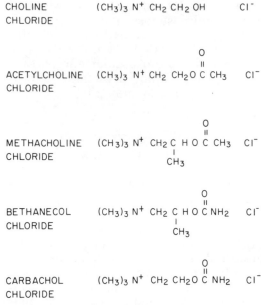

Figure 5.3.   Chemical formulae of acetylcholine and the choline esters.

group which contributes a pair of electrons to form a bond between the esteratic site and the ester group of actylcholine. Choline is then split off, leaving the acetylated enzyme. The acetyl enzyme then reacts with water to produce the regenerated active enzyme and acetic acid (Figs. 5.4 and 5.5). Thus, the products of the hydrolysis of acetylcholine are free

---

Figures 5.4 and 5.5.   Hydrolysis of acetylcholine by acetylcholinesterase. The substrate acetylcholine combines with an active unit of the enzyme acetylcholinesterase to form a complex by electrostatic attraction between the quaternary H^+ atom of the choline moiety and the anionic site of the enzyme, and by interaction between the electrophilic C atom of the carbonyl group and the serine hydroxyl group of the esteratic site. Choline is then split off, leaving the acetylated enzyme. The acetylated enzyme then reacts rapidly with water to produce acetic acid and the regenerated active enzyme. (Adapted with permission from Koelle CB. Anticholinesterase agents. In Goodman LS, Gilman A (eds): *The Pharmacological Basis of Therapeutics,* ed 5. New York, Macmillan, 1975, p 448.)

choline, acetic acid, and the enzyme regenerated for further use.

THE ANTICHOLINESTERASES

Drugs that bind to either the anionic or esteratic sites of acetylcholinesterase or both will inhibit the hydrolysis of acetylcholine, because they prevent the access of acetylcholine to the active sites of the enzyme. Drugs that inhibit or inactivate cholinesterase are called **anticholinesterases.** Most of these drugs inhibit both acetylcholinesterase and pseudocholinesterase. They cause acetylcholine to accumulate at cholinergic receptors throughout the body, and their effects can be predicted to some extent from a

knowledge of the physiology and pharmacology of the autonomic nervous system described earlier in this chapter.

Anticholinesterases have been divided into two types, depending on whether they inhibit the anionic or esteratic sites of acetylcholinesterase. Drugs that inhibit the *anionic* site are called *prosthetic, reversible competitive inhibitors,* because inhibition is due to competition between the anticholinesterase and acetylcholine for the anionic site. Thus, acetylcholine can compete with edrophonium for access to the active site on the enzyme in a concentration-dependent manner. Anticholinesterase drugs in this group therefore tend to have a brief duration of action. Quaternary ammonium compunds, e.g., tetraethylammonium ion, inhibit the enzyme reversibly by binding to the anionic site. Edrophonium, which has a short duration of action, is primarily an anionic site inhibitor, but in addition, combines with the imidazole nitrogen atom of histidine at the esteratic site by hydrogen bonding.

The other group of anticholinesterases are those which inhibit the *esteratic* site of acetylcholinesterase, called *acid-transferring inhibitors.* These drugs include carbamates, such as neostigmine, pyridostigmine, and physostigmine and the organophosphorus inhibitors. Ecothiophate, a quaternary organophosphorus compound, combines at both the esteratic and anionic sites. The reaction between the acid-transferring inhibitors and acetylcholinesterase is similar to that between acetylcholine and acetylcholinesterase; but the reaction between the carbamylated enzyme and water to release the regenerated enzyme takes much longer, and until regenerated enzyme is released, the active sites of the enzyme are not available for the further hydrolysis of acetylcholine. Acetylcholine cannot compete with these anticholinesterases for the active site on the enzyme until the carbamylated enzyme is regenerated. The half-life of the acetyl enzyme is measured in microseconds, the half-life of the carbamyl enzyme in minutes, and the phosphoryl enzyme in weeks or months. Thus, the half-life of the acetylated enzyme in the case of the pysiological substrate acetylcholine is 42 microseconds, while the half-life of dimethylcarbamyl-acetylcholinesterase formed by the reaction with the carbamyl ester, neostigmine, is 30 minutes. Thus, it is the difference in the mechanism of inhibition produced by edrophonium ("reversible") and neostigmine ("acid-transferring") which accounts for the longer duration of action associated with neostigmine and pyridostigmine.

The organophosphorus insecticides have been termed "irreversible" anticholinesterases because the phosphorylated esteratic site of acetylcholinesterase undergoes regeneration at an extremely slow rate. However, it is important to understand that the mechanism of action of the carbamyl esters and the organophosphorus insecticides is essentially the same, and that they both react with the enzyme acetylcholinesterase in a similar manner as the natural substrate, acetylcholine, but regeneration of the enzyme takes substantially longer to occur.

STRUCTURE-ACTIVITY RELATIONSHIPS

The chemical formulae of the important anticholinesterases are given in Figure 5.6. Physostigmine and neostigmine, which both possess a carbamyl group, are carbamate inhibitors. Edrophonium which does not possess a carbamyl group is less potent and shorter acting, since it produces reversible inhibition of acetylcholinesterase. The presence of a quaternary nitrogen atom, while not essential for anticholinesterase activity, confers increased potency. Thus, neostigmine, which possesses a quarternary nitrogen atom, is a much more potent anticholinesterase than the tertiary amine, physostigmine.

INDIVIDUAL ANTICHOLINESTERASE DRUGS

The pharmacological effects of the anticholinesterase drugs can be predicted from a knowledge of the sites where acetylcholine is the neurotransmitter (Table 5.1). Thus, the anticholinesterases may produce the following effects:

1. Cholinergic stimulation of muscarinic receptors, bradycardia, miosis, salivation, in-

creased oropharyngeal secretions, sweating, bronchospasm, increased peristaltic activity, micturition, and defecation;
2. Stimulation (followed by depression at higher doses) of nicotinic receptors at autonomic ganglia and the skeletal neuromuscular junction;
3. Stimulation, followed by depression of cholinoceptive receptors in the central nervous system.

In addition to the inhibition of acetylcholinesterase, anticholinesterase drugs have presynaptic and postsynaptic effects at the motor nerve terminal that may also contribute to the antagonism of neuromuscular blockade.

Neostigmine

Neostigmine is a carbamyl ester acid-transferring cholinesterase inhibitor. Its chemical structure is given in Figure 5.6.

CARDIOVASCULAR SYSTEM

The effects of neostigmine on the cardiovascular system are complex and depend on the relative degree of nicotinic or muscarinic stimulation. Peripheral accumulation of acetylcholine may cause profound bradycardia due to vagal stimulation. In addition, vasodilation and hypotension may occur. Cardiac arrhythmias and even cardiac arrest have been reported following the administration of the combination of atropine and neostigmine to reverse neuromuscular blockade at the termination of anesthesia. Occasionally, when the muscarinic effects are blocked by atropine, or when large doses are used, the blood pressure and heart rate may rise due to stimulation of autonomic ganglia and release of epinephrine from the adrenal medulla (nicotinic effect). The comparative cardiovascular effects of neostigmine, pyridostigmine, and edrophonium are discussed later in this chapter.

RESPIRATORY SYSTEM

Bronchoconstriction may occur due to contraction of bronchial smooth muscle, and there may be increased oropharyngeal and bronchial gland secretion.

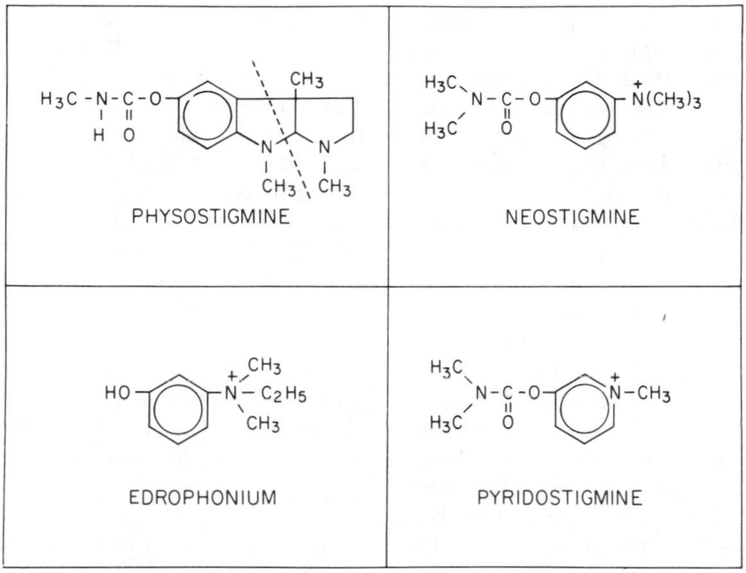

Figure 5.6. Chemical formulae of the important anticholenesterases.

NEUROMUSCULAR JUNCTION

Neostigmine is routinely used during anesthesia to reverse the action of the nondepolarizing neuromuscular blocking agents. Neostigmine, by inhibiting acetylcholinesterase, allows acetylcholine to accumulate at the neuromuscular junction and so increases the depolarizing action of acetylcholine by the competitive displacement of *d*-tubocurarine from the cholinergic receptor. A small dose of neostigmine, therefore, increases skeletal muscle contractility and reverses a competitive neuromuscular block.

It is important for the anesthesiologist to understand that the reversal of a competitive neuromuscular block by neostigmine is limited in nature and that once the enzyme is fully inhibited, increasing doses of neostigmine will not reduce the block any further. Indeed, very large doses of neostigmine, by allowing the accumulation of high concentrations of acetylcholine or by a direct effect, cause neuromuscular blockade. This is rarely seen in clinical practice, except following poisoning with organophosphorous insecticides or as a "cholinergic crisis" in patients with myasthenia gravis who have received excessive anticholinesterase therapy.

The interaction between neostigmine and depolarizing muscle relaxants is complex. In general, neostigmine in clinical doses intensifies a depolarizing block, but antagonizes a competitive nondepolarizing block. Acetylcholine and succinylcholine act as cholinergic agonists at the cholinergic receptors, and so both depolarize the post-junctional membrane and produce additive effects. Therefore, one would expect neostigmine to augment a depolarizing block. However, when repeated doses of succinylcholine are given such that a phase II block occurs, a nondepolarization stage results where all the classical signs of a competitive block are present and, in this case, administration of an anticholinesterase drug causes a reduction in neuromuscular blockade.

GASTROINTESTINAL TRACT

Neostigmine increases gastric contractility and secretions. It also increases large and small bowel motility and peristalsis. This may be painful to the patient and may be attenuated by the administration of atropine.

PHARMACOKINETICS

Neostigmine contains a quaternary ammonium group making it relatively polar, and therefore it does not cross the blood-brain barrier to any significant extent and is poorly absorbed from the gastrointestinal tract. Oral doses required for the treatment of myasthenia gravis are therefore much higher than those used parenterally by the anesthesiologist. The oral bioavailability of neostigmine has been estimated to be about 20%.

The distribution and elimination of neostigmine have been investigated in patients undergoing anesthesia. Renal excretion accounts for 50% of the clearance of neostigmine; nonrenal mechanisms for the elimination of neostigmine are unclear, but possible modes of elimination include hepatic uptake and metabolism, biliary excretion, and hydrolysis of neostigmine by acetylcholinesterase. Neostigmine is metabolized to a number of metabolites, the major one being 3-hydroxy phenyltrimethylammonium. This metabolite has one-tenth the antagonist activity of neostigmine but does not appear to contribute to antagonism of neuromuscular blockade in laboratory experiments. Other metabolites probably exist but have not yet been identified.

Neostigmine is rapidly eliminated from the plasma following intravenous administration. The distribution half-life $(t_{1/2\alpha})$ varies between 1 and 3.5 minutes, while the elimination half-life $(t_{1/2\beta})$ has been reported as ranging from 15 to 80 minutes (Table 5.3).

Since myasthenia gravis does not impair renal or hepatic function, there are no indications that the elimination of anticholinesterases is impaired in this disease, and comparisons of pharmacokinetics in patients with myasthenia gravis, healthy subjects, or anesthetized patients have revealed no differences. The metabolism and excretion of neostigmine (2.0 mg intramuscularly) have been investigated in patients with myasthenia gravis, when the half-life $(t_{1/2\beta})$ was estimated to be 72 minutes, the volume of distribution, 50.0 L, and the plasma clearance ranged from 434 to 549 ml/min. Approximately 80% of the drug was eliminated in the urine within 24 hours; 50% as unchanged neostigmine; 15% as 3-hydroxyphenyl trimethylammonium; and 15% as other metabolites.

PHARMACODYNAMICS

In clinical practice, the magnitude of antagonism and time to onset of action of the anticholinesterases are dependent on the amount of spontaneous recovery of muscle twitch at the time of drug administration. Therefore, the potencies of the three anticholinesterases neostigmine, pyridostigmine, and edrophonium have been compared during halothane anesthesia and a tubocurarine infusion that maintained a stable 90% depression of muscle twitch tension. The dose of antagonist producing 50% antagonism (ED_{50}) gives potency ratios showing that neostigmine is 4.4 times more potent than pyridostigmine and 5.7 times more potent than edrophonium (Fig. 5.7). However, it should be noted that the dose-response curve for edrophonium is not parallel to the curves for neostigmine and pyridostigmine, and so potency ratios vary depending on whether the compar-

Table 5.3.
Comparative Pharmacokinetics of Neostigmine, Edrophonium, and Pyridostigmine

	Volume of distribution (V_{dss}, L/kg)	Distribution half-life ($t_{1/2\alpha}$, min)	Elimination half-life ($t_{1/2\beta}$, min)	Clearance (Cl, ml/kg/min)
Neostigmine (5.0 mg)	0.7	3.5	80	9.0
Edrophonium (0.5–1.0 mg/kg)	1.1	7.2	110	9.6
Pyridostigmine (0.35 mg/kg)	1.1	6.8	112	8.6

Note that the pharmacokinetic parameters are very similar for all three drugs. (Data with permission from Cronnelly R, Morris RB: Antagonism of neuromuscular blockade. *Br J Anaesth* 54:183–194, 1982.)

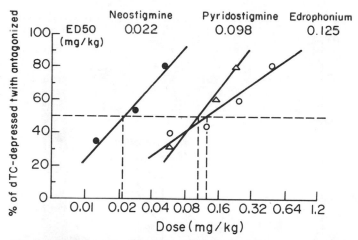

Figure 5.7. Dose-response curves for neostigmine, pyridostigmine, and edrophonium in anesthetized patients. Edrophonium, 0.5 mg/kg (○), was equipotent on the basis of antagonizing d-tubocurarine (dTC)-induced twitch depression to neostigmine, 0.043 mg/kg (●), or pyridostigmine, 0.22 mg/kg (△). (With permission from Cronnelly R, Morris RB, Miller RD: Edrophonium: duration of action and atropine requirement in humans during halothane anesthesia. *Anesthesiology* 57:261–266, 1982.)

ison is made at the ED_{25}, ED_{50}, or ED_{75} point. The dose of edrophonium that corresponds to the usual clinical dose of neostigmine (3.0 mg/70 kg) and pyridostigmine (15 mg/70 kg) is commonly quoted as 0.5 mg/kg or 35 mg/70 kg. The fact that the dose-response curve for edrophonium does not parallel the curves for neostigmine and pyridostigmine has been attributed by some workers to the different mechanism of action of edrophonium.

The time to onset of action (i.e., time from drug administration to peak effect) for equipotent doses of neostigmine, pyridostigmine, and edrophonium is illustrated in Figure 5.8. The time to onset of action is 1.2 minutes for edrophonium (0.5 mg/kg), 7.1 minutes neostigmine (3.0 mg/70 kg), and 12.2 minutes for pyridostigmine (15 mg/70 kg). Thus, pyridostigmine has the slowest and edrophonium the most rapid onset of action. The duration of action of neostigmine is similar to that of edrophonium (about 60 minutes), but the duration of antagonism produced by pyridostigmine is about 40% longer than that produced by the two other anticholinesterases (Fig. 5.9).

RENAL DISEASE

Renal function has a marked effect on the elimination of neostigmine, and $t_{1/2\beta}$ is increased from 80 minutes in healthy anesthetized patients to 183 minutes in anephric patients. In addition, the plasma clearance is decreased from 9.0 ml/kg/min in the normal subject to 3.4 ml/kg/min in anephric patients. There was no change in the volume of distribution (Vd_{ss}) at steady state. Therefore, in the absence of renal function, the plasma clearance of neostigmine is decreased, and the elimination half-life is increased. This has also been shown to be true for d-tubocurarine and pancuronium and may be advantageous, in that although prolonged neuromuscular blockade may occur in patients with abnormal renal function due to delayed elimination of relaxants, the elimination of the anticholinesterase reversal agent is also delayed and may prevent the occurrence of recurarization. Pharmacokinetic parameters for neostigmine in patients who have received a functioning renal transplant are similar to those estimated in patients with normal renal function, indicating that the elimination of neostigmine returns to

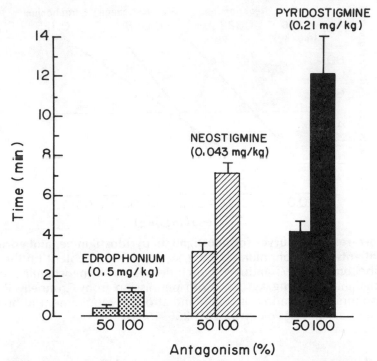

Figure 5.8.   Comparison of the onset of action of edrophonium, neostigmine, and pyridostigmine.   The time from administration of the antagonist to its peak effect is 0.8 to 2.0 minutes for edrophonium, 7 to 11 minutes for neostigmine, and 12 to 16 minutes for pyridostigmine. Thus, onset of action of edrophonium is faster than that of neostigmine or pyridostigmine. (With permission from Cronnelly R, Morris RB, Miller RD: Edrophonium: duration of action and atropine requirement in humans during halothane anesthesia. *Anesthesiology* 57:261–266, 1982.

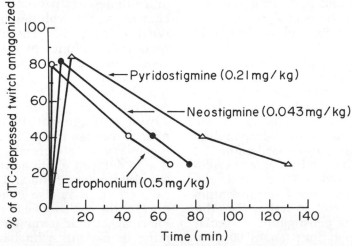

Figure 5.9.   Duration of action of neostigmine, pyridostigmine, and edrophonium.   The durations of action of neostigmine and edrophonium are similar, but both are shorter than pyridostigmine. (With permission from Cronnelly R, Morris RB, Miller RD: Edrophonium: duration of action and atropine requirement in humans during halothane anesthesia. *Anesthesiology* 57:261–266, 1982.)

normal with successful renal transplantation.

AGE

This disposition of neostigmine has also been defined in different age groups. Investigators have compared the pharmacokinetics of neostigmine in small infants and children with those of adults. Distribution half-lives and volumes were similar for infants, children, and adults; however, the elimination half-life was shorter in infants (approximately 39 minutes) and children (48 minutes) compared with adults in whom $t_{1/2\beta}$ was reported to be 67 minutes. Plasma clearance values were therefore slightly higher in children. The time course for onset and duration of antagonism of neuromuscular blockade by neostigmine is similar for infants, children, and adults, but it is interesting that the dose of neostigmine required to antagonize tubocurarine-induced neuromuscular blockade is lower in infants and children than adults; i.e., the dose-response curve for neostigmine in infants and children is shifted to the left of the curve for adults. The dose of neostigmine which produces 50% antagonism of tubocurarine-induced neuromuscular depression (ED_{50}) is 13.1 $\mu g/kg$ in infants, 15.5 $\mu g/kg$ in children, and 22.9 $\mu g/kg$ in adults. Thus, pediatric patients do not require larger doses than adults to reverse neuromuscular blockade, but actually require about half that recommended for adults. Pharmacokinetic parameters for neostigmine in elderly patients are similar to those of young adults, but the duration of antagonism appears to be longer in elderly patients.

DRUG INTERACTIONS

Neostigmine inhibits both acetylcholinesterase and pseudocholinesterase activity. Red cell acetylcholinesterase activity has been shown to be inhibited within 2 to 3 minutes of the intravenous injection of clinical doses of neostigmine, and the enzyme activity is only 55% of control values 60 minutes later. Similarly, it has been demonstrated that pseudocholinesterase activity is decreased after the administration of neostigmine.

The neuromuscular blocking effect of succinylcholine is significantly prolonged by both neostigmine and pyridostigmine due to inhibition of pseudocholinesterase, the enzyme responsible for the hydrolysis of succinylcholine.

SUGGESTED DOSAGE AND ADMINISTRATION

Neostigmine bromide is available for oral use in 15-mg tablets and neostigmine methylsulfate for parenteral use in ampuls and vials containing 0.25 mg, 0.5 mg, or 1.0 mg/ml. Atropine or an anticholinergic agent should always be given with neostigmine to protect against the potentially dangerous cardiovascular muscarinic effects. A dose of 40 to 45 $\mu g/kg$ of neostigmine and 15 to 20 $\mu g/kg$ of atropine is recommended to reverse neuromuscular blockade in adults. A dose of 2.5 to 3.0 mg of neostigmine accompanied by 1.2 mg of atropine may therefore be safely administered to reverse nondepolarizing neuromuscular blockade at the termination of anesthesia in the adult patient. A dose of more than 5.0 mg is unlikely to be beneficial and may be even dangerous.

Controversy existed as to the proper sequence of injection of the anticholinergic and anticholinesterase agents to reverse neuromuscular blockade. One group of anesthetists were taught to give atropine first, wait for an increase in heart rate, and then give neostigmine; while other anesthetists commonly administered atropine and neostigmine simultaneously. Case reports of extreme bradycardia and cardiac arrest following the simultaneous administration of atropine and neostigmine appeared in the literature, and it was suggested that this was due to the synergistic effect of central vagal stimulation by atropine and the cholinergic effect of neostigmine. However, it has been demonstrated that atropine only produces a bradycardia when given in very small doses and that, when atropine and neostigmine are administered together, it nearly always produces a biphasic response, i.e., an initial tachycardia followed by a bradycardia (Fig. 5.10). If atropine is given before neostigmine, the degree of tachycardia is almost twice as

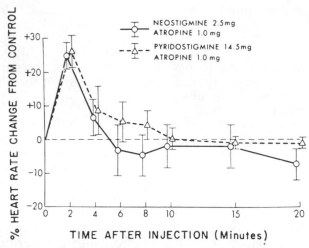

**Figure 5.10.   Heart rate changes during antagonism of *d*-tubocurarine-induced neuro-
muscular blockade by neostigmine and pyridostigmine with atropine, 1.0 mg.**   (With permission from Fogdall RP, Miller RD: Antagonism of *d*-tubocurarine and pancuronium-induced neuromuscular blockades by pyridostigmine in man. *Anesthesiology* 39:504–509,
1973.)

great as when atropine and neostigmine
are given together. Therefore, it is today
considered good practice to administer
atropine and neostigmine simultaneously, when the direct vagolytic effects of
atropine usually precede the muscarinic
effects of neostigmine by 1 to 2 minutes.

The peak effect of antagonism following neostigmine is not reached clinically
until 7 to 11 minutes of administration. It
is important to appreciate that the degree
of neuromuscular blockade at the time of
attempted reversal determines the time
of onset of action and extent of the antagonistic effect of neostigmine. Clinical
studies have demonstrated that, when
twitch height is more than 20% of control, time from neostigmine administration (2.5 mg) to attainment of control
twitch height is 3 to 14 minutes. However, when the twitch height is less than
20% of control, recovery may take as long
as 8 to 29 minutes. The duration of action
of neostigmine is between 40 and 60
minutes.

TOXICITY, PRECAUTIONS, AND CONTRAINDICATIONS

Atropine should always be given when
neostigmine is administered parenterally
to attenuate the muscarinic actions, and
the heart rate should be monitored postoperatively. Neostigmine should be used
cautiously in patients with asthma and
heart disease.

Pyridostigmine

Pyridostigmine is a pyridine analogue
of neostigmine being the dimethyl car-
bamic ester of 3-hydroxyl-1-methylpyri-
dinium bromide. Its chemical structure is
given in Figure 5.6. It is an acetylcholinesterase inhibitor that is used clinically
by anesthesiologists to antagonize nondepolarizing neuromuscular blockade. It
has been suggested that pyridostigmine
might possess certain advantages over-
neostigmine in that it has a longer duration of action and fewer muscarinic side
effects. It is also used in the management
of myasthenia gravis.

CARDIOVASCULAR SYSTEM

Gyermek showed that when atropine
and neostigmine are administered together, there is usually an initial tachycardia (due to the more rapid onset of atropine) followed by a bradycardia. In
addition, he demonstrated that when

pyridostigmine was substituted for neo-stigmine in the mixture with atropine, the occurrence of the initial tachycardia was higher but the bradycardia following the initial tachycardia was less frequent with pyridostigmine (43% of cases) than with neostigmine (62% of cases). The higher incidence of tachycardia associated with atropine and pyridostigmine is probably due to the slower onset of action of pyridostigmine. The incidence of arrhythmias was also less with pyrido-stigmine than with neostigmine. However, Fogdall and Miller found no difference between the cardiac muscarinic effects of neostigmine and pyridostig-mine (Fig. 5.10) and suggest that there is no advantage in administering pyrido-stigmine in preference to neostigmine in terms of cardiac muscarinic effects. They did not investigate other muscarinic side effects, such as oropharyngeal secretions. Thus, equivalent doses of pyridostigmine and neostigmine require the same amount of atropine (i.e., 15 μg/kg) to prevent bradycardia.

It has been suggested that the combination of glycopyrrolate and pyridostig-mine might possess certain advantages over the conventional atropine-neostig-mine combination. Regimens for the reversal of neuromuscular blockade usually consist of an anticholinesterase agent and a parasympatholytic anticho-linergic agent which blocks the undesirable muscarinic side effects of the anti-cholinesterase, such as bradycardia, salivation, and increased exocrine secretions. In addition, the different time courses of the onset and duration of action of the various anticholinergic and anticholinesterase drug combinations have proved to be a problem. Glycopyr-rolate (see Chapter 6), a synthetic quaternary ammonium anticholinergic agent, which has a slower onset of anticholin-ergic action than atropine, has been investigated as a substitute for atropine with both neostigmine and pyridostig-mine. An ideal parasympathetic blocking agent should match the onset and duration of the anticholinesterase agent and, therefore, produce a mirror image of the bradycardic effect of the anticholinester-

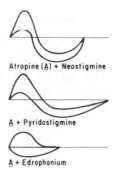

Figure 5.11. Schematic patterns (effect versus time) of changes in heart rate when atropine is combined with different anti-cholinesterase agents for the reversal of neuromuscular blockade. (With permission from Gyermek L: The glycopyrrolate-pyridostigmine combination. *Anesthesiol Rev* 5:19–22, 1978.)

ase, as illustrated in Figures 5.11 and 5.12 where the heart rate changes obtained with combinations of atropine and gly-copyrrolate with neostigmine, pyridostig-mine, and edrophonium are depicted. Thus, the onset of action of neostigmine and especially pyridostigmine is slow as compared to edrophonium, which possesses a relatively fast but short duration of action. The combination of a rapidly acting anticholinesterase (edrophonium) and a slower but longer acting anticho-

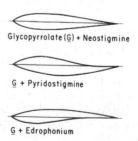

Figure 5.12. Schematic patterns (effect versus time) of changes in heart rate when glycopyrrolate is combined with different anticholinesterase agents for the reversal of neuromuscular blockade. (With permission from Gyermek L: The glycopyrro-late-pyridostigmine combination. *Anesthesiol Rev* 5:19–22, 1978.)

linesterase (pyridostigmine) has also proved satisfactory. Figures 5.11 and 5.12 also indicate that glycopyrrolate produces a "better mirror image" for both neostigmine and pyridostigmine than atropine, due to its slower onset of action.

PHARMACOKINETICS

The pharmacokinetic parameters of pyridostigmine have been examined in patients with normal and without renal function (Table 5.3). Distribution of pyridostigmine following intravenous administration (0.35 mg/kg) is rapid, resulting in a distribution half-life ($t_{1/2\alpha}$) of 6.8 minutes. This is approximately 2-fold greater than that for neostigmine and may explain the similar difference in onset time reported for the two drugs. The main route of excretion of neostigmine and pyridostigmine is via the kidneys. The elimination half-life ($t_{1/2\beta}$) is 112 minutes in patients with normal renal function, while the clearance is 8.6 ml/kg/min. However, anephric patients have a longer elimination half-life (379 minutes) and a reduced clearance (2 ml/kg/min), indicating that renal function plays an important role in the elimination of pyridostigmine. Renal excretion can be calculated to account for 75% of the clearance of pyridostigmine and, thus, 25% is dependent on nonrenal mechanisms such as metabolism. Pyridostigmine has been shown to be metabolized to a number of metabolites, one of which is the hydrolysis product 3-hydroxy-N-methylpyridinium, which is then rapidly glucuronidated. Pharmacokinetic values for pyridostigmine in patients who have undergone renal transplantation are the same as those derived in patients with normal renal function. The oral bioavailability of pyridostigmine is low and has been estimated to be about 10%.

PHARMACODYNAMICS

The time to onset of antagonism and duration of effect for pyridostigmine are discussed earlier in the section describing the pharmacodynamics of neostigmine (see Figs. 5.8 and 5.9). The onset of action is delayed when compared with

neostigmine and edrophonium, while the duration of effect is longer, being approximately 90 minutes.

SUGGESTED DOSAGE AND ADMINISTRATION

Pyridostigmine may be given by mouth, intramuscularly, or intravenously. It is a standard anticholinesterase drug for the treatment of myasthenia gravis, when it is usually administered orally. It is available as tablets, pyridostigmine bromide, 60 mg, and timed release, 180 mg, of which 60 mg is released immediately and 120 mg over several hours. Pyridostigmine bromide is also available for parenteral use, 5 mg/ml.

Pyridostigmine is used during anesthesia for the reversal of neuromuscular blockade, the usual dose being 10 to 15 mg/70 kg intravenously, when atropine or glycopyrrolate should also be given to mitigate the potentially dangerous cardiac muscarinic effects. The dose of atropine required to be given with pyridostigmine is 15 to 20 μg/kg. Gyermek has advocated the combined use of edrophonium and pyridostigmine for more rapid reversal of neuromuscular blockade and, when this combination is administered, the following doses are suggested: edrophonium, 0.2 to 0.4 mg/kg; pyridostigmine, 0.1 to 0.16 mg/kg; and glycopyrrolate, 0.004 to 0.006 mg/kg.

The onset and duration of action of pyridostigmine are longer than those of neostigmine. The peak effects of antagonism are not reached until 12 to 16 minutes after administration of pyridostigmine in contrast to 7 to 11 minutes for neostigmine and 0.8 to 2.0 minutes for edrophonium, indicating that it should be given 5 minutes sooner than one would normally give neostigmine. The duration of action of pyridostigmine is approximately 40% longer than that of neostigmine when equivalent antagonistic doses are administered.

Edrophonium

Edrophonium is an anticholinesterase agent that also possesses a direct action on the neuromuscular junction similar to that of acetylcholine. Its chemical structure is given in Figure 5.6. It has a fast onset but short duration of action and, in addition, has weak muscarinic effects. Edrophonium is used in the diagnosis of myasthenia gravis, the differentiation of myasthenic or cholinergic crisis, to routinely reverse neuromuscular blockade at the termination of anesthesia, and to assess residual neuromuscular paralysis following anesthesia.

CARDIOVASCULAR SYSTEM

Edrophonium has weak muscarinic effects, and it might be expected that atropine requirements to prevent heart rate changes would be less than those for neostigmine. The cardiovascular effects of edrophonium and atropine have been compared to those of neostigmine and atropine and are shown in Figure 5.13. The simultaneous administration of edropho-

nium (0.5 µg/kg) and atropine (7.0 µg/kg) produces minimal changes in heart rate and blood pressure in contrast to the heart rate changes associated with neostigmine (0.043 mg/kg) and atropine (15 µg/kg). Thus, edrophonium requires less atropine to prevent bradycardia than does neostigmine. However, high doses of atropine combined with edrophonium result in prolonged tachycardia and a rise in blood pressure. Thus, in summary, equipotent doses of neostigmine and pyridostigmine require equal doses of atropine (15 µg/kg) to prevent associated heart rate changes, while edrophonium requires 50% less (7 µg/kg) atropine to prevent bradycardia and attenuate the tachycardic response.

The slower onset of the cardiac vagal effects of glycopyrrolate is well matched by the slower onset of action of pyridostigmine and neostigmine (see Figs. 5.11 and

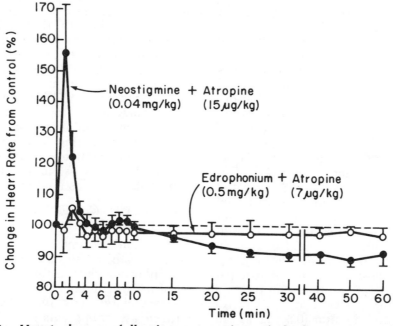

Figure 5.13. Heart changes following antagonism of *d*-tubocurarine neuromuscular blockade by neostigmine and edrophonium with atropine. Note the atropine requirement for equipotent doses of neostigmine (0.04 mg/kg) and edrophonium (0.5 mg/kg). Compared to neostigmine and atropine (15 µg/kg), the simultaneous administration of edrophonium and atropine (7.0 µg/kg) produced minimal changes in heart rate. (With permission from Cronnelly R, Morris RB, Miller RD: Edrophonium: duration of action and atropine requirement in humans during halothane anesthesia. *Anesthesiology* 57:261–266, 1982.)

5.12), but the more rapid onset of action of atropine is better matched with edrophonium, since the combination of edrophonium and glycopyrrolate is more likely to result in bradycardia. In addition, the duration of action of atropine and edrophonium is similar.

PHARMACOKINETICS

The pharmacokinetics of edrophonium in healthy patients are compared with those for neostigmine and pyridostigmine in Table 5.3. In patients with renal failure, the elimination half-life ($t_{1/2\beta}$) is increased from 110 to 206 minutes, and the plasma clearance is decreased from 9.6 to 2.7 ml/kg/min. Volumes of distribution are unaffected by renal disease. The disposition of edrophonium is normal in patients who have undergone successful renal transplantation.

Edrophonium is metabolized to the inactive metabolite, edrophonium glucuronide. Renal excretion accounts for 70% of the total clearance of edrophonium, and 40% of the clearance is therefore presumed to be dependent on extrarenal mechanisms such as metabolism.

The disposition of edrophonium has been investigated in small infants and children in a similar manner to that described earlier for neostigmine. Elimination half-lives and distribution volumes for edrophonium (1.0 mg/kg) are similar in infants, children, and adults. However, plasma clearance is greater in infants (17.8 ml/kg/min) when compared with children (14.2 ml/kg/min) and adults (8.3 ml/kg/min). Dose requirements for edrophonium are not different for adults, children, or small infants, in contrast to the lower dose requirements reported for neostigmine in pediatric patients; the dose of edrophonium producing equivalent antagonism to that reported for edrophonium (0.5 mg/kg) in adults is 0.6 mg/kg in infants, and 0.9 mg/kg in children. Large interindividual variation in dose-response occurs in pediatric patients. Thus it is important to monitor neuromuscular function, and doses as high as 1.0 mg/kg may be required in some patients. Onset times for edrophonium are similar for pediatric and adult patients and faster than those

associated with neostigmine administration. In pediatric patients, as in adults, the dose of atropine required to minimize heart rate changes is less than that recommended for neostigmine. It is important to administer atropine (10 μg/kg) at least 30 seconds before edrophonium to prevent edrophonium-induced bradycardia.

At the other extreme of life, the elimination half-life ($t_{1/2\beta}$) is prolonged and the clearance decreased in elderly patients, probably reflecting the reduced renal function seen in this age group. The onset time and duration of effect of edrophonium are both unaffected by aging.

PHARMACODYNAMICS

The dose-response curve for edrophonium is shown in Figure 5.7. The dose of edrophonium that produced 50% antagonism of neuromuscular blockade (ED_{50}) was 0.125 mg/kg compared to values of 0.098 and 0.022 for pyridostigmine and neostigmine, respectively. However, as discussed earlier in this chapter, the dose-response curve for edrophonium is not parallel to those for neostigmine and pyridostigmine, and this has been attributed to the different mechanism of inhibition produced by edrophonium. The onset of action of edrophonium, assessed as time from administration to peak effect, is very rapid (Fig. 5.8), while the duration of action (about 60 minutes) is similar to that of neostigmine but shorter than that of pyridostigmine (Fig. 5.9).

SUGGESTED DOSAGE AND ADMINISTRATION

Edrophonium is now routinely used by many anesthesiologists to reverse neuromuscular blockade at the termination of anesthesia. Although the duration of action associated with its use in patients with myasthenia gravis is said to be relatively short acting, it does appear to be safe and effective in anesthetic practice. However, it is important to note that the antagonism produced by edrophonium may be unpredictable if spontaneous recovery has not occurred, such that four responses to train of four stimulation are not visible, implying that at profound degrees of neuromuscular blockade, edrophonium may be slow to produce antagonism.

Edrophonium is available for parenteral use, 10 mg/1.0 ml in 15-ml vials. The suggested dose for reversal of neuromuscular blockade at the termination of anesthesia is 0.5 mg/kg, but the dose should be increased to 1.0 mg/kg when neuromuscular blockade is profound. The usual commencement dose for an adult patient is thus 10 mg, and the dosage may be repeated to a maximum total dose of 40 mg. Atropine, 7.0 μg/kg, should also be administered with edrophonium in this situation.

Edrophonium may be used to detect the type of neuromuscular blockade in a patient developing prolonged apnea following the use of muscle relaxants, when 10 to 20 mg is administered intravenously preceded by atropine. If the block is competitive, improvement in muscle power and respiration may occur, but if the block is of the depolarizing type, there will either be no improvement or worsening of the paralysis.

Edrophonium is used in the diagnosis of myasthenia gravis, when 2 mg is given intravenously followed by up to 8 mg 1 minute later if the first dose causes no improvement. Edrophonium may also be given to confirm the optimal oral dose of anticholinesterase therapy. In addition, it is used to differentiate between a cholinergic crisis and myasthenic weakness. A cholinergic crisis results from overdose with anticholinesterase agents which produce a depolarization blockade; and the excessive weakness that occurs may be clinically mistaken for a myasthenic crisis. A myasthenic crisis is due to inadequate anticholinesterase therapy or to exacerbation of the disease. When edrophonium, 1 mg followed by 1 mg 1 minute later, is cautiously administered, patients in cholinergic crisis exhibit an increase in weakness, while those with myasthenic weakness improve.

Physostigmine

Physostigmine is an alkaloid obtained from the calabar bean of West Africa. It is a tertiary amine (Fig. 5.6) and not possessing a quaternary ammonium group, it crosses the blood-brain barrier and is readily absorbed from the gastrointestinal tract and mucous membranes. It has a greater effect on the central nervous system and cardiovascular system than neostigmine and possesses prominent muscarinic activity. Physostigmine is destroyed in the body by hydrolysis at the ester linkage by cholinesterase and is usually eliminated within 2 hours of administration. It has a short elimination half-life of 20 to 30 minutes. Plasma concentrations of 3 to 5 μg/L are necessary to antagonize drug-induced postoperative sedation. Renal excretion appears to play a minor role in the disposition of physostigmine.

Its uses include the treatment of glaucoma, atropine intoxication, and tricyclic antidepressant poisoning. Physostigmine has recently been used to reverse some of the sedative effects of central nervous system depressants, such as hyoscine, phenothiazines, benzodiazepines, and the tricyclic antidepressants. It has also been suggested that it is useful in the treatment of postoperative somnolence or disorientation, when the adult dose is 0.5 to 2.0 mg, injected intravenously.

Some patients encounter side effects due to the inhibition of peripheral cholinesterases by physostigmine, such as nausea, pallor, sweating, and bradycardia. Use of anticholinergic drugs which are quaternary amines (e.g., glycopyrrolate) and which do not cross the blood-brain barrier is recommended to prevent the peripheral side effects of physostigmine. The administration of physostigmine in this situation should be carried out under electrocardiographic monitoring and, in addition, it is important to ensure that the patient does not relapse into pretreatment status once the action of physostigmine wears off.

Echothiophate

Echothiophate is a long-acting anticholinesterase agent that is used in the treatment of glaucoma. Succinylcholine should be avoided in patients receiving this drug because impaired hydrolysis of succinylcholine due to depression of plasma cholinesterase may result in prolonged apnea.

4-AMINOPYRIDINE

4-Aminopyridine has been proposed as an antagonist of nondepolarizing neuromuscular blockade. It is not an acetylcholinesterase inhibitor, but increases both evoked and spontaneous release of acetylcholine from the motor nerve terminal, thereby increasing the force of muscle contration. In addition, it has been shown to antagonize the neuromuscular blockado produced by many antibiotics and to be relatively free of muscarinic side effects. 4-Aminopyridine potentiates the antagonist activity of neostigmine and pyridostigmine and decreases the dose of anticholinesterase needed. Therefore, the requirement for atropine is reduced by 60 to 70%. Unfortunately, 4-aminopyridine readily crosses the blood-brain barrier, and the doses necessary for complete antagonism (>1 mg/kg) may cause central nervous symptoms such as postoperative restlessness and confusion.

ORGANOPHOSPHORUS INHIBITORS

Organic esters of phosphoric acid were first shown to inhibit acetylcholinesterase in 1937 and were subsequently used as insecticides in agriculture and as "nerve gases" during World War II. These drugs have toxicological rather than therapeutic importance, but a brief description will be included here because the anesthesiologist may be required to treat anticholinesterase intoxication or poisoning in the intensive care unit.

The organophosphorus anticholinesterases are said to be "irreversible" inhibitors of acetylcholinesterase because recovery takes weeks or months to occur. Diisopropyl phosphorofluoridate (DFP) and Parathion are two well known examples of such agents. The accidental or suicidal intoxication by organophosphorus anticholinesterases may lead to death due to muscarinic and nicotinic effects causing central nervous system symptoms, respiratory paralysis due to peripheral neuromuscular blockade, and circulatory effects such as pulmonary edema, hypotension, and bradycardia. The cause of death is usually respiratory failure accompanied secondarily by cardiovascular failure. Atropine should be administered in large doses, although it only antagonizes the muscarinic effects and not the nicotinic effects.

The phosphorylated esteratic sites of acetylcholinesterase undergo regeneration at an extremely slow rate, so that recovery depends on either the formation of new enzyme which may take weeks to occur, or the regeneration of cholinesterase by cholinesterase reactivators. The oxime *pralidoxime* has been successfully used as a cholinesterase reactivator in the treatment of anticholinesterase poisoning. It rapidly reverses the neuromuscular blockade which is not antagonized by the administration of atropine.

PSEUDOCHOLINESTERASE OR PLASMA CHOLINESTERASE

Plasma cholinesterase is found in the plasma but not in the red cell. In addition, it is also present in many tissues, including the liver, brain, kidney, intestine, and pancreas. The physiological function of this enzyme is not known, but it hydrolyzes a large number of choline and other esters and, thus, is less specific than true acetylcholinesterase. It is synthesized in the liver. A number of drugs of importance to the anesthesiologist are metabolized by plasma cholinesterase. These include succinylcholine and some of the local anesthetics, such as procaine, 2-chloroprocaine, and tetracaine, which are esters of benzoic acid derivatives.

HYDROLYSIS OF SUCCINYLCHOLINE

Succinylcholine is the dicholine ester of succinic acid (Fig. 5.14), and it basically consists of two acetylcholine molecules joined by their acetate groups. The short duration of action of succinylcholine is due to the rapid inactivation of succinylcholine by pseudocholinesterase (Fig. 5.15). The hydrolysis takes place in two steps. Firstly, succinylcholine is hydrolyzed to succinylmonocholine and choline. The second step, which occurs

$$CH_3 - COO - CH_2 - CH_2 - N^+(CH_3)_3$$

ACETYLCHOLINE

$$CH_2 - COO - CH_2 - CH_2 - N^+(CH_3)_3$$
$$|$$
$$CH_2 - COO - CH_2 - CH_2 - N^+(CH_3)_3$$

SUCCINYLCHOLINE

Figure 5.14. Chemical formulae of acetylcholine and succinylcholine.

much more slowly, is the hydrolysis of succinylmonocholine to succinic acid and choline. The intermediate, succinyl-monocholine, possesses only weak neuromuscular blocking activity, and therefore the inactivation of succinylcholine occurs extremely rapidly.

ABNORMAL PLASMA CHOLINESTERASE ACTIVITY

Plasma cholinesterase activity may be abnormal due to (a) acquired or (b) genetic enzyme defects.

Acquired Enzyme Defect. In the newborn, serum cholinesterase is slightly lower than the adult, but reaches adult levels by 2 to 6 months. Plasma cholinesterase is synthesized in the liver, and the levels are therefore reduced in patients suffering from liver disease, such as acute hepatitis and hepatic metastases. Levels are also lower in pregnant patients in the last trimester and early postpartum period. Other acquired causes of decreased plasma cholinesterase activity include collagen disease (progressive muscular dystrophy, congenital myotonia, derma-

tomyositis), carcinoma, chronic debilitating disease, chronic anemia, uremia, malnutrition, and myxedema. Plasma cholinesterase levels are also low in burned patients. Anticholinesterases inhibit plasma cholinesterase activity, and consequently low levels are found following treatment with echothiophate eyedrops and accidental organophosphorus insecticide poisoning. Other drugs that have been shown to reduce plasma cholinesterase activity include neostigmine, monoamine oxidase inhibitors, anticancer drugs, oral contraceptives, propanidid, chlorpromazine, and pancuronium. Increased levels are associated with obesity and toxic goiter.

Inherited Enzyme Defect. Two varieties of plasma cholinesterase exist: the common or normal type and the rare abnormal or atypical type. The common type of plasma cholinesterase is able to hydrolyze succinylcholine at concentrations that occur in the blood of anesthetized patients. Ordinary quantitative laboratory estimations of plasma cholinesterase do not differentiate between the two types. The atypical enzyme is less active than the normal enzyme in hydrolyzing other substrates, such as acetylcholine and benzoylcholine, and is unable to hydrolyze therapeutic concentrations of succinylcholine at a normal rate. In addition, the atypical enzyme is more resistant to the effects of certain cholinesterase inhibitors, and this pharmacological effect has led to the development of the dibucaine "number." Kalow and Genest found that the local anesthetic dibucaine (cinchocaine) inhibits normal plasma cholinesterase to a much greater extent than the atypical enzyme. They showed that a 10^{-5} molar concentration inhibits the normal enzyme by about 80% and the

STEP I   SUCCINYLCHOLINE $\xrightarrow{\text{Pseudocholinesterase}}$ SUCCINYLMONOCHOLINE + CHOLINE

STEP II   SUCCINYLMONOCHOLINE $\xrightarrow{\text{Pseudocholinesterase}}$ SUCCINIC ACID + CHOLINE
Specific Liver Esterase

Figure 5.15. Enzymatic hydrolysis of succinylcholine.

Table 5.4.
Dibucaine Number

Dibucaine number (% of inhibition)	Genotype	Incidence in population
70–85	Normal homozygote (NN)	96.2%
50–65	Heterozygote (ND)	3.8%
16–25	Abnormal homozygote (DD)	1/3000

atypical enzyme by 20%, and the term "dibucaine number" (DN) represents the percentage of inhibition of plasma cholinesterase activity by dibucaine under standardized conditions. Thus, the dibucaine number distinguishes between the reduced ability of pseudocholinesterase to hydrolyze succinylcholine due to an acquired defect or a genetic defect. In addition the dibucaine number enables the genotype to be determined. The homozygote group of patients possesses only abnormal enzyme and has a dibucaine number of 20%. A dibucaine number of 80% found in the majority of the population indicates the presence of only normal enzyme. Heterozygotes possessing normal and abnormal enzyme have a dibucaine number that varies between 50 and 65% (Table 5.4).

Other cholinesterase variants have also been described and are as follows.

Fluoride-resistant Enzyme. Harris and Whittaker have described a rare variant of plasma cholinesterase that can be identified using sodium fluoride as an inhibitor in the same manner as dibucaine. They have called the percentage inhibition of plasma cholinesterase activity produced by a given concentration of fluoride, the fluoride number. This variant has a decreased ability to hydrolyze succinylcholine.

The Silent Gene. Homozygotes for this silent cholinesterase gene have almost no pseudocholinesterase activity and are, therefore, extremely sensitive to succinylcholine.

Other genetic variants of pseudocholinesterase may also exist. A pseudocholinesterase variant called C_5 has been identified by electrophoresis. Pseudocholinesterase usually migrates as four bands, C_1–C_4, during electrophoresis, but plasma from patients that possess the C_5 variant has an additional pseudocholinesterase component that migrates as a fifth band, the C_5 band. Patients possessing the C_5 variant are not sensitive to succinylcholine but, rather, have elevated pseudocholinesterase activity. This variant is nonallelic to the other genes described and is situated at another locus on the chromosome.

Thus, in summary, four allelic genes for plasma cholinesterase are recognized:

1. The normal gene;
2. The atypical or dibucaine-resistant gene;
3. The fluoride-resistant gene;
4. The silent gene.

The four genes were originally designated as: N (normal); D (dibucaine resistant or atypical); F (fluoride resistant); and S (silent), so that individuals who have two normal genes (NN) are homozygotes, those with two atypical dibucaine-resistant genes (DD) are homozygotes, and heterozygotes for the atypical gene are designated (ND). Therefore, there are four types of homozygotes (NN, DD, FF, SS) and six combinations of heterozygotes (ND, NF, NS, DF, DS, and FS). Another classification proposed by Motulsky that is also commonly used recognizes the four allelic genes as normal gene E_1^u, atypical or dibucaine-resistant gene E_1^a, silent gene E_1^s, and the fluoride-resistant gene E_1^f, which again gives rise to 10 recognized genotypes designated as E_1^u, E_1^u, E_1^u, E_1^s, E_1^u, E_1^f, and so on.

The differential diagnosis and management of prolonged response to succinylcholine are further discussed in Chapter 10.

BIBLIOGRAPHY

General

Aquilonius SM, Hartvig P: Clinical pharmacokinetics of cholinesterase inhibitors. *Clin Pharmacokinet* 11:236–249, 1986.

Cronnelly R, Morris RB: Antagonism of neuromuscular blockade. *Br J Anaesth* 54:183–194, 1982.

Donati F, Ferguson A, Bevan DR: Twitch, depression, and train of four ratio after antagonism of pancuronium with edrophonium, neostigmine, or pyridostigmine. *Anesth Analg* 62:314–316, 1983.

Ferguson A, Egerszegi P, Bevan DR: Neostigmine, pyridostigmine, and edrophonium as antagonists of pancuronium. *Anesthesiology* 53:390–394, 1980.

Gyermek L: Clinical pharmacology of the reversal of neuromuscular block. *Int J Clin Pharmacol Biopharm* 15:356–362, 1977.

Hall GM, Wood GJ, Paterson JL: Half-life of plasma cholinesterase. *Br J Anaesth* 56:903–904, 1984.

Kanto J, Klotz U: Pharmacokinetic implications for the clinical use of atropine, scopolamine, and glycopyrrolate. *Acta Anaesthesiol Scand* 32:69–78, 1988.

Kitz RJ: Molecular pharmacology of acetylcholinesterase. In Featherstone RM (ed): *A Guide to Molecular Pharmacology and Toxicology.* New York, Marcel Dekker, 1977, pp 333–374.

Miller RD: Antagonism of neuromuscular blockade. *Anesthesiology* 44:318–329, 1976.

Mirakhur RK, Ferres CJ, Lavery TD: Plasma cholinesterase levels following pancuronium and vecuronium. *Acta Anaesthesiol Scand* 27:451–453, 1983.

Owen H, Hunter AR: Heterozygotes for atypical cholinesterase. *Br J Anaesth* 55:315–318, 1983.

Silk E, King J, Whittaker M: Assay of cholinesterase in clinical chemistry. *Ann Clin Biochem* 16:57–75, 1979.

Sunew KY, Hicks RG: The effects of neostigmine and pyridostigmine on duration of succinylcholine action and pseudocholinesterase activity. *Anesthesiology* 49:188–191, 1978.

Whittaker M: Plasma cholinesterase variants and the anaesthetist. *Anaesthesia* 35:174–197, 1980.

Williams FM: Clinical significance of esterases in man. *Clin Pharmacokinet* 10:392–403, 1985.

Neostigmine

Blitt CD, Moon BJ, Kartchner CD: Duration of action of neostigmine in man. *Can Anaesth Soc J* 23:80–84, 1976.

Calvey TI, Wareing M, Williams NE, Chan K: Pharmacokinetics and pharmacological effects of neostigmine in man. *Br J Clin Pharmacol* 7:149–155, 1979.

Cronnelly R, Stanski DR, Miller RD, Sheiner LB, Sohn YJ: Renal function and the pharmacokinetics of neostigmine in anesthetized man. *Anesthesiology* 51:222–226, 1979.

Fisher DM, Cronnelly R, Miller RD, Sharma M: The neuromuscular pharmacology of neostigmine in infants and children. *Anesthesiology* 59:220–225, 1983.

Hennis PJ, Cronnelly R, Sharma M, Fisher DM, Miller RD: Metabolites of neostigmine and pyridostigmine do not contribute to antagonism of neuromuscular blockade in the dog. *Anesthesiology* 61:534–539, 1984.

Katz RL: Neuromuscular effects of d-tubocurarine, edrophonium, and neostigmine in man. *Anesthesiology* 28:327–336, 1967.

Lawson JI: Cardiac arrest following the administration of neostigmine. *Br J Anaesth* 28:333–337, 1956.

Meakin G, Sweet PT, Bevan JC, Bevan DR: Neostigmine and edrophonium as antagonists of pancuronium in infants and children. *Anesthesiology* 59:316–321, 1983.

Miller RD, Larson CP, Way WL: Comparative antagonism of d-tubocurarine, gallamine, and pancuronium induced neuromuscular blockades by neostigmine. *Anesthesiology* 37:503–509, 1972.

Miller RD, VanNyhuis LS, Eger E III, Vitez TS, Way WL: Comparative times to peak effect and durations of action of neostigmine and pyridostigmine. *Anesthesiology* 41:27–33, 1974.

Morris R, Cronnelly R, Miller RD: Pharmacokinetics of edrophonium and neostigmine when antagonizing d-tubocurarine neuromuscular blockade in man. *Anesthesiology* 54:399–402, 1981.

Somani SM, Chan K, Dehghan A, Calvey TN: Kinetics and metabolism of intramuscular neostigmine in myasthenia gravis. *Clin Pharmacol Ther* 28:64–68, 1980.

Williams NE, Calvey TN, Chan K: Clearance of neostigmine from the circulation during the antagonism of neuromuscular block. *Br J Anaesth* 50:1065–1067, 1978.

Young WL, Backus W, Matteo RS, Ornstein E, Diaz J: Pharmacokinetics and pharmacodynamics of neostigmine in the elderly. *Anesthesiology* 61:A300, 1984.

Pyridostigmine

Breyer-Pfaff U, Maier U, Brinkmann AM, Schumm F: Pyridostigmine kinetics in healthy subjects and patients with myasthenia gravis. *Clin Pharmacol Ther* 37:495–501, 1985.

Cronnelly R, Stanski DR, Miller RD, Sheiner LB: Pyridostigmine kinetics with and without renal function. *Clin Pharmacol Ther* 28:78–81, 1980.

Fogdall RP, Miller RD: Antagonism of d-tubocurarine and pancuronium induced neuromuscular blockades by pyridostigmine in man. *Anesthesiology* 39:504–509, 1973.

Gyermek L: The glycopyrrolate-pyridostigmine combination. Is it the ultimate development in reversing nondepolarizing neuromuscular block. *Anesthesiol Rev* 5:19–22, 1978.

Katz RL: Pyridostigmine (Mestinon) as an antagonist of d-tubocurarine. *Anesthesiology* 28:528–534, 1967.

Lippmann M, Rogoff RC: A clinical evaluation of pyridostigmine bromide in the reversal of pancuronium. *Anesth Analg* 53:20–23, 1974.

Miller RD, VanHyhuis LS, Eger EI, Vitez TS, Way WL: Comparative times to peak effect and durations of action of neostigmine and pyridostigmine. *Anesthesiology* 41:27–33, 1974.

Ravin MB: Pyridostigmine as an antagonist of d-tubocurarine-induced and pancuronium-induced neuromuscular blockade. *Anesth Analg* 54:317–321, 1975.

Sunew KY, Hicks RG: Effects of neostigmine and pyridostigmine on duration of succinylcholine action and pseudocholinesterase activity. *Anesthesiology* 49:188–191, 1978.

Williams NE, Calvey TN, Chan K: Plasma concentrations of pyridostigmine during the antagonism of neuromuscular block. *Br J Anaesth* 55:27–31, 1983.

Winnie AP, Mahor RA, Shaker MH, Ramamurthy S: Pyridostigmine for reversal. *Anesthesiol Rev* 10:16–24, 1977.

Edrophonium

Azar I, Pham AN, Karambelkar DJ, Lear E: The heart rate following edrophonium-atropine and edrophonium-glycopyrrolate mixtures. *Anesthesiology* 59:139–141, 1983.

Bevan DR: Reversal of pancuronium with edrophonium. *Anaesthesia* 34:614–619, 1979.

Caldwell JE, Robertson EN, Baird WLM: Antagonism of vecuronium and atracurium: comparison of neostigmine and edrophonium administered at 5% twitch height recovery. *Br J Anaesth* 59:478–481, 1987.

Cronnelly R, Miller RD: Edrophonium: dose-response, onset, and duration of antagonism in elderly patients. *Anesthesiology* 61:A303, 1984.

Cronnelly R, Morris RB, Miller RD: Edrophonium: duration of action and atropine requirement in humans during halothane anesthesia. *Anesthesiology* 57:261–266, 1982.

Fisher DM, Cronnelly R, Sharma M, Miller RD: Clinical pharmacology of edrophonium in infants and children. *Anesthesiology* 61:428–433, 1984.

Kopman AF: Edrophonium antagonism of pancuronium-induced neuromuscular blockade in man: a reappraisal. *Anesthesiology* 51:139–142, 1979.

Meakin G, Sweet PT, Bevan JC, Bevan DR: Neostigmine and edrophonium as antagonists of pancuronium in infants and children. *Anesthesiology* 59:316–321, 1983.

Miller RD, Cronnelly R: Editorial: a new look at an old drug. *Anesthesiology* 59:84–85, 1983.

Mirakhur RK: Antagonism of the muscarinic effects of edrophonium with atropine or glycopyrrolate. *Br J Anaesth* 57:1213–1216, 1985.

Morris RB, Cronnelly R, Miller RD, Stanski DR, Fahey MR: Pharmacokinetics of edrophonium in anephric and renal transplant patients. *Br J Anaesth* 53:1311–1314, 1981.

Morris RB, Cronnelly R, Miller RD, Stanski DR, Fahey MR: Pharmacokinetics of edrophonium and neostigmine when antagonizing d-tubocurarine neuromuscular blockade in man. *Anesthesiology* 54:399–402, 1981.

Osserman KE, Genkins G: Critical reappraisal of the use of edrophonium (Tensilon) chloride tests in myasthenia gravis and significance of clinical classification. *Ann NY Acad Sci* 135:312–326, 1966.

Rupp SM, McChristian JW, Miller RD, Taboada JA, Cronnelly R: Neostigmine and edrophonium antagonism of varying intensity neuromuscular blockade induced by atracurium, pancuronium, or vecuronium. *Anesthesiology* 64:711–717, 1986.

Silverberg PA, Matteo RS, Ornstein E, Young WL, Diaz J: Pharmacokinetics and pharmacodynamics of edrophonium in the elderly. *Anesth Analg* 65:S142, 1986.

Physostigmine

Avant GR, Speeg KV Jr, Freemon FR, Schenker S, Berman ML: Physostigmine reversal of diazepam-induced hypnosis: a study in human volunteers *Ann Intern Med* 91:53–55, 1979.

Baraka A: Antagonism of neuromuscular block by physostigmine in man. *Br J Anaesth* 50:1075–1077, 1978.

Bourke DL, Rosenberg M, Allen PD: Physostigmine: effectiveness as an antagonist of respiratory depression and psychomotor effects caused by morphine or diazepam. *Anesthesiology* 61:523–528, 1984.

Brebner J, Hadley L: Experiences with physostigmine in the reversal of adverse post-anaesthetic effects. *Can Anaesth Soc J* 23:574–581, 1976.

Hill GE, Stanley TH, Sentker CR: Physostigmine reversal of postoperative somnolence. *Can Anaesth Soc J* 24:707–711, 1977.

Larson GF, Hurlbert JB, Wingard DW: Physostigmine reversal of diazepam-induced depression. *Anesth Analg* 56:348–351, 1977.

Nilsson E, Himberg JJ: Physostigmine for post-operative somnolence after diazepam-nitrous oxide anaesthesia. *Acta Anaesthesiol Scand* 26:9–14, 1982.

Salmenpera M, Nilsson E: Comparison of physostigmine and neostigmine for antagonism of neuromuscular blockade. *Acta Anaesthesiol Scand* 2:387–390, 1981.

Spaulding BC, Choi DS, Gross JB, Apfelbaum JL, Broderson H: The effect of physostigmine on diazepam-induced ventilatory depression: a double blind study. *Anesthesiology* 61:551–554, 1984.

4-Aminopyridine

Miller RD, Booij LHDJ, Agoston S, Crul JF: 4-Aminopyridine potentiates neostigmine and pyridostigmine in man. *Anesthesiology* 50:416–420, 1979.

Miller RD, Dennissen PAF, VanDerPol F, Agoston S, Booij LHD, Crul J: Potentiation of neostigmine and pyridostigmine by 4-aminopyridine in the rat. *Pharm Pharmacol* 30:699–702, 1978.

Wirtavuori K, Salmenpera M, Tammisto T: Antagonism of d-tubocurarine-induced neuromuscular blockade with a mixture of 4-aminopyridine and neostigmine in man. *Can Anaesth Soc J* 31:624–630, 1984.

Metoclopramide

Jones MJ, Mitchell RWD, Hindocha: Effects on the lower oesophageal sphincter of cisapride given before the combined adminsitration of atropine and neostigmine. *Br J Anaesth* 62:124–128, 1989.

Manchikanti L, Marrero TC, Roush JR: Preanesthetic cimetidine and metoclopramide for acid aspiration prophylaxis in elective surgery. *Anesthesiology* 61:48–54, 1984.

Pinder RM, Brogden RN, Sawyer PR, Speight TM, Avery GS: Metoclopramide: a review of its pharmacological properties and clinical use. *Drugs* 12:81–131, 1976.

Rao TLK, Madhavareddy S, Chinthagada M, El-Etr AA: Metoclopramide and cimetidine to reduce gastric fluid pH and volume. *Anesth Analg* 63:1014–1016, 1984.

Rowbotham DJ, Nimmo WS: Effect of cisapride on morphine-induced delay in gastric emptying. *Br J Anaesth* 59:536–539, 1987.

Schulze-Delrieu K: Metoclopramide. *N Engl J Med* 305:28–33, 1981.

Solanki DR, Suresh M, Ethridge HC: The effects of intravenous cimetidine and metoclopramide on gastric volume and pH. *Anesth Analg* 63:599–602, 1984.

6

Anticholinergic Drugs; Anesthetic Premedication

MARGARET WOOD

PHYSIOLOGY OF THE CHOLINERGIC NERVOUS SYSTEM

Acetylcholine is the neurotransmitter or chemical mediator at a large number of sites in the peripheral and central nervous systems of many vertebrates, including humans. It is traditional to refer to nerves that release acetylcholine from their terminals as cholinergic nerves. Cholinergic or cholinomimetic drugs act at sites in the body where acetylcholine is the chemical transmitter of the nerve impulse.

The autonomic nervous system is divided into two divisions—sympathetic and parasympathetic. The preganglionic fibers of the sympathetic nervous system arise from the thoracolumbar segments of the spinal cord, while the corresponding preganglionic fibers of the parasympathetic nervous system have a craniosacral origin. These preganglionic fibers synapse in autonomic ganglia from which arise postganglionic fibers that then innervate either adrenergic or cholinergic receptors situated throughout the body. The autonomic or involuntary nervous system innervates the heart, blood vessels, glands, viscera, and smooth muscle and, therefore, controls and integrates the autonomic functions of the body. Nerve impulses are transmitted across the synapses and neuroeffector junctions of the autonomic nervous system by means of specific chemical agents called neurotransmitters. The neurotransmitter for the adrenergic receptor is norepinephrine and that for the cholinergic receptor is acetylcholine. The neurotransmitter of all preganglionic autonomic nerve fibers, all postganglionic parasympathetic fibers, and a few postganglionic sympathetic fibers (e.g., sweat glands) is acetylcholine. Acetylcholine is also the transmitter at the motor neuromuscular junction.

Acetylcholine and cholinergic drugs may therefore act at the following sites:

1. **Parasympathetic nervous system**
   autonomic ganglia
   postganglionic nerve terminals
2. **Sympathetic nervous system**
   autonomic ganglia
   some postganglionic nerve endings, e.g., sweat glands
3. **Neuromuscular junction**
4. **Central nervous system**
5. **Blood vessels**
   Acetylcholine has a direct vasodilator action on arterioles.

Cholinergic receptors have been divided into two types, "muscarinic" and "nicotinic" because muscarine and nicotine were found to stimulate them selectively. The peripheral actions of acetylcholine are 2-fold: the effects of its release at parasympathetic postganglionic fibers are mimicked by the action of muscarine and are, therefore, called muscarinic effects. Nicotinic effects of the transmitter are seen at the skeletal neuromuscular junction and autonomic ganglia and are mimicked by nicotine. It should be noted that muscarinic receptors may exist in the absence of cholinergic innervation, for example, in blood vessels and the placenta.

The physiology and pharmacology of the cholinergic nervous system are further discussed in Chapter 5.

ANTICHOLINERGIC DRUGS

Drugs which oppose the actions of acetylcholine may be divided into three groups.

1. **Antimuscarinic drugs** (e.g., atropine) which antagonize the actions of acetylcholine on autonomic effectors innervated by postganglionic cholinergic (parasympathetic) nerves (site 2 in Fig. 6.1). Their effect is due to the blockade of the access of endogenous acetylcholine or exogenously administered cholinomimetic agents to the muscarinic receptor, i.e., competitive antagonism. The antagonism can be overcome by the administration of sufficiently high concentrations of acetylcholine or anticholinesterase agents which increase acetylcholine levels at the receptor site.

2. **Ganglionic blocking drugs** (site 1 in Fig. 6.1).

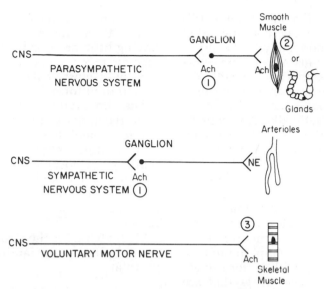

Figure 6.1.   Autonomic nervous system—anticholinergic drugs   Site 1 is blocked by ganglionic blocking agents and stimulated by nicotine and large doses of some choline esters and anticholinesterases. Site 2 is blocked by atropine and stimulated by some choline esters and the increase in acetylcholine produced by anticholinesterases. *Ach,* acetylcholine; *NE,* norepinephrine; *CNS,* central nervous system.

3. **Neuromuscular blocking agents** (site 3 in Fig. 6.1).

Atropine and other antimuscarinic drugs have little or no effect on nicotinic receptors at autonomic ganglia or the neuromuscular junction. In the central nervous system, cholinergic neurons have predominantly either nicotinic (spinal cord) or muscarinic (thalamus, cerebral cortex) receptors. Therefore, many of the central nervous system effects of atropine and related antimuscarinic drugs at therapeutic doses are probably due to their central anticholinergic actions. At high or toxic doses (for example, poisoning), the central effects consist of stimulation followed by depression. Atropine and scopolamine are tertiary amines which cross the blood-brain barrier. Recently, compounds with a quaternary ammonium structure have been developed as anticholinergic agents. Since quaternary ammonium compounds do not readily penetrate the blood-brain barrier, antimuscarinic drugs of this type do not usually exhibit central nervous system effects.

The pharmacological effects of the antimuscarinic drugs can be predicted from a knowledge of the sites innervated by postganglionic cholinergic nerve fibers. Thus, antimuscarinic drugs may produce the following effects:

1. **Exocrine glands.** Small doses depress salivary and bronchial secretion and sweating.
2. **Eye.** Mydriasis occurs, accommodation of the eye is inhibited, and intraocular pressure rises.
3. **Cardiovascular system.** Heart rate is increased due to a reduction in vagal tone.
4. **Gastrointestinal system.** Large doses decrease the tone and motility of the gut. Gastric secretion and motility are decreased.
5. **Bladder.** Large doses inhibit parasympathetic control of the bladder, and urinary retention can occur.

STRUCTURE-ACTIVITY RELATIONSHIP

Belladonna alkaloids are widely distributed in nature, particularly in the deadly nightshade (*Atropa belladonna*) which yields the alkaloid atropine (*dl*-hyoscyamine). The alkaloid scopolamine (*l*-hyoscine) is found chiefly in the shrub henbane (*Hyoscyamus niger*). The naturally occurring alkaloids are organic esters, formed by the combination of tropic acid with organic bases such as tropine or scopine. The synthetic alkaloids contain mandelic acid rather than tropic acid, and homatropine is a semisynthetic compound formed by combining the base tropine with mandelic acid. The synthetic anticholinergic drug, glycopyrrolate, also contains mandelic acid rather than tropic acid. Synthetic substitutes, often with a quaternary ammonium structure, have been developed in an attempt to produce antimuscarinic drugs with a more selective effect, for example, drugs that are capable of selectively inhibiting gastric secretion without undesirable antimuscarinic effects on other organs. Drugs with a quaternary ammonium structure are unreliably absorbed when given orally and do not usually possess central effects due to their poor penetration of the blood-brain barrier. In general, compounds with a quaternary ammonium structure usually have a greater ganglion blocking action than atropine because of their greater potency at nicotinic receptors. Thus, overdosage with quaternary ammonium compounds of this nature causes acetylcholine blockade at muscarinic receptors, but in addition ganglionic and even neuromuscular blockade may be evident. Central nervous system involvement is not usually a feature. An asymmetric carbon atom in tropic acid makes the compound optically active.

Scopolamine (*l*-hyoscine) is much more active than the *d*-isomer, *d*-hyoscine, having little or no activity. Atropine is a racemic mixture of *d*- and *l*-hyoscyamine and owes most of its antimuscarinic action to the *l*-form.

The sensitivity of the various muscarinic receptors to the effects of atropine and scopolamine is different. Small doses may inhibit salivation and sweating, while large doses are required to elicit cardiovascular and gastrointestinal effects. In addition, ocular effects tend to be later in onset and persist for longer periods.

Figure 6.2 gives the structural formulae of atropine, scopolamine, and glycopyrrolate.

INDIVIDUAL ANTICHOLINERGIC DRUGS

Atropine

Atropine is an ester of the organic base tropine, and its structural formula is given in Figure 6.2. The mechanism of action of atropine and other antimuscarinic agents is due to competitive antagonism of the actions of acetylcholine at the muscarinic receptor, which can be overcome by increasing the concentration of acetylcholine at the receptor site. Although atropine is a highly selective antagonist at muscarinic receptors situated in smooth muscle, cardiac muscle, and the exocrine glands, as with many drug-receptor interactions, this selectivity is not absolute, and very large doses may block nicotinic receptors result-

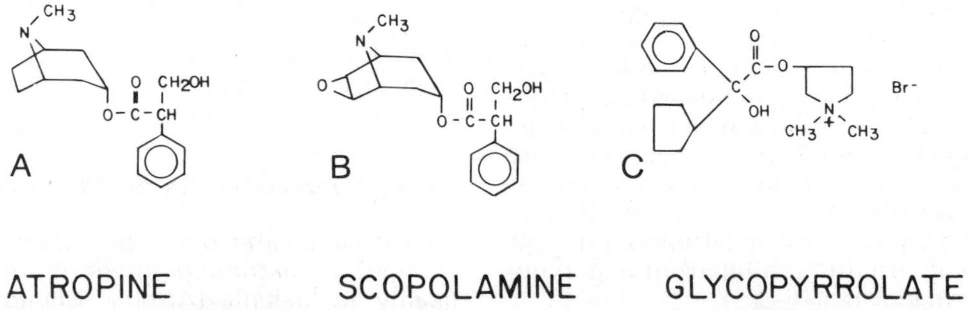

ATROPINE   SCOPOLAMINE   GLYCOPYRROLATE
Figure 6.2.   Structural formulae of atropine, scopolamine, and glycopyrrolate.

ing in ganglionic and neuromuscular blockade.

CENTRAL NERVOUS SYSTEM

Atropine is a tertiary amine and, thus, may cross the blood-brain barrier. High doses of atropine stimulate and then depress medullary and higher cerebral centers. However, clinical doses (0.5 mg) usually only produce transient central vagal stimulation with subsequent cardiac slowing. (This central effect is overshadowed by peripheral muscarinic blockade resulting in tachycardia.) In humans, excitement due to atropine is particularly evident after toxic doses leading to restlessness, irritability, mental excitement, mania, delirium, hallucinations, and hyperthermia—"central anticholinergic syndrome." After very large doses, stimulation is followed by depression and coma, and medullary depression and death ensue.

CARDIOVASCULAR SYSTEM

Small doses of atropine (0.2 to 0.3 mg) cause a transient fall in heart rate, which disappears as soon as the peripheral muscarinic blockade is fully established. This is believed to be due to stimulation of the medullary cardioinhibitory center, although other workers have suggested that the response of the S-A node itself is biphasic, slowing with small doses and accelerating with larger doses of atropine. Larger doses (0.6 to 1.2 mg intravenously) usually cause an increase in heart rate due to peripheral vagal blockade of the S-A node. Tachycardia occurs more rapidly if large doses of atropine are administered and may mask the bradycardia. These effects are less evident in the elderly in whom vagal tone is low. Arrhythmias such as A-V dissociation, A-V block, and nodal rhythm may occur. Ventricular ectopic beats have also been reported. However, A-V conduction time may be decreased and certain types of heart block improved. Therapeutic doses of atropine generally have little effect on arterial blood pressure, although if large doses (more than 2 mg) are used, there may be a small fall in blood pressure due to the shortened diastolic filling time of

the heart. Atropine in therapeutic doses is capable of blocking the peripheral vasodilation and hypotension produced by acetylcholine and other choline esters. However, atropine itself has no significant effect on peripheral blood vessels in clinical doses, but in poisoning, vasodilation with a characteristic red flush to the skin may be evident.

RESPIRATORY SYSTEM

Atropine inhibits secretions of the mouth, pharynx, and bronchi and, in addition, the smooth muscle of the bronchi is relaxed. Airway resistance is decreased and anatomical and physiological dead space is increased. Atropine is a more potent bronchodilator than scopolamine, but both atropine and scopolamine appear to reduce the incidence of laryngospasm during the induction of anesthesia, possibly due to reduced respiratory tract secretions. However, atropine and glycopyrrolate are equally effective as bronchodilators in normal subjects.

GASTROINTESTINAL SYSTEM

Antimuscarinic agents such as atropine affect both gastrointestinal secretion and motility. Atropine almost completely abolishes salivary secretion with the result that the mouth becomes dry and talking and swallowing become uncomfortable. Gastric secretion is only affected when doses are administered that also produce other antimuscarinic side effects such as an increase in heart rate. Secretion during both psychic and gastric phases is reduced but not abolished by 1.0 mg of atropine. Volume is usually reduced, but hydrogen ion concentration may be unaltered. The intestinal phase of gastric secretion may also be reduced. Relatively large doses (1.2 mg) of atropine reduce but do not completely abolish the fasting secretion of gastric acid and, in addition, histamine-, alcohol-, or caffeine-induced secretion is inhibited but not completely abolished in humans. Atropine administration may decrease the secretion (mucin and enzymes) of the gastric cells which are partly under vagal control.

Anticholinergics, in doses used by anesthesiologists for premedication, do not affect gastric fluid pH or volume at the time of anesthetic induction. In addition, atropine and glycopyrrolate have no effect on gastric fluid volume after 2 hours of fentanyl, enflurane, or halothane-nitrous oxide anesthesia. Likewise, anticholinergics are ineffective in raising gastric pH after fentanyl anesthesia. In contrast, the use of atropine or glycopyrrolate as a premedicant appears to raise gastric fluid pH after 2 hours of halothane anesthesia; the magnitude of this increase in pH is greater after glycopyrrolate than after atropine. It is important to emphasize that cimetidine (see Chapter 23) and ranitidine are considerably more effective in raising gastric pH than is the anticholinergic group of drugs.

Atropine in therapeutic doses inhibits gastrointestinal tone and motility, and peristalsis is reduced. In addition, atropine antagonizes the increased tone and motility produced by parasympathomimetic drugs and anticholinesterase agents. This is of importance to the anesthesiologist who routinely administers atropine with neostigmine at the termination of anesthesia to alleviate unwanted muscarinic side effects such as increased gastrointestinal tone and excessive bradycardia. Atropine and hyoscine possess antiemetic action, although hyoscine is more potent. In addition, atropine reduces the opening pressure of the lower esophageal sphincter and, thus, increases the risk of passive regurgitation. However, neostigmine produces the opposite effect, so that when atropine and neostigmine are administered simultaneously, there is an initial decrease in the pressure differential between the lower esophagus and stomach, which returns to previous levels 2 minutes later when the effect of neostigmine becomes evident.

EYE

The muscle which causes constriction of the pupil—constrictor pupillae—is supplied by parasympathetic fibers from the third cranial nerve (oculomotor). Under normal circumstances, atropine, therefore, causes pupillary dilation (mydriasis) since it leaves the iris under the unopposed influence of the sympathetic nervous system. The oculomotor nerve also supplies the ciliary muscle of the lens, and atropine thus causes paralysis of accommodation (cycloplegia). Distant vision remains good, but near vision is indistinct. Pupillary dilation results in photophobia. Atropine administration also blocks constrictor reflexes, such as that provoked by shining a light in the eye. Therapeutic doses of atropine which are routinely administered as part of a premedication regimen (0.4 to 0.6 mg of atropine) usually have little ocular effect, while equal doses of scopolamine cause mydriasis and loss of accommodation.

Atropine raises intraocular pressure due to pupillary dilation thickening the peripheral part of the iris with a consequent narrowing of the irido-corneal angle. This restricts drainage of the aqueous humor while secretion continues, and the pressure therefore rises. This is usually not important except in patients with narrow-angle glaucoma, where a dangerous rise in pressure may result. Atropine-like drugs can usually be safely used in wide-angle glaucoma.

OTHER EFFECTS

Small doses of atropine prevent sweat secretion, and the skin becomes hot and dry. Large doses may cause a rise in body temperature. Atropine dilates the ureters and bladder and decreases ureter and bladder contractions. Urinary retention can occur. The administration of atropine to mothers undergoing cesarean section has been reported to produce loss of fetal heart rate variability, although other workers have shown that fetal heart rate is not affected by either atropine or glycopyrrolate administration to the mother.

PHARMACOKINETICS

Atropine is absorbed from the gastrointestinal tract and other mucosal surfaces. The duodenum and jejunum are the main sites of absorption following oral administration. The total absorption following oral administration is in the region of 10 to 25% of the administered dose. Following intravenous administration (1.35- and 2.15-mg atropine base), atropine elimination follows first-order kinetics, with an initial distribution half-life $(t_{1/2\alpha})$ of 1.0 minute and an elimination half-life $(t_{1/2\beta})$ of 140 minutes. The steady-state volume of distribution is large, 210 L. Atropine is broken down by enzymatic hydrolysis to yield tropine and tropic acid, but some atropine is excreted unchanged by the kidney. Urinary excretion of unchanged drug is about 57% of the dose, while urinary excretion of tropine amounts to about 30% of the administered dose. Renal clearance of atropine is urine flow dependent, and active tubular secretion probably occurs. Following the administration of ^{14}C-labeled atropine, up to 80% of the dose is excreted in the urine during the first 8 hours and up to 94% during the first 24 hours. The plasma protein binding of atropine is about 50%.

The rectal administration of premedication is often preferred for children; the peak plasma concentration of atropine reached after 15 minutes of rectal administration (0.02 mg/kg) was 0.7 ng/ml compared with 2.4 ng/ml reached 5 minutes following intramuscular injection of the same dose. Thus, atropine concentrations following rectal administration are only 30% of the peak plasma concentrations attained after intramuscular injection.

Postoperative delirium or the central anticholinergic syndrome appears to be related to elevated plasma atropine concentrations. It is interesting that the central anticholinergic syndrome is more common in elderly patients. Age-related changes in response to atropine are well recognized, and relatively more atropine is required to increase heart rate in both very young and elderly patients. The clearance of atropine is reduced in the elderly, leading to a prolonged elimination half-life. For children under 2 years of age compared with older children, clearance values remain unchanged, but volume of distribution is increased leading to a prolonged elimination half-life in very young children.

Atropine rapidly crosses the placenta to reach the fetus. Maternal pharmacokinetic values for intravenous atropine in pregnant female patients are similar to those described for normal subjects $(t_{1/2\alpha}$, 1.02 minutes; $t_{1/2\beta}$, 2.56 hours). The concentrations of atropine in the umbilical vein 1 to 2 minutes after maternal intravenous injection are about 25% of maternal values, and equilibrium is reached in about 6 minutes.

SUGGESTED DOSAGE AND ADMINISTRATION

The usual dose of atropine for premedication is 0.4 to 0.6 mg. The dose of atropine for children is 0.02 mg/kg intravenously at induction or intramuscularly 30 minutes prior to surgery with a maximum dose of 0.6 mg. For infants below 5 kg, the dose is 0.05 to 0.1 mg. The use of atropine with an anticholinesterase agent to reverse residual neuromuscular blockade is discussed in Chapter 5. Atropine is administered under these circumstances to antagonize unwanted muscarinic side effects, when a dose of 0.6 to 1.2 mg is usually administered to the adult patient. Atropine (0.02 mg/kg) is administered with the anticholinesterase drug (neostigmine, 0.05 mg/kg) to pediatric patients to reverse nondepolarizing neuromuscular blocking agents.

TOXICITY, PRECAUTIONS, AND CONTRAINDICATIONS

Atropine should be avoided as part of a preanesthetic drug regimen when there is marked tachycardia, such as in hyperthyroidism and cardiovascular disease, when scopolamine may be a better choice, since atropine in therapeutic doses blocks the cardiac vagus nerve more than equivalent doses of scopolamine. Atropine and other antimuscarinic agents should be avoided in narrow-angle glaucoma for the reasons outlined earlier in this chapter.

Atropine poisoning presents with the predicted peripheral effects of dry mouth, mydriasis, blurred vision, hot dry skin, hyperpyrexia, restlessness, anxiety, hallucinations, delirium, and mania, all of which may lead eventually to central nervous system depression and coma.

Many H_1-histamine receptor blocking compounds, such as the phenothiazines and tricyclic antidepressants, have antimuscarinic activity, and poisoning with these drugs may cause clinical features that resemble atropine toxicity. Atropine poisoning may occur in children who have eaten berries of deadly nightshade or henbane or who have ingested atropine eye drops. The treatment of atropine intoxication consists of sedation (diazepam) and the administration of physostigmine (an anticholinesterase agent) which crosses the blood-brain barrier and therefore may reverse both the central nervous system and peripheral effects.

Scopolamine

Scopolamine is the ester of the organic base scopine, and its structural formula is given in Figure 6.2. Scopolamine is an alkaloid whose peripheral actions resemble those of atropine. It antagonizes the action of acetylcholine at cholinergic postganglionic nerve endings. However, atropine and scopolamine differ quantitatively in their antimuscarinic effects. Scopolamine has a strong effect on the eye and exocrine glands and is a more powerful antisialogogue than atropine. It is a more rapidly acting mydriatic and cycloplegic than atropine, but its effect pass off more quickly. Scopolamine is an effective agent in preventing motion sickness, but the high incidence of side effects and short duration of action preclude widespread use, either orally or parenterally.

The effects of scopolamine on the heart rate are less strong than atropine, although a short lasting tachycardia, followed by a secondary bradycardia, has been observed. Small doses of both atropine and scopolamine decrease heart rate, while larger doses increase heart rate. Stroke volume is generally unaffected by both drugs, and large doses decrease total peripheral resistance. Low doses of scopolamine (0.1 and 0.2 mg) cause more cardiac slowing than atropine, and usual premedicant doses

of scopolamine given intramuscularly cause a decrease or no change in heart rate. The cardiac slowing is probably due to central stimulation of the vagus.

Scopolamine is a tertiary amine and, thus, may cross the blood-brain barrier and enter the central nervous system. It differs from atropine in its central nervous system effects in that it has a more marked and longer lasting sedative effect, therapeutic doses causing drowsiness, euphoria, amnesia, and fatigue. However, occasionally scopolamine may cause restlessness, hallucinations, and delirium. This syndrome, known as the central anticholinergic syndrome, occurs more often in the elderly. Physostigmine is usually highly effective in reversing the central effects of scopolamine. Scopolamine readily crosses the placenta.

Scopolamine (0.4 mg intravenously) produces plasma concentrations that decline biexponentially, with an elimination half-life $(t_{-1/2\beta})$ of 1.6 to 3.3 hours. Volume of distribution varies between 1.2 and 2.7 L/kg, and the systemic clearance is reported to vary between 0.4 and 0.9 L/kg/h. Bioavailability is 21 to 26%. The percentage of the administered dose excreted as unchanged scopolamine is 1.7 to 5.9%.

SUGGESTED DOSAGE AND ADMINISTRATION

Scopolamine is generally used by anesthesiologists as a premedicant when its central sedative effects and smaller rise in heart rate are desired. The adult parenteral dose is 0.2 to 0.6 mg. In some cases, particularly in the elderly and young, scopolamine produces confusion and restlessness. For this reason, scopolamine is usually used as a premedicant in combination with a narcotic analgesic.

Scopolamine may also be administered by the transdermal route, using a patch containing a reservoir of the drug that is placed on the postauricular skin. The absorption process is controlled and, thus, the rate of drug entry into the systemic circulation resembles a low-dose intravenous infusion. Scopolamine has been given to patients by this route to treat motion sickness in an attempt to prevent adverse side effects and prolong the duration of therapeutic effect. Transdermal scopolamine has also been used by anesthesiologists both as a premedicant and to control postoperative nausea and vomiting. Although transdermal scopolamine may reduce the incidence of nausea and vomiting, the effect is short lived (only 24 hours), and the drug does not appear to provide prolonged protection. Other studies have failed to show an improvement and, in one study in children, there was an unacceptably high incidence of adverse effects, such as agitation and hallucinations. Transdermal scopolamine contains a drug reservoir of 1.5 mg of scopolamine and is designed to deliver 0.5 mg of scopolamine over a 72-hour period. An initial priming dose of 140 μg is provided, and the remainder is released at 5 μg/h.

Glycopyrrolate

Glycopyrrolate is an anticholinergic drug which has been used in the treatment of peptic ulcer for a number of years and has recently been introduced into anesthetic practice. It is a synthetic quaternary ammonium compound, and its structural formula is given in Figure 6.2. There are several important differences between glycopyrrolate and the belladonna alkaloids, atropine and scopolamine. Glycopyrrolate has been shown to possess potent antisialogogue activity of long duration. Wyant and Kao compared the effect of glycopyrrolate with that of atropine and showed that, on a weight-for-weight basis, glycopyrrolate is twice as potent an antisialogogue as atropine, while Mirakhur has shown it to be 4 or 5 times as potent as atropine. Glycopyrrolate is a quaternary ammonium compound making its passage across the blood-brain and placental barriers poor. It is, therefore, without the potential undesirable central nervous system effects associated with the tertiary compounds.

It is well recognized that the morbidity and mortality following aspiration of gastric contents depend upon the pH of the aspirate, less serious sequelae resulting if the pH is above 2.5. Anticholinergic drugs reduce both gastric acid secretion and volume. However, as discussed previously in this chapter, the value of anticholinergic premedication in raising gastric fluid pH is questionable. Some studies have suggested that premedication with glycopyrrolate results in a pH above 2.5 at induction in most cases, but other investigators have failed to confirm these findings. The effect of glycopyrrolate on gastric acidity has been investigated in parturients undergoing cesarean section. In patients receiving no anticholinergic premedication, gastric juice is markedly acidic. Premedication with atropine does not increase gastric juice pH to safe levels, while premedication with glycopyrrolate can raise the pH above the critical level of 2.5, suggesting that glycopyrrolate premedication can be used in the obstetric patient as an additional safety measure against Mendelson's syndrome. The use of atropine or glycopyrrolate prior to halothane anesthesia in surgical patients increases gastric fluid pH during anesthesia, the magnitude of the increase being greater after glycopyrrolate than after atropine. This is probably due to the longer duration of action of glycopyrrolate.

mine or pyridostigmine for the reversal of neuromuscular blockade is discussed in Chapter 5. It protects against bradycardia without causing marked tachycardia and, in addition, the duration of action of glycopyrrolate (6 to 8 hours) is longer than that of neostigmine and pyridostigmine. Atropine and scopolamine when given as anesthetic premedication are associated with a high incidence of dysrhythmias, while glycopyrrolate premedication produces small changes in heart rate and a low incidence of cardiac dysrhythmias. Slowing or no change in heart rate may follow the administration of 0.1 and 0.14 mg. This is similar to the effect of atropine which, when administered intravenously in small doses, causes bradycardia. The fact that glycopyrrolate causes bradycardia in some instances is surprising, because one would not expect

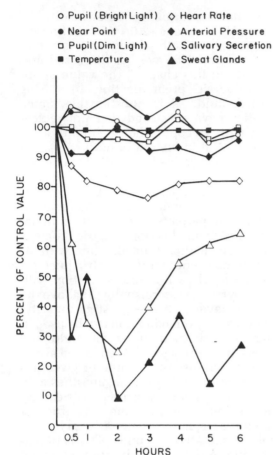

Figure 6.3. **The effects of glycopyrrolate on postganglionic cholinergic function.** In clinically useful doses, salivation and sweat gland activity appear to be selectively affected. (Adapted from Mirakhur RK: Anticholinergic drugs. *Br J Anaesth* 51:671–679, 1979.)

this drug (a quaternary ammonium compound) to possess such a central effect. Tachycardia is usually only associated with doses larger than 0.2 mg intravenously.

Figure 6.3 illustrates the selective effect of glycopyrrolate on parasympathetic activity. Its predominant effect on salivary and sweat gland secretion should be noted. Table 6.1 compares the pharmacological effects of the anticholinergic drugs atropine, scopolamine, and glycopyrrolate.

SUGGESTED DOSAGE AND ADMINISTRATION

The usual adult dose for premedication is 0.1 to 0.2 mg intramuscularly, or 0.1 mg intravenously at induction. For children, the preanesthetic dose is 0.002 to 0.004 mg per pound of body weight or 0.004 to 0.008 mg/kg intramuscularly. The recommended pediatric dose intraoperatively is 0.002 mg per pound of body weight intravenously not to exceed 0.1 mg in a single dose. The recommended doses when they are administered with neostigmine and pyridostigmine for the reversal of neuromuscular blockade are given in Chapter 5.

Ipratropium

Ipratropium bromide, a derivative of methylatropine, is an anticholinergic agent which is used by aerosol inhalation in the treatment of asthma and chronic obstructive pulmonary disease. Its principal difference from atropine is that it is much less lipid soluble than atropine and, therefore, is not well absorbed into the systemic circulation after either oral administration or by inhalation. Thus, the very low, and frequently undetectable, plasma concentrations are much less likely to produce the adverse anticholinergic side effects associated with atropine. Inhalation of ipratropium bromide by either puffs of a metered dose inhaler (usual dose, 2 to 4 puffs of 20 µg/puff) or nebulized solution of 50 to 125 µg results in blockade of the cholinergically mediated bronchomotor tone. In asthmatic patients and patients with chronic airways obstruction, this results in bronchodilation. In asthmatics, ipratropium bromide appears less potent than adrenergic agents and methylxanthines (see Chapter 19); however, its potency may be similar to these agents in patients with chronic obstructive pulmonary disease. A particularly useful indication for this drug is in patients who develop bronchospasm in response to β blocker administration. The ability of adrenergic agonists to reverse the bronchospasm is severely impaired during β blockade; however,

Table 6.1.
The Anticholinergic Drugs

Effect	Atropine	Glycopyrrolate	Scopolamine
Chemical structure	Tertiary amine	Quaternary ammonium compound	Tertiary amine
Duration of action	Short	Long	Short[a]
Salivation	Reduced+	Reduced++	Reduced++
Heart rate	Decreased with low doses Increased with high doses	Small increase	Little effect
Dysrhythmias during anesthesia	++	+	++
Central nervous system	Stimulation	−	Depression

[a]Central nervous system effects are longer lasting.

ipratropium, because of its anticholinergic effects, can still reverse the bronchospasm.

Very little (less than 1%) of the dose is absorbed following inhalation, so that its effects are virtually confined to the bronchial tree; systemic and central nervous system effects associated with the other anticholinergic drugs are rarely seen.

THERAPEUTIC USES

The clinical uses of anticholinergic drugs are many. Their use as part of an anesthetic premedication regimen has been discussed. Their effects on the central nervous system have been used to treat the rigidity and tremor of Parkinsonism (see later in this chapter). They are used as antiemetics and as sedatives (scopolamine). Their peripheral actions (atropine, homatropine, cyclopentolate) are utilized by ophthalmologists to dilate the pupil and paralyze ocular accommodation. Although the anticholinergic drugs have been used to treat gastrointestinal disease, their efficacy is limited and their use has declined due to the introduction of the H_2-receptor blocking agents (see Chapter 23). Anticholinergic agents (atropine) have been used in the treatment of cardiovascular arrhythmias. During anesthesia, atropine is often used in the treatment of reflex-mediated bra-

dycardia. Anticholinergic drugs in general are bronchodilators, and ipratropium, a derivative of methylatropine, is administered by inhalation as an aerosol in the treatment of asthma and obstructive airway disease. In cholinergic poisoning (anticholinesterase or mushroom), large doses of atropine (see Chapter 5) are required to antagonize the central nervous, parasympathomimetic, and vasodilator effects. It has no effect at the neuromuscular junction and will not prevent skeletal muscle paralysis. Atropine is an antidote for the rapid type of mushroom poisoning due to the alkaloid muscarine found in *Amanita muscaria*. It is of no value in the delayed type of mushroom poisoning due to the toxins of *A. phalloides*. Atropine is also used to antagonize the muscarinic effects of neostigmine and other anticholinesterase agents administered in the treatment of myasthenia gravis.

Drug Treatment of Parkinsonism

The basal ganglia contain high concentrations of two neurotransmitters, dopamine and acetylcholine. The function of the basal ganglia is to control movement by a balance between the dopaminergic system (inhibitory; neurotransmitter, dopamine) and the cholinergic system (excitatory; neurotransmitter, acetylcholine). Any imbalance between these two systems produces specific disorders of movement, and it has been shown that there is a marked deficiency of the dopaminergic component of the basal ganglia in Parkinson's disease. The relative deficiency of dopamine produces the classical features of tremor, rigidity, and hypokinesia. Thus, the aim in the treatment of Parkinson's disease is to restore functional balance between the two systems by:

1. Reduction in cholinergic activity;
2. Enhancement of dopaminergic function.

ANTICHOLINERGIC DRUGS

Synthetic anticholinergic drugs can reduce tremor and rigidity and are often administered with levodopa to cause a further reduction in symptoms. In addition, they are sometimes useful in the treatment of Parkinsonism induced by the neuroleptic group of drugs. Examples of anticholinergic drugs available for the treatment of Parkinsonism include trihexyphenidyl, procyclidine, benztropine, and ethopropazine. Certain antihistamine drugs have central anticholinergic-like properties that are also useful in the treatment of Parkinson's disease; these include diphenhydramine, orphenadrine, and chlorphenoxamine. Anticholinergics have a modest effect and improve the clinical features of the disease by about 10 to 25%.

LEVODOPA

Levodopa is formed from L-tyrosine as an intermediate compound in the synthesis of the catecholamines (see Chapter 13). Dopamine is then synthesized from levodopa under the influence of the enzyme, L-amino acid decarboxylase. Much of the exogenously administered levodopa is quickly converted into dopamine in peripheral tissue by decarboxylation so that only a small amount of levodopa enters the central nervous system to be converted into dopamine at the site where it is needed to produce its therapeutic effect. Dopamine does not cross the blood-brain barrier; thus, large doses

of levodopa are required to allow the accumulation of levodopa in the brain where decarboxylation converts it to dopamine, causing a rise in the concentration of dopamine in the basal ganglia. The dose of levodopa must be increased gradually to allow tolerance to develop. Levodopa reduces hypokinesia and rigidity and may benefit tremor in some cases. It also has psychic effects, causing a marked improvement in emotional outlook. Adverse effects include nausea, postural hypotension, and cardiac arrhythmias. It is therefore important to exercise caution in the administration of levodopa to patients with angina, cardiac arrhythmias, and cerebrovascular disease. Monoamine oxidase inhibitors, such as phenelzine and isocarboxazid, interfere with the breakdown of dopamine and other catecholamines and, thus, may potentiate the effects of levodopa.

Decarboxylation of levodopa to dopamine is catalyzed by the pyridoxine-dependent enzyme, L-amino acid decarboxylase. Excessive doses of pyridoxine increase the decarboxylation of levodopa to dopamine in the periphery and thus reduce the amount of levodopa available to enter the central nervous system. Thus, pyridoxine may reverse or reduce the therapeutic effect of levodopa. It has been reported that the amount of pyridoxine present in some multivitamin preparations has been sufficient to exert an antagonistic effect in some cases.

Caution should be exercised when inhalational anesthetics are administered to patients receiving levodopa since hypo- and hypertensive reactions have been reported. If levodopa is being administered in conjunction with a peripheral decarboxylase inhibitor, levodopa should be administered up to and on the morning of surgery and restarted as soon as possible postoperatively to prevent deterioration in mobility.

CARBIDOPA

Although levodopa is the most effective single drug in the treatment of Parkinson's disease, the side effects have always been a serious clinical problem.

Levodopa is often administered with an inhibitor of the enzyme aromatic L-amino acid decarboxylase which facilitates the conversion of levodopa to dopamine; this combination allows the dose of levodopa required to produce the same central nervous system effects to be reduced by 60 to 80%. The L-amino acid inhibitor **carbidopa** reduces the decarboxylation of levodopa in the periphery and thus allows a greater amount of levodopa to enter the central nervous sytem, allowing the dosage to be reduced. *Benserazide* is another decarboxylase inhibitor that has similar clinical effects as carbidopa, but is only available in Europe.

AMANTADINE

Amantadine is an antiviral agent that has been found to be beneficial in the treatment of Parkinson's disease. It may act by releasing dopamine from dopaminergic terminals in the nigrostriatum of patients with Parkinson's disease. Amantadine improves the clinical features of Parkinson's disease to about the same or slightly greater extent than the anticholinergics; thus, it effects are not as great as those of levodopa.

BROMOCRIPTINE

Bromocriptine is a directly acting dopaminergic agonist, with preference for D_2 receptors (see page 400) now in widespread use for the treatment of Parkinson's disease. Adverse effects are similar to those of levodopa and include nausea, vomiting, and postural hypotension. Bromocriptine is often used in combination with levodopa.

ANESTHETIC PREMEDICATION

The aims of anesthetic premedication are:

1. To allay anxiety and to sedate the patient;
2. To aid in the induction of anesthesia;
3. To reduce the overall dose of anesthetic required.

In addition, premedicant drugs may be given for special purposes, e.g., to aid in the production of induced hypotension or hypothermia and as part of preopera-

tive steroid therapy when necessary. Certain groups of patients may be singled out as requiring special attention: the young; the elderly; patients suffering from certain disease states (respiratory and cardiac disease, porphyria); and those receiving drug medication prior to anesthesia and surgery. It has been estimated that over a third of patients coming to the operating room are receiving medication that might adversely affect the outcome of surgery and anesthesia.

Many patients are anxious, although much of their fear and apprehension can be relieved by the preoperative visit and a talk with the anesthesiologist. However, some patients require sedation especially if their surgery is late in the day. Thus, patients are often premedicated with a sedative-hynotic, narcotic analgesic, or tranquilizer with or without an anticholinergic drug. The sedative and narcotic drugs most commonly used are morphine, meperidine, and the benzodiazepines. The phenothiazines are also used, for both their tranquilizing and antiemetic actions. Narcotic analgesics and sedative drugs may reduce overall anesthetic requirements. It has been shown that premedication with 8 to 15 mg of morphine decreases halothane minimum alveolar concentration (MAC) required to prevent the response to skin incision in 50% of subjects by 7%. Diazepam and midazolam also reduce halothane MAC in humans. The great drawback to the use of powerful narcotic drugs as premedicants is the production of postoperative nausea and vomiting, and these drugs are frequently administered in conjunction with an antiemetic.

The benzodiazepines (diazepam, midazolam, and lorazepam) have all been used as part of a premedicant regimen, when they produce anxiolysis, sedation, and amnesia. Lorazepam produces more profound and more prolonged sedation and amnesia than diazepam, but its onset of action is less rapid. Midazolam is also a useful sedative-anxiolytic drug; it has a rapid onset of action and perhaps a more rapid recovery than diazepam when administered intramuscularly.

The main reason given by anesthesiologists for the use of anticholinergic drugs as part of a premedication regimen are the inhibition of salivation and the protection against vagal reflexes. In addition, they partially inhibit gastric secretion, decrease gastrointestinal motility, and produce a limited degree of bronchodilation. They may also reduce the incidence of laryngeal spasm, cough, and hiccough associated with the administration of intravenous barbiturate induction agents. The routine use of anticholinergic drugs as part of a premedication regimen has been criticized by many workers. Atropine and other antimuscarinic drugs decrease opening pressure of the lower esophageal sphincter, increasing the likelihood of regurgitation, and in addition, they may be associated with the production of cardiac dysrhythmias during anesthesia, especially on laryngoscopy and intubation. In the days when irritating inhalational anesthetics were used, the drying effect of the anticholinergic drugs was necessary. However, modern nonirritating anesthetics do not require the routine use of antisialogogue drugs, and many studies have demonstrated that general anesthesia may be carried out safely without the use of anticholinergic drugs. The maximal effect of atropine given by subcutaneous or intramuscular injection is apparent 30 minutes after injection, and it is thus more logical to give atropine intravenously at induction if its cardiac effects are desired. Many anesthesiologists therefore do not routinely prescribe these drugs in premedication, but administer them intravenously on induction if required, thus sparing the patient the unpleasant sensations of thirst and a dry mouth. However, neonates and small infants still require anticholinergic premedication both to reduce secretions in small airways and to reduce the cholinergic influence on the heart. Atropine-induced tachycardia can make deliberate hypotension more difficult to achieve, and scopolamine or glycopyrrolate is a more logical choice in this situation.

Antacids and the histamine H_2-receptor blocking agents, cimetidine and ranitidine, are often administered during the prospective period to patients considered to be at increased risk for pulmonary aspiration of gastric contents. Patients with a gastric pH of less than 2.5 and a gastric fluid volume greater than 25 ml are generally thought to be at increased risk for developing the acid aspiration syndrome. Thus, agents that increase gastric fluid pH and reduce gastric fluid volume are often administered to reduce the risk of developing aspiration pneumonitis. Histamine H_2-receptor blocking agents increase gastric fluid pH (see Chapter 23), and it is useful to administer an agent of this kind on the evening prior to surgery and again on the morning of surgery to decrease gastric acidity and volume. Parenteral administration is more effective than the oral route when a rapid onset of effect is required. Cimetidine, 150 to 300 mg, and ranitidine, 50 to 100 mg, increase gastric fluid pH within 1 hour of parenteral administration. Antacids are also administered to neutralize gastric acid. Antacid suspensions can themselves produce adverse pulmonary effects when aspirated, and therefore the nonsuspension antacid, sodium citrate, is often administered to increase gastric pH; unfortunately it also increases gastric fluid volume.

Certain disease states require special attention to premedication. Hyperthyroid patients should be made euthyroid before surgery whenever possible; sedation is of great importance in these patients, and scopolamine is a logical choice as an anticholinergic agent, for both its minimal effect on heart rate and its amnesic sedative action. Patients receiving monoamine oxidase inhibitors may present for anesthesia and surgery. It would be wise to avoid meperidine or other narcotic agents in this group of patients, although it has been shown that adverse reactions do not always occur.

Patients suffering from Parkinson's disease receiving levodopa should not receive butyrophenone drugs (droperidol and haloperidol) as part of their preanesthetic drug regimen. Butyrophenones antagonize the effects of dopamine within the central nervous system and may precipitate Parkinsonian rigidity in these patients (the development of extrapyramidal rigidity is a well-recognized

Table 6.2.
Drug Doses in Pediatric Anesthetic Premedication

Atropine	0.02 mg/kg i.v. at induction or i.m. 30 minutes preoperatively. Maximum dose = 0.6 mg. Neonates and infants under 5 kg: dose = 0.1mg
Scopolamine	0.008 mg/kg i.m.
Glycopyrrolate	0.004 mg/kg to 0.008 mg/kg i.m. 30 minutes preoperatively
Morphine	0.05 to 0.2 mg/kg i.m. 60 minutes, preoperatively
Meperidine	1.0 to 1.5 mg/kg i.m. 60 minutes, preoperatively
Pentazocine	0.5 mg/kg i.m. 60 minutes, preoperatively
Diazepam	0.2 to 0.4 mg/kg orally 1 to 2 hours preoperatively to older children. Maximum dose, 10 mg.
Droperidol	0.1 to 0.15 mg/kg i.m.
Promethazine	0.5 mg/kg i.m.
Hydroxyzine	0.5 to 1.0 mg/kg i.m.
Pentobarbital	2 mg/kg i.m. 2 hours, preoperatively
Secobarbital	2 mg/kg i.m.

side effect of droperidol; see Chapter 20). Many patients may be receiving corticosteroids prior to their anesthesia. Cardiovascular and respiratory collapse from adrenocortical suppression is unlikely to occur more than 2 months after cessation of a course of treatment; routine cover therefore need only be considered in patients who have received significant doses of steroids during the 2 months preceding surgery. A scheme for the administration of hydrocortisone during surgery is given in Chapter 19.

The seriously ill patient should not be premedicated in his room. Patients suffering from shock, hypovolemia, or severe chronic pulmonary disease should rarely be premedicated on the ward. In contrast, there are certain patients who require heavy premedication. These include those patients in whom balanced anesthesia with nitrous oxide, analgesics, and muscle relaxants is planned and patients with ischemic heart disease and hypertension where fear and anxiety may increase myocardial work with potentially serious results.

Premedication in Children

Although the use of anticholinergic drugs in premedication may be criticized in adults, infants and small children should be considered separately. The presence of secretions in small airways may cause an increase in airway resistance, respiratory obstruction, and laryngeal spasm, and many anesthesiologists prefer to routinely administer atropine to infants. In addition, atropine is frequently administered in relatively large doses to prevent the vagal reflexes which are readily elicited in pediatric patients.

Sedation in neonates and small infants is usually considered unnecessary, and premedication to patients under 1 year of age should be limited to atropine alone or not at all, while infants with cyanotic congenital heart disease weighing over 10 kg may be given morphine preoperatively. For pediatric patients over 1 year of age, sedation may be achieved by the administration of morphine, meperidine, or diazepam.

The doses of drugs commonly employed in pediatric anesthetic practice are given in Table 6.2.

BIBLIOGRAPHY

General

Abboud T, Raya J, Sadri S, Grobler N, Stine L, Miller F: Fetal and maternal cardiovascular effects of atropine and glycopyrrolate. *Anesth Analg* 62:426–430, 1983.

Conner JT, Bellville JW, Wender R, Schehl D, Dorey F, Katz RL: Morphine, scopolamine, and atropine as intravenous surgical premedicants. *Anesth Analg* 56:606–614, 1977.

Eger EI: Atropine, scopolamine, and related compounds. *Anesthesiology* 23:365–383, 1962.

Eger EI, Kraft ID, Keasling HH: A comparison of atropine, or scopolamine, plus pentobarbital, meperidine, or morphine as pediatric preanesthetic premedication. *Anesthesiology* 22:962–969, 1961.

Gravenstein JS, Anderson TW, DePadua CB: Effects of atropine and scopolamine on the cardiovascular system in man. *Anesthesiology* 25:123–130, 1964.

Greenan J: Cardiac dysrhythmias and heart rate changes at induction of anaesthesia: a comparison of two intravenous anticholinergics. *Acta Anaesthesiol Scand* 28:182–184, 1984.

Herxheimer A: A comparison of some atropine-like drugs in man, with particular reference to their end-organ specificity. *Br J Pharmacol* 13:184–192, 1958.

Hey VMF, Phillips K, Woods I: Pethidine, atropine, metoclopramide, and the lower oesophageal sphincter. *Anaesthesia* 38:650–653, 1983.

Kantelip JP, Alatienne M, Gueorguiev G, Duchene-Marullaz P: Chronotropic and dromotropic effects of atropine and hyoscine methobromide in unanaesthetized dogs. *Br J Anaesth* 57:214–219, 1985.

Kongsrud F, Sponheim S: A comparison of atropine and glycopyrrolate in anaesthetic practice. *Acta Anaesthesiol Scand* 26:620–625, 1982.

Korttila K, Kauste A, Auvinem J: Comparison of domperidone, droperidol, and metoclopramide in the prevention and treatment of nausea and vomiting after balanced general anesthesia. *Anesth Analg* 58:396–400, 1979.

Manchikanti L, Rousch JR: Effects of preanesthetic glycopyrrolate and cimetidine on gastric fluid pH and volume in outpatients. *Anesth Analg* 63:40–46, 1984.

Meyers EF, Tomeldan SA: Glycopyrrolate compared with atropine in prevention of the oculocardiac reflex during eye-muscle surgery. *Anesthesiology* 51:350–352, 1979.

Mirakhur RK: Anticholinergic drugs. *Br J Anaesth* 51:671–679, 1979.

Mirakhur RK, Briggs LP, Clarke RSJ, Dundee JW, Johnston HML: Comparison of atropine and glycopyrrolate in a mixture with pyridostigmine for the antagonism of neuromuscular block. *Br J Anaesth* 53:1315–1320, 1981.

Mirakhur RK, Clarke RJJ, Elliott J, Dundee JW: Atropine and glycopyrronium premedication. *Anaesthesia* 33:906–912, 1978.

Mirakhur RK, Dundee JW: Glycopyrrolate: pharmacology and clinical use. *Anaesthesia* 38:1195–1204, 1983.

Mirakhur RK, Dundee JW, Connolly JDR: Studies of drugs given before anaesthesia. XVII. Anticholinergic premedicants. *Br J Anaesth* 51:339–345, 1979.

Mirakhur RK, Jones CJ, Dundee JW: Effects of intravenous administration of glycopyrrolate and atropine in anaesthetised patients. *Anaesthesia* 35:277–281, 1980.

Mirakhur RK, Reid J, Elliott J: Volume and pH of gastric contents following anticholinergic premedication. *Anaesthesia* 34:453–457, 1979.

Opie JC, Chaye H, Steward DJ: Intravenous atropine rapidly reduces lower esophageal sphincter pressure in infants and children. *Anesthesiology* 67:989–990, 1987.

Preiss D, Berguson P: Dose-response studies on glycopyrrolate and atropine in conscious cardiac patients. *Br J Clin Pharmacol* 16:523–527, 1983.

Roper RE, Salem MG: Effects of glycopyrrolate and atropine combined with antacid on gastric acidity. *Br J Anaesth* 53:1277–1280, 1981.

Rumack BH: Anticholinergic poisoning: treatment with physostigmine. *Pediatrics* 52:449–451, 1973.

Salem MR, Wong AY, Mani M, Bennett EJ, Toyama T: Premedicant drugs and gastric juice pH and volume in pediatric patients. *Anesthesiology* 44:216–219, 1976.

Shutt LE, Bowes JB: Atropine and hyoscine. *Anaesthesia* 34:476–490, 1979.

Simpson KH, Smith RJ, Davies LF: Comparison of the effects of atropine and glycopyrrolate on cognitive function following general anaesthesia. *Br J Anaesth* 59:966–969, 1987.

Smith TC, Stephen GW, Zeiger L, Wollman H: Effects of premedicant drugs on respiration and gas exchange in man. *Anesthesiology* 28:883–890, 1967.

Stoelting RK: Responses to atropine, glycopyrrolate, and riopan of gastric fluid pH and volume in adult patients. *Anesthesiology* 48:367–369, 1978.

Stoelting, RK: Gastric fluid volume and pH after fentanyl, enflurane, or halothane-nitrous oxide anesthesia with or without atropine or glycopyrrolate. *Anesth Analg* 59:287–290, 1980.

Thorburn JR, James MFM, Feldman C, Moyes DG, DuToit PS: Comparison of the effects of atropine and glycopyrrolate on pulmonary mechanics in patients undergoing fiberoptic bronchoscopy. *Anesth Analg* 65:1285–1289, 1986.

Tune LE, Damlouji NF, Holland A, Gardner TJ, Folstein MF, Coyle JT: Association of postoperative delirium with raised serum levels of anticholinergic drugs. *Lancet* 2:651–652, 1981.

Atropine

Adams RG, Verma P, Jackson AJ, Miller RL: Plasma pharmacokinetics of intravenously administered atropine in normal human subjects. *J Clin Pharmacol* 22:477–481, 1982.

Bejersten A, Olsson GL, Palmer L: The influence of body weight on plasma concentration of atropine after rectal administration in children. *Acta Anaesthesiol Scand* 29:782–784, 1985.

Dauchot P, Gravenstein JS: Effects of atropine on the electrocardiogram in different age groups. *Clin Pharmacol Ther* 12:274–280, 1971.

Fielder DL, Nelson DC, Anderson TW, Gravenstein JS: Cardiovascular effects of atropine and neostigmine in man. *Anesthesiology* 30:637–641, 1969.

Gal TJ, Suratt PM: Atropine and glycopyrrolate effects on lung mechanics in normal man. *Anesth Analg* 60:85–90, 1981.

Gillick JS: Atropine toxicity in a neonate. *Br J Anaesth* 46:793–794, 1974.

Hayes AH, Copelan HW, Ketchum JS: Effects of large intramuscular doses of atropine on cardiac rhythm. *Clin Pharmacol Ther* 12:482–486, 1971.

Hinderling PH, Gundert-Remy U, Schmidlin O: Integrated pharmacokinetics and pharmacodynamics of atropine in healthy humans. I. Pharmacokinetics. *J Pharm Sci* 74:703–710, 1985.

Jones RE, Deutsch S, Turndorf H: Effects of atropine on cardiac rhythm in conscious and anesthetized man. *Anesthesiology* 22:67–73, 1961.

Kanto J, Virtanen R, Iisalo E, Maenpaa K, Liukko P: Placental transfer and pharmacokinetics of atropine after a single maternal intravenous and intramuscular administration. *Acta Anaesthesiol Scand* 25:85–88, 1981.

Longo VG: Behavioral and electroencephalographic effects of atropine and related compounds. *Pharmacol Rev* 18:965–966, 1966.

Murrin KR: A study of oral atropine in healthy adult subjects. *Br J Anaesth* 45:475–480, 1973.

Olsson GL, Bejersten A, Feychting H, Palmer L, Pettersson B-M. Plasma concentrations of atropine after rectal administration. *Anaesthesia* 38:1179–1182, 1983.

Turner DAB, Smith G: Evaluation of the combined effects of atropine and neostigmine on the lower oesophageal sphincter. *Br J Anaesth* 57:956–959, 1985.

Virtanen R, Kanto J, Iisalo E, Iisalo EUM, Salo M, Sjovall S: Pharmacokinetic studies on atropine with special reference to age. *Acta Anaesth Scand* 26:297–300, 1982.

Scopolamine

Aronson JK, Sear JW: Transdermal hyoscine (scopolamine) and postoperative vomiting. *Anaesthesia* 41:1–3, 1986.

Clissold SP, Heel RC: Transdermal hyoscine (scopolamine). *Drugs* 29:198–207, 1985.

List WF, Gravenstein JS: Effects of atropine and scopolamine on the cardiovascular system in man. II. Secondary bradycardia after scopolamine. *Anesthesiology* 26:299–304, 1965.

Ostfeld AM, Arguete A: Central nervous system effects of hyoscine in man. *J Pharmacol Exp Ther* 137:133–139, 1962.

Putcha L, Tsui J, Cintron NM, Vanderploeg JM, Kramer WG: Pharmacokinetics of scopolamine in normal subjects. *Clin Pharmacol Ther* 37:222, 1985.

Uppington J, Dunnet J, Blogg CE: Transdermal hyoscine and postoperative nausea and vomiting. *Anaesthesia* 41:16–20, 1986.

Glycopyrrolate

Baraka A, Saab M, Salem MR, Winnie AP: Control of gastric acidity by glycoyrrolate premedication in the parturient. *Anesth Analg* 56:642–645, 1977.

Brock-Utne JG, Rubin J, Welman S, Dimopoulos GE, Moshal MG, Downing JW: The effect of glycopyrrolate (Robinul) on the lower oesophageal sphincter. *Can Anaesth Soc J* 25:144–146, 1978.

Meyers EF, Charles P: Glycopyrrolate compared with atropine in patients undergoing intraocular operations with local anesthesia. *Anesthesiology* 49:370–371, 1978.

Mirakhur RK: Intravenous administration of glycopyrronium: effects on cardiac rate and rhythm. *Anaesthesia* 34:458–462, 1979.

Mirakhur RK, Dundee JW: Glycopyrrolate: pharmacology and clinical use. *Anaesthesia* 38:1195–1204, 1983.

Sengupta A, Gupta PK, Pandey K: Investigation of glycopyrrolate as a premedicant durg. *Br J Anaesth* 51:513–516, 1980.

Warran P, Radford P, Manford MLM: Glycopyrrolate in children. *Br J Anaesth* 53:1273–1276, 1981.

Wyant GM, Kao E: Glycopyrrolate methobromide. I. Effect on salivary secretions. *Can Anaesth Soc J* 21:230–241, 1974.

Young R, Sun DCH: Effect of glycopyrrolate on antral motility, gastric emptying and intestinal transit. *Ann NY Acad Sci* 99:174–178, 1962.

Ipatropium

Gross NJ: Ipratropium bromide. *N Engl J Med* 319:486–494, 1988.

Parkinsonism

Bevan DR, Monks, PS, Calne DB: Cardiovascular reactions to anaesthesia during treatment with levodopa. *Anaesthesia* 28:29–31, 1973.

Cedarbaum JM: Clinical pharmacokinetics of anti-Parkinsonian drugs. *Clin Pharmacokinet* 13:141–178, 1987.

Goldberg LI: Anesthetic management of patients treated with antihypertensive agents or levodopa. *Anesth Analg* 51:625–632, 1972.

Ngai SH: Parkinsonism, levodopa, and anesthesia. *Anesthesiology* 37:344–351, 1972.

Quinn NP: Anti-Parkinsonian drugs today. *Drugs* 28:236–262, 1984.

Severn AM: Parkinsonism and the anaesthetist. *Br J Anaesth* 61:761–770, 1988.

Anesthetic Premedication

Kanto J: Benzodiazepines as oral premedicants. *Br J Anaesth* 53:1179–1188, 1981.

Leighton KM, Sanders HD: Anticholinergic premedication. *Can Anaesth Soc J* 23:563–566, 1976.

Madej TH, Paasuke RT: Anaesthetic premedication: aims, assessment, and methods. *Can Anaesth Soc J* 34:259–273, 1987.

White PF: Pharmacologic and clinical aspects of preoperative medication. *Anesth Analg* 65:963–974, 1986.

7

Opioid Agonists and Antagonists

MARGARET WOOD

CLASSIFICATION OF ANALGESICS

OPIATE OR OPIOID RECEPTORS

ENDOGENOUS OPIOID PEPTIDES

CHEMICAL STRUCTURE OF THE OPIOID ANALGESICS

INDIVIDUAL OPIOID ANALGESICS

Morphine	Fentanyl
Codeine	Alfentanil
Heroin	Sufentanil
Hydromorphone	Pentazocine
Oxycodone	Butorphanol
Oxymorphone	Nalbuphine
Meperidine	Buprenorphine

DRUG INTERACTIONS

MANAGEMENT OF POSTOPERATIVE PAIN

OPIOID ANTAGONISTS

Nalorphine
Naloxone
Naltrexone
Nalmefene

CLASSIFICATION OF ANALGESICS

Analgesic drugs may be divided into two main groups based on their potency:

1. The strong analgesics;
2. The mild or simple analgesics.

In addition, the strong analgesics may be further subdivided into **opioid** or **narcotic** and **nonnarcotic** subgroups.

Opium is the dried powdered mixture of alkaloids obtained from the unripe seed capsules of the poppy plant, *Papaver somniferum*. There are many alkaloids in opium, but morphine is the chief constituent and is considered to be representative of the opiates as a group. Although morphine can be synthesized in the laboratory, it is still prepared commercially from purified opium. Semisynthetic compounds have been made by modifying morphine and related molecules. Although **opiate** is the term originally used to describe drugs derived from opium, the term **opioid** refers to all drugs, natural and synthetic, that have morphine-like properties and, therefore, bind to opioid receptors to produce some agonist effect. **Narcotic** is derived from the Greek "Narko" (to be numb) and is also used to refer to potent morphine-like agonist drugs.

The opioid analgesics have also been classified into groups which, although possessing similar pharmacological properties, are structurally quite different.

1. Natural alkaloids or opium—morphine, codeine;
2. Semisynthetic derivatives—diacetylmorphine (heroin), hydromorphone, oxymorphone, hydrocodone, oxycodone;
3. Synthetic derivatives
   a. Phenylpiperidines—meperidine, fentanyl
   b. Benzmorphans—pentazocine, phenazocine, cyclazocine
   c. Morphinans—levorphanol
   d. Propionanilides—methadone.

Opioids are frequently used in anesthetic practice for a variety of reasons; for pain relief; premedication; supplementation of general anesthetics; supplementation of regional anesthetics and local procedures; and as primary anesthetics themselves, when they may be given as the sole agent.

OPIATE OR OPIOID RECEPTORS

History

In 1915, Pohl demonstrated that N-allylnorcodeine not only antagonized the effects of morphine and heroin but also possessed direct respiratory stimulant activity. However, it was many years later (1951) before nalorphine was synthesized and shown to antagonize the effects of morphine, to precipitate an abstinence syndrome in morphine-dependent subjects, and in addition to be a potent analgesic. In 1956, another narcotic antagonist, levallorphan, was introduced into clinical practice. It soon became evident that nalorphine and levallorphan possessed certain properties similar to morphine, but that they could antagonize the respiratory depression produced by large doses of narcotics, while augmenting and increasing the respiratory depression due to low doses of narcotics. Further, nalorphine and levallorphan could produce respiratory depression when administered alone without prior narcotic medication. These observations stimulated the search for a narcotic antagonist which could be used as a potentially nonaddicting analgesic drug.

Although nalorphine possesses some agonist effects that are similar to morphine (analgesia, miosis, respiratory depression), it also has some quite different agonist effects, such as dysphoria and hallucinations, and because of these psychotomimetic effects, nalorphine is not a clinically acceptable analgesic. Two benzmorphan compounds—pentazocine and cyclazocine—were later studied and found to have antagonistic properties. Since then, pentazocine has achieved wide acceptance as an analgesic drug for the treatment of moderate to severe pain.

The situation became more confused when it was noted that cyclazocine and nalorphine differed in their agonist actions not only from morphine, but also from each other; e.g., cyclazocine produced gross ataxia while nalorphine produced only slight ataxia. The physiological effects of morphine and cyclazocine physical dependence were also shown to be different. Thus, at this point, there were conflicting data which could not be readily explained on the basis of a single opioid receptor.

The theory of multiple receptors and receptor dualism was proposed by Martin to explain this conflict. He suggested that there were two distinguishable receptors, one responsible for the analgesic effects of morphine and the other responsible for the analgesic effects of nalorphine and cyclazocine—a morphine receptor and a nalorphine receptor. Nalorphine and cyclazocine were thus thought to be competitive antagonists of morphine at the morphine receptor, to which they bind but do not stimulate and agonists at the nalorphine receptor where they produce stimulation. Martin called this situation receptor dualism and suggested that a drug could be a strong agonist, a partial agonist, or a competitive antagonist at either or both of these receptor subtype sites.

Progress in the understanding of how narcotic drugs act was provided by the synthesis of naloxone, which was shown to have no morphine, nalorphine, or cyclazocine-like agonist action. Thus, naloxone is almost a pure antagonist; i.e., when it binds to the receptor, no pharmacological effect is produced. Naloxone was shown to be less potent in antagonizing the agonist actions of cyclazocine than the agonist actions of morphine and less potent in precipitating a withdrawal syndrome in pentazocine-dependent than morphine-dependent subjects.

Classification of Opioid Receptors

Studies of the binding of the opioid drugs and peptides to specific receptor sites in the central nervous system and other organs such as the mouse vas deferens and guinea pig ileum have now demonstrated that it is no longer tenable to think of a simple opioid receptor, or even two opioid receptors, and that a number of different populations of opioid receptors exist in the brain and the peripheral tissues. In the central nervous system, four receptors, designated mu (μ), kappa (κ), delta (δ), and sigma (σ) have been described.

1. **Mu receptor (morphine).** Stimulation of this receptor causes supraspinal analgesia, feelings of wellbeing, euphoria, respiratory depression, and a morphine-type physical dependence. Morphine acts as an agonist at this receptor, and beta endorphin is an endogenous ligand. Naloxone is a selective antagonist.

2. **Kappa receptor.** Ketocyclazocine is the prototype agonist for the kappa receptor. Stimulation of the kappa receptor causes spinal analgesia, sedation and anesthesia, and a cyclazocine-type physical dependence. Morphine also acts as an agonist at this receptor. Dynorphin is an endogenous agonist, and naloxone is a selective antagonist.

3. **Sigma receptor.** This receptor is responsible for feelings of dysphoria, hallucinations, mydriasis, and respiratory stimulation.

4. **Delta receptor.** Some of the in vitro pharmacological effects of the enkephalins and endorphins on the mouse vas deferens are due to another opioid receptor, designated the delta receptor. The enkaphalin analog D-Ala,D-Leuenkephalin (DADL) is the prototype agonist. Although the function of the delta receptor in humans is not clear, the delta receptor may be responsible for modulation of the activity of mu receptors.

Another opioid receptor, the ϵ-receptor (epsilon), has been described using in vitro binding studies in a rat vas deferens preparation. The proposed endogenous agonist is β-endorphin and the selective antagonist, naloxone. This receptor is not well characterized at present.

Thus, multiple opioid receptor subtypes have been identified and classified (Table 7.1). The morphine (mu) receptor has been subdivided into mu_1 and mu_2 receptors; mu_1 receptors bind with high affinity both morphine and the enkephalins, mu_2 receptors selectively bind morphine, and delta receptors bind most enkephalins (Fig. 7.1). It is interesting that

Table 7.1.
Classification of Opioid or Opiate Receptors

Receptor	Prototype agonist	Effect
mu_1	Opioids and most opioid peptides— enkephalin, beta endorphin, morphine	Supraspinal analgesia, morphine-like dependence
mu_2	Morphine	Respiratory depression, inhibition of gastrointestinal tract motility, and most cardiovascular effects (e.g., bradycardia)
delta	Enkephalins, DADL	Spinal analgesia
kappa	Cyclazocine, dynorphin	Spinal analgesia, inhibition of antidiuretic hormone release, sedation, miosis
sigma	N-Allylnormetazocine	Dysphoria, hallucinations
epsilon	beta endorphin	?

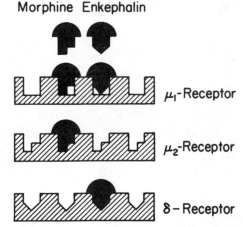

Morphine Enkephalin

μ_1-Receptor

μ_2-Receptor

δ-Receptor

Figure 7.1. A schematic model of morphine and enkephalin binding to opioid receptors. Morphine and the enkephalins label three classes of opiate receptors in the brain. In addition to sites selective for morphine (mu_2) or the enkephalins (delta), a mu_1 site has been identified which binds opiates and enkephalins equally well and with very high affinity. Thus, morphine activates mu_1 and mu_2 receptors while most enkephalins activate mu_1 and delta receptors. (From Pasternak GW, Wood PJ: Multiple mu opiate receptors. *Life Sci* 38:1889–1898, 1986.)

morphine and the enkephalins appear to bind to mu_1 sites with greater potency (high affinity) than to their selective receptor sites, mu_2 and delta, respectively. The mu_2 receptor thus exhibits low affinity. The most important mu_1-mediated opiate effect is supraspinal analgesia, while effects that are related to the mu_2 receptor include respiratory depression, inhibition of gastrointestinal tract motility, and cardiovascular effects such as bradycardia. Thus, the development of a selective mu_1 agonist drug might be an important advance.

Drugs acting at the opioid receptors can thus be divided into three groups:

1. **Opioid agonists,** e.g., morphine, act as agonists at the mu and kappa receptors. The relative affinity of morphine for the mu receptor is 200 times greater than for the kappa receptor. Opioid agonists also include drugs such as meperidine, fentanyl, sufentanil, and alfentanil.
2. **Competitive antagonists,** drugs that act as competitive antagonists at opioid receptors but are devoid of any agonist effect, e.g., naloxone. Naloxone is a pure opioid antagonist but is 10 times more effective at the mu receptor than at other receptors.
3. **Agonist-antagonists,** opioid analgesics can act as agonists at one receptor and antagonists at another receptor. Opioid agonist-antagonist drugs include pentazocine, bu-

torphanol, nalorphine, buprenorphine, nalbuphine, bremazocine, and dezocine. Most of the agonist-antagonist group of opioids are partial agonists at the kappa and sigma receptors and antagonists at the mu receptor.

Thus, it can be seen that morphine acts as an agonist at the mu and kappa receptors, while nalorphine is a competitive antagonist at the mu receptor, a partial agonist at the kappa receptor, and a sigma receptor agonist. Naloxone is an antagonist at the mu and kappa receptors, but has greater affinity for the mu receptor, and is devoid of any agonist activity. Pentazocine is considered a weak competitive antagonist at the mu receptor, a strong kappa receptor agonist, and a sigma receptor agonist. Nalorphine is a partial kappa agonist, whereas cyclazocine is a kappa agonist, which explains the difference in degree of ataxia noted previously between these two drugs. Butorphanol does not have an effect (agonist or antagonist) at the mu receptor but is an agonist at the kappa and sigma receptors. Buprenorphine is a partial agonist at the mu receptor. Table 7.2 lists the important narcotic agonist and antagonists and their action at the various opioid receptor subtypes.

What is a **partial agonist?** (See Chapter 3.) Buprenorphine has been shown to be a partial agonist at the mu receptor, while nalbuphine is a partial agonist at the kappa receptor. Receptor theory

states that drugs have two independent properties at receptor sites:

1. **affinity,** the ability of a drug to bind to the receptor and to form a stable complex;
2. **intrinsic activity** or **efficacy,** the ability of the drug-receptor complex to initiate a pharmacological effect. Therefore, an agonist and antagonist may have the same affinity for the receptor site, but an agonist has high intrinsic activity, whereas the antagonist has low or no intrinsic activity and thus can antagonize the effect of the agonist by preventing its access to the receptor site. Drugs that produce less than maximal response and therefore have a lowered intrinsic activity are called partial agonists. This concept implies that partial agonists should also have antagonistic properties because, by occupying receptor sites yet only producing weak effects due to their low intrinsic activity, they block the access of full agonists to these receptor sites.

Partial agonist drugs exhibit certain characteristic pharmacological properties:

1. The slope of the dose-response curve for a partial agonist is less than for a full agonist.
2. The dose-response curve exhibits a ceiling effect, giving a plateau-shaped curve with the maximum response being lower than that of a strong agonist (see Fig. 3.10).
3. A partial agonist can partially antagonize the effects of large doses of stronger agonists and reduce the effect of the full ago-

Table 7.2.
Actions of Opioid Agonists and Antagonists at Opioid Receptor Subtypes

	Receptor subtype		
Drug	mu	kappa	sigma
Morphine	Agonist	Agonist	
Pentazocine	Antagonist	Agonist	Agonist
Butorphanol		Agonist	Agonist
Nalbuphine	Antagonist	Partial agonist	Agonist
Buprenorphine	Partial agonist		
N-Allyl-normetazocine	Antagonist		Agonist
Nalorphine	Antagonist	Partial agonist	Agonist
Naloxone	Antagonist	Antagonist	Antagonist
Naltrexone	Antagonist		

nist to the maximum effect of the partial agonist.

ENDOGENOUS OPIOID PEPTIDES

Opioid receptors have been found in the brain, particularly in the limbic system (amygdaloid and septal nuclei), medial thalamic nuclei, the periaqueductal gray area and midline reticular formation of the midbrain, and the periventricular gray areas in the medulla. Within the spinal cord, opioid receptors have been localized in the substantia gelatinosa. It is interesting that opioid receptors are thought to be concentrated in the area postrema which contains the chemoreceptor trigger zone, the site at which opioids are thought to induce nausea and vomiting.

When these opioid receptors were discovered, it was wondered why the brain should possess receptors that were able to respond to exogenous morphine-like substances, and it was suggested that the brain might manufacture its own morphine-like compounds.

The enkephalins were the first endogenous ligands to be isolated and purified from the brain. The two pentapeptides, methionine enkephalin (met-enkephalin) and leucine enkephalin (leu-enkephalin), were identified by Hughes in 1974 and shown to possess opioid-like activity. The peptides *leu*-enkephalin (tyr–gly–gly–phe–*leu*) and *met*-enkephalin (tyr–gly–gly–phe–*met*) are so named because of their terminal amino acid residues. It is thought that the enkephalins are neurotransmitters that mediate integration of sensory information related to pain and emotional behavior. Regional variation in enkephalin levels parallels the distribution of opioid receptors.

The peptide methionine enkephalin is contained within the 91 amino acid beta-lipotropin which was isolated from the pituitary in 1965 by C. H. Li. The amino acid sequence of methionine enkephalin corresponds to residues 61-65 of beta lipotropin. Beta-endorphin, the most potent of the endorphins, corresponds to residues 61-91 of the lipotropin molecule

and accounts for much of the pituitary's opioid activity. Alpha and gamma-endorphins have also been isolated. Dynorphin, a potent opioid peptide commencing with the leu-enkephalin sequence, is also found in the pituitary and is a ligand for the kappa receptor subtype.

Thus, three families of endogenous opioid peptides have been identified: the enkephalins; the endorphins; and the dynorphins. They are derived from precursor polypeptides; proenkephalin (proenkephalin A); pro-opiomelanocortin (POMC); and prodynorphin (proenkephalin B). Pro-opiomelanocortin contains the amino acid sequence for melanocyte-stimulating hormone (MSH), adrenocorticotropin (ACTH), and beta lipotropin. Leu-enkephalin and other opioid peptides result from both proenkephalin and prodynorphin.

Opioid peptides have been detected in the pituitary gland, and this organ is an important location for peptides formed from pro-opiomelanocortin. Although the term endorphin is sometimes used to designate any endogenous substance with morphine-like activity, it is most often applied to the opioid peptides of the pituitary gland.

CHEMICAL STRUCTURE OF THE OPIOID ANALGESICS

Morphine, codeine, and thebaine are all phenanthrene alkaloids of opium. Codeine is methylmorphine, the methyl substitution being on the phenolic OH group. Semisynthetic compounds are obtained by producing small changes in the structure of the naturally occurring alkaloids. Diacetylmorphine (heroin), e.g., is made from morphine by the acetylation of both the phenolic and alcoholic OH groups. Dihydrocodeine, hydromorphine, oxymorphine, and oxycodone are other semisynthetic compounds. Figure 7.2 and Table 7.3 show the chemical structures of morphine and other opioid analgesics, while Table 7.4 shows the dose and duration of action of the important opioid analgesic agents.

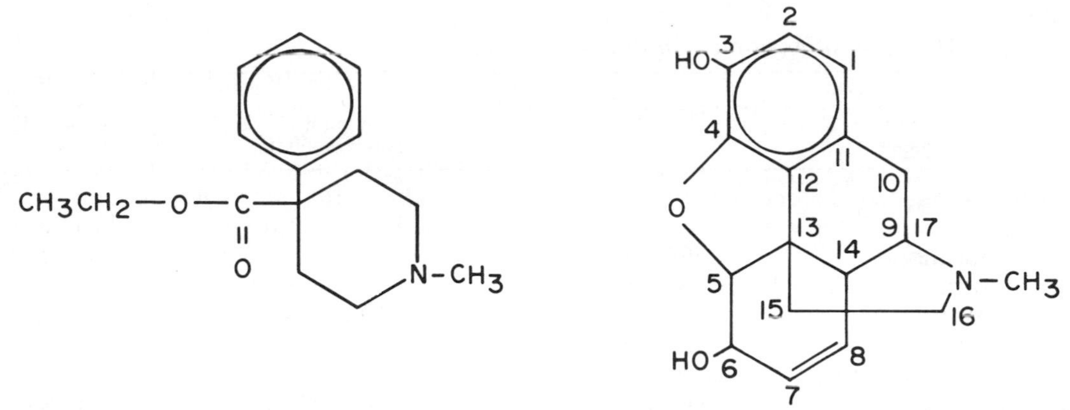

MEPERIDINE   MORPHINE

Figure 7.2. Chemical structure of morphine and meperidine.

Alkaloids of Opium

MORPHINE

Morphine is the standard opioid ago-nist against which all other opioids are compared. The chemical synthesis of morphine is difficult, and therefore the

drug today is still obtained from opium. The chemical structure is given in Figure 7.2.

Central Nervous System. Morphine both depresses and excites the central ner-vous system. In humans, morphine causes depression of the central nervous system leading to analgesia, respiratory

Table 7.3.
Structures of the Opioid Analgesics and Opioid Antagonists

	Substitutions on the morphine molecule*			
Name	3	6	17	Other changes†
Morphine	—OH	—OH	—CH₃	
Heroin	—OCOCH₃	—OCOCH₃	—CH₃	
Hydromorphone	—OH	=O	—CH₃	(1)
Oxymorphone	—OH	=O	—CH₃	(1)(2)
Levorphanol	—OH	—H	—CH₃	(1)
Codeine	—OCH₃	—OH	—CH₃	
Hydrocodone	—OCH₃	=O	—CH₃	(1)
Oxycodone	—OCH₃	=O	—CH₃	(1)(2)
Nalorphine	—OH	—OH	—CH₂CH=CH₂	(1)(2)
Naloxone	—OH	=O	—CH₂CH=CH₂	(1)(2)
Naltrexone	—OH	=O	—CH₂ ◁	(1)(2)
Buprenorphine	—OH	—OCOH₃	—CH₂ ◁	(1)(2)(4)
Butorphanol	—OH	—H	—CH₂ ◇	(2)(3)
Nalbuphine	—OH	—OH	—CH₂ ◇	(1)(2)

From Goodman LS, Gilman AG, Rall TW, Murad F (eds): *The Pharmacological Basis of Therapeutics,* ed. 7. New York, MacMillan, 1985.
*Numbers 3, 6, and 17 refer to positions on the morphine molecule as shown in Figure 1.
†Other changes in the morphine molecule are as follows: (1), single instead of double bond between C7 and C8; (2), OH added to C14; (3), no oxygen between C4 and C5; (4) endoetheno bridge between C6 and C14; 1-hydroxy-1,2,2-trimethylpropyl substitution on C7.

Table 7.4.
Dose and Duration of Action of Opioid Analgesics

Generic name	Trade name	Equipotent dose parenteral (mg)	Duration of action (hr)
Morphine		10	4–5
Heroin		3	3–4
Hydromorphone	Dilaudid	1.5	4–5
Oxymorphone	Numorphan	1.0–1.5	4–5
Codeine*		120 (10–30)	(4–6)
Hydrocodone* (dihydrocodeinone)	Hycodan	(5–10)	(4–8)
Oxycodone	Percodan	10–15	4–5
Methadone	Dolophine	7.5–10	3–5
Meperidine	Demerol	80–100	2–4
Fentanyl	Sublimaze	100 μg	0.5
Sufentanil	Sufenta	15 μg	0.5
Alfentanil	Alfenta	750 μg	0.25
Pentazocine	Talwin	45–60 (25–100)	3
Buprenorphine	Buprenex	0.4	4–6
Butorphanol	Stadol	2–3	4–5
Nalbuphine	Nubain	10	4–5

*Numbers in parentheses, doses and duration of action for oral doses.

depression, depression of the cough reflex, reduced levels of consciousness, and eventual sleep. However, it can also stimulate and excite the central nervous system causing nausea, vomiting, and miosis. The balance between excitation and depression varies according to the species studied. In cats and pigs, e.g., excitation predominates and may result in increased motor activity and hyperthermia. However, in humans, the excitatory effects are much less obvious.

The most clinically important use of morphine is as an opioid analgesic. When small to moderate amounts of morphine (5 to 10 mg, intramuscularly) are administered to patients in pain, analgesia usually occurs without loss of consciousness, although with the relief of tension and anxiety, drowsiness may result. The analgesia obtained with this drug is said to be due to several mechanisms, including an altered perception and response to the pain stimulus, the euphoria and sleep that occur, and an elevation in pain threshold. However, clinical investigations determining pain thresholds during morphine administration are extremely

difficult to conduct and have shown variable results. Mood changes, such as euphoria and a general feeling of well-being, also contribute to the reduction of pain. In normal subjects under stressful conditions and in patients suffering from discomfort and pain, morphine definitely produces a feeling of well-being which may change the patient's attitude toward his pain. When morphine is given to pain-free subjects, however, they may show the opposite effect and exhibit dysphoria, as well as increased fear and anxiety. Mental clouding, drowsiness, lethargy, an inability to concentrate, and sleep may all occur. Morphine produces changes in the electroencephalogram, namely, a shift toward increased voltage and a lowered frequency of wave patterns.

The two most important excitatory effects of morphine seen in humans are those of nausea, vomiting and the production of miosis. The miotic effects of morphine are due to the stimulation and facilitation of the nucleus of Edinger and Westphal of the 3rd nerve. Following overdose with morphine, miosis is marked. Asphyxia and severe arterial hypoxemia can, however, produce mydriasis. The nausea and vomiting that is seen with morphine administration is due to stimulation of the chemoreceptor trigger zone. In addition, stimulation of the vestibular nerve may be important, and morphine-induced nausea is said to be more common in the ambulatory patient. High doses may produce convulsions. Excitatory effects are also said to be responsible for the muscular rigidity, especially of the chest wall, encountered by anesthesiologists during the use of high-dose morphine and other opioid (e.g., fentanyl) anesthetic regimens.

Morphine has been associated with raised cerebrospinal fluid pressure, but this is not seen if patient ventilation is controlled and arterial carbon dioxide tension (P_aCO_2) is maintained within normal limits. The elevation in cerebrospinal fluid pressure is, therefore, probably a response to respiratory depression and

an elevation in P_aCO_2. Opioids in the absence of respiratory depression have been shown to decrease cerebral blood flow and reduce intracranial pressure. Morphine should be used with caution in patients with head injury and should be avoided as premedication in neurosurgical patients where elevated intracranial pressure is likely.

Respiratory System. Morphine depresses respiration, principally by reducing the sensitivity of the brainstem respiratory centers to P_aCO_2. Initially, respiratory rate is affected more than tidal volume, but as the dose of morphine is increased, periodic breathing and apnea occur. The normal clinical dosage of 10 mg of morphine causes respiratory tidal volume and frequency to be reduced, and the resting P_aCO_2 rises about 3 mm Hg in normal healthy subjects. P_aCO_2/ventilation response curves before and after the administration of large doses of morphine (2 mg/kg) show a displacement to the right

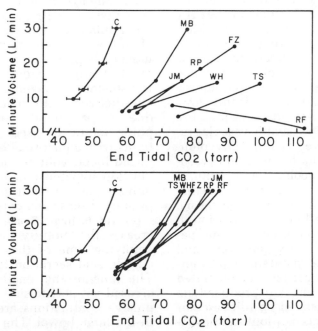

Figure 7.3. Individual ventilation response curves to carbon dioxide before and after morphine, 2 mg/kg. Response curves after morphine are labeled with the subject's *initials,* while *curve C* is the averaged control prior to the administration of morphine. *A* (above), prenaloxone; *B* (below), after antagonism by naloxone. (From Johnstone RE, Jobes DR, Kennell EM, Behar MG, Smith TC: Reversal of morphine anesthesia with naloxone. *Anesthesiology* 41:361–367, 1974.)

and reduction of the slope of the curve which can be partially reversed by the opioid antagonist, naloxone (Fig. 7.3). Although a patient's respiration may be depressed by morphine if he is conscious, the subject will usually breathe on command showing that voluntary control is still maintained. Morphine is dangerous in patients with respiratory insufficiency and should be used cautiously in asthmatic patients. The cough reflex is depressed by a central action. Elderly patients may be more "sensitive" to the ventilatory depressant effects of morphine. Although morphine (10 mg/kg) does not appear to cause greater ventilatory depression in older subjects as assessed by elevation in end-tidal carbon dioxide tension, they have evidence of increased apneic periods, periodic breathing, and paradoxical breathing, and therefore dose should be titrated to effect and older patients given morphine should be carefully monitored.

Cardiovascular System. Clinical doses of morphine produce very little effect on the cardiovascular system in healthy normovolemic supine subjects. Morphine (0.125 mg/kg) during cardiac catheterization has no effect on cardiac index, left ventricular stroke work index, pulmonary arterial pressure, pulmonary vascular resistance, but significantly lowers systolic and diastolic blood pressure due to a decrease in systemic vascular resistance. Therefore, postural hypotension may occur due to peripheral vasodilation, venous pooling, and reduced venous return to the heart. Even at the doses used in cardiovascular anesthesia, there is said to be limited depression of circulatory function provided the patient's ventilation, oxygenation, and blood volume are maintained. Lowenstein and his colleagues demonstrated that morphine (1 mg/kg) produced no significant changes in cardiovascular function in subjects without cardiovascular disease and that there was a slight improvement in function in patients with aortic valvular disease. Morphine may improve myocardial function in patients with elevated left ventricular end diastolic pressures due to dilation of venous capacitance vessels. Studies investigating the response of the peripheral circulation to morphine (0.5 mg/kg and 1.0 mg/kg) have shown that morphine decreases peripheral vascular resistance and increases venous capacitance (Fig. 7.4). In some patients hypotension may occur; this is most commonly attributed to histamine release, since the administration of an H_1- and H_2-receptor antagonist together (diphenhydramine and cimetidine) attenuates the decrease in systemic vascular resistance and cardiac index, although morphine-induced histamine release still occurs and plasma histamine levels are elevated. The failure of naloxone to inhibit morphine-induced histamine release in human skin mast cells suggests that histamine release by narcotics is not dependent on opioid receptor binding or activation.

The direct myocardial effects of morphine are not significant in humans, and there does not seem to be a primary depressant effect. A sinus bradycardia may occur due to central vagal excitation that is abolished by atropine.

Patients anesthetized with large doses of intravenous morphine for cardiopulmonary bypass have increased requirements for intravenous fluids and blood transfusions as compared to patients anesthetized with halothane, probably due to peripheral venodilation. Morphine should be used cautiously in patients with a history of blood loss and reduced blood volume, because they may develop hypotension. In addition, morphine is dangerous in patients with respiratory disease and corpulmonale.

Gastrointestinal Tract. Morphine decreases the motility and increases the emptying time of the stomach. Hydrochloric acid secretion is also decreased. The tone of the small intestine is increased yet peristalsis is decreased. Propulsive contractions are also decreased in the large bowel. The tone in the anal and ileocolic sphincters is increased. Morphine causes spasm of the sphincter of Odi, and marked rises in biliary tract pressure may occur causing severe biliary colic. Delay in the passage of intestinal contents results in the increased ab-

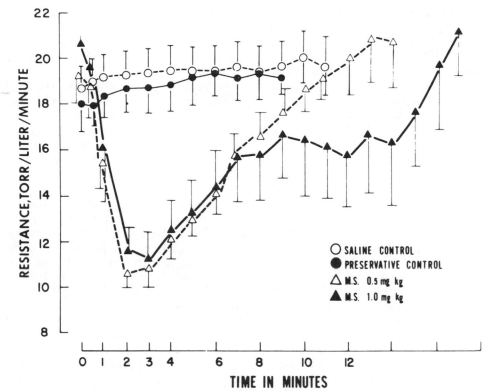

Figure 7.4.   Effect of morphine on peripheral vascular resistance.   Morphine, 0.5 and 1.0 mg/kg, decreased peripheral vascular resistance while the injection of saline solution or the preservatives in morphine solution (*M.S*) did not (*P* < 0.01). *Points,* mean; *bars,* SEM. (From Hsu HD, Hickey RF, Forbes AR: Morphine decreases peripheral vascular resistance and increases capacitance in man. *Anesthesiology* 50:98–102, 1979.)

sorption of water, causing the contents of the bowel to become viscous and desiccated. All these factors contribute to the development of constipation.

Morphine inhibits gastric emptying and therefore will influence the absorption of most if not all orally administered drugs. Morphine also decreases lower esophageal pressure and increases the severity of reflux in patients with preexisting spontaneous reflux. This may make regurgitation and aspiration of gastric contents more likely during anesthesia.

Genitourinary System. Ureteric tone and contractions are increased. The tone of the detrusor muscle of the bladder is augmented by morphine as is the tone of the vesicular sphincter, causing difficulty in urination. In addition, morphine has an antidiuretic effect. Large doses of morphine may prolong labor, but there is lit-

tle experimental evidence to suggest that morphine has a direct depressant action on the myometrium.

Pharmacokinetics of Morphine. After the intravenous administration of morphine (10 mg) to healthy volunteers, morphine distribution is rapid and extensive with a short distribution half-life ($t_{1/2\alpha}$ = 1.65 minutes) and a large volume of distribution (3.2 L/kg). The elimination half-life ($t_{1/2\beta}$) is 177 minutes and clearance is 14.7 ml/min/kg. This relatively short elimination half-life of less than 4 hours is consistent with the duration of analgesic action of between 3 and 4 hours. The high hepatic extraction ratio (0.70) means that morphine undergoes extensive first-pass metabolism (see Chapter 1), and only 30% of an orally administered dose reaches the systemic circulation, causing relatively poor systemic availability after oral administration. The first-pass effect probably explains the poor and unpredictable effectiveness of oral morphine. However, following intramuscular injection, absorption is 90% complete within 45 minutes.

The kinetics of high-dose intravenous morphine in cardiac surgery patients who received a constant rate infusion of morphine (total dose, 1.0 mg/kg by infusion at 5 mg/min) yields values of 0.9 minute for the distribution half-life $(t_{1/2\alpha})$, 137 minutes for the terminal elimination half-life $(t_{1/2\beta})$, 1.02 L/kg for the volume of distribution, and a total clearance of 378 ml/min. Thus, morphine distribution is again rapid, and the elimination half-life is similar to those reported for smaller doses of morphine. The pharmacokinetics of morphine is therefore probably independent of dose (see page 9). Plasma protein binding is about 35%. The pharmocokinetics of morphine during enflurane-nitrous oxide anesthesia has been determined by Murphy and Hug, when the terminal elimination half-life $(t_{1/2\beta})$ was found to be 104 minutes, while the clearance was 23 ml/min/kg. The volume of distribution was 3.4 L/kg. For all the kinetic studies, morphine plasma clearance approaches or exceeds hepatic plasma flow values, suggesting firstly that hepatic blood flow is the rate-limiting step for morphine elimination and sec-

ondly that extrahepatic metabolism also occurs.

Table 7.5 describes the pharmacokinetics of morphine and other important opioid agonists.

Biotransformation and Excretion. The major pathway for the metabolism of morphine is conjugation with glucuronic acid in the liver to yield morphine 3-glucuronide (M3G) and morphine 6-glucuronide (M6G) (Fig. 7.5). Morphine also undergoes demethylation to normorphine, but this is a secondary pathway. The conjugates are mainly excreted in the urine and partially excreted in the bile (7 to 10%). Thus, hepatic biotransformation is the major route of morphine elimination, with less tha 10% of the administered dose of morphine being excreted unchanged (free morphine) in the urine in 24 hours. Larger amounts of conjugated morphine are found in the urine, primarily as morphine 3-glucuronide. Although traces of both free and conjugated morphine are found in the urine up to 48 hours after administration, 90% of the total excretion occurs in the first 24 hours.

Factors Affecting Morphine Pharmacokinetics. Disease states may affect the disposition of morphine. The elimination of morphine is unaffected by moderate to severe *cirrhosis*, in keeping with the lack of impairment of glucuronidation in liver

Table 7.5.
Pharmacokinetics of Opioid Agonists

Drug	Protein binding (% bound)	Distribution elimination half-life (min)	Terminal elimination half-life (hr)	Volume of distribution (L/kg)	Clearance (ml/kg/min)
Morphine	35	1.65	3.0	3.2	15.0
Meperidine	65	4–11	3–8	4.4	7.5–16.0
Fentanyl	79–86	13	3.6	4.0	13.0
Alfentanil	88–92	11.6	1.6	0.86	6.4
Sufentanil	92	17.7	2.7	1.7	13.0
Pentazocine	60		3.3–5.7	4.3–5.6	10.9–17.8
Butorphanol	80	5.0	2.6		High
Buprenorphine	96		3–5.0		12.8–18.0
Nalbuphine	25–40		2.0–3.5	2.9	15.6–22

Some of the values quoted in the literature for volume of distribution and clearance have been adjusted for a 70-kg subject. See bibliography for data sources.

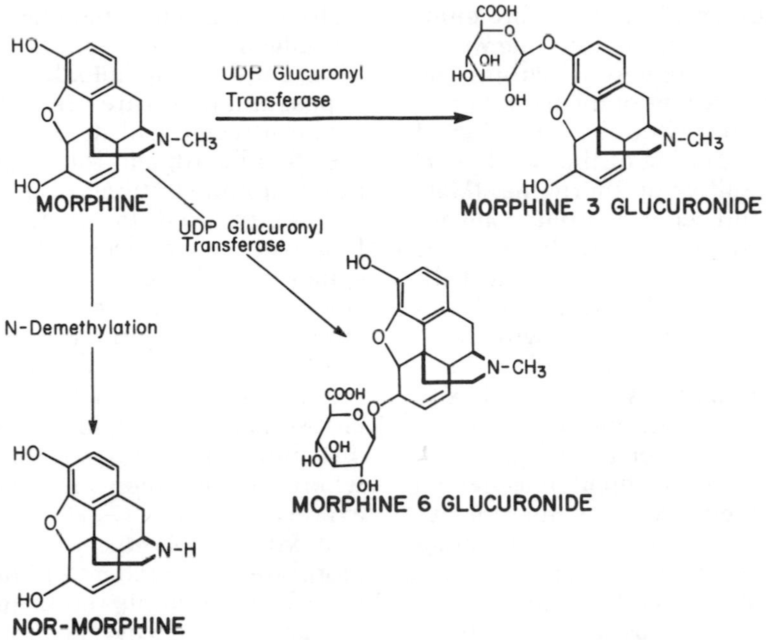

Figure 7.5.   Metabolic pathways for morphine.

disease in contrast to the reduction in oxidation seen in this disease state (see Chapter 1). The elimination of the metabolite morphine 3-glucuronide is also relatively unaffected by cirrhosis. However, in other studies of patients with perhaps more severe liver disease, the elimination half-life has been shown to be longer, accompanied by a reduced clearance, and no change in volume of distribution. Oral bioavailability is increased in cirrhotic patients. Plasma protein binding of morphine is decreased in liver disease, presumably as a consequence of abnormal protein synthesis. Thus, cautious morphine administration is required in patients with hepatic cirrhosis.

Numerous clinical case reports exist describing respiratory depression after morphine administration in chronic renal failure, suggesting that *renal failure* may significantly prolong the effects of morphine in some patients. However, studies describing the kinetics of morphine in patients with renal failure have failed to show important alterations in morphine disposition.

Morphine has been administered to patients with chronic renal failure on hemodialysis when plasma concentrations were found to be higher for the first 15 minutes after administration, resulting in a longer distribution half-life ($t_{1/2\alpha}$ for normal patients = 0.47 minute; $t_{1/2\alpha}$ for renal failure patients = 1.07 minute) and a reduced volume of distribution at steady state (V_{dss} for normal patients = 2.8 L/kg; V_{dss} for renal failure patients = 1.81 L/kg). However, there was no difference in either terminal elimination half-life ($t_{1/2}$ for normal patients = 209 minutes; $t_{1/2}$ for renal failure patients = 190 minutes) or plasma clearance, (Cl for normal patients = 11.5 ml/min/kg; Cl for renal failure patients = 10.3 ml/min/kg). In another study, also showing no change in elimination half-life or clearance, the volume of distribution of the central compartment (V_1 or V_c) was shown to be reduced. The plasma protein binding of morphine is reduced in renal disease. Thus, the higher plasma concentrations and smaller distribution volumes immediately after injection might result in increased effects of morphine in the immediate postinjection period.

The metabolites of morphine are eliminated by the kidney, and thus one would predict that, in chronic renal failure, the plasma concentrations of the parent compound, morphine, would be unaffected but that accumulation of the renally excreted metabolites of morphine (M3G and M6G) would occur. Morphine metabolites are undetectable 12 hours after morphine administration in patients with normal renal function but are still elevated at 36 hours in patients with renal failure. The elimination half-life of M3G is 49.6 hours in patients with uremia and about 4.0 hours in patients with normal renal function. Although morphine 3-glucuronide has been reported as having no pharmacological activity, there is evidence in animals that morphine 6-glucuronide may be more potent than morphine and may account for the greater effect of morphine in patients with renal failure. It is interesting that, in some patients undergoing renal transplantation, morphine elimination is reduced during surgery and is resumed when renal function returns and the transplanted kidney demonstrates the ability to clear creatinine.

Age-related changes in both the pharmacokinetics and pharmacodynamics of morphine are important to anesthesiologists. Morphine kinetics in children are similar to those described for adults. In addition, there does not seem to be any difference between children of different ages in their sensitivity to morphine. However, in infants under 4 weeks of age, the conjugating capacity of the liver is not fully developed, and increased sensitivity to morphine has been described for the newborn infant. Thus, morphine should be avoided or used cautiously in neonates and very young infants. At the other extreme of life, opioid toxicity and reduced dosage requirements have been demonstrated in elderly patients. In the elderly, the volume of distribution both at steady state (V_{dss}) and of the central compartment (V_c) is approximately half that seen in younger patients, resulting in higher initial plasma concentrations in elderly patients. Clearance was also reduced in older subjects.

Pharmacokinetics—Intrathecal and Epidural Administration. Animal experiments have shown that opioid receptors (mu, kappa, and delta) are present in the dorsal horn region (substantia gelatinosa) of the spinal cord, and intrathecal and epidural administration of opioids is now frequently used to produce analgesia. However, pharmacokinetic studies of spinal opioids in humans are difficult since (like local anesthetics) diffusion, absorption, and elimination take place simultaneously. After epidural or intrathecal morphine administration, morphine is absorbed by the epidural veins and redistributed to the systemic circulation, where it is then metabolized and excreted.

Maximum plasma concentrations of morphine are found 5 to 10 minutes after intrathecal administration (0.3 mg) and average about 4.5 ng/ml. Since therapeutic analgetic concentrations in plasma are in the range of 20 to 40 ng/ml, the low plasma concentrations after intrathecal morphine must contribute little to the analgesia produced. In contrast, maximum cerebrospinal fluid (CSF) concentrations are very high (6410 ng/ml), and the CSF elimination half-life for morphine is about 90 minutes. Large interindividual variation in CSF morphine kinetics exists, making prediction of dose and effect difficult. Similarly when morphine is given epidurally (3 mg), it rapidly appears in the plasma, and maximum concentrations of 33 to 40 ng/ml are achieved within 5 minutes. The terminal plasma half-life is about 87 to 91 minutes. Morphine crosses the dura relatively slowly, and maximal CSF concentrations are usually seen 60 to 90 minutes postinjection. About 3.6% of the morphine dose crosses the dura to reach the CSF. CSF morphine concentrations decline biexponentially after the initial rise due to diffusion, with half-life values of 73 to 369 minutes, respectively. Morphine is more hydrophilic than meperidine (see Table 7.6), and this physicochemical property is responsible for the more prolonged duration of action associated with epidural morphine in comparison to meperidine. The more lipo-

Table 7.6.
Physicochemical Properties of Some Important Opioid Agonists

Drug	pKa	% Ionized at pH 7.4	Plasma protein binding (% bound)	Partition coefficient (n-octanol:water)* at pH 7.4
Morphine	7.9	76	35	1.4
Meperidine	8.7	95	65	39
Fentanyl	8.4	91	79–86	860
Alfentanil	6.5	11	88–92	130
Sufentanil	8.0	80	92	1778
Lofentanil	7.8	73	94	1450

*Note that fentanyl and sufentanil are highly lipid soluble and that morphine has lower lipid solubility.

philic meperidine diffuses across the dura more rapidly, resulting in peak CSF drug concentrations 4 times sooner than for the more hydrophilic drug morphine. Similarly, CSF meperidine concentrations decrease 4 times faster than CSF morphine concentrations. Figure 7.6 shows comparative morphine plasma and CSF concentrations following epidural and intrathecal administration.

Pharmacodynamics. Studies describing the relationship between plasma morphine concentrations and effect are limited, but there appears to be a poor correlation between plasma concentration and analgesic effect or respiratory de-

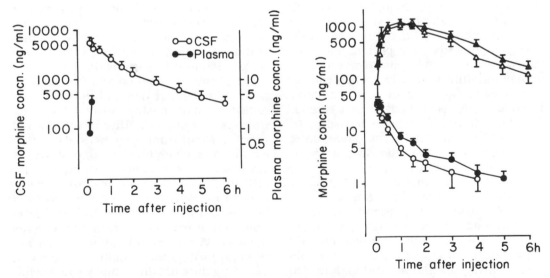

Figure 7.6. Plasma and CSF morphine concentrations after intrathecal and epidural administration. *Left,* mean CSF (O) and plasma (●) concentrations of morphine following an intrathecal bolus of 0.3 mg. *Right,* mean morphine CSF concentrations (△, group I; ▲, group II) and plasma concentrations (O, group I; ●, group II) after epidural administration of morphine, 3 mg in 1 ml (group I) and 10 ml (group II). (From Sjostrom S, Hartvig P, Persson MP, Tamsen A: Pharmacokinetics of epidural morphine and meperidine in humans. *Anesthesiology* 67:877–888, 1987; and Sjostrom S, Tamsen A, Persson MP, Hartvig P: Pharmacokinetics of intrathecal morphine and meperidine in humans. *Anesthesiology* 67:889–895, 1987.)

pression. One reason for this poor correlation might lie in the fact that, since morphine has low lipid solubility and does not readily cross the blood-brain barrier, there is a delay in CSF peak concentrations compared to plasma concentrations and thus a poor correlation between plasma concentrations and analgesic effect. The minimum effective analgesic concentration (MEAC) of morphine in plasma to provide pain relief after major abdominal surgery was 16 ± 9 ng/ml in a group of 10 patients receiving patient-controlled analgetic therapy.

Suggested Dosage and Administration. Morphine is available as morphine sulfate and hydrochloride. In adults, 10 mg/70 kg of body weight is the usual dose, given by subcutaneous or intramuscular injection. The dose should be modified according to the age and disease of the patient. The oral dose is 8 to 20 mg, but as stated previously, oral administration is unreliable and, therefore, the parenteral route is preferred in anesthetic practice. However, oral morphine sulfate slow release tablets (30 mg) are used for the relief of moderate to severe chronic pain for patients who require repeated dosing of opioids over periods of more than a few days. Morphine may be administered intravenously to control severe postoperative pain, cardiac pain, and in certain cases of pulmonary edema. The dose should be titrated according to effect and given slowly, the usual adult dose being 4 to 10 mg. As morphine causes respiratory depression, it is important that the patient's ventilation is carefully monitored during this procedure. Respiratory depression following morphine administration usually occurs about 7 minutes after intravenous administration and up to 30 minutes following intramuscular administration.

Morphine should be avoided in patients with respiratory disease, such as asthma. It should not be given to neurosurgical patients with raised intracranial pressure because it may elevate carbon dioxide tension, thereby increasing cerebral blood flow and resulting in increased intracranial pressure. Morphine and other opioids should be used cau-

tiously in the elderly and in patients who have a reduced blood volume because of the risks of hypotension. Morphine should also be avoided in patients with liver or kidney disease. It should not be administered to neonates except in special circumstances (e.g., congenital cyanotic heart disease) and avoided as routine premedication for children under 1 year of age. The dose of morphine for infants and children is 0.1 to 0.2 mg/kg.

Morphine is today most often used by anesthesiologists for premedication and to manage postoperative pain. With the advent of fentanyl and its analogs, morphine is less frequently used in high doses as part of a "balanced" anesthetic technique. High-dose morphine "anesthesia" usually involves doses as high as 0.5 to 3.0 mg/kg administered intravenously during ventilation with 100% oxygen. Problems associated with high-dose morphine anesthesia include occasional histamine-related reactions (cutaneous flushing, hypotension, bronchoconstriction), increases in perioperative blood and fluid requirements, delayed postoperative respiratory depression, and occasional cardiovascular instability manifest as bradycardia and hypotension or hypertension.

Morphine can also be administered by patient-controlled demand delivery systems to provide postoperative pain relief; there is a wide variability in the dose of morphine consumed by patients, but it averaged 2.6 mg/hour in one study. A loading intravenous dose (0.5 mg) is usually prescribed by the anesthesiologist, and a unit dose (0.5 to 2.0 mg) can then be injected by the patient. Safety limitations are programmed into the various devices. When morphine infusions are used for postoperative pain management, a loading dose of 5 to 15 mg is usually followed by a maintenance infusion of 1 to 3 mg/hour.

Morphine administration via the epidural or intrathecal route is now advocated for the treatment of pain, when it is said to produce a form of highly selective spinal analgesia. The term "selective spinal analgesia" was suggested by Cousins and Mather to denote the delivery of opioids directly to specific receptors in the spinal cord, thus providing relief of pain without interfering with efferent motor activity or obtunding other sensory modalities. The onset of analgesia of epidural morphine (15 to 60 minutes) is longer than that of meperidine (5 to 10 minutes), reflecting its lower lipid solubility. Similarly, the duration of analgesia of epidural morphine exceeds that of the other opioids, varying between 12 and 20 hours. Respiratory depression is a complication that may occur up to 24 hours after intrathecal or epidural morphine administration. Other side effects include nausea, vomiting, pruritus, sedation, and urinary retention.

The respiratory effects of intraspinal opioids correlate with CSF concentrations that spread rostrally to reach the medullary respiratory center. As stated earlier, the lipid-soluble drugs (meperidine, fentanyl) are more rapidly absorbed, whereas opioid agonists with poor lipid solubility (morphine) are absorbed more slowly. Therefore, in general, lipid-soluble agents tend to have more rapid onset and brief duration of action, while poorly lipid-soluble agents have a slow onset and longer duration of effect and are associated with delayed onset of adverse effects, such as respiratory depression. Early ventilatory depression usually reflects systemic absorption of opioid and is more likely to occur with lipid-soluble agents.

Preservative-free morphine sulfate is now available for epidural and intrathecal injection. The epidural adult dosage is an initial injection of 5.0 mg in the lumbar region, which may provide analgesia for up to 24 hours. If adequate pain relief is not obtained within 60 minutes, incremental doses of 1 to 2 mg may be given. No more than 10 mg per 24 hours should be administered.

Intrathecal adult dosage is usually $\frac{1}{10}$ that of the epidural dosage. A single injection of 0.2 to 1.0 mg is usually recommended. Respiratory depression has occurred more frequently following intrathecal administration. Intrathecal and epidural opioid administration is still at an investigational stage, and it is likely that the lipophilic opioids, such as fentanyl and meperidine, may have advantages over morphine.

Pantopon is a mixture of purified opium alkaloids, including morphine. It has no special advantages over morphine. Dosage (intramuscular, subcutaneous) for adults is 5 to 20 mg.

CODEINE

Although codeine is one of the alkaloids found in opium and is subject to drug control, it is classified as a simple or mild analgesic. Codeine is commonly used in low doses as an oral analgesic. It has antitussive and constipating properties. Codeine is approximately two-thirds as effective when given orally compared to parenterally. It is metabolized by the liver and excreted in the urine, chiefly in the inactive form. Ten percent of the administered dose is demethylated to form morphine, and consequently the urine may contain free and conjugated forms of codeine, norcodeine, and morphine.

Suggested Dosage and Administration. Codeine phosphate (and sulfate) is available as tablets of 15, 30, and 60 mg and for injection as a solution of 30 mg/ml. Codeine may be given by mouth in a dose of 10 to 60 mg. It is used as a simple analgesic, to suppress the cough reflex (antitussive), and in the treatment of diarrhea.

SEMISYNTHETIC OPIOIDS

This group of drugs comprises all of those which are made by simple modification of the morphine molecule and includes heroin, oxymorphone, oxycodone, and hydromorphine.

HEROIN (DIAMORPHINE, DIACETYLMORPHINE)

Diacetylmorphine has very similar pharmacological properties to morphine. It is a strong analgesic and will produce respiratory depression. However, there is said to be a slightly lower incidence of nausea and vomiting after the administration of heroin. It causes drug addiction, and its manufacture and medicinal use are illegal in the United States, but not in some other countries. Heroin is rapidly hydrolyzed to monoaceytlmorphine, which is then hydrolyzed to morphine.

HYDROMORPHONE

Hydromorphone is a semisynthetic modification of morphine that is pharmacologically similar to morphine. Two mg of hydromorphone are equivalent to 10 mg of morphine. It is effective when administered orally but is still more effective when given parenterally.

OXYCODONE

Oxycodone is a semisynthetic narcotic analgesic with pharmacological actions similar to those of morphine. It is administered orally for the relief of moderate to moderately severe pain.

OXYMORPHONE

Oxymorphone is also a semisynthetic derivative of morphine that has similar pharmacological effects to morphine.

SYNTHETIC OPIOIDS

The analgesics in this group do not necessarily have the same chemical structure as morphine, but do have similar pharmacological activity.

MEPERIDINE

Meperidine is a synthetic analgesic drug whose structure is given in Figure 7.2. It is a piperidine derivative and was first described by Eisleb and Schaumann (1939) as being a compound derived from a series of potential atropine-like spasmolytic compounds, but having morphine-like analgesic activity. Meperidine is approximately one-tenth as potent an analgesic as morphine. The clinical actions of meperidine on the major organ systems are similar to morphine. There are two main uses of meperidine: (*a*) as a premedicant drug prior to anesthesia; and (*b*) as an analgesic in the treatment of acute or chronic pain.

Central Nervous System. Meperidine is a central nervous system depressant producing analgesia, sedation, euphoria, and respiratory depression. Meperidine abolishes the corneal reflex. It stimulates the chemoreceptor trigger zone and thus causes nausea and vomiting. Meperidine is a strong analgesic, producing relief of pain within 10 minutes of intramuscular injection, but after parenteral injection, the duration of action (2 to 4 hours) is shorter than that of morphine. More frequent administration is thus required with the use of meperidine than morphine. Quantitatively, 80 to 100 mg of meperidine intramuscularly are equianalgesic to approximately 10 mg of morphine intramuscularly.

Respiratory System. Meperidine produces as much respiratory depression as morphine when given in equivalent analgesic doses, but tends to affect respiratory rate less, having a greater effect on tidal volume. The respiratory depression can be antagonized by naloxone.

Cardiovascular System. Meperidine, when administered in analgesic doses, has no significant effect on the cardiovascular system. Intravenous meperidine causes a small increase in peripheral blood flow and a decrease in peripheral arterial and venous resistance that may lower blood pressure in some instances. In contrast to fentanyl, meperidine in high doses causes serious cardiovascular depression; meperidine is 20 times more likely to depress myocardial contractility in the isolated cat papillary muscle than morphine. Meperidine causes a tachycardia, rarely a bradycardia. Meperidine is therefore not a suitable opioid agonist for use in high doses as part of an anesthetic technique in patients with cardiovascular disease.

Smooth Muscle. Meperidine causes less smooth muscle spasm and rise in intrabiliary pressure than morphine and is the analgesic of choice in the treatment of biliary or renal colic. Like morphine, gastric motility is decreased, and the gastric emptying time of the stomach is increased after meperidine administration.

The kinetics of acetaminophen following oral administration has been used to study the rate of gastric emptying in women during labor, who required analgesics such as meperidine. Gastric emptying was shown to be normal in patients who had not received narcotic analgesics, but markedly delayed in women given meperidine or pentazocine. The inhibitory effect of meperidine on gastric emptying was not reversed by metoclopramide. Delayed gastric emptying is of concern to the anesthesiologist who may have to administer an emergency general anesthetic, and the fact that gastric emptying is almost totally inhibited by the administration of opioid analgesics, such as meperidine, is a serious hazard in obstetric anesthetic practice.

Pharmacokinetics. Studies of plasma concentrations following intramuscular injection (100 mg) have shown considerable variability, especially in surgical patients, and probably reflect differences in physiologic status, such as vasoconstriction, that alter absorption from the intramuscular site. In contrast, the intramuscular (deltoid) injection of meperidine (25 mg) in healthy human volunteers resulted in complete, reproducible, and rapid absorption of the drug. Thus, the site of injection, dose, and type of patient may affect the intramuscular absorption of meperidine.

Following intravenous injection, meperidine elimination is multiphasic with rapid and extensive extravascular distribution which is essentially complete within 30 to 45 minutes and a terminal half-life between 3 and 8 hours. Plasma clearance is relatively high (700 to 1300 ml/min), and only 5% of the administered dose is excreted unchanged in the urine, most of the clearance being extrarenal and presumably hepatic. Meperidine is moderately bound to plasma proteins, the free fraction, i.e., the fraction not bound to plasma proteins being only about 36%.

Oral bioavailability is about 45 to 75% due to presystemic elimination during the drug's passage through the liver, and peak plasma concentrations occur 2 hours after the oral administration of meperidine. With intramuscular injection, absorption is essentially complete with maximum meperidine concentrations occurring within 20 minutes.

Meperidine is metabolized in the liver. It first undergoes N-demethylation to normeperidine, which is then hydrolyzed to normeperidinic acid, which is partly excreted unchanged in the urine and partially conjugated and then excreted. Meperidine is also hydrolyzed to meperidinic acid, which is then partially conjugated. About one-third of the administered dose of meperidine is N-demethylated. Very little meperidine is excreted unchanged in the urine. Normeperidine is only one-half as active as meperidine as an analgesic, but twice as active a convulsant agent as meperidine. Enzyme induction increases the metabolic conversion of meperidine to normeperidine, which may lead to enhanced sedative effects. After intramuscular or intravenous doses of meperidine, approximately 5% of the dose is excreted in the urine as unchanged drug. Urinary excretion of unchanged meperidine is dependent on urine pH and is increased if the urine is acidified. However, this does not significantly affect plasma levels. Normeperidine can be detected in blood, and concentrations as high as 100 ng/ml occur after single doses of meperidine.

Disease and age may affect the pharmacokinetics of meperidine, and the dose should be adjusted according to the clinical condition of the patient. Renal failure may cause the accumulation of active metabolites, and patients with renal failure tend to have higher plasma normeperidine/meperidine ratios. Cirrhosis and acute viral hepatitis cause a decrease in plasma clearance (about 50%) and an increased elimination half-life and bioavailability. Elderly patients have twice as high plasma concentrations when given intramuscular meperidine compared to young subjects, probably due to decreased plasma clearance and altered protein binding. Therefore, it is wise to reduce the dose of meperidine in the elderly. The pharmacokinetics of meperidine in the perioperative period has been extensively studied in surgical patients. Although only one study has examined meperidine elimination during surgery and several days later in the same patients, overall, the data suggest that meperidine clearance is reduced by about 25% in the perioperative period.

When meperidine (30 mg) is administered into the epidural space, maximum

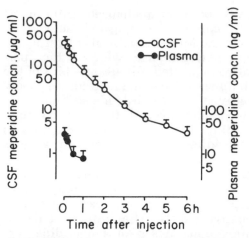 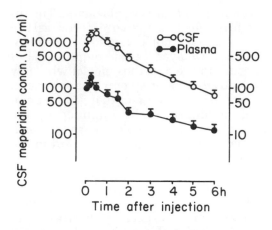

Figure 7.7.   Plasma and CSF meperidine concentrations after intrathecal and epidural administration.   *Left,* mean CSF (O) and plasma (●) concentrations of meperidine following an intrathecal bolus of 10 mg. *Right,* mean meperidine CSF concentrations (O) and plasma concentrations (●) after epidural administration of meperidine (30 mg). (From Sjostrom S, Hartvig P, Persson MP, Tamsen A: Pharmacokinetics of epidural morphine and meperidine in humans. *Anesthesiology* 67:877–888, 1987; and Sjostrom S, Tamsen A, Persson MP, Hartvig P: Pharmacokinetics of intrathecal morphine and meperidine in humans. *Anesthesiology* 67:889–895, 1987.)

plasma concentrations are usually detected 10 or 15 minutes after injection and average about 196 ng/ml, with a terminal plasma elimination half-life of 124 minutes. In contrast to morphine, meperidine crosses the dura relatively quickly, and maximum CSF concentrations are attained 15 to 30 minutes post injection. About 3.7% of the injected dose crosses the dura. The early half-life in CSF for meperidine is about 71 minutes, and the late half-life is 982 minutes. Intrathecal meperidine (10 mg) administration results in low maximum plasma concentrations (36 ng/ml) compared with high maximum CSF concentrations (364 μg/ml). The disappearance of meperidine from the CSF is faster than that of morphine by either intrathecal or epidural administration; this may reduce the risk of cephalad spread and supraspinal adverse effects such as respiratory depression. Figure 7.7 shows the pharmacokinetics of meperidine following intrathecal and epidural administration.

Pharmacodynamics. The relationship between plasma concentrations of meperi-

dine and its effects is illustrated in Figure 7.8. Unfortunately, respiratory depression occurs at plasma concentrations required to produce analgesia, and some depression of ventilation occurs at steady-state plasma concentrations below those associated with moderate analgesia in postoperative patients (0.4 mg/L). As with other opioid agonists, there is considerable interpatient variability in the plasma concentration required for analgesia; however, the minimum effective analgesic concentration (MEAC), i.e., the concentration at which the patient notes a change from some pain to effective analgesia, is 0.46 mg/L, while meperidine concentrations of 0.7 mg/L produce effective analgesia in 95% of patients, Postoperative pain relief may be more logically achieved by a continuous infusion, and a loading dose followed by a maintenance infusion of 0.4 mg/min produces mean steady-state plasma meperidine concentrations of 0.67 mg/L in patients undergoing intraabdominal surgery. This regimen produced constant effective analgesia (Fig. 7.9), in contrast to

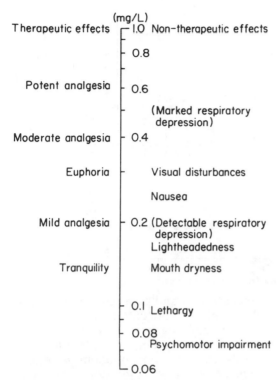

Figure 7.8. Correlation between meperidine concentrations (mg/L) with pharmacologic effect (therapeutic and nontherapeutic). (From Mather LE, Meffin PF: Clinical pharmacokinetics of pethidine. *Clin Pharmacokinet* 3:352–369, 1978.)

the episodic pain control produced by intramuscular injection (Fig. 7.10).

Pregnancy and the Neonate. Meperidine is commonly used for pain control during labor and crosses the placenta where it can cause respiratory depression in the newborn. Umbilical cord/maternal blood concentration ratios vary between 0.8 and 1.0, but this ratio may exceed unity in some individuals. The longer the interval (up to 5 hours) between administration of the meperidine to the mother and the delivery of the baby, the more meperidine and normeperidine are found in the neonate's urine. In addition, the greater the interval between maternal meperidine administration and delivery, the greater the cord/maternal concentration ratio. Thus, neonatal depression is more likely if meperidine is administered to the mother more than 1 hour before delivery than if less than 1 hour elapses before delivery. Therefore, significant amounts of meperidine cross the placenta to reach the fetus over a period of several hours during labor. Although metabolites of meperidine might contribute to neonatal depression, the concentrations of normeperidine in umbilical cord plasma are low, in keeping with its lower lipid solubility, and as discussed previously, normeperidine has only one-third to one-half the analgesic potency of meperidine so that the low concentrations of normeperidine in neonates seem unlikely to contribute to neonatal depression. The time required for neonatal elimination of meperidine is much greater than the adult and is highly dependent on urine flow. Three to 6 days may be required by neonates following maternal administration to eliminate the drug completely. The elimination half-life in the neonate is approximately 24 hours, i.e., approximately 7 times longer than in adults. The use of meperidine during labor and delivery is further discussed in Chapter 12.

Suggested Dosage and Administration. In adults, 75 to 100 mg of meperidine intramuscularly may be required for patients in severe pain, and the dose may need to be repeated every 3 hours. Meperidine infusions of 0.5 to 1.5 mg/kg given over 30 to 60 minutes as a loading dose followed by a maintenance infusion of 0.25 to 0.75 mg/min have been used to treat postoperative pain. The maintenance infusion must be titrated to clinical effect. Meperidine may also be administered by a programmable pump controlled by the patient. Meperidine (0 to 50 mg) is given by the anesthesiologist as a loading dose, and a unit dose of 5 to 20 mg of meperidine is injected by the patient.

Adverse effects produced by meperidine include respiratory depression, hallucinations, nausea, vomiting, drowsiness, and syncope. Meperidine causes constipation less frequently than morphine. The precautions and contraindications are the same as for morphine. Overdose of meperidine causes respira-

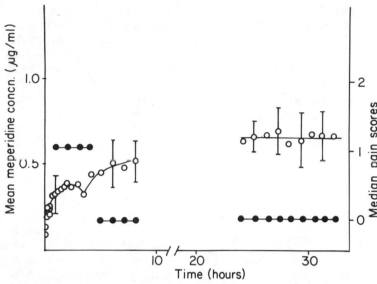

Figure 7.9.   Relationship between meperidine concentration and pain relief with continuous intravenous infusion of meperidine.   Blood meperidine concentrations (○) and median pain scores (●) measured during the two 8-hour sampling periods of the infusion, which was given for 48 hours. Pain was assessed with a scale ranging from 0 to 2 (0 = no pain; 1 = moderate pain; 2 = severe pain). Mean steady-state concentrations were 0.67 μg/ml. Median pain scores were moderate for the first 4 hours of the infusion but fell to 0 (pain free) after a therapeutic blood concentration of 0.46 μg/ml was achieved. (From Stapleton JV, Austin KL, Mather LE: A pharmacokinetic approach to postoperative pain: continuous infusion of pethidine. *Anaesth 7:25–32, 1979.*)

tory depression, cardiovascular collapse, coma, and convulsions. In addition, large doses of meperidine produce muscle tremors, dilated pupils, hyperactive reflexes, and convulsions.

FENTANYL

Fentanyl is a synthetic opioid related to the phenylpiperidines. The structural formula of fentanyl is given in Figure 7.11. Fentanyl is 1000 times more potent than meperidine and 50 to 100 times more potent than morphine. Fentanyl has a rapid onset and a brief duration of action when given in small intravenous doses (Table 7.4).

Central Nervous System. Fentanyl is a central nervous system depressant, producing marked analgesia, respiratory depression, and at high doses, sedation and unconsciousness. Although fentanyl is structurally related to meperidine, it is largely devoid of hypnotic and sedative activity at low doses (1 to 2μg/kg), but at

high doses (50 to 150 μg/kg), sedation and unconsciousness result. However, awareness has been reported in some patients following fentanyl anesthesia (72 and 90 μg/kg), and adjuvant drugs are required to minimize the incidence of awareness. In high doses, fentanyl may cause chest wall rigidity which can make ventilation difficult. Naloxone antagonizes the analgesic and respiratory depressant effects of fentanyl. Fentanyl causes progressive slowing of the electroencephalogram (EEG) in humans characterized by high-voltage, slow delta waves.

Respiratory System. Although fentanyl is much more potent than morphine and meperidine, in equianalgesic doses it produces approximately the same degree of respiratory depression, 200 μg of fentanyl causing a significant reduction of ventilation in the adult. Fentanyl (1 to 2 μg/kg) results in respiratory rate decreases and a compensatory increase in

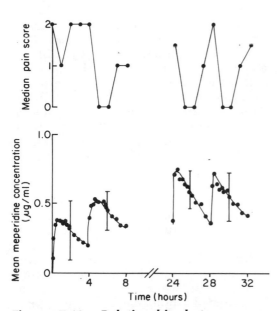

Figure 7.10. Relationship between meperidine concentration and pain relief with intramuscular meperidine. Mean meperidine blood concentrations following intramuscular meperidine at time 0, 4, 20, 24, and 28 hours. The minimum effective analgesic concentration (MEAC) was 0.5 µg/ml, but blood concentrations fluctuated above and below this value, and analgesic concentrations were achieved only 35% of the time. (From Austin KL, Stapleton JV, Mather LE: Multiple intramuscular injections: a source of variability in analgesic response to meperidine. *Pain* 8:47–62, 1980.)

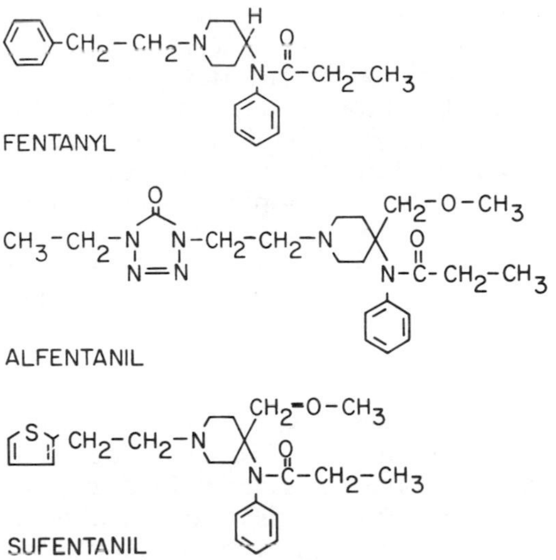

Figure 7.11. Chemical structures of fentanyl, alfentanil, and sufentanil.

Table 7.7.
Relationship between Fentanyl Plasma Concentration and Effect

Plasma fentanyl concentration (ng/ml)	Pharmacological effect
>1	Slight analgesia, minimal ventilatory depression
1–3	Analgesia; 50% decrease in the ventilatory response to carbon dioxide
4–10	Analgesia for surgery if combined with nitrous oxide
>20	Unconsciousness; satisfactory anesthesia if used as sole agent

tidal volume. However, at larger doses (>3 µg/kg) of fentanyl, both respiratory rate and tidal volume decrease, accompanied by a moderate decrease in heart rate and blood pressure. The dose-response curve to carbon dioxide is shifted to the right, as it is with morphine (see Fig. 7.3), so that a plasma fentanyl concentration of 3 ng/ml causes a 50% depression of the CO_2 response curve and an elevation of P_aCO_2 (45 to 49 mm Hg). As a plasma concentration of 3 ng/ml is required for complete analgesia in the majority of patients, there is unfortunately little separation between the plasma concentration producing analgesia and ventilatory depression (Table 7.7).

There have been reports of postoperative respiratory depression following the administration of intravenous fentanyl during general anesthesia despite its brief duration of action, even at lower dosage regimens (1 to 2 µg/kg). It has been suggested that this delayed respiratory depression in the postoperative period might be due to secondary increases in plasma fentanyl concentrations (see later in the chapter). However, recurrence of respiratory depression may also be the consequence of too early extubation at the termination of surgery; or the stimulation from oropharyngeal suctioning, awakening, transfer to the recovery room, etc., may have masked residual fentanyl-induced respiratory depression which only becomes manifest once the patient is later "settled" in the recovery room.

Cardiovascular System. Even when fentanyl is administered in large doses, provided ventilation is maintained, cardiovascular stability is good. Although laboratory studies have demonstrated dose-related negative inotropic effects, very high concentrations are required to produce these effects. Concentrations of 5000 ng/ml are needed to cause a 30% depression of myocardial contractility, while high-dose fentanyl anesthesia (75 to 100 μg/kg) produces plasma concentrations of around only 100 ng/ml. There are now many clinical reports attesting to the hemodynamic stability of high-dose fentanyl for both cardiac and noncardiac surgery, and the position of fentanyl in cardiovascular anesthesia is well established. Cardiovascular variables change very little in patients with coronary artery disease and valvular heart disease during fentanyl anesthesia. The addition of diazepam to fentanyl causes significant decreases in stroke volume, cardiac output, and arterial blood pressure as well as increases in central venous pressure (see also page 199), and the combination of a benzodiazepine and opioid agonist should be used with caution in patients with cardiovascular disease. It should also be noted that, in many patients, although high-dose fentanyl anesthesia does not depress the cardiovascular system, it often fails to attenuate the hypertension and tachycardia that may occur due to noxious stimuli during anesthesia and surgery. Thus, in healthy patients with good left ventricular function and coronary artery disease, intraoperative hypertension may fail to respond to supplemental doses of fentanyl

and adjuvant anesthetic agents (such as nitrous oxide, diazepam, low doses of inhalational anesthetics), and vasodilators may be required to modify the hemodynamic response during high-dose fentanyl anesthesia. On the other hand, in patients who are dependent on sympathetic tone for preservation of blood pressure (e.g., cardiac failure), the administration of even small doses of fentanyl (50 to 200 μg) can cause a marked reduction in peripheral vascular resistance and arterial blood pressure; in this situation, fentanyl should be administered slowly and the dose carefully titrated (25-μg increments) to clinical effect.

Profound bradycardia may occur during high-dose fentanyl anesthesia; atropine is usually effective in treating opioid-induced bradycardia, and prior pancuronium administration attenuates not only the bradycardia but also the muscular rigidity associated with fentanyl administration. Thus, in contrast to morphine, fentanyl rarely causes hypotension. Although the etiology of hypotension secondary to morphine administration is multifactorial, histamine release is probably important (see earlier in chapter). Fentanyl rarely causes histamine release (Fig. 7.12) and, unlike morphine, causes minimal peripheral vascular effects.

Endocrine System. The well-recognized hormonal and metabolic responses to surgical trauma include increases in plasma concentrations of catecholamines, cortisol, antidiuretic hormone (ADH), human growth hormone, glucose, lactate, and pyruvate. Severe trauma and major surgery, such as cardiac surgery with cardiopulmonary bypass, are associated with the greatest hormonal changes. High-dose fentanyl anesthesia has been shown to abolish or modify the "stress" response to anesthesia and surgery; fentanyl (50 μg/kg) abolishes the hyperglycemic response and reduces plasma cortisol and growth hormone levels compared with halothane and nitrous oxide anesthesia, while aldosterone, ADH, and renin increases are prevented by fentanyl (60 to 100 μg/kg) anesthesia. Fentanyl (50 to 60 μg/kg) attenuates

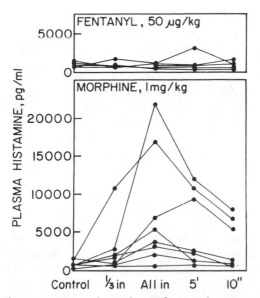

Figure 7.12. Histamine release after morphine and fentanyl administration.
Arterial plasma histamine concentrations in patients exposed to morphine (1 mg/kg) or fentanyl (50 μg/kg). Individual data for plasma histamine concentrations at the following times: control; after administration of ⅓ of total narcotic dose; and 0 (all in), 5, and 10 minutes following drug infusion. (From Rosow CE, Moss J, Philbin DM, Savarese JJ: Histamine release during morphine and fentanyl anesthesia. *Anesthesiology* 56:93–96, 1982.)

plasma catecholamine release during cardiac surgery pre-bypass, although marked increases still occur when cardiopulmonary bypass is commenced. Thus, fentanyl in high doses usually ablates or inhibits the metabolic response to surgical trauma—so-called "stress-free anesthesia."

Pharmacokinetics. When fentanyl was introduced into clinical practice in the 1960s, single intravenous doses of 100 to 200 μg were usually administered which resulted in a short duration of action and rapid recovery. However, it soon became evident in the 1970s that the use of multiple and large doses of fentanyl, administered as part of a narcotic anesthetic regimen, was associated with delayed recovery and prolonged respiratory depression. Since that time, pharmacokinetic

studies describing the disposition of fentanyl have shown that the effect of a single dose of fentanyl is terminated by redistribution, not elimination, in a fashion analogous to that seen with thiopental (see page 182). Thus, the short duration of action of a single dose of fentanyl reflects the rapid tissue uptake and rapid decline in plasma concentration of fentanyl. However, following multiple or large doses of fentanyl as the tissue depots (such as fat and muscle) are filled, drug accumulates and the decline in plasma concentration is slower with a prolongation of effect because the decline now reflects elimination, not distribution.

Since fentanyl is so highly lipid soluble, it is rapidly and extensively distributed to tissues. High concentrations are rapidly achieved in the well-perfused tissues, such as heart, brain, kidney, and lung, while maximum concentrations occur in fat about 30 minutes after injection. Although fat has a very high affinity for fentanyl, it has a limited blood supply so that accumulation of fentanyl by fat requires the sustained plasma concentrations produced by repeated administration or continuous intravenous infusion.

Although there is considerable interstudy variability in the calculated pharmacokinetic parameters for fentanyl, Murphy and Hug reported that, following [³H]fentanyl administration to volunteers, fentanyl concentrations declined rapidly with distribution half-life ($t_{1/2\alpha}$) of 13 minutes. The volume of distribution was large (4.0 L/kg) indicating extensive tissue uptake, while the initial volume of distribution of the central compartment (V_c) was 0.36 L/kg. The terminal elimination half-life was 219 minutes, and plasma clearance for fentanyl equals or approaches hepatic blood flow (13.0 ml/kg/min) (Table 7.5). Fentanyl has a high hepatic extraction ratio, and clearance is primarily dependent on hepatic blood flow. Eighty-five percent of the dose was recovered in urine and feces in 72 hours; less than 8% was recovered as unchanged fentanyl. Fentanyl plasma protein binding is high (Table 7.5). Fentanyl avidly binds to alpha$_1$-acid glycoprotein and is also bound to albumin (see Chapter 1).

Fentanyl is metabolized in the liver to polar inactive metabolites which are then excreted in the bile and urine. It is thought that fentanyl is metabolized by N-dealkylation to norfentanyl and by hydroxylation to hydroxpropionyl fentanyl and hydroxpropionyl norfentanyl.

The delayed-onset respiratory depression that occurs in some patients receiving fentanyl has been attributed to secondary peaks of plasma fentanyl concentration occurring about 45 minutes after apparent recovery from anesthesia. It is postulated that fentanyl undergoes gastric secretion, is sequestered in the acid gastric fluid, and that recycling of fentanyl between gastric juice and the plasma might then be responsible for these secondary peaks. Fentanyl is thus reabsorbed back into the circulation from the more alkaline contents of the small bowel to cause a secondary elevation of plasma fentanyl concentration and consequently a recurrence of depression of ventilation.

Factors Affecting Fentanyl Pharmacokinetics. Most pharmacokinetic studies are carried out in healthy subjects, but fentanyl is most commonly administered to surgical patients, often with concomitant disease states. Thus, following fentanyl (100 μg/kg) given to patients undergoing major abdominal aortic surgery, fentanyl pharmacokinetics was found to be very different from previously determined values in healthy volunteers described in the previous section or in patients having perhaps less major nonvascular surgery. Total drug clearance was 9.8 ml/min/kg compared with the previously reported estimates that range from 12 to 15 ml/min/kg. Volume of distribution at steady state ($V_{d_{ss}}$) was 5.4 L/kg, while the termination elimination half-life ($t_{1/2\beta}$) was markedly prolonged (8.7 hours) compared to other reported values between 1.7 and 4.4 hours. It is interesting that other studies have reported fentanyl elimination half-lives of 5.2 and 7.0 hours in patients undergoing cardiac surgery with cardiopulmonary bypass. Thus, when fentanyl is administered in anes-

thetic practice, when other factors may alter disposition such as fluid shifts, altered hemodynamic status, and hypothermia, it is difficult to predict plasma concentrations from established pharmacokinetic parameters.

Fentanyl elimination may be reduced in elderly patients; an increased elimination half-life (15.8 hours) and decreased fentanyl clearance (4.0 ml/min/kg) have been demonstrated in a small number of elderly patients undergoing intraabdominal surgery. However, other studies have shown similar clearances for young and elderly patients, but a smaller volume of distribution at steady state and higher plasma concentrations immediately following administration. In neonates, fentanyl disposition is highly variable, but the terminal elimination half-life tends to be prolonged and the volume of distribution larger.

Fentanyl disposition is relatively unaffected by cirrhosis. Fentanyl does not exhibit zero-order kinetics in dogs, even for doses as high as 640 μg/kg, and there is no evidence that increasing the dose leads to zero-order kinetics in clinical practice. The route of administration affects the pharmacokinetics of fentanyl. When fentanyl is administered by the transdermal route using a patch, absorption and elimination occur simultaneously, leading to a longer elimination half-life. Patches that deliver fentanyl at rates of 50, 75, and 100 μg/hour produce plasma concentrations of about 1.0, 1.5, and 2.0 ng/ml. It takes at least 8 hours or longer to achieve constant analgesic fentanyl concentrations, and so when the patch is first placed on the skin, an intravenous dose of fentanyl is also administered. The patch is usually left on the skin for 24 hours and provides a depot of fentanyl in the skin that is subsequently absorbed once the patch is removed.

Pharmacodynamics. Table 7.7 shows the relationship between plasma concentration and pharmacological effect. Effective analgesic concentrations are between 1 and 3 ng/ml, while concentrations of 1.5 to 3.0 ng/ml result in a 50% decrease in the ventilatory response to carbon dioxide. Respiratory effects are probably unimportant at plasma fentanyl concentrations below 0.7 ng/ml. It is not possible to correlate plasma fentanyl concentrations with hemodynamic response, but generally "anesthetic" concentrations appear to be in the range of 20 to 30 ng/ml. When combined with nitrous oxide, adequate anesthetic conditions are obtained with plasma concentrations of 5 to 10 ng/ml. Patients become responsive when plasma concentrations drop below 8.0 ng/ml.

Scott and Stanski have used the EEG to measure opioid pharmacodynamic effect in a similar manner to that for thiopental and other anesthetic induction agents (see Fig. 8.7). Although no significant change was found in the pharmacokinetics of fentanyl with age, they were able to show that the decreased dose requirement of fentanyl in the elderly was due to an increase in brain sensitivity. The steady-state fentanyl concentration producing half the EEG effect (IC_{50}, i.e., an index of brain sensitivity to fentanyl) decreased with age (Fig. 7.13).

Suggested Dosage and Administration. Fentanyl may be given as an analgesic during balanced general anesthesia with nitrous oxide and as part of the tech-

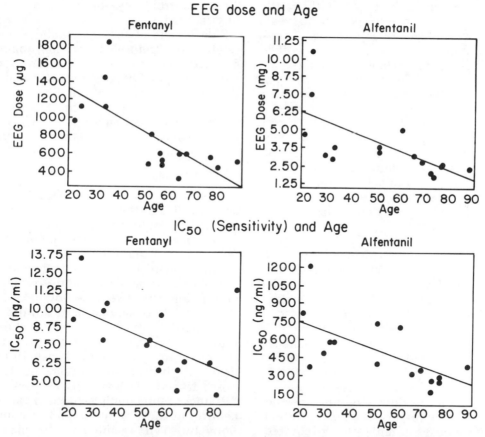

Figure 7.13. Decreased fentanyl and alfentanil dose requirements with age. The decreased dose requirement for fentanyl and alfentanil in the elderly is due to an increase in brain sensitivity. *Top,* EEG dose versus age for fentanyl and alfentanil. The dose administered when delta waves appear in the EEG *(EEG dose)* is plotted against age. Note the decline in IC_{50} (an index of brain sensitivity to fentanyl and alfentanil) with age *(bottom).* (From Scott JC, Stanski DR: Decreased fentanyl and alfentanil dose requirements with age. A simultaneous pharmacokinetic and pharmacodynamic evaluation. *J Pharmacol Exp Ther* 240:159–166, 1987.)

nique of neurolept analgesia when it is often combined with the butyrophenone, droperidol. The combination of a neuroleptic with a potent analgesic produces mental apathy, psychomotor inhibition, and physical immobility. Nitrous oxide is then added to induce and maintain unconsciousness. Droperidol is able to block alpha-adrenergic receptors and thus vasodilatation may occur. The cardiovascular stability that occurs with this technique is extremely useful, and if hypotension does occur, it is usually easily corrected by the administration of appropriate fluids.

Large doses of fentanyl have been employed during major surgery, either with nitrous oxide and oxygen or oxygen alone. Advantages of high doses of fentanyl are said to be "stress-free" anesthesia, cardiovascular stability, and a reduction in the catabolic response to trauma. However, respiratory depression may persist for several hours after anesthesia. Postoperative ventilatory depression can be corrected by naloxone, but this antagonist can cause a rebound effect seen as acute arousal, psychomotor agitation, elevation in plasma catecholamine concentrations, hypertension, and even the precipitation of myocardial ischemia and pulmonary edema.

Fentanyl is available for injection, 50 μg/ml. It is also available combined with droperidol as a fixed 50:1 mixture of droperidol and fentanyl (2.5 mg of droperidol and 50 μg of fentanyl in 1 ml). Fentanyl may be administered as part of a low-dose regimen in small doses for short surgical procedures as part of a "balanced" anesthetic technique, 2 μg/kg or 100 to 200 μg being the usual dose in the adult. The dose may need to be repeated every 30 to 60 minutes during general anesthesia. For major surgery of longer duration, moderate doses of fentanyl are required; 2 to 20 μg/kg and ventilation must be controlled. Postoperative depression of respiration is likely at these dose regimens. High-dose fentanyl anesthesia (with nitrous oxide/oxygen or oxygen alone), e.g., 50 to 150 μg/kg, has been employed for cardiac surgery and long sur-

gical procedures. Maintenance incremental bolus doses ranging from 25 to 100 μg may be required. Postoperative ventilation should be routinely employed when high doses are administered. Fentanyl may be administered by continuous intravenous infusion for the management of postoperative pain, when following a loading dose of fentanyl (approximately 50 to 150 μg) a maintenance infusion of 0.5 to 1.5 μg/kg/hour is given. Transdermal administration of fentanyl using a patch has recently been shown to produce stable postoperative fentanyl concentrations. Disadvantages of this system include a slow onset of action and "less control" by both patient and physician.

Side effects of fentanyl include dose-related respiratory depression, nausea and vomiting due to stimulation of the chemoreceptor trigger zone located in the area postrema in the floor of the fourth ventricle close to the respiratory center, decreased gastrointestinal motility, delayed gastric emptying, and constipation.

ALFENTANIL

Alfentanil is a synthetic potent opioid agonist, structurally related to fentanyl (Fig. 7.11). In humans, alfentanil is between 5 and 10 times less potent than fentanyl on a mg-dose basis. It is a mu-receptor agonist, and its effects such as morphine-like analgesia and ventilatory depression can be reversed by naloxone. It has a rapid onset and brief duration of action. Its duration of action is shorter than fentanyl by about two-thirds. Alfentanil is used by anesthesiologists in high doses to induce anesthesia, in small doses to provide analgesia as part of a "balanced" anesthetic especially for procedures of short duration, and by continuous intravenous infusion for maintenance of anesthesia either as a sole agent or with nitrous oxide. It has also been used by continuous intravenous infusion to provide pain relief after operation.

Alfentanil produces dose-related analgesia, sedation, and unconsciousness. As with other opioids, alfentanil causes muscular rigidity of the chest wall, trunk, and extremities. Nausea and vomiting are also side effects of alfentanil administration. Alfentanil depresses respiration in a dose-dependent fashion; 6.4 μg/kg of alfentanil depress the ventilatory response to carbon dioxide acutely, but no effects are seen 30 to 50 minutes later, indicating the transient nature of ventilatory depression at this dosage. Alfentanil infusion (50 or 100 μg/kg/hour) to supplement nitrous oxide anesthesia, followed by 20 μg/kg/hour to provide postoperative pain relief, produces satisfactory analgesia but depresses the carbon dioxide response curve to 50% of its preoperative value. However, this depression in carbon dioxide responsiveness is accompanied by only moderate changes in minute volume and P_aCO_2. In comparison to fentanyl, recovery of respiratory depression is more rapid. It is important to remember that the administration of even small doses of alfentanil can lead to apnea in some patients, albeit very short-lived, and careful monitoring is essential.

Alfentanil has been found to give good cardiovascular stability when used as an induction agent, and there are few hemodynamic differences between fentanyl (60 to 70 μg/kg) and alfentanil (125 μg/kg) during induction and endotracheal intubation. Very high doses of alfentanil have also been shown to maintain cardiovascular stability comparable to that of fentanyl during cardiac surgery for ischemic and valvular heart disease; a small reduction in heart rate and blood pressure occur. However, in contrast to fentanyl, the cardiovascular effects of high-dose alfentanil (120 μg/kg bolus) are evident for only a short period of time, about 20 minutes, and therefore for long operations, alfentanil must be given by continuous infusion. Indeed, the high incidence of hypertension resulting from stressful surgical stimuli, such as sternotomy associated with high-dose bolus injection, can be reduced by the administration of alfentanil by continuous infusion.

Alfentanil causes significant inhibition of gastric emptying and increases common bile duct pressure, although fentanyl has a longer duration of effect on biliary pressure.

Pharmacokinetics and Dynamics. Table 7.5 gives the comparative pharmacokinetics of alfentanil and fentanyl. The terminal elimination half-life for alfentanil is very short and is only half that of fentanyl (1.6 hours versus 3.1 hours for fentanyl). However, the clearance of alfentanil in only 238 ml/min, while that of fentanyl is much larger (1500 ml/min). Thus, the short elimination half-life of alfentanil is due to its very small volume of distribution. The large fentanyl steady-state distribution volume is a result of its higher lipid solubility and its extensive uptake by muscle and fat, described earlier in the chapter. In contrast, alfentanil with comparatively low lipid solubility does not distribute into these tissues nearly as rapidly. The initial volume of distribution of the central compartment (V_1 or V_c) of alfentanil is therefore much smaller than that of fentanyl, 11 L compared to 60 L for fentanyl. However, as alfentanil is a weak base and therefore 89% of the unbound drug in plasma is unionized (Table 7.6), rapid access to the central nervous system occurs since it is unionized molecules that rapidly cross the blood-brain barrier. Alfentanil is extensively metabolized in the liver by N-deaklylation and O-demethylation, and little parent drug is excreted unchanged.

When equipotent doses of fentanyl (10 μg/kg) and alfentanil (50 μg/kg) are given as a single intravenous bolus injection, the initial plasma concentrations achieved by alfentanil are 100- to 150-fold higher, because of its smaller initial distribution volume (V_1), reflecting reduced peripheral tissue uptake (Fig. 7.14). The alfentanil concentrations then decline more rapidly to levels below the therapeutic threshold relative to fentanyl.

Using spectral analysis of the EEG (see page 189), the effect of fentanyl and alfentanil on the spectral edge (EEG frequency) has been used to measure their

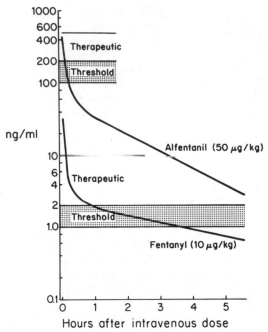

Figure 7.14. Computerized simulation of the plasma concentration decay after intravenous administration of equipotent doses of fentanyl and alfentanil. Note that plasma concentrations compatible with satisfactory spontaneous ventilation will be reached 3 hours and 7.2 hours after discontinuation of alfentanil and fentanyl, respectively. (From Stanski DR, Hug CC: Alfentanil—a kinetically predictable narcotic analgesic. *Anesthesiology* 57:435–438, 1982.)

central nervous system (CNS) effects. For fentanyl, there is a distinct time lag of 3 to 5 minutes between the fentanyl plasma concentration and EEG effect (Fig. 7.15) so that the peak effect on the EEG occurs 3 to 5 minutes after peak plasma fentanyl concentrations are achieved. In contrast, following alfentanil the peak EEG effect is closely associated with peak plasma concentrations, and there is rapid equilibration between alfentanil plasma concentration and the EEG effect. Thus, the half-time of plasma/brain equilibration is 6.4 minutes for fentanyl but only 1.1 minutes for alfentanil. Although alfentanil is less lipid soluble than fentanyl and exhibits somewhat greater plasma protein binding, it is thought that penetration of the blood-brain barrier is rapid because of its low degree of ionization at physiological pH (see Table 7.6). A plasma concentration-potency ratio of 75:1 for fentanyl/alfentanil has been shown using EEG criteria. However, as stated previously, the clinical potency ratio of an intravenous bolus (mg) dose is approximately 7:1.

Marked differences in plasma alfentanil concentrations are required to provide analgesia and ablate reflex responses to different perioperative stimuli; for example, higher plasma con-

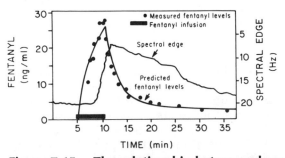

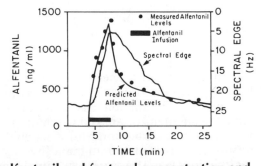

Figure 7.15.   The relationship between plasma alfentanil and fentanyl concentration and EEG (spectral edge) effect.   Fentanyl and alfentanil were infused at rates of 150 μg/min and 1500 μg/min, respectively. Note the distinct delay or lag between the fentanyl plasma concentration and EEG effect, while for alfentanil, spectral edge changes closely parallel serum concentrations. This difference in time lag between concentration and effect may be due to the larger brain-blood coefficient (lipid solubility) of fentanyl. (From Scott JC, Ponganis KV, Stanski DR: EEG quantitation of narcotic effect: the comparative pharmacodynamics of fentanyl and alfentanil. *Anesthesiology* 62:234–241, 1985.)

centrations are required for endotracheal intubation than incision and, as one might expect, lower concentrations are required for skin closure than incision (Fig. 7.16). Similarly, different types of surgery exhibit different plasma concentration requirements, with upper abdominal surgery needing higher plasma concentrations than breast or lower abdominal surgery. Plasma alfentanil concentrations of 200 to 500 ng/ml are required for anesthesia with nitrous oxide, while plasma alfentanil concentrations comparable with recovery of spontaneous ventilation are approximately 100 to 200 ng/ml. Depression of

the carbon dioxide ventilatory response curve by 50% is associated with plasma alfentanil concentrations in the range of 100 to 120 ng/ml; the comparable plasma fentanyl concentration is about 2 to 3 ng/ml, indicating that fentanyl is 40 times more potent in depressing the CO_2 response. The differences in potency ratios for fentanyl and alfentanil based on mg-dose and plasma concentration data are thought to be due to the different pharmacokinetic properties of alfentanil and fentanyl.

It is important to remember that a large interindividual variation in the pharmacokinetics of alfentanil exists, and there

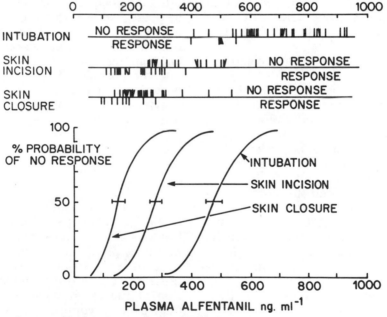

Figure 7.16.   Plasma alfentanil concentrations required to supplement nitrous oxide anesthesia.   Relationship between alfentanil plasma concentrations and their effects for three events—intubation, skin incision, and skin closure. The diagrams in the *upper part* show the alfentanil plasma concentrations of every patient associated with (downward deflection) or without (upward deflection) a response to each of these three stimuli. The plasma concentration-effect curves were then defined for these stimuli. The alfentanil induction dose was 150 mg/kg, followed by an infusion that varied between 25 and 150 μg/kg/hour. $C_{p_{50}}$ (the alfentanil plasma concentration that results in a 50% probability of a response) was 475 $\pm$ 28 ng/ml for tracheal intubation, 279 $\pm$ 20 ng/ml for skin incision, and 150 $\pm$ 23 ng/ml for skin closure. $C_{p_{50}}$ for breast surgery was 270 $\pm$ 63 ng/ml, lower abdominal surgery was 309 $\pm$ 44 ng/ml, and upper abdominal surgery was 412 $\pm$ 135 ng/ml. $C_{p_{50}}$ for spontaneous ventilation was 223 $\pm$ 13 ng/ml. (From Ausems ME, Hug CC, Stanski DR, Burm AGL: Plasma concentrations of alfentanil required to supplement nitrous oxide anesthesia for general surgery. *Anesthesiology* 65:362–373, 1986.)

is a wide range of plasma concentrations that can result from the same alfentanil dose. This is reflected in a 30 to 50% variability for the pharmacokinetic parameters for alfentanil. Thus, as always in anesthetic practice, it is important to titrate the rate of alfentanil infusion to patient response.

Age and disease may modify the pharmacokinetics and pharmacodynamics of alfentanil. In children aged 5 to 10 years, the terminal elimination half-life is shorter than that of adults due to a decreased volume of distribution, while the elderly have an increased elimination half-life and a slightly reduced clearance. The elderly patient exhibits an increased sensitivity to alfentanil, and lower plasma concentrations are required to cause EEG slowing (Fig. 7.13). Thus, the dose of alfentanil should be reduced in the elderly.

In uremic patients, alfentanil clearance is unaltered, but volumes of distribution may change depending on whether a change in protein binding occurs. Thus, although the elimination of alfentanil is unaffected by renal disease, changes in protein binding may affect drug distribution. Patients with cirrhosis have a lower plasma clearance of alfentanil (1.6 ml/min/kg) compared to normal patients (3.1 ml/min/kg) and a prolonged elimination half-life (220 minutes in cirrhosis compared to 90 minutes in noncirrhotic patients). Plasma protein binding is decreased. The delayed elimination kinetics of alfentanil may result in prolongation of alfentanil's effects in liver disease.

Suggested Dosage and Administration. The dose of alfentanil required depends on whether alfentanil is being used as an induction agent, to provide intraoperative analgesia or as the sole anesthetic agent. The pharmacokinetics of alfentanil makes it an attractive agent to administer by continuous intravenous infusion. During the induction period, for surgery of 30-minute duration or less, a loading dose of 8 to 20 μg/kg is given followed by a bolus increment of 3 to 5 μg/kg if required. Alternatively, an infusion of 0.5 to 1.0 μg/kg/min can be given. For sur-

gery lasting 30 to 60 minutes, an initial dose of 20 to 50 μg/kg, followed by increments of 5 to 15 μg/kg, is given. A preintubation dose of 50 μg/kg attenuates the cardiovascular response to endotracheal intubation, while 7 to 14 μg/kg may be needed to suppress the response to stimulation during surgery. For longer operations, a continuous infusion is recommended: a loading dose of 50 to 70 μg/kg followed by 0.5 to 3.0 μg/kg/min titrated to patient response. The average infusion rate is usually in the region of 1 to 1.5 μg/kg/min, when used to supplement nitrous oxide/oxygen anesthesia. For anesthetic induction, the dose may be 150 μg/kg or higher. During anesthesia, the infusion should be at the lowest rate that provides adequate analgesia and should be decreased or terminated 15 to 20 minutes before the end of surgery. In addition, alfentanil infusions at lower rates (0.33 μg/kg/min) have been continued into the postoperative period to provide postoperative analgesia. Infusion rates to provide sedation in the intensive care unit vary from 2.5 μg/kg/min to 0.8 μg/kg/min. The dose of alfentanil should be reduced in elderly and debilitated patients.

SUFENTANIL

Sufentanil is a potent fentanyl derivative (Fig. 7.11) with analgesic potency in humans 5 to 10 times that of fentanyl. It produces predictable opioid effects such as analgesia, sedation, respiratory depression, bradycardia, miosis, stimulation of the chemoreceptor trigger zone (nausea and vomiting), smooth muscle spasm, and truncal rigidity. These effects are reversed by naloxone. Sufentanil produces excellent cardiovascular stability for patients undergoing cardiac surgery; moderate decreases in blood pressure and bradycardia have been reported similar to those for fentanyl. However, the incidence of hypertensive episodes in response to surgical stimulation such as sternotomy may be less for sufentanil. In some patients, hypotension has been reported, especially when sufentanil is used as an anesthetic induction agent, leading to the belief that the vasodilatory effects of sufentanil may be greater than those of fentanyl. Sufentanil attenuates or ablates the endocrine stress response to surgery. Like fentanyl, sufentanil does not cause histamine release. Sufentanil has a rapid onset of action compared to fentanyl and a slightly shorter duration of action.

The pharmacokinetic parameters of sufentanil are given in Table 7.5. The volume of distribution is slightly smaller and the elimination half-life shorter than fentanyl. Both fentanyl and sufentanil have a high hepatic extraction ratio, and plasma clearances are similar. Sufentanil is rapidly and extensively metabolized in the liver by N-dealkylation and O-demethylation. Sufentanil is highly lipid soluble which allows the rapid passage across the blood-brain barrier and production of unconsciousness. Sufentanil is bound extensively to plasma proteins (92.5%) and, like fentanyl and alfentanil, the principal binding protein is alpha$_1$-acid glycoprotein. Sufentanil disposition is unchanged in patients with chronic renal failure, but more interpatient variability is seen, so that the sufentanil dose must be carefully titrated to effect in these patients.

In children undergoing cardiac surgery, sufentanil (15 μg/kg) produces excellent cardiovascular stability. Cardiac surgery, hypothermia, and cardiopulmonary bypass all modify the disposition of sufentanil and, though the data in this situation are limited, children and infants tend to have an increased clearance, while hypothermia markedly prolongs the elimination half-life of sufentanil. Similarly in elderly patients, pharmacokinetic results are also variable but generally, no marked changes have been demonstrated.

Suggested Dosage and Administration. Sufentanil, 1 to 2 μg/kg, produces analgesia when given as part of a nitrous oxide/oxygen muscle-relaxant technique, while doses of 2 to 8 μg/kg may be required for more major surgical procedures. High-dose sufentanil (8 to 30 μg/kg) is administered with oxygen for major surgery, such as cardiovascular surgery, when postoperative ventilation is required. If

sufentanil is used for induction of anesthesia, it should be carefully and slowly titrated to effect since hypotension and bradycardia may occur in some patients. Side effects of sufentanil are similar to those described for fentanyl and alfentanil.

PENTAZOCINE

Phenazocine is an analgesic drug of similar potency to morphine. The N-allyl derivative of phenazocine, pentazocine, has weak opioid antagonist but strong opioid agonist properties, being an agonist at the kappa and sigma opioid receptors and a weak antagonist at the mu receptor. Following its introduction into clinical practice, it became a widely used analgesic, but more recently, its use may have declined with the advent of new agonist-antagonist opioid drugs that have a very low incidence of psychotomimetic side effects. In animal studies, pentazocine was approximately ⅕ to ⅙ as potent an analgesic as nalorphine but only ⅟₅₀ to ⅟₂₀₀ as potent as a narcotic antagonist. It is a benzmorphan derivative, and the chemical formula is shown in Figure 7.17. Pentazocine is a racemic mixture of its D- and L-isomers with the L-isomer completely responsible for its analgesic properties.

When pentazocine was first introduced into clinical practice, it was said to have low abuse potential, but since then it has been realized that this is not so, and the drug is now controlled by narcotic regulations. It is indicated for the relief of moderate to severe pain, and 30 mg of pentazocine are said to be equivalent to 10 mg of morphine or 100 mg of meperidine.

Central Nervous System. Although drowsiness may occur, one does not see the euphoria and sense of well-being that is associated with morphine. Analgesia following intramuscular pentazocine is comparable to that obtained from morphine. The onset of analgesia occurs in under 20 minutes following intramuscular injection and 2 to 3 minutes after intravenous administration. The duration of analgesia is 3 to 4 hours. There is said to be less nausea and vomiting with pen-

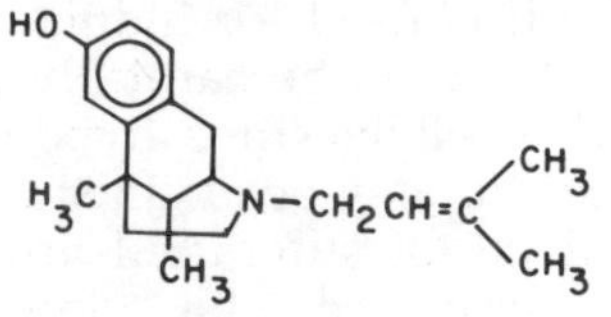

PENTAZOCINE

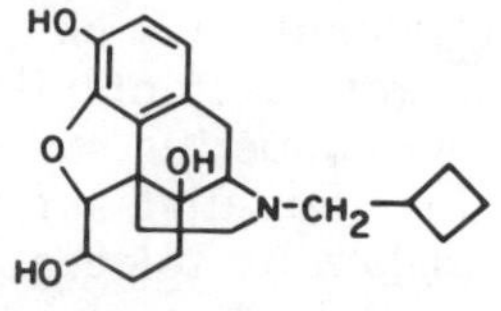

NALBUPHINE

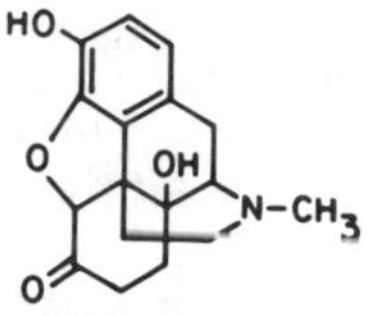

OXYMORPHONE

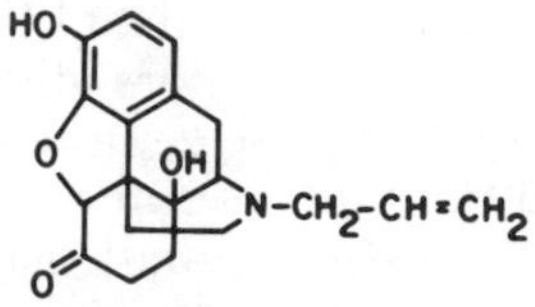

NALOXONE

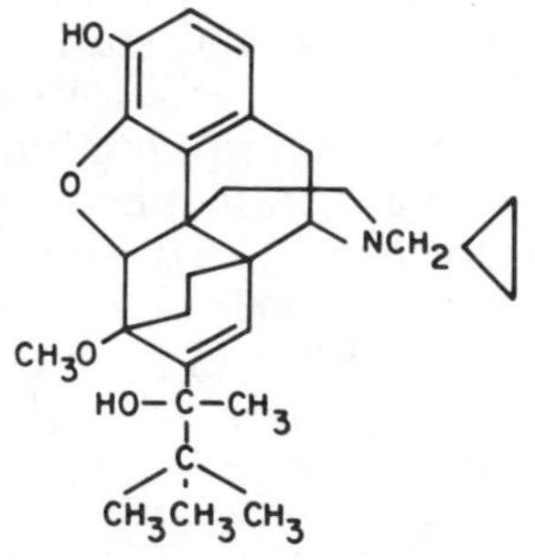

BUPRENORPHINE

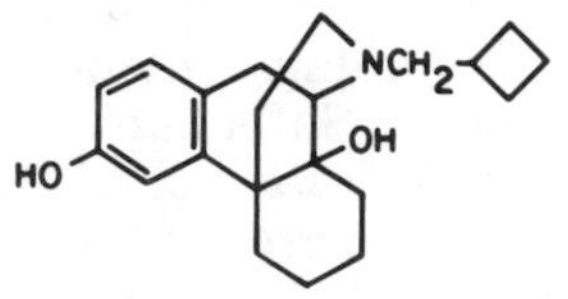

BUTORPHANOL

Figure 7.17. Chemical structures of the opioid agonist-antagonists.

tazocine than with equianalgesic doses of morphine.

Respiratory System. It was originally hoped that pentazocine would be as effective an analgesic as morphine, but with less risk of respiratory depression and addiction. However, pentazocine produces a similar degree of respiratory depression when compared with equianalgesic doses of other opioid drugs. Increasing the dose of pentazocine beyond 30 mg does not usually produce a further proportionate increase in respiratory depression, and the dose-response curve is therefore plateau shaped (Fig. 7.18). Clinical studies have suggested that the respiratory depression induced by pentazocine reaches a ceiling at 60 mg in the adult 70-kg man. However, it is important to monitor the patient for respiratory depression and apnea, which can be reversed by naloxone but not by nalorphine or levallorphan.

Cardiovascular System. Pentazocine differs from morphine in that it does not produce hypotension or bradycardia. A slight rise in blood pressure and heart rate has been observed following its administration, suggesting that pentazocine might increase cardiac workload. In patients with myocardial infarction, pentazocine has been shown to cause a significant increase in pulmonary artery pressure and therefore should be used

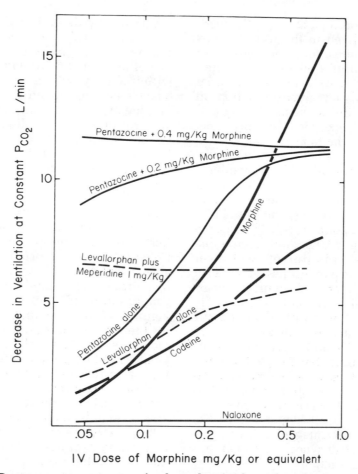

Figure 7.18.   Dose-response curves of selected opioids.   The *abscissa* scale is for morphine sulfate or the equianalgesic multiple of the other opioids assuming codeine is ¹⁄₁₀ as potent as morphine, levallorphan 10 times as potent, and pentazocine ½ as potent. The *ordinate* is change in ventilation at a constant controlled alveolar carbon dioxide tension. Note the ceiling effect with pentazocine compared with the proportionate decrease in ventilation seen with increasing dose of morphine. (From Smith TC: Pharmacology of respiratory depression. *Int Anesthesiol Clin* 9:125–142, 1971.)

with caution in patients with myocardial ischemia and elevated left ventricular end-diastolic pressure. Plasma catecholamines also rise with the administration of pentazocine which may account for its effects on the cardiovascular system.

Gastrointestinal System. As with other opioid drugs, pentazocine causes a delay in gastric emptying and reduction in the propulsive motility of the small intestine.

Pharmacokinetics. Pentazocine may be administered by the oral, intramuscular, or intravenous routes, but there is considerable interindividual variation in blood concentrations. Peak blood levels are reached 15 to 60 minutes following intramuscular administration (45 mg) but not until 1 to 3 hours following oral administration (75 mg). Comparable plasma levels are achieved by 75 mg orally and 40 mg intramuscularly. The plasma elimination half-life of pentazocine is about 2.5 to 3.0 hours after intravenous or intramuscular injection and plasma clearance approximately 1250 ml/min. The peak analgesic effect occurs within 1 hour of intramuscular administration (45 mg) and within 15 minutes after intravenous administration (20 mg.). Pentazocine is metabolized in the liver by oxidation and conjugation, and only 2 to 12% of the administered dose is excreted unchanged. After oxidation of terminal methyl groups and glucuronidation in the liver, both the unchanged drug and metabolites are excreted in the urine. Sixty percent of the total dose appears in the urine within 24 hours of administration. There is considerable intersubject variation in hepatic biotransformation which may account for the individual variation in analgesic response. Oral bioavailability is about 18 to 20%. Plasma protein binding is 60%. Pentazocine disposition is altered in patients with liver disease; cirrhotic patients have increased terminal half-lives and reduced clearance values. Bioavailability is markedly increased in patients with alcoholic cirrhosis, and values as high as 70% have been reported. Table 7.5 gives the pharmacokinetic parameters for pentazocine.

Addiction and Physical Dependence. Although pentazocine does have a low abuse potential, it can cause both psychological and physical dependence. Because it is a weak antagonist, it can provoke a withdrawal syndrome in patients with narcotic addiction.

Suggested Dosage and Administration. Pentazocine is available for injection, 30 mg/ml, and as tablets, 50 mg. Pentazocine (30 to 50 mg) is approximately equianalgesic to 10 mg of morphine when given parenterally. Pentazocine may be administered intramuscularly when the usual adult dose is 30 mg, and 50 mg may be administered orally every 3 to 4 hours. A dose of 50 mg of oral pentazocine results in analgesia equivalent to that produced by 60 mg of codeine.

Side Effects, Toxicity, and Precautions. Similar precautions should be observed as for morphine and meperidine. Pentazocine may cause respiratory depression, sedation, dizziness, and nausea and should be used with caution in the presence of raised intracranial pressure and respiratory and liver disease. Hallucinations or psychotomimetic effects ("active thoughts," dreaming, feelings of impending doom, depersonalization) have been

reported, especially at higher dosages. It may cause dysphoria rather than euphoria. As pentazocine is a narcotic antagonist of low potency, it may provoke mild withdrawal symptoms in patients previously receiving opioid drugs. As stated previously, it also has abuse potential and can produce addiction. Pentazocine crosses the placenta, but to a lesser extent than meperidine, and thus may cause fetal depression.

BUTORPHANOL

Butorphanol is a synthetic agonist-antagonist opioid drug with similar properties to pentazocine. It is about 3.5 to 5 times as potent as morphine, and the analgesia is comparable with that produced by morphine and meperidine. The chemical structure of butorphanol is given in Figure 7.17. Butorphanol has low affinity for the mu receptor (antagonistic effect), moderate affinity for the kappa receptor (analgesic effect), and minimal affinity for the sigma receptor so that the incidence of dysphoric reactions, such as hallucinations, is low. Central nervous system effects include analgesia and sedation.

Respiratory System. Butorphanol causes respiratory depression; however, in common with other agonists-antagonists, the dose-response curve for respiratory depression is plateau like (ceiling effect), and increasing doses do not produce further respiratory-depressant effects. When compared with equianalgesic doses of morphine, butorphanol produces similar rightward displacement of the carbon dioxide dose-response curve, but at higher doses of butorphanol, comparatively less respiratory depression is produced by butorphanol than by morphine. The respiratory depression can be reversed with naloxone.

Cardiovascular System. Systemic arterial pressure is slightly decreased and, like pentazocine, butorphanol markedly increases pulmonary artery pressure during cardiac catheterization, causing increased myocardial work and oxygen demand. Under these circumstances, systemic blood pressure and cardiac output may also rise.

Pharmacokinetics. Pharmacokinetic data

for butorphanol are limited, and Table 7.5 lists tentative pharmacokinetic parameters for the drug. Butorphanol is well absorbed following oral or intramuscular administration. In healthy subjects, the distribution half-life is about 5 minutes, and the terminal elimination half-life is around 160 minutes, with a high plasma clearance. Butorphanol is about 80% bound to plasma proteins. However, oral bioavailability is low (17%) due to extensive first-pass metabolism as might be expected from its high plasma clearance. Butorphanol is metabolized in the liver mainly to hydroxybutorphanol and, also, to norbutorphanol (10%). The major route of elimination in humans is renal (75%) with biliary elimination accounting for about 15% of the dose. Neither of the metabolites appears to have analgesic activity. Butorphanol crosses the placenta, and neonatal serum levels may rise above maternal serum levels.

Suggested Dosage and Administration. Butorphanol is indicated for moderate to severe pain; the onset of analgesia occurs less than 30 minutes after intramuscular injection, and the duration of analgesia is 3 to 4 hours. Butorphanol is available only for parenteral use in solutions containing 1 or 2 mg/ml.

The recommended intramuscular dose is 1 to 2 mg every 3 to 4 hours. The usual intravenous dose for an adult is 0.5 to 2.0 mg. The same precautions should be observed as with the administration of other opioids. Side effects include sedation, hallucinations, increase or decrease in blood pressure, nausea and vomiting, and respiratory depression.

NALBUPHINE

Nalbuphine is an opioid agonist-antagonist structurally related to oxymorphone and the pure narcotic antagonist naloxone (Fig. 7.17). Nalbuphine is primarily a partial agonsit at the kappa receptor, has minimal effects at the sigma receptor, but is a potent antagonist at the mu receptor. It is therefore less likely to produce dysphoric side effects than is pentazocine. Its analgesic potency is comparable to that of morphine.

Central Nervous System. The analgesic effect of 10 mg of nalbuphine is approximately equal to that of 10 mg of morphine. Analgesia begins within 2 to 3 minutes of intravenous injection and within 15 minutes of intramuscular injection. The duration of analgesia is from 3 to 6 hours, which is comparable to morphine.

Respiratory System. At the adult dose of 10 mg/70 kg, nalbuphine causes respiratory depression approximately as frequently as equianalgesic doses of morphine. However, in contrast to morphine, increased doses of nalbuphine do not produce proportional increases in respiratory depression; i.e., the dose-response curve exhibits a plateau or ceiling effect, which is paralleled by its limited analgesic effect to experimental pain with increasing dosage. In anesthetized patients, butorphanol causes greater respiratory depression as assessed by effects on CO_2 ventilation response curves, than nalbuphine. Nalbuphine-induced respiratory depression can be reversed by naloxone.

Cardiovascular System. No significant hemodynamic changes have been observed after nalbuphine administration in patients undergoing cardiac catheterization, cardiac surgery, or after myocardial infarction. In contrast to other agonist-antagonist analgesics, such as pentazocine and butorphanol, increases in pulmonary artery pressure have not been observed.

Pharmacokinetics. Peak concentrations of nalbuphine occur 30 minutes following intramuscular injection, and an elimination half-life of about 2 to 3.5 hours has been reported in healthy subjects (Table 7.5). Extensive first-pass biotransformation occurs, and the oral bioavailability of nalbuphine is about 10%. An inactive glucuronide conjugate is the major metabolite. Fecal excretion from biliary secretion of nalbuphine and its metabolites is the primary route of elimination in laboratory animals. In humans, 7% of a single dose is excreted in the urine as unchanged nalbuphine and metabolites.

Suggested Dosage and Administration. Nalbuphine is indicated for the treatment of moderate to severe pain. The precautions and contraindications are the same for nalbuphine as for any opioid drug, and nalbuphine can cause adverse effects such as sedation, dizziness, nausea, and vomiting.

Psychotomimetic effects such as hallucinations and feelings of depersonalization have occurred, but are said to be less than those seen with pentazocine administration. Cardiovascular stability is good with nalbuphine, and the workload of the heart is not increased. This contrasts with the increased workload of the heart produced by two other agonist-antagonist drugs, butorphanol and pentazocine. Nalbuphine is therefore the preferred opioid agonist-antagonist drug to provide analgesia and sedation in patients with heart disease. Nalbuphine can precipitate withdrawal symptoms in patients who are physically dependent on narcotics, and nalbuphine (15 μg/kg) can antagonize the postoperative depression of ventilation due to large doses of fentanyl administered during cardiac surgery.

Suggested Dosage and Admininstration. Nalbuphine is available only for parenteral use; the usual intramuscular or intravenous adult dose is 10 mg every 3 to 6 hours as required.

BUPRENORPHINE

Buprenorphine belongs to the narcotic agonist-antagonist group of drugs but, in contrast to the other three important compounds in this class, pentazocine, butorphanol, and nalbuphine, which are primarily kappa (and sigma) receptor agonists, buprenorphine is a partial agonist at the mu receptor. Its chemical structure is given in Figure 7.17; it is a highly lipophilic derivative of the opium alkaloid, thebaine.

Central Nervous System. Buprenorphine produces morphine-like effects, such as analgesia, euphoria, sedation, and miosis. Since it is a partial agonist at the mu receptor, it has a significant pharmacological effect when given alone and is additive with small to moderate doses of other opioid agonists, but like other partial agonists, buprenorphine partially reverses the effects of relative large doses of full agonists, such as morphine. Buprenorphine, 0.3 mg, is equivalent to 10

mg of morphine. Following intramuscular injection, the onset of analgesia occurs in about 30 minutes, and the duration of effect is about 8 hours and may persist up to 24 hours. Thus, buprenorphine has a more prolonged duration of action than morphine. Because it is not a sigma receptor agonist, it does not cause dysphoria and hallucinations. Nausea and vomiting are side effects of buprenorphine administration, and the incidence is similar to that seen with meperidine and morphine.

Respiratory System. Buprenorphine causes dose-related respiratory depression and, as with other narcotic agonist-antagonist drugs, a ceiling or plateau effect has been described. There is no completely reliable specific antagonist available to reverse the respiratory depression produced by buprenorphine, since even very high doses of naloxone may only produce partial reversal.

Cardiovascular System. Hemodynamic studies suggest that buprenorphine produces small dose-related reductions in heart rate and blood pressure. The cardiovascular effects appear to be similar to those produced by morphine. Buprenorphine has been given to surgical patients and patients who have undergone myocardial infarction, when a small (5 to 10%) reduction in heart rate and decrease in systolic (10 to 25%) and diastolic (10 to 25%) pressure occurred.

Pharmacokinetics. Pharmacokinetic data for buprenorphine obtained from anesthetized patients and postoperative patients indicate that buprenorphine has a terminal elimination half-life of about 3 to 5 hours and a clearance ranging from 901 to 1275 ml/min. Buprenorphine is metabolized in humans by N-dealkylation and conjugation of N-dealkylbuprenorphine and conjunction of N-dealkylbuprenorphine and the parent drug, but most of the drug is excreted unchanged in the feces.

Buprenorphine dissociates slowly from the mu receptor, and this may be partly responsible for buprenorphine's greater duration of effect than would be predicted from its plasma half-life.

Suggested Dosage and Administration. Buprenorphine can be given intramuscularly or intravenously, and the usual dose of 0.3 mg (equivalent to 10 mg of morphine) can be repeated at 6-hour intervals. Adverse effects include sedation, vomiting, and respiratory depression. As with morphine and other opioid drugs, caution should be exercised in patients with impaired respiratory function. Buprenorphine has also been given by the sublingual route, and 0.4 to 0.8 mg of the drug provide good analgesia in postoperative patients. It has been suggested that the potential for abuse with buprenorphine is less than that of morphine.

OTHER OPIOID AGONIST-ANTAGONIST DRUGS

Meptazinal is an agonist-antagonist opioid that is less potent ($\frac{1}{10}$) than morphine as an analgesic. It has been suggested that, as meptazinol is a selective mu_1 receptor agonist, it would be less likely to cause respiratory depression than other opioids, such as morphine and meperidine. However, early clinical reports suggest that meptazinol (1 mg/kg) does cause some degree of ventilatory depression.

Dezocine is another agonist-antagonist with similar potency to that of morphine. Dezocine causes ventilatory depression, but increasing doses produces a ceiling effect. The incidence of dysphoric effects is low.

Bremazocine is an agonist-antagonist drug that is thought to be a selective kappa agonist. The degree of respiratory depression may be low.

DRUG INTERACTIONS AND THE STRONG ANALGESICS

Monoamine Oxidase Inhibitors (MAOI)

Severe reactions may occur if meperidine is administered to patients receiving drugs of the monoamine oxidase inhibitor group. Excitation, convulsions, hyperpyrexia, respiratory depression, and hypotension may result. Patients may become comatose, and deaths have occurred. The mechanism is unclear, but one suggestion is that the marked degree of potentiation may be due to inhibition of the biotransformation of meperidine

by hepatic microsomal enzymes. A second type of interaction between meperidine and MAOI is characterized by potentiation of meperidine, and thus respiratory depression, hypotension, and depressed consciousness might occur. Interaction with other opioids is uncertain, but it is probably safer to withhold opioid drugs from patients who are receiving monoamine oxidase inhibitors.

MAOIs, their effects on the sympathetic nervous system, and interactions with vasopressors are discussed on page 390, while the clinical pharmacology of MAOIs and anesthesia are discussed in detail in Chapter 21.

MANAGEMENT OF POSTOPERATIVE PAIN

From the preceding sections of this chapter, it is evident that opioids are being administered in new ways to improve the relief of postoperative pain, since traditional intermittent intramuscular administration of a narcotic every 4 hours is ineffective in a large number of patients. Alternative methods include the administration of narcotic agonist-antagonist drugs such as butorphanol and nalbuphine that can be administered in larger doses with a "ceiling effect" on their ventilatory and analgesic effects, regional analgesia using intrathecal or epidural opioids, continuous infusions of narcotic analgesics to maintain constant therapeutic blood levels, and finally the use of devices that allow the patient to control his own narcotic administration in relation to his need for pain relief—patient-controlled analgesia (PCA).

Intrathecal and epidural opioid administration may provide routine postoperative analgesia in the future in some patients. Mather and Cousins have developed the concept of MEAC, the minimum effective analgesic concentration in plasma of drug that the anesthesiologist should attempt to achieve to relieve postoperative pain (Table 7.8). Knowledge of the desired plasma concentration range then allows the calculation of a loading dose followed by a maintenance infusion regimen for the postoperative period.

Table 7.8.
Minimum Effective Analgesic Concentration (MEAC) and Calculated Infusion Regimens for the Management of Postoperative Pain

Drug	MEAC (ng/ml)	Loading dose (mg)* (given over 15–60 min)	Maintenance infusion†
Meperidine	300–650	50–100	25–40 mg/hr
Morphine	10–24	5–15	1–6 mg/hr
Fentanyl	1–3	0.05–0.15	30–100 ng/hr

*Loading dose = MEAC × volume of distribution, since $D = C_p \times V_d$ (see page 5).
†Maintenance infusion = clearance × MEAC, since infusion rate = clearance × steady-state concentration (see page 10).

OPIOID ANTAGONISTS

Drugs in this group include levallorphan, nalorphine, naloxone, and naltrexone, although naloxone is the most widely used drug. Nalorphine and levallorphan have antagonist and agonist actions, while naloxone is a pure antagonist and is devoid of agonist action. Their chemical structures are given in Figure 7.19.

NALORPHINE

Nalorphine (N-allylnormorphine) will antagonize opioid-induced respiratory depression. It is closely related to morphine and has similar but weaker effects. It was hoped that nalorphine would be the first nonaddictive opioid analgesic, but unforunately it was soon realized that it caused marked dysphoria and hallucinations. Nalorphine has been super-

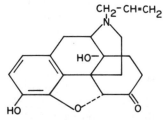

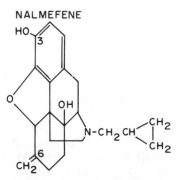

Figure 7.19.   Chemical structures of the opioid antagonists.   Both nalorphine and levallorphan are N-allyl derivatives of narcotics. They are obtained by substituting an allyl ($-CH_2-CH=CH_2$) group for the methyl (CH_3-) on the basic nitrogen of morphine and levorphan, respectively. Naloxone is the N-allyl-substituted analog of the narcotic oxymorphone. It is synthesized by substituting the allyl ($-CH_2-CH=CH_2$) group for a methyl group (CH_3).

seded by the introduction of naloxone and is no longer available in the United States.

NALOXONE

Naloxone, the N-allyl derivative of the narcotic analgesic oxymorphone, is different from the other N-allyl narcotic antagonists in that it possesses almost no agonist activity. Naloxone is a competitive antagonist at mu, delta, kappa, and sigma opioid receptors. Naloxone is more effective in reversing the effects of mu receptor agonists than kappa or sigma agonists and is therefore said to have the highest affinity for the mu receptor. It has gained widespread use in anesthesia for the purpose of reversing opioid-induced respiratory depression and sedation in the postoperative period. If administered in the absence of opioid drugs, it produces almost no clinical effect, very high doses causing only slight drowsiness. Naloxone antagonizes the effects of pure opioid agonists and also those drugs with antagonist-agonist activity, such as pentazocine and butorphanol. A single intravenous dose of naloxone, 0.4 mg, wil antagonize the effects of morphine (respiratory depression, miosis) for only 30 to 45 minutes. Thus, the agonist action of morphine outlasts the antagonist effect of a single dose of naloxone, and either repeated doses or a continuous infusion may be required for effective reversal. New and experimental therapeutic roles for naloxone are evolving; for example, studies in animals suggest that naloxone will attenuate the hypotension associated with septic and hypovolemic shock. However, studies in humans have been disappointing. Naloxone may cause an "overshoot" phenomenon; antagonism of opioid effects by naloxone causes hypertension and tachycardia, and the respiratory rate may become even higher than before opioid administration. There have also been reports of ventricular dysrhythmia, hypertension, and pulmonary edema following an intravenous bolus of naloxone, 0.4 mg. The underlying mechanism is postulated to be due to "nonspecific acute arousal," leading to centrally mediated catecholamine release. Nalox-

one precipitates a withdrawal syndrome in subjects who are dependent on morphine-like opioids that occurs within minutes of naloxone administration.

Serum naloxone concentrations rapidly decline following intravenous administration (0.8 mg) so that 90% of the administered dose has left the plasma by about 5 minutes, with a terminal elimination half-life of about 1.0 to 2.5 hours (Table 7.9). Clearance of naloxone is very high (27 to 35 ml/kg/min) and exceeds hepatic blood flow, suggesting that hepatic metabolism is not the only route of elimination. Naloxone has a high hepatic extraction ratio and undergoes extensive first-pass metabolism, so that the oral dose is about $\frac{1}{50}$ as effective as the same dose given systemically. Naloxone crosses the placenta rapidly to reach the fetus. Naloxone is metabolized in the liver, and the major urinary metabolite is naloxone -3- glucuronide.

Naloxone has a rapid onset but very short duration of action. Its rapid onset of

Table 7.9.
Comparative Pharmacokinetics of the Opioid Antagonists

	Naloxone	Nalmefene
Terminal elimination half-life $t_{1/2\beta}$ (hr)	1.0–2.5	8–9
Clearance (Cl) (ml/min)	2100–2700	1000
Steady-state volume of distribution (V_{dss}, L)	252	480–515

Most of the data from Rawal N, Schott U, Dahlstrom B, Inturrisi CE, Tandon B, Sjostrand U, Wennhager M: Influence of naloxone infusion on analgesia and respiratory depression following epidural morphine. *Anesthesiology* 64:194–210, 1986; Aitkenhead AR, Derbyshire DR, Pinnock CA, Achola K, Smith G: Pharmacokinetics of intravenous naloxone in healthy volunteers. *Anesthesiology* 61:A381, 1984; Ngai SH, Berkowitz BA, Yang JC, Hempstead J, Spector S: Pharmacokinetics of naloxone in rats and in man; basis for its potency and short duration of action. *Anesthesiology* 44:398–401, 1976; Dixon R, Howes J, Gentile J, Hsu HB, Hsiao J, Garg D, Weidler D, Meyer M, Tuttle R: Nalmefene: intravenous safety and kinetics of a new opioid antagonist. *Clin Pharmacol Ther* 39:49–53, 1986.

action may be related to its high lipid solubility. The analgesic and respiratory effects of morphine outlast the duration of effect of naloxone, and thus multiple dosing or a continuous intravenous infusion is required.

Suggested Dosage and Administration. Naloxone is the drug of choice in the treatment of opioid-induced respiratory and cardiovascular depression. It is also used in the treatment of postanesthetic depression caused by large doses of narcotics, especially fentanyl, that have been used to supplement nitrous oxide anesthesia. It is usually given in doses of 0.1 to 0.4 mg intravenously. A large dose may suddenly arouse the patient, and therefore the drug should be administered slowly in small intravenous increments, titrating the dose against the reversal of respiratory depression and the maintenance of analgesia. The duration of action of naloxone is said to be longer when given by intramuscular injection, 20 to 70 μg/kg. Naloxone may also be administered by intravenous infusion. Naloxone infusions of 5 to 10 μg/kg/hour have been administered to prevent respiratory depression following epidural morphine. Naloxone is also used for the neonatal reversal of the depressant effects of meperidine received by the mother during labor. The usual initial dose in neonates is 0.01 mg/kg administered intravenously or intramuscularly. Repeated doses may need to be administered. Naloxone is also very useful in small doses for differentiating between coma and ventilatory depression due to narcotics and other causes.

NALMEFENE

Nalmefene is a pure narcotic antagonist, devoid of agonist effects, that is structurally similar to naloxone and naltrexone (Fig. 7.19). The exocyclic methylene (CH_2) group increases potency at the opioid receptor and is also thought to enhance bioavailability so that the drug may be effective when given by the oral route. It is capable of antagonizing opioid-induced analgesia and respiratory depression for a prolonged period of time. The antagonistic effects of 2 mg of nalmefene are evident for more than 8 hours, while an even lower dose of 0.5 mg produces antagonism lasting 3 to 4 times that of naloxone. Thus, the duration of action of nalmefene is considerably longer than that of naloxone when given to reverse fentanyl-induced ventilatory depression. In addition, a dose-related effect is seen when nalmefene is given in increasing doses of 0.5, 1.0, or 2.0 mg intravenously, while increasing the dose of naloxone above 0.1 mg does not prolong its effect.

The explanation for the different pharmacodynamic profile of nalmefene compared to naloxone lies in the fact that nalmefene has a longer terminal elimination half-life relative to naloxone (Table 7.9). Immediately after intravenous administration, nalmefene undergoes an initial rapid distribution of only a few minutes, followed by a slower distribution phase of about 1.0 hour. Nalmefene has a larger volume of distribution than naloxone, further indicating the extensive distribution of the drug. The long duration of effect reflects its terminal elimination half-life of 8.6 hours; for example, the effect of 1 mg of naloxone in reversing fentanyl-induced respiratory depression is lost by 90 minutes after administration, while the same dose of nalmefene exhibits its antagonistic effects for at least 8.0 hours. Naloxone has a very high clearance which exceeds hepatic blood flow, while nalmefene's clearance is about 1000 ml/min, approximately 70% of hepatic blood flow.

Five percent of the dose is excreted in the urine as unchanged drug; conjugation represents a major route of metabolism.

NALTREXONE

Naltrexone is a long-acting narcotic antagonist that is used in the treatment of narcotic addiction. It is available as tablets (50 mg) and is used in large oral doses to prevent the effects of opioid agonists for periods as long as 24 hours.

BIBLIOGRAPHY

General

Bovill JG: Which potent opioid? Important criteria for selection. *Drugs* 33:520–530, 1987.

Bovill JG, Sebel PS, Stanley TH: Opioid analgesics in anesthesia: with special reference to their use in cardiovascular anesthesia. *Anesthesiology* 66:731–755, 1984.

Bovill JG, Warren PJ, Schuller JL, van Wezel HB, Hoeneveld MH: Comparison of fentanyl, sufentanil, and alfentanil anesthesia in patients undergoing valvular heart surgery. *Anesth Analg* 63:1081–1086, 1984.

Bromage PR: The price of intraspinal narcotic analgesia: basic constraints. *Anesth Analg* 60:461–463, 1981.

Bullingham RES: Optimum management of postoperative pain. *Drugs* 29:376–386, 1985.

Bullingham RES, McQuay HF, Moore RA: Clinical pharmacokinetics of narcotic agonist-antagonist drugs. *Clin Pharmacokinet* 8:332–343, 1983.

Cahalan MK, Lurz FW, Eger EI, Schwartz LA, Beaupre PN, Smith JS: Narcotics decrease heart rate during inhalational anesthesia. *Anesth Analg* 66:166–170, 1987.

Coltart DJ, Malcolm AD: Pharmacological and clinical importance of narcotic antagonists and mixed antagonists—use in cardiology. *Br J Clin Pharmacol* 7:309S–313S, 1979.

Cousins MJ: Comparative pharmacokinetics of spinal opioids in humans: a step toward determination of relative safety. *Anesthesiology* 67:875–876, 1987.

Cousins MJ, Mather LE: Intrathecal and epidural administration of opioids. *Anesthesiology* 61:276–310, 1984.

DeCastro J: Use of narcotic antagonists in anaesthesia. *Br J Clin Pharmacol* 7:319S–321S, 1979.

Duthie DJR, Nimmo WS: Adverse effects of opioid analgesic drugs. *Br J Anesth* 58, 61–77, 1987.

Editorial: Patient-controlled analgesia. *Lancet* 1:289–290, 1980.

Editorial: Epidural opiates. *Lancet* 1:962–963, 1980.

Editorial: Analgesia and the metabolic response to surgery. *Lancet* 1:1018–1019, 1985.

Flacke JW, Bloor BC, Kripke BJ, Flacke WE, Warneck CM, Van Etten AP, Wong DH, Katz RL: Comparison of morphine, meperidine, fentanyl, and sufentanil in balanced anesthesia: a double-blind study. *Anesth Analg* 64:897–910, 1985.

Flacke JW, Flacke WE, Bloor BC, Van Etten AP, Kripke BJ: Histamine release by four narcotics: a double-blind study in humans. *Anesth Analg* 66:723–730, 1987.

Fragen RJ, Caldwell N: Comparison of dezocine (WY 16,225) and meperidine as postoperative analgesics. *Anesth Analg* 57:563–566, 1978.

Freye E, Hartung E, Schenk GK: Bremazocine: an opiate that induces sedation and analgesia without respiratory depression. *Anesth Analg* 62:483–488, 1983.

Gal TJ, DiFazio CA: Ventilatory and analgesic effects of dezocine in humans. *Anesthesiology* 61:716–722, 1984.

Graves DA, Foster TS, Batenhorst RL, Bennett RL, Baumann TJ: Patient-controlled analgesia. *Ann Intern Med* 99:360–366, 1983.

Hermens JM, Ebertz JM, Hanifin JM, Hirshman CA: Comparison of histamine release in human skin mast cells induced by morphine, fentanyl, and oxymorphone. *Anesthesiology* 62:124–129, 1985.

Houde RW: Analgesic effectiveness of the narcotic agonist-antagonists. *Br J Clin Pharmacol* 7:297S–308S, 1979.

Hug CC: Improving analgesic therapy. *Anesthesiology* 53:441–443, 1980.

Kitahata LM, Collins JG: Spinal action of narcotic analgesics. *Anesthesiology* 54:153–163, 1981.

Knill RL, Clement JL, Thompson WR: Epidural morphine causes delayed and prolonged ventilatory depression. *Can Anaesth Soc J* 28:537–543, 1981.

Loan WF, Morrison JD: Strong analgesics: pharmacological and therapeutic aspects. *Drugs* 5:108–143, 1973.

Lowenstein E, Philbin DM: Narcotic "anesthesia" in the eighties. *Anesthesiology* 55:195–197, 1981.

Martin WR: Pharmacology of opioids. *Pharmacol Rev* 35:285–323, 1984.

Meuldermans WEG, Hurkmans RMA, Heykants JJP: Plasma protein binding and distribution of fentanyl, sufentanil, alfentanil, and lofentanil in blood. *Arch Int Pharmacodyn Ther* 257:4–19, 1982.

Nimmo WS, Wilson J, Prescott LF: Narcotic analgesics and delayed gastric emptying during labour. *Lancet* 1:890–893, 1975.

Parry JWL: The evaluation of analgesic drugs. *Anaesthesia* 34:468–475, 1979.

Rance MJ: Animal and molecular pharmacology of mixed agonist-antagonist analgesic drugs. *Br J Clin Pharmacol* 7:281S–286S, 1979.

Rendig SV, Amsterdam EA, Henderson GL, Mason DT: Comparative cardiac contractile actions of six narcotic analgesics: morphine, meperidine, pentazocine, fentanyl, methadone, and l-alpha-acetylmethadol (LAAM). *J Pharmacol Exp Ther* 215:259–263, 1980.

Rothbard RL, Schreiner BF, Yu PN: Hemodynamic and respiratory effects of dezocine, ciramadol, and morphine. *Clin Pharmacol Ther* 38:84–88, 1985.

Rowlingson JC, Moscicki JC, DiFazio CA: Anesthetic potency of dezocine and its interaction with morphine in rats. *Anesth Analg* 62:899–902, 1983.

Scott JC, Ponganis KV, Stanski DR: EEG quantitation of narcotic effect: the comparative pharmacodynamics of fentanyl and alfentanil. *Anesthesiology* 62:234–241, 1985.

Shaw FH, Bentley G: Morphine antagonism. *Nature (Lond.)* 169:4304:712–713, 1952.

Slattery PJ, Boas RA: Newer methods of delivery of opiates for relief of pain. *Drugs* 30:539–551, 1985.

Smith NT, Dec-Silver H, Sanford TJ, Westover CJ, Quinn ML, Klein F, Davis DA: EEGs during high-dose fentanyl-, sufentanil-, or morphine-oxygen anesthesia. *Anesth Analg* 63:386–393, 1984.

Smith TC: Pharmacology of respiratory depression. *Int Anesth Clin* 9:3:125–142, 1971.

Swerdlow BN, Holley FO: Intravenous anaesthetic agents: pharmacokinetic-pharmacodynamic relationships. *Clin Pharmacokinet* 12:79–110, 1987.

Wilkinson DJ, O'Connor SA, Dickson GR, Drake HF: Meptazinol—a cause of respiratory depression in general anesthesia. *Br J Anaesth* 57:1077–1084, 1985.

Yaksh TL, Rudy TA: Analgesia mediated by a direct spinal action of narcotics. *Science (Wash DC)* 192:1357–1358, 1976.

Yaksh TL, Wilson PR, Kaiko RF, Inturrisi CE: Analgesia produced by a spinal action of morphine and effects on parturition in the rat. *Anesthesiology* 51:386–392, 1979.

Opioid Receptors

Martin WR: History and development of mixed opioid agonists, partial agonists, and antagonists. *Br J Clin Pharmacol* 7:273S–279S, 1979.

Pleuvry BJ: An update on opioid receptors. *Br J Anaesth* 55:143S–146S, 1983.

Snyder SH: Opiate receptors in the brain. *N Engl J Med* 296:266–271, 1977.

Stoelting RK: Opiate receptors and endorphins: their role in anesthesiology. *Anesth Analg* 59:874–880, 1980.

Endogenous Opioid Peptides

Beaumont A, Hughes J: Biology of opioid peptides. *Annu Rev Pharmacol Toxicol* 19:245–267, 1979.

Editorial: Searching for the endogenous analgesic. *Lancet* 2:665–666, 1976.

Lord JAH, Waterfield AA, Hughes J, Kosterlitz HW: Endogenous opioid peptides: multiple agonists and receptors. *Nature (Lond)* 267:495–499, 1977.

Stoelting RK: Opiate receptors and endorphins: their role in anesthesiology. *Anesth Analg* 59:874–880, 1980.

Morphine

Aithkenhead AR, Vater M, Achola K, Cooper CMS, Smith G: Pharmacokinetics of a single-dose i.v. morphine in normal volunteers and patients with end-stage renal failure. *Br J Anaesth* 56:813–819, 1984.

Arunasalam K, Davenport HT, Painter S, Jones JG: Ventilatory response to morphine in young and old subjects. *Anaesthesia* 38:529–533, 1983.

Ball M, Moore RA, Fisher A, McQuay HJ, Allen MC, Sear J: Renal failure and the use of morphine in intensive care. *Lancet* 1:784–786, 1985.

Berkowitz BA, Ngai SH, Yang JC, Hempstead J, Spector S: The disposition of morphine in surgical patients. *Clin Pharmacol Ther* 17:629–635, 1975.

Chauvin M, Sandouk P, Scherrmann JM, Farinotti R, Strumza P, Duvaldestin P: Morphine pharmacokinetics in renal failure. *Anesthesiology* 66:327–331, 1987.

Dahlstrom B, Bolme P, Feychting H, Noack G, Paalzow L: Morphine kinetics in children. *Clin Pharmacol Ther* 26:354–365, 1979.

Dahlstrom B, Tamsen A, Paalzow L, Hartvig P: Patient-controlled analgesic therapy. Part IV. Pharmacokinetics and analgesic plasma concentrations of morphine. *Clin Pharmacokinet* 7:266–279, 1982.

Daykin AP, Bowen DJ, Saunders DA, Norman J: Respiratory depression after morphine in the elderly. *Anaesthesia* 41:910–914, 1986.

Drew JH, Dripps RD, Comroe JH: Clinical studies on morphine. II. The effect of morphine upon the circulation of man and upon the circulatory and respiratory responses to tilting. *Anesthesiology* 7:44–61, 1946.

Dundee JW, Clarke RSJ, Loan WB: Comparison of the sedative and toxic effects of morphine and pethidine. *Lancet* 2:1262–1263, 1965.

Hsu HO, Hickey RF, Forbes AR: Morphine decreases peripheral vascular resistance and increases capacitance in man. *Anesthesiology* 50:98–102, 1979.

Jacqz E, Ward S, Johnson R, Schenker S, Gerkens J, Branch RA: Extrahepatic glucuronidation of morphine in the dog. *Drug Metab Dispos* 14:627–631, 1986.

Kafer ER, Brown JT, Scott D, Findlay JWA, Butz R, Teeple E, Ghia JN: Biphasic depression of ventilatory responses to CO_2 following epidural morphine. *Anesthesiology* 58:418–427, 1983.

Laitinen L, Kanto J, Vapaavuori M, Viljanen MK: Morphine concentrations in plasma after intramuscular injection. *Br J Anaesth* 47:1265–1267, 1975.

Lasagne L: The clinical evaluation of morphine and its substitutes as analgesics. *Pharmacol Rev* 16:47–83, 1964.

Mazoit J-X, Sandouk P, Zetlaoui P, Scherrmann J-M: Pharmacokinetics of unchanged morphine in normal and cirrhotic subjects. *Anesth Analg* 66:293–298, 1987.

McDermott RW, Stanley TH: Cardiovascular effects of low concentrations of nitrous oxide during morphine anesthesia. *Anesthesiology* 41:89–91, 1974.

Moore A, Sear J, Baldwin D, Allen M, Hunniset A, Bullingham R, McQuay H: Morphine kinetics during and after renal transplantation. *Clin Pharmacol Ther* 35:641–645, 1984.

Murphy MR, Hug CC: Pharmacokinetics of intravenous morphine in patients anesthetized with enflurane-nitrous oxide. *Anesthesiology* 54:187–192, 1981.

Nishitateno K, Ngai SH, Finck AD, Berkowitz A: Pharmacokinetics of morphine: concentrations in the serum and brain of the dog during hyperventilation. *Anesthesiology* 50:520–523, 1979.

Nordberg G, Hedner T, Mellstrand T, Dahlstrom B: Pharmacokinetic aspects of epidural morphine analgesia. *Anesthesiology* 58:545–551, 1983.

Nordberg G, Hedner T, Mellstrand T, Dahlstrom B: Pharmacokinetic aspects of intrathecal morphine. *Anesthesiology* 60:448–454, 1984.

Owen H, Reekie RM, Clements JA, Watson R, Nimmo WS: Analgesia from morphine and ketamine. *Anaesthesia* 42:1051–1056, 1987.

Owen JA, Sitar DS, Berger L, Brownell L, Duke PC, Mitenko PA: Age-related morphine kinetics. *Clin Pharmacol Ther* 34:364–368, 1983.

Patwardhan RV, Johnson RF, Hoyumpa A, Sheehan JJ, Desmond PV, Wilkinson GR, Branch RA, Schenker S: Normal metabolism of morphine in cirrhosis. *Gastroenterology* 81:1006–1011, 1981.

Philbin DM, Moss J, Akins CW, Rosow CE, Kono K, Schneider RC, VerLee TR, Savarese JJ: The use of H_1 and H_2 histamine antagonists with morphine anesthesia: a double-blind study. *Anesthesiology* 55:292–296, 1981.

Rigg JRA: Ventilatory effects and plasma concentration of morphine in man. *Br J Anaesth* 50:759–765, 1978.

Rosow CE, Moss J, Philbin DM, Savarese JJ: Histamine release during morphine and fentanyl anesthesia. *Anesthesiology* 56:93–96, 1982.

Sjostrom S, Hartvig P, Persson MP, Tamsen A: Pharmacokinetics of epidural morphine and meperidine in humans. *Anesthesiology* 67:877–888, 1987.

Sjostrom S, Tamsen A, Persson MP, Hartvig P: Pharmacokinetics of intrathecal morphine and meperidine in humans. *Anesthesiology* 67:889–895, 1987.

Stanski DR, Greenblatt DJ, Lappas DG, Koch-Weser J, Lowenstein E: Kinetics of high-dose intravenous morphine in cardiac surgery patients. *Clin Pharmacol Ther* 19:752–756, 1976.

Stanski DR, Greenblatt DJ, Lowenstein E: Kinetics of intravenous and intramuscular morphine. *Clin Pharmacol Ther* 24:52–59, 1978.

Vandenberghe H, MacLeod S, Chinyanga H, Endrenyi L, Soldin S: Pharmacokinetics of intravenous morphine in balanced anesthesia: studies in children. *Drug Metab Rev* 14:887–903, 1983.

Way EL, Adler TK: The pharmacological implications of the fate of morphine and its surrogates. *Pharmacol Rev* 12:383–446, 1960.

Way WL, Costley EC, Way EL: Respiratory sensitivity of the newborn infant to meperidine and morphine. *Clin Pharmacol Ther* 6:454–461, 1965.

Wong KC, Martin WE, Hornbein TF, Freund FG, Everett J: The cardiovascular effects of morphine sulfate with oxygen and with nitrous oxide in man. *Anesthesiology* 38:542–549, 1973.

Yaksh TL, Wilson PR, Kaiko RF, Inturrisi CE: Analgesia produced by a spinal action of morphine and effects upon parturition in rat. *Anesthesiology* 51:386–392, 1979.

Yrjola H: Comparison of haemodynamic effects of morphine and fentanyl in patients with coronary artery disease. *Acta Anaesthesiol Scand* 27:117–122, 1983.

Meperidine

Austin KL, Stapleton JV, Mather LE: Relationship between blood meperidine concentrations and analgesic response: a preliminary report. *Anesthesiology* 53:460–466, 1980.

Austin KL, Stapleton JV, Mather LE: Pethidine clearance during continuous intravenous infusions in postoperative patients. *Br J Clin Pharmacol* 1:25–30, 1981.

Edwards DJ, Svensson CK, Visco JP, Lalka D: Clinical pharmacokinetics of pethidine: 1982. *Clin Pharmacokinet* 7:421–433, 1982.

Glynn CJ, Mather LE, Cousins MJ, Graham JR, Wilson PR: Peridural meperidine in humans: analgetic response, pharmacokinetics, and transmission into CSF. *Anesthesiology* 55:520–526, 1981.

Klotz U, McHorse TS, Wilkinson GR, Schenker S: The effect of cirrhosis on the disposition and elimination of meperidine in man. *Clin Pharmacol Ther* 16:667–675, 1974.

Koska AJ, Kramer WG, Romangnoli A, Keats AS, Sabawala PB: Pharmacokinetics of high-dose meperidine in surgical patients. *Anesth Analg* 60:8–11, 1981.

Kuhnert BR, Kuhnert PM, Prochaska AL, Sokol RJ: Meperidine disposition in mother, neonate, and nonpregnant females. *Clin Pharmacol Ther* 27:486–491, 1980.

Mather LE, Lindop MJ, Tucker FT, Pflug AE: Pethidine revisited: plasma concentrations and effects after intramuscular injection. *Br J Anaesth* 47:1269–1275, 1975.

Mather LE, Meffin PJ: Clinical pharmacokinetics of pethidine. *Clin Pharmacokinet* 3:352–368, 1978.

Nimmo WS, Heading RC, Wilson J, Tothill P, Prescott LF: Inhibition of gastric emptying and drug absorption by narcotic analgesics. *Br J Clin Pharmacol* 2:509–513, 1975.

Nimmo WS, Wilson J, Prescott LF: Narcotic analgesics and delayed gastric emptying during labour. *Lancet* 1:890–893, 1975.

Pond SM, Tong T, Benowitz NL, Jacob P, Rigod J: Presystemic metabolism of meperidine to normeperidine in normal and cirrhotic subjects. *Clin Pharmacol Ther* 30:183–188, 1981.

Priano LL, Vatner SF: Generalized cardiovascular and regional hemodynamic effects of meperidine in conscious dogs. *Anesth Analg* 60:649–654, 1981.

Rees HA, Muir AL, MacDonald HR, Lawrie DM, Burton JL, Donald KW: Circulatory effects of pethidine in patients with acute myocardial infarction. *Lancet* 2:863–866, 1967.

Rigg JRA, Ilsley AH, Vedig AE: Relationship of ventilatory depression to steady-state blood pethidine concentrations. *Br J Anaesth* 53:613–620, 1981.

Shnider SM, Moya F: Effects of meperidine on the newborn infant. *Am J Obstet Gynecol* 89:1009–1015, 1964.

Tamsen A, Hartvig P, Fagerlund C, Dahlstrom B: Patient-controlled analgesic therapy. Part I. Pharmacokinetics of pethidine in the pre- and postoperative periods. *Clin Pharmacokinet* 7:149–163, 1982.

Tamsen A, Hartvig P, Fagerlund C, Dahlstrom B: Patient-controlled analgesic therapy. Part II. Individual analgesic demand and analgesic plasma concentrations of pethidine in postoperative pain. *Clin Pharmacokinet* 7:164–175, 1982.

Verbeeck RK, Branch RA, Wilkinson GR: Meperidine disposition in man: influence of urinary pH and route of administration. *Clin Pharmacol Ther* 30:619–628, 1981.

Way WL, Costley EC, Way EL: Respiratory sensitivity of the newborn infant to meperidine and morphine. *Clin Pharmacol Ther* 6:454–461, 1965.

Fentanyl

Arndt JO, Mikat M, Parasher C: Fentanyl's analgesic, respiratory, and cardiovascular actions in relation to dose and plasma concentration in unanesthetized dogs. *Anesthesiology* 61:355–361, 1984.

Bazaral MG, Wagner R, Abi-Nader E, Estafanous FG: Comparison of the effects of 15 and 60 µg/kg fentanyl used for induction of anesthesia in patients with coronary artery disease. *Anesth Analg* 64:312–318, 1985.

Bennett GM, Stanley TH: Cardiovascular effects of fentanyl during enflurane anesthesia in man. *Anesth Analg* 58:179–182, 1979.

Bent JM, Paterson JL, Mashiter K, Hall GM: Effects of high-dose fentanyl anaesthesia on the established metabolic and endocrine response to surgery. *Anaesthesia* 39:19–23, 1984.

Cahalan MK, Lurz FW, Eger EI, Schwartz LA, Beaupre PN, Smith JS: Narcotics decrease heart rate during inhalational anesthesia. *Anesth Analg* 66:166–170, 1987.

Cartwright P, Prys-Roberts C, Gill K, Dye A, Stafford M, Gray A: Ventilatory depression related to plasma fentanyl concentrations during and after anesthesia in humans. *Anesth Analg* 62:966–974, 1983.

Craft JB, Coaldrake LA, Bolan JC, Mondino M, Mazel P, Gilman RM, Shokes LK, Woolf WA: Placental passage and uterine effects of fentanyl. *Anesth Analg* 62:894–898, 1983.

DeLange S, Boscoe MJ, Stanley TH, deBruijin N, Philbin DM, Coggins CH: Antidiuretic and growth hormone responses during coronary artery surgery with sufentanil-oxygen and alfentanil-oxygen anesthesia in man. *Anesth Analg* 61:434–438, 1982.

Duthie DJR, Rowbotham DJ, Wyld R, Henderson PD, Nimmo WS: Plasma fentanyl concentrations during transdermal delivery of fentanyl to surgical patients. *Br J Anaesth* 60:614–618, 1988.

Editorial: High-dose fentanyl. *Lancet* 1:81–82, 1979.

Foldes FF: Neurolept anesthesia for general surgery. *Int Anesth Clin* 11:1–35, 1973.

Goromaru T, Matsuura H, Yoshimura N, Miyawaki T, Sameshima T, Miyao J, Furuta T, Baba S: Identification and quantitative determination of fentanyl metabolites in patients by gas chromatography-mass spectrometry. *Anesthesiology* 61:73–77, 1984.

Haberer JP, Schoeffler P, Couderc E, Duvaldestin P: Fentanyl pharmacokinetics in anaesthetized patients with cirrhosis. *Br J Anaesth* 54:1267–1270, 1982.

Holley FO, Van Steennis C: Postoperative analgesia with fentanyl: pharmacokinetics and pharmacodynamcs of constant-rate i.v. and transdermal delivery. *Br J Anaesth* 60:608–613, 1988.

Hudson RJ, Thomson IR, Cannon JE, Friesen RM, Meatherall RC: Pharmacokinetics of fentanyl in patients undergoing abdominal aortic surgery. *Anesthesiology* 64:334–338, 1986.

Hug CC, Murphy MR: Fentanyl disposition in cerebrospinal fluid and plasma and its relationship to ventilatory depression in dog. *Anesthesiology* 50:342–349, 1979.

Kissin I, Fournier SE, Smith LR, Reves JG: Additive negative inotropic effect of a combination of diazepam and fentanyl. *Anesth Analg* 63:97–100, 1984.

Klingstedt C, Giesecke K, Hamberger B, Jarnberg P-O: High- and low-dose fentanyl anaesthesia: circulatory and plasma catecholamine responses during cholecystectomy. *Br J Anaesth* 59:184–188, 1987.

Koehntop DE, Rodman JH, Brundage DM, Hegland MG, Buckley JJ: Pharmacokinetics of fentanyl in neonates. *Anesth Analg* 65:227–232, 1986.

Lehmann KA, Freier J, Daub D: Fentanyl-Pharmacokinetik und postoperative Atemdepression. *Anaesthesist* 31:111–118, 1982.

Lehtinen A-H, Fyhrquist F, Kivalo I: The effect of fentanyl on arginine vasopressin and cortisol secretion during anesthesia. *Anesth Analg* 63:25–30, 1984.

Mather LE: Clinical pharmacokinetics of fentanyl and its newer derivatives. *Clin Pharmacokinet* 8:422–446, 1983.

McClain DA, Hug CC: Intravenous fentanyl kinetics. *Clin Pharmacol Ther* 28:106–114, 1980.

Meuldermans W, Hurkmans R, Heykants J: Plasma protein bindling and distribution of fentanyl, sufentanil, alfentanil, and lofentanil in blood. *Arch Int Pharmacodyn Ther* 257:4–19, 1982.

Murkin JM, Moldenhauer CC, Hug CC: High-dose fentanyl for rapid induction of anaesthesia in patients with coronary artery disease. *Can Anaesth Soc J* 32:320–325, 1985.

Murphy MR, Olson WA, Hug CC: Pharmacokinetics of ^{3}H-fentanyl in the dog anesthetized with enflurane. *Anesthesiology* 50:13–19, 1979.

Nimmo WS, Todd JG: Fentanyl by constant rate i.v. infusion for postoperative analgesia. *Br J Anaesth* 57:250–254, 1985.

Pathak KS, Brown RH, Nash CL, Cascorbi HF: Continuous opioid infusion for scoliosis fusion surgery. *Anesth Analg* 62:841–845, 1983.

Reilly CS, Wood AJJ, Wood M: Variability of fentanyl pharmacokinetics in man. *Anaesthesia* 40:837–843, 1984.

Rucquoi M, Camu F: Cardiovascular responses to large doses of alfentanil and fentanyl. *Br J Anaesth* 55:223S–230S, 1983.

Scott JC, Stanski DR: Decreased fentanyl and alfentanil dose requirements with age. A simultaneous pharmacokinetic and pharmacodynamic evaluation. *J Pharmacol Exp Ther* 240:159–166, 1987.

Sebel PS, Bovill JG, Schellenkens APM, Hawker CD: Hormonal responses to high-dose fentanyl anaesthesia. *Br J Anaesth* 53:941–948, 1981.

Sebel PS, Bovill JG, Wauquier A, Rog P: Effects of high-dose fentanyl anesthesia on the electroencephalogram. *Anesthesiology* 55:203–211, 1981.

Singleton MA, Rosen JI, Fisher DM: Pharmacokinetics of fentanyl in the elderly. *Br J Anaesth* 60:619–622, 1988.

Sonntag H, Larsen R, Hilfiker O, Kettler D, Brockschnieder B: Myocardial blood flow and oxygen consumption during high-dose fentanyl anesthesia in patients with coronary artery disease. *Anesthesiology* 56:417–422, 1982.

Stoekel H, Hengstmann JH, Schuttler J: Pharmacokinetics of fentanyl as a possible explanation for recurrence of respiratory depression. *Br J Anaesth* 51:741–745, 1979.

Waller JL, Hug CC, Nagle DM, Craver JM: Hemodynamic changes during fentanyl-oxygen anesthesia for aortocoronary bypass operation. *Anesthesiology* 55:212–217, 1981.

Weiskopf RB, Reid IA, Fisher DM, Holmes MA, Rosen JI, Keil LC: Effects of fentanyl on vasopressin secretion in human subjects. *J Pharmacol Exp Ther* 242:970–973, 1987.

White PF: Use of continuous infusion versus intermittent bolus administration of fentanyl or ketamine during outpatient anesthesia. *Anesthesiology* 59:294–300, 1983.

White PF, Dworsky WA, Horai Y, Trevor AJ:

Comparison of continuous infusion fentanyl or ketamine versus thiopental—determining the mean effective serum concentrations for outpatient surgery. *Anesthesiology* 59:564–569, 1983.

Wynands JE, Wong P, Whalley DG, Sprigge JS, Townsend GE, Patel YC: Oxygen-fentanyl anesthesia in patients with poor left ventricular function: hemodynamics and plasma fentanyl concentrations. *Anesth Analg* 62:476–482, 1983.

Alfentanil

Andrews CJH, Sinclair M, Prys-Roberts C, Dye A: Ventilatory effects during and after continuous infusion of fentanyl or alfentanil. *Br J Anaesth* 55:211S–216S, 1983.

Arndt JO, Bednarski B, Parasher C: Alfentanil's analgesic, respiratory, and cardiovascular actions in relation to dose and plasma concentration in unanesthetized dogs. *Anesthesiology* 64:345–352, 1986.

Ausems ME, Hug CC: Plasma concentrations of alfentanil required to supplement nitrous oxide anaesthesia for lower abdominal surgery. *Br J Anaesth* 55:191S–197S, 1983.

Ausems ME, Hug CC, DeLange S: Variable rate infusion of alfentanil as a supplement to nitrous oxide anesthesia for general surgery. *Anesth Analg* 62:982–986, 1983.

Ausems ME, Hug CC, Stanski DR, Burm AGL: Plasma concentrations of alfentanil required to supplement nitrous oxide for general surgery. *Anesthesiology* 65:362–373, 1986.

Ausems ME, Stanski DR, Hug CC: An evaluation of the accuracy of pharmacokinetic data for the computer assisted infusion of alfentanil. *Br J Anaesth* 57:1217–1225, 1985.

Black E, Kay B, Healy TEJ: The analgesic effect of a low dose of alfentanil. *Anaesthesia* 39:546–548, 1984.

Bovill JG, Sebel PS, Blackburn CL, Heykants J: The pharmacokinetics of alfentanil (R39209): a new opioid analgesic. *Anesthesiology* 57:439–443, 1982.

Bower S, Hull JC: Comparative pharmacokinetics of fentanyl and alfentanil. *Br J Anaesth* 54:871–877, 1982.

Camu F, Gepts E, Rucquoi M, Heykants J: Pharmacokinetics of alfentanil in man. *Anesth Analg* 61:657–661, 1982.

Chauvin M, Bonet F, Montembault C, Levron JC, Viars P: The influence of hepatic plasma flow on alfentanil plasma concentration plateaus achieved with an infusion model in humans: measurement of alfentanil hepatic extraction coefficient. *Anesth Analg* 65:999–1003, 1986.

Chauvin M, Lebrault C, Levron JC, Duvaldestin P: Pharmacokinetics of alfentanil in chronic renal failure. *Anesth Analg* 66:53–56, 1987.

Chauvin M, Salbaing J, Perrin D, Levron JC, Viars P: Clinical assessment and plasma pharmacokinetics associated with intramuscular or extradural alfentanil. *Br J Anaesth* 57:886–891, 1985.

Cookson RF, Niemegeers CJE, Bussche GV: The development of alfentanil. *Br J Anaesth* 55:147S–155S, 1983.

DeLange S, deBruijn NP: Alfentanil-oxygen anaesthesia: plasma concentrations and clinical effects during variable-rate continuous infusion for coronary artery surgery. *Br J Anaesth* 55:183S–189S, 1983.

DeLange S, Stanley TH, Boscoe MJ: Alfentanil-oxygen anaesthesia for coronary artery surgery. *Br J Anaesth* 53:1291–1296, 1981.

Ferrier C, Marty J, Bouffard Y, Haberer JP, Levron JC, Duvaldestin P: Alfentanil pharmacokinetics in patients with cirrhosis. *Anesthesiology* 62:480–484, 1985.

Fisher DM: Are the pharmacokinetics of alfentanil really predictable? *Anesthesiology* 59:256–257, 1983.

Fragen RJ, Booij LHDJ, Braak GJJ, Vree TB, Heykants J, Crul JF: Pharmacokinetics of the infusion of alfentanil in man. *Br J Anaesth* 55:1077–1081, 1983.

Grevel J, Whiting B: The relevance of pharmacokinetics to optimal intravenous anesthesia. *Anesthesiology* 66:1–2, 1987.

Helmers H, Peer AV, Woestenborghs R, Noorduin H, Heykants J: Alfentanil kinetics in the elderly. *Clin Pharmacol Ther* 36:239–243, 1984.

Hug CC: Lipid solubility, pharmacokinetics, and the EEG: are you better off today than you were four years ago? *Anesthesiology* 62:221–226, 1985.

Hull CJ: The pharmacokinetics of alfentanil in man. *Br J Anaesth* 55:157S–164S, 1983.

Hynynen MJ, Turunen MT, Korttila KT: Effects of alfentanil on common bile duct pressure. *Anesth Analg* 65:370–372, 1986.

Kay B: Alfentanil. *Br J Anaesth* 54:1011–1013, 1982.

Kay B, Pleuvry B: Human volunteer studies of alfentanil (R39209), a new short-acting narcotic analgesic. *Anaesthesia* 35:952–956, 1980.

Maitre PO, Vozeh S, Heykants J, Thomson DA, Stanski DR: Population pharmacokinetics of alfentanil: the average dose-plasma concentration relationship and interindividual variability in patients. *Anesthesiology* 66:3–12, 1987.

Martin WR: Pharmacology of opioids. *Pharmacol Rev* 35:283–323, 1984.

McDonnell TE, Bartkowski RR, Bonilla FA, Henthorn TK, Williams JJ: Nonuniformity of alfentanil pharmacokinetics in healthy adults. *Anesthesiology* 57:A236, 1982.

Meistelman C, Saint-Maurice C, Lepaul M, Levron J-C, Loose J-P, MacGee K: A comparison of alfentanil pharmacokinetics in children and adults. *Anesthesiology* 66:13–16, 1987.

Meuldermans W, Woestenborghs R, Noorduin H, Camu F, Van Steenberge A, Heykants J: Protein binding of the analgesics alfentanil and sufentanil in maternal and neonatal plasma. *Eur J Clin Pharmacol* 30:217–219, 1986.

Nauta J, DeLange S, Koopman D, Spierdijk J, VanKleef J, Stanley TH: Anesthetic induction with alfentanil: a new short-acting narcotic analgesic. *Anesth Analg* 61:267–272, 1982.

Nauta J, Stanley TH, DeLange S, Koopman D, Spierdijk J, VanKleef J: Anesthetic induction with alfentanil: comparison with thiopental, midazolam, and etomidate. *Can Anaesth Soc J* 30:53–60, 1983.

O'Connor M, Escarpa A, Prys-Roberts C: Ventilatory depression during and after infusion of alfentanil in man. *Br J Anaesth* 55:217S–221S, 1983.

Roure P, Jean N, LeClerc A-C, Cabanel N, Levron J-C, Duvaldestin P: Pharmacokinetics of alfentanil in children undergoing surgery. *Br J Anaesth* 59:1437–1440, 1987.

Scamman FL, Ghoneim MM, Korttila K: Ventilatory and mental effects of alfentanil and fentanyl. *Acta Anaesthesiol Scand* 28:63–67, 1984.

Scott JC, Ponganis KV, Stanski DR: EEG quantitation of narcotic effect: the comparative pharmacodynamics of fentanyl and alfentanil. *Anesthesiology* 62:234–241, 1985.

Sebel PS, Bovill JG, Van der Haven A. Cardiovascular effects of alfentanil anaesthesia. *Br J Anaesth* 54:1185–1189, 1982.

Shafer A, Sung M-L, White PF: Pharmacokinetics and pharmacodynamics of alfentanil infusions during general anesthesia. *Anesth Analg* 65:1021–1028, 1986.

Stanski DR, Hug CC: Alfentanil—a kinetically predictable narcotic analgesic. *Anesthesiology* 7:435–438, 1982.

Van Peer A, Vercauteren M, Noorduin H, Woestenborghs R, Heykants J: Alfentanil kinetics in renal insufficiency. *Eur J Clin Pharmacol* 30:245–247, 1986.

Welchew EA, Hosking J: Patient-controlled postoperative analgesia with alfentanil. *Anaesthesia* 40:1172–1177, 1985.

White PF, Coe V, Shafer A, Sung ML: Comparison of alfentanil with fentanyl for outpatient anesthesia. *Anesthesiology* 64:99–106, 1986.

Yate PM, Thomas D, Short SM, Sebel PS, Morton J: Comparison of infusions of alfentanil or pethidine for sedation of ventilated patients on the ITU. *Br J Anaesth* 58:1091–1099, 1986.

Sufentanil

Bovill JG, Sebel PS, Blackburn CL, Oei-Lim V, Heykants JJ: The pharmacokinetics of sufentanil in surgical patients. *Anesthesiology* 61:502–506, 1984.

Bovill JG, Sebel PS, Fiolet JWT, Touber JL, Kok K, Philbin DM: The influence of sufentanil on endocrine and metabolic responses to cardiac surgery. *Anesth Analg* 62:391–397, 1983.

Davis PJ, Cook DR, Stiller RL, Davin-Robinson KA: Pharmacodynamics and pharmacokinetics of high-dose sufentanil in infants and children undergoing cardiac surgery. *Anesth Analg* 66:203–208, 1987.

Davis PJ, Stiller RL, Cook DR, Brandom BW, Davin-Robinson KA: Pharmacokinetics of sufentanil in adolescent patients with chronic renal failure. *Anesth Analg* 67:268–271, 1988.

De Lange S, Boscoe MJ, Stanley TH, Page N: Comparison of sufentanil-O_2 and fentanyl-O_2 for coronary artery surgery. *Anesthesiology* 56:112–118, 1982.

De Lange S, Stanley TH, Boscoe MJ, deBruijn N, Berman L, Green O, Robertson D: Catecholamine and cortisol responses to sufentanil-O_2 and alfentanil-O_2 anaesthesia during coronary artery surgery. *Can Anaesth Soc J* 30:248–254, 1983.

Flezzani P, Alvis MJ, Jacobs JR, Schilling MM, Bai S, Reves JG: Sufentanil disposition during cardiopulmonary bypass. *Can J Anaesth* 34:566–569, 1987.

Greeley WJ, deBruijn NP: Changes in sufentanil pharmacokinetics within the neonatal period. *Anesth Analg* 67:86–90, 1988.

Greeley WJ, deBruijn NP, Davis DP: Sufentanil pharmacokinetics in pediatric cardiovascular patients. *Anesth Analg* 66:1067–1072, 1987.

Hickey PR, Hansen DD: Fentanyl- and sufentanil-oxygen-pancuronium anesthesia for cardiac surgery in infants. *Anesth Analg* 63:117–124, 1984.

Monk JP, Beresford R, Ward A: Sufentanil. A review of its pharmacological properties and therapeutic use. *Drugs* 36:286–313, 1988.

Rosow CE, Philbin DM, Keegan CR, Moss J: Hemodynamics and histamine release during induction with sufentanil or fentanyl. *Anesthesiology* 60:489–491, 1984.

Sebel PS, Bovill JG: Cardiovascular effects of sufentanil anaesthesia. *Anesth Analg* 61:115–119, 1982.

Wiggum DC, Cork RC, Weldon ST, Gandolfi AJ, Perry DS: Postoperative respiratory depression and elevated sufentanil levels in a patient with chronic renal failure. *Anesthesiology* 63:708–710, 1985.

Pentazocine

Beckett AH, Taylor JF: Blood concentrations of pethidine and pentazocine in mother and infant at time of birth. *J Pharm Pharmacol* 19:50S–52S, 1967.

Brogden RN, Speight TM, Avery GS: Pentazocine: a review of its pharmacological properties, therapeutic efficacy, and dependence liability. *Drugs* 5:6–91, 1973.

Jewitt DE, Maurer GJ, Hubner PJB: Increased pulmonary arterial pressures after pentazocine in myocardial infarction. *Br Med J* 1:795–796, 1970.

Lal S, Savidge RS, Chabra GP: Cardiovascular and respiratory effects of morphine and pentazocine in patients with myocardial infarction. *Lancet* 1:379–381, 1969.

Schmucker P, VanAckern K, Franke N, Noisser H, Militzer H, Peter K, Kreuzer E, Turk R: Hemodynamic and respiratory effects of pentazocine. Studies on surgical cardiac patients. *Anaesthesist* 29:475–480, 1980.

Butorphanol

Heel RC, Brogden RN, Speight TM, Avery GS: Butorphanol: a review of its pharmacological properties and therapeutic efficacy. *Drugs* 16:473–505, 1978.

Stanley TH, Reddy P, Gilmore S, Bennett G: The cardiovascular effects of high-dose butorphanol-nitrous oxide anaesthesia before and during operation. *Can Anaesth Soc J* 30:337–341, 1983.

Vandam LD: Butorphanol. *N Engl J Med* 302:381–384, 1980.

Nalbuphine

Errick JK, Heel RC: Nalbuphine: a preliminary review of its pharmacological properties and therapeutic efficacy. *Drugs* 26:191–211, 1983.

Gal TJ, DiFazio CA, Moscicki J: Analgesic and respiratory depressant activity of nalbuphine: a comparison with morphine. *Anesthesiology* 57:367–374, 1982.

Lee G, Low RI, Amsterdam EA, DeMaria AN, Huber PW, Mason DT: Hemodynamic effects of morphine and nalbuphine in acute myocardial infarction. *Clin Pharmacol Ther* 29:576–581, 1981.

Sear JW, Keegan M, Kay B: Disposition of nalbuphine in patients undergoing general anaesthesia. *Br J Anaesth* 59:572–575, 1987.

Buprenorphine

Heel RC, Brogden RN, Speight TM, Avery GS: Buprenorphine: a review of its pharmacological properties and therapeutic efficacy. *Drugs* 17:81–110, 1979.

Drug Interactions

El-Ganzouri AR, Ivankovich AD, Braverman B, McCarthy R: Monoamine oxidase inhibitors: should they be discontinued preoperatively? *Anesth Analg* 64:592–596, 1985.

Evans-Prosser CDG: The use of pethidine and morphine in the presence of monoamine oxidase inhibitors. *Br J Anaesth* 40:279–282, 1968.

London DR, Milne MD: Danger of monoamine oxidase inhibitors. *Br Med J* 2:1752–1753, 1962.

MacKenzie JE, Frank LW: Influence of pretreatment with monoamine oxidase inhibitor (phenelzine) on the effects of buprenorphine and pethidine in the conscious rabbit. *Br J Anaesth* 60:216–221, 1988.

Michaels I, Serrins M, Shier NQ, Barash PG: Anesthesia for cardiac surgery in patients receiving monoamine oxidase inhibitors. *Anesth Analg* 63:1041–1044, 1984.

Palmer H: Potentiation of pethidine. *Br Med J* 2:944, 1960.

Rogers KJ, Thornton JA: The interaction between monoamine oxidase inhibitors and narcotic analgesics in mice. *Br J Pharmacol* 36:470–480, 1969.

Shee JC: Dangerous potentiation of pethidine by iproniazid, and its treatment. *Br Med J* 2:507–508, 1960.

Sides CA: Hypertension during anaesthesia with monoamine oxidase inhibitors. *Anaesthesia* 42:633–635, 1987.

Stack CG, Rogers P, Linter SPK: Monoamine oxidase inhibitors and anaesthesia. *Br J Anaesth* 60:222–227, 1988.

Taylor DC: Alarming reaction to pethidine in patients on phenelzine. *Lancet* 2:401–402, 1962.

Vigran IM: Dangerous potentiation of meperidine hydrochloride by pargyline hydrochloride. *JAMA* 187:163–164, 1964.

Opioid Antagonists

Aitkenhead AR, Derbyshire DR, Pinnock CA, Achola K, Smith G: Pharmacokinetics of intravenous naloxone in healthy volunteers. *Anesthesiology* 61:A381, 1984.

Arndt JO, Freye E: Perfusion of naloxone through the fourth cerebral ventricle reverses the circulatory and hypnotic effects of halothane in dogs. *Anesthesiology* 51:58–63, 1979.

Azar I, Turndorf H: Severe hypertension and multiple atrial premature contractions following naloxone administration. *Anesth Analg* 58:524–525, 1979.

Chiang CN, Hollister LE, Kishimoto A, Barnett G: Kinetics of a naltrexone sustained-release preparation. *Clin Pharmacol Ther* 36:704–708, 1984.

Dixon R, Howes J, Gentile J, Hsu H-B, Hsiao J, Garg D, Weidler D, Meyer M, Tuttle R: Nalmefene: intravenous safety and kinetics of a new opioid antagonist. *Clin Pharmacol Ther* 39:49–53, 1986.

Estilo AE, Cottrell JE: Hemodynamic and catecholamine changes after administration of naloxone. *Anesth Analg* 61:349–353, 1982.

Evans JM, Hogg MIJ, Lunn JN, Rosen M: Degree and duration of reversal by naloxone of effects of morphine in conscious subjects. *Br Med J* 2:589–591, 1974.

Faden AI, Holaday JW: Opiate antagonists: a role in the treatment of hypovolemic shock. *Science (Wash DC)* 205:317–318, 1979.

Faden AI, Jacobs TP, Holaday JW: Opiate antagonist improves neurologic recovery after spinal injury. *Science (Wash DC)* 211:493–494, 1981.

Frame WT, Allison RH, Moir DD, Nimmo WS: Effect of naloxone on gastric emptying during labour. *Br J Anaesth* 56:263–266, 1984.

Freye E, Hartung E, Kaliebe S: Prevention of late fentanyl-induced respiratory depression after the injection of opiate with antagonists naltrexone and S-20682: comparison with naloxone. *Br J Anaesth* 55:71–77, 1983.

Gal TJ, DiFazio CA: Prolonged antagonism of opioid action with intravenous nalmefene in man. *Anesthesiology* 64:175–180, 1986.

Gal TJ, DiFazio CA, Dixon R: Prolonged blockade of opioid effect with oral nalmefene. *Clin Pharmacol Ther* 40:537–542, 1986.

Groeger JS, Carlson GC, Howland WS: Naloxone in septic shock. *Crit Care Med* 11:650–654, 1983.

Gurll NJ, Reynolds DG, Vargish T, Lechner R: Naloxone without transfusion prolongs survival and enhances cardiovascular function in hypovolemic shock. *J Pharmacol Exp Ther* 220:621–624, 1982.

Gurll NJ, Reynolds DG, Vargish T, Lechner R: Naltrexone improves survival rate and cardiovascular function in canine hemorrhagic shock. *J Pharmacol Exp Ther* 220:625–628, 1982.

Hibbard BM, Rosen M, Davies D: Placental transfer of naloxone. *Br J Anaesth* 58:45–48, 1986.

Johnstone RE, Jobes DR, Kennell EM, Behar MG, Smith TC: Reversal of morphine anesthesia with naloxone. *Anesthesiology* 41:361–367, 1974.

Kraynack BJ, Gintautas JG: Naloxone: analeptic action unrelated to opiate receptor antagonism? *Anesthesiology* 56:251–253, 1982.

McNicholas LF, Martin WR: New and experimental therapeutic roles for naloxone and related opioid antagonists. *Drugs* 27:81–93, 1984.

Milne B, Jhamandas K: Naloxone: new therapeutic roles. *Can Anaesth Soc J* 31:272–278, 1984.

Ngai SH, Berkowitz BA, Yang JC, Hempstead J, Spector S: Pharmacokinetics of naloxone in rats and in man. Basis for its potency and short duration of action. *Anesthesiology* 44:398–401, 1976.

Peters WP, Johnson WM, Friedman PA, Mitch WE: Pressor effect of naloxone in septic shock. *Lancet* 1:529–532, 1981.

Peterson BT, Ross JC, Brigham KL: Effect of naloxone on the pulmonary vascular responses to graded levels of intracranial hypertension in anesthetized sheep. *Am Rev Respir Dis* 128:1024–1029, 1983.

Rawal N, Schott U, Dahlstrom B, Inturrisi CE, Tandon B, Sjostrand U, Wennhager M: Influence of naloxone infusion on analgesia and respiratory depression following epidural morphine. *Anesthesiology* 64:194–201, 1986.

Smith G, Pinnock C: Naloxone—paradox or panacea? *Br J Anaesth* 57:547–549, 1985.

Yaksh TL, Howe JR: Opiate receptors and their definition by antagonists. *Anesthesiology* 56:246–249, 1982.

8

Intravenous Anesthetic Agents

MARGARET WOOD

The first effective intravenous anesthetic induction agent was hexobarbital which was introduced into clinical practice in Germany in 1932. Soon after, in 1934, thiopental was studied in the United States by Lundy and Waters and rapidly achieved widespread acceptance as a useful intravenous induction agent. Although a large number of nonbarbiturate drugs have undergone clinical trials since that time, thiopental remains the most widely used intravenous induction agent. The intravenous induction agents may be classified as follows:

I. BARBITURATES
   Thiopental and methohexital
II. NONBARBITURATES
   1. Dissociative Anesthetics—ketamine
   2. Benzodiazepines—diazepam, midazolam
   3. Neuroleptanalgesics and neuroleptanesthetics—droperidol and fentanyl
   4. Imidazole derivatives—etomidate
   5. Phenol derivatives—propofol
   6. Eugenols—propanidid
   7. Steroids—althesin

BARBITURATE INTRAVENOUS ANESTHETICS

Chemical Structure

Barbituric acid is obtained from the condensation of malonic acid and urea to form barbituric acid and water (Fig. 8.1). The structural formula of barbituric acid is given in Fig. 8.2. All the barbiturates used clinically are substituted water-soluble sodium salts of barbituric acid.

Table 8.1 shows the clinical formulae and substitutions of some of the commonly used barbiturates in the United States.

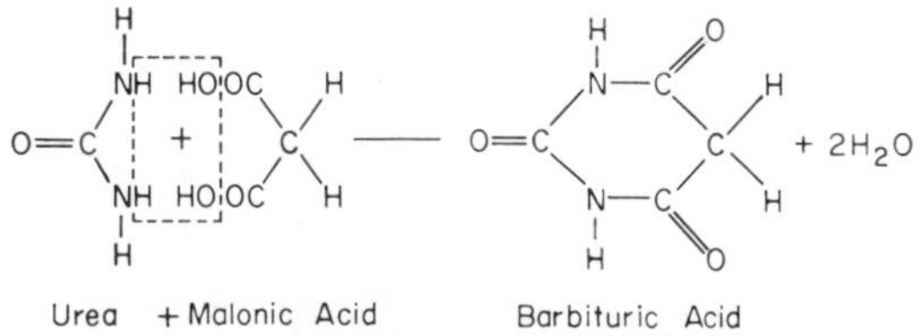

Figure 8.1. Reaction between urea and malonic acid.

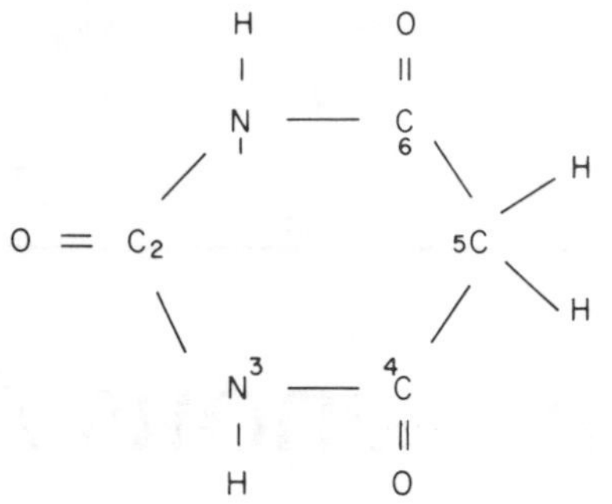

Figure 8.2. Structural formula of barbituric acid. The keto form that is shown can convert to the enol form by transition of the hydrogens at positions 1 or 3 in the ring to oxygen at position 2.

Barbiturates are almost insoluble in water, but possess weak acidic properties because they exist as an equilibrium mixture of keto ($-CO-NH-$) and enol ($-C(OH):N-$) forms, as shown in Fig. 8.3. Most barbiturates tend to exist in the enol form and therefore act as weak acids. Sodium can be substituted for the hydrogen of the enol form to make soluble salts which can be administered intravenously.

Structure-Activity Relationships

Barbituric acid is not itself a central nervous system depressant, and substitution of the hydrogens on the carbon atom at position 5 with alkyl or aryl groups is essential for hypnotic or sedative activity. A phenyl group on C5 or one of the nitrogens of the barbituric acid ring confers anticonvulsant activity on the compound (e.g., phenobarbital). Thus, hypnotic and anticonvulsant activities are relatively independent, and phenobarbital may be used as an anticonvulsant drug at nonhypnotic doses. Increase

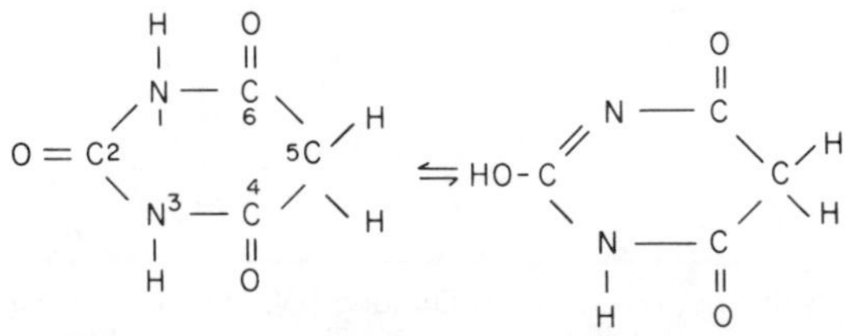

Figure 8.3. Keto - enol tautomerization.

Table 8.1.
Chemical Structure of Some Important Barbiturates

Barbiturate	Trade name	R_1	R_2	R_3	X
Amobarbital	Amytal	Ethyl	Isopentyl	H	O
Barbital	Neuronidia	Ethyl	Ethyl	H	O
Butabarbital	Butisol	Ethyl	sec-Butyl	H	O
Hexobarbital	Sombulex	Methyl	1-Cyclohexen-1-yl	CH_3	O
Methohexital	Brevital	Allyl	1-Methyl-2-pentynyl	CH_3	O
Pentobarbital	Nembutal	Ethyl	1-Methylbutyl	H	O
Phenobarbital	Luminal	Ethyl	Phenyl	H	O
Secobarbital	Seconal	Allyl	1-Methylbutyl	H	O
Thiamylal	Surital	Allyl	1-Methylbutyl	H	S
Thiopental	Pentothal	Ethyl	1-Methylbutyl	H	S

Adapted from Harvey SC: Chapter 17. In Goodman AG, Goodman L, Gilman A (eds): *Hypnotics and Sedatives in the Pharmacological Basis of Therapeutics.* New York, Macmillan, 1980, p 351.

in length of one or both of the alkyl side chains at C5 increases hypnotic potency, but if the side chains are increased to more than five or six carbons, hypnotic activity is reduced and convulsant properties may result.

The barbiturates have been divided into four groups according to their chemical structure as follows (Table 8.2):

1. Barbiturates (oxybarbiturates);
2. Methylated oxybarbiturates;

Table 8.2.
Structure-Activity Relationship of the Barbiturates

Group	Position 1*	Position 2*	Group characteristics when given
Oxybarbiturates	H	O	Delay in onset of action, hypnotic potency depends on side chains at C5, prolonged duration of action
Methylated barbiturates	CH_3	O	Usually rapid onset of action, rapid recovery, high incidence of excitatory phenomena
Thiobarbiturates	H	S	Rapid, smooth onset of action, rapid recovery
Methylated thiobarbiturates	CH_3	S	Rapid onset of action, high incidence of excitatory phenomena precludes clinical use

With permission from Dundee JW, Wyant GM: *Barbiturates: Chemistry and Pharmacokinetics in Intravenous Anaesthesia.* Edinburgh, Churchill-Livingstone, 1974, Chap 5.
*Position numbers refer to numbering in Figure 8.2.

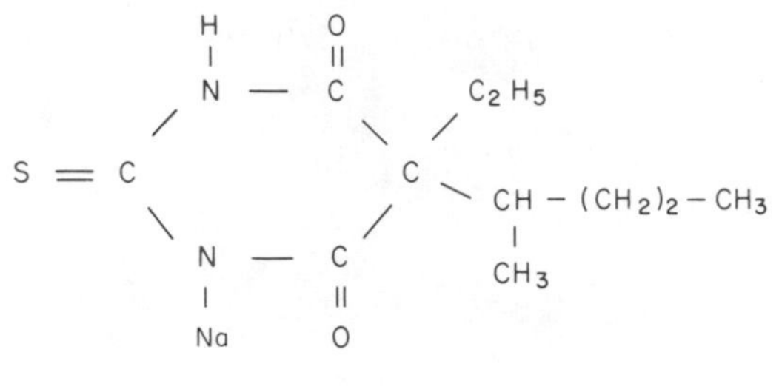

THIOPENTAL

Figure 8.4. Structural formula of thiopental.

3. Thiobarbiturates;
4. Methylated thiobarbiturates.

Compounds having a barbituric acid ring (oxygen at C2) are commonly called oxybarbiturates, while barbiturates in which the oxygen at C2 is replaced by sulfur are called thiobarbiturates. This substitution usually results in a lipid-soluble, rapidly acting hypnotic drug that may be used as an intravenous induction agent. Thiopental is the thioanalog of pentobarbital; substitution of the oxygen at C2 by sulfur converts the relatively slow acting pentobarbital into thiopental, a rapidly acting compound (Fig. 8.4). The introduction of a methyl (CH_3) or ethyl (C_2H_5) group on the nitrogen at position 1 of the barbituric acid ring also produces rapidly acting compounds, but in addition a high incidence of excitatory phenomena, such as tremor, hypertonus, and spontaneous involuntary movement. Methohexital is an oxybarbiturate whose rapidity of action is due to methylation at position 1 on the barbituric acid ring (Fig. 8.5).

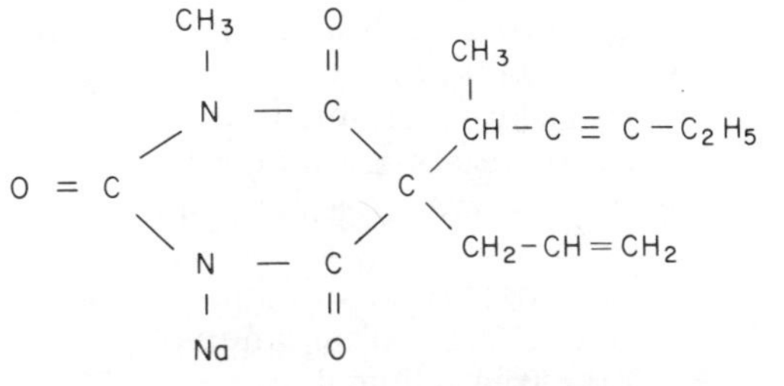

METHOHEXITAL

Figure 8.5. Structural formula of methohexital.

Classification of Barbiturates

Traditionally, the barbiturates have been classified as long, medium, and short acting, but it is now recognized that there are probably not any important clinical differences among the three groups. In addition, another group "ultrashort acting" has been defined which comprises the intravenous barbiturate induction agents.

The traditional classification is as follows:

	Elimination Half-Life
1. **Long acting** e.g., phenobarbital	Half-life = 24–96 hours
2. **Medium acting** e.g., pentobarbital	Half-life = 21–42 hours
3. **Short acting** e.g., secobarbital	Half-life = 20–28 hours
4. **Ultrashort acting** e.g., thiopental	Half-Life = 10–12 hours

The "ultrashort" acting compounds act briefly because, following intravenous injection, rapid redistribution occurs which terminates their action. However, excretion takes much longer and continues for many hours after the anesthetic effect has worn off. Although these drugs are termed "ultrashort acting," thiopental, e.g., has a half-life of elimination of around 10 to 12 hours.

The "ultrashort" acting barbiturates are used principally as intravenous anesthetic agents, while the short and medium acting barbiturates are mainly prescribed as sedative-hypnotic agents. However, the barbiturates have been largely replaced as sedative-hypnotic agents by the safer benzodiazepines (see Chapter 20). The long acting drugs, e.g., phenobarbital, are especially useful in the management of epilepsy as anticonvulsant agents.

Pharmacokinetics

The distribution, metabolism, and elimination of the barbiturates and, especially, thiopental have been carefully studied. It cannot be overemphasized that the clinical recovery from the intravenous administration of thiopental is due to redistribution (and to some extent metabolism), which is accompanied by a rapid fall in plasma concentration so that the patient awakes even though most of the administered dose still remains in the body.

Distribution

In order for a drug to produce the rapid onset of unconsciousness, it must be capable of pentrating the blood-brain barrier relatively quickly and producing high local concentrations within the brain. The rapid penetration of the blood-brain barrier by thiopental is due to its high lipid solubility and low degree of ionization.

DEGREE OF IONIZATION

The degree of ionization has an important influence on drug distribution and, in particular, on the onset and duration of drug action because it is only the unionized form that readily crosses cell membranes and, therefore, penetrates the blood-brain barrier. The rate at which a drug crosses the blood-brain barrier depends on both the lipid solubility of the unionized form and the degree of ionization at plasma pH, which determines the proportion of the unionized form present in the blood. Knowledge of the dissociation constant (pKa), which is the pH at which a weak acid is 50% ionized, and of its nature as a base or acid allows prediction of the effect of pH on the degree of ionization (see Chapter 1, page 23). For example, a weak acid will become more ionized as pH increases. The barbiturates are weak acids with pKa values that are slightly higher than 7.4 so that ionization is maximal at high pH. Thiopental has a pKa of 7.6 and is 61% unionized at normal body pH; methohexital is 75% unionized at pH 7.4, and phenobarbital with a pKa lower than 7.4 is 40% unionized at physiological pH.

The degree of ionization can change with physiological or pathological variation in acid-base balance. Brodie has shown in dogs that, by experimentally decreasing the plasma pH to 6.8, the plasma concentration of thiopental fell considerably, probably due to altered distribution, because the fall in plasma pH caused the proportion of unionized thiopental to rise, thereby allowing more to cross cell membranes resulting in increased penetration into the brain and other tissues. Acidosis, therefore, favors the passage of thiopental across the blood-brain barrier, and alkalosis will have the opposite effect. The intracerebral thiopental concentration will therefore be increased by lowering and decreased by elevating plasma pH.

In the stomach (low pH), barbiturates exist mainly in the nonionized form and, therefore, are absorbed according to their lipid solubility. Highly lipid-soluble drugs are rapidly absorbed after oral administration. The degree of ionization also affects the renal excretion of barbiturates. Any unionized drug in the glomerular filtrate can diffuse back into the circulation through the renal tubules, thus reducing renal excretion. This diffusion will be less if the drug is highly ionized, and forced alkaline diuresis has been used in the treatment of phenobarbital overdose or poisoning to enhance renal excretion of phenobarbital.

LIPID SOLUBILITY

It is the highly lipid-soluble drugs that have a rapid onset and duration of action. The rapidly acting intravenous barbiturate induction agents are relatively unionized at plasma pH 7.4, so passage of these drugs into the brain depends on their lipid solubility. Thiopental, which is very highly lipid soluble, easily penetrates the blood-brain barrier, and brain concentrations equal maximal plasma concentrations extremely quickly, causing the rapid induction of unconsciousness. In contrast, phenobarbital of relatively low lipid solubility penetrates the blood-brain barrier slowly, and sleep may take over 15 minutes to occur when this drug is given intravenously.

PROTEIN BINDING

Plasma binding is important as it is the unbound or free fraction that is available for crossing cell membranes and for exerting pharmacological effect. The barbiturates are bound to the plasma proteins, chiefly albumin. The plasma binding of thiopental has been reported to vary between 65 and 86%. Competitive displacement of thiopental from its binding sites by a number of drugs, e.g., sulfisoxazole, may increase the free fraction and enhance its pharmacological activity. In addition, thiopental binding is decreased in disease states such as uremia and hepatic cirrhosis.

PLACENTAL TRANSFER

Factors controlling transplacental drug transfer are the same as those controlling passage across other cell membranes, namely, lipid solubility, protein binding, and degree of ionization (see Chapter 1). Thiopental is highly lipid soluble and therefore readily crosses the placenta. Maximum barbiturate concentrations have been demonstrated in fetal blood within 3 minutes of the intravenous injection of thiopental to the mother (see Chapter 12).

Uptake and Redistribution

The termination of the action of the barbiturates is due to redistribution, metabolism, and renal excretion. In the case of thiopental, metabolism is too slow (10 to 15%/hour) to account for its short duration of action, and the rapid return of consciousness is due to two factors: (*a*) the bolus injection of barbiturate mixing within the circulating blood; and (*b*) physical redistribution from the brain to other tissue compartments.

When thiopental is given intravenously, maximal plasma arterial concentrations are achieved rapidly, and sleep occurs within 10 to 20 seconds. Cerbral blood flow constitutes about one-sixth of the cardiac output, and therefore a large mass or bolus of lipid-soluble and largely unionized drug reaches the brain within one circulation time. Peak plasma arterial thiopental concentrations of around 175 mg/L are achieved withing 30 seconds of the intravenous administration of 350 mg of thiopental, while peak internal

jugular venous concentrations are much lower (75 mg/L). Blood thiopental levels then fall rapidly due to dilution and mixing within the circulation and also to redistribution to other tissues.

The relative rate at which the various organs and tissues take up thiopental will depend upon their blood flow or the proportion of the cardiac output that they receive (Fig. 8.6). Organs that are very highly perfused (vessel-rich group, VRG), such as brain, heart, liver, and kidney, rapidly achieve concentrations equal to peak plasma concentrations. The brain achieves maximal concentrations of thiopental within 30 seconds of intravenous administration, and loss of consciousness therefore quickly ensues. Because of its high blood flow, the heart initially receives a large proportion of the dose of thiopental, accounting for the speed with which cardiovascular depression often follows intravenous administration. As the drug is taken up by the heart, liver, and kidney, the plasma concentration starts to fall, and thiopental passes out of the brain along a concentration gradient. The blood flow to the muscles is less than that to the vessel-rich group (20% of the cardiac output), and 15 to 30 minutes are required for the concentration of thiopental in muscle to equilibrate with the plasma and reach maximal concentration. This is achieved by redistribution of the drug from the highly perfused tissues. Muscle, because of its large mass, is an important reservoir for drug storage. Thus, as muscle concentration rises, brain concentration falls and the patient may awaken within 5 to 15 minutes of intravenous injection. Although thiopental has a very high affinity for fat, because of its very poor blood supply, it take several hours for distribution to this tissue to occur. Therefore, the decline in plasma concentration in the first 30 minutes after intravenous administration is due to redistribution to muscle and, after that, redistribution to fat and metabolism become important. Fig. 8.6 shows diagramatically the distribution of thiopental to the various tissues following a single intravenous injection.

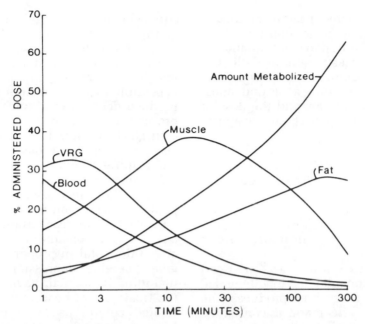

Figure 8.6.   Uptake and redistribution of an intravenous bolus of thiopental. Following an intravenous bolus, the amount of thiopental in the blood rapidly decreases as drug moves from blood to body tissues. Time to attainment of peak tissue levels is a direct function of tissue capacity for barbiturate relative to blood flow. Thus, a larger capacity or smaller blood flow is related to a longer time to a peak tissue level. Initially, most thiopental is taken up by the VRG (vessel-rich group) because of its high blood flow. Subsequently, drug is redistributed to muscle and to a lesser extent to fat. Throughout this period, small but substantial amounts of thiopental are removed by the liver and metabolized. Unlike removal by the tissues, this removal is cumulative. The rate of metabolism equals the early rate of removal by fat. The sum of this early removal by fat and metabolism is the same as the removal by muscle. (With permission from Saidman LJ: Uptake, distribution, and elimination of barbiturates. In Eger EJ (ed): *Anesthetic Uptake and Action*. Baltimore, Williams & Wilkins, 1974, pp 264–284.)

Metabolism

In general, the barbiturates are metabolized in the liver to inactive water-soluble metabolites that are then excreted in the urine. Very little thiopental is excreted unchanged in the urine. Brodie has calculated that only 10 to 15% of thiopental is metabolized per hour. Other workers have demonstrated that the liver removes up to 50% of the thiopental presented to it in hepatic arterial blood and, thus, although redistribution to muscle plays the most important role in the rapid fall of plasma arterial concentrations, metabolism may have a more significant effect than has previously been recognized.

Renal Excretion

Renal elimination of the intravenous barbiturates occurs extremely slowly due to their high lipid solubility and relatively low degree of ionization.

Cumulation and Prolonged Administration

Because thiopental remains in the body for hours after apparent clinical recovery, cumulative effects may be seen after intermittent repeated doses or prolonged continuous intravenous administration, and the dose required to maintain unconsciousness becomes progressively less as time proceeds. Caution is required if the patient should require a second anesthetic on the same day, and the dose of intravenous barbiturate should be appropriately reduced.

INDIVIDUAL BARBITURATE INTRAVENOUS ANESTHETICS

THIOPENTAL

Thiopental is the sulfur analog of pentobarbital, and its chemical structure is given in Fig. 8.4.

Central Nervous System. *Sleep.* The rapid injection of thiopental (3.5 to 4.0 mg/kg) over 10 to 20 seconds produces the smooth onset of sleep and unconsciousness, which is usually unaccompanied by spontaneous movement or respiratory excitatory phenomena. Sleep is often preceded by one or more deep breaths. Prior to loss of consciousness, the patient may exhibit hypersensitivity to external stimuli, such as touch or pain, and increased sensitivity of the pharyngeal and laryngeal reflexes may also occur.

Analgesia. Barbiturates in general are poor analgesics unless they are used in doses that alter the level of consciousness, and small doses may even increase sensitivity to pain—"antanalgesia" or "hyperalgesia." Antanalgesia associated with thiopental is usually evident at low plasma concentrations and, thus, is more likely to be manifest as postoperative restlessness when the plasma concentration has fallen or, to be seen after the administration of small doses, such as 25 to 100 mg. Children who have been premedicated with barbiturates may also show these features.

Anesthesia. The classical signs and stages of ether anesthesia are not seen with thiopental, because induction is so rapid. The clinical level of anesthesia produced by thiopental is related to the intensity of surgical stimulation as well as the degree of cerebral depression. Thiopental usually produces short-lived surgical anesthesia within 1 or 2 minutes of injection. However, if the patient is then stimulated surgically, laryngeal spasm may occur, abdominal relaxation may be lost, and the patient may move. It is possible to give sufficient thiopental to produce deep surgical anesthesia in the presence of external stimulation, such as a surgical incision, but these doses may also produce dangerous cardiovascular and respiratory depression.

Anticonvulsant Activity. In common with other barbiturates used clinically, thiopental possesses anticonvulsant activity.

Cerebral Metabolism. Brain metabolism and oxygen consumption are reduced after thiopental in proportion to the degree of cerebral depression. Barbiturates, including thiopental, have been used in the treatment of head injuries and other related conditions to reduce ischemic brain damage. The rationale is that reduction in oxygen demand will bring oxygen consumption into balance with the inadequate blood supply.

Cerebral Circulation. Thiopental produces profound cerebral vasoconstriction in humans in a dose-dependent fashion. However, alterations in arterial carbon dioxide tensions also have well-recognized effects on the cerebral circulation with elevation in $Paco_2$ causing an increase in cerebral blood flow. Therefore, in the absence of controlled ventilation and normocapnia, thiopental may increase cerebral blood flow due to raised arterial carbon dioxide tensions secondary to thiopental-induced respiratory depression.

Cardiovascular System. Hypotension nearly always follows the administration of thiopental, the degree depending on the dose, speed of injection, and clinical status of the patient. In the past direct myocardial depression has been consistently demonstrated after thiopental in isolated mammalian heart preparations. However, recently it has been shown in dogs that thiopental at clinical plasma concentrations causes minimal direct cardiac depression, but that a significant depression occurs at high levels.

In humans, hemodynamic effects include a fall in cardiac index, stroke volume, systemic blood pressure, and either an increase or decrease in total systemic vascular resistance. In patients with intact cardiovascular reflexes, the initial fall in cardiac output and blood pressure is usually compensated for by increased sympathetic activity mediated by baroreceptor reflexes, and this compensatory activity may account for the reported increases in systemic peripheral vascular resistance and heart rate. In patients suffering from hypovolemia, shock, or severe cardiac disease, where baroreceptor sensitivity may be decreased or adequate compensation cannot occur, severe uncompensated falls in cardiac output may follow even small doses of thiopental. Thiopental causes a reduction in the tone of systemic capacitance vessels, leading to peripheral pooling of blood. This may cause a reduction in left ventricular diastolic filling and stroke volume. Myocardial depression also occurring in this situation might, however, result in an elevation in end-diastolic and atrial pressures due to an inability of the heart to eject blood in normal amounts. The effect on central venous pressure and heart rate is variable. Ventricular arrhythmias have been observed but may be due to other factors, such as hypercarbia.

Thiopental has been shown in dogs and humans to increase myocardial blood flow and oxygen utilization. If the balance between myocardial oxygen demand and delivery is not maintained, however, impaired myocardial contractility, cardiac output, and reduced coronary perfusion result. These effects would be extremely hazardous for the patient with ischemic heart disease, and it is probably wise to avoid the use of thiopental in patients with coronary disease and evidence of impaired ventricular contractility.

Respiratory System. Thiopental is a potent central respiratory depressant. Following the slow injection of an induction dose of thiopental, the patient will often take a few deep breaths, followed by a transient period of apnea. Respiration then returns with a reduction in tidal volume and rate that depends on the dose adminstered. The respiratory depression is potentiated by narcotic premedication. Barbiturates reduce the sensitivity of the central respiratory center to carbon dioxide.

Laryngeal reflexes are not usually depressed until deep levels of thiopental anesthesia are reached, and stimulation such as attempted intubation or excess secretions during light thiopental anesthesia may provoke laryngeal spasm.

Other General Effects. Renal, hepatic, and gastrointestinal functions are all said to be depressed by intravenous barbiturates, but these are rarely of clinical importance.

Local Effects. Solutions of thiopental are alkaline and, therefore, are extremely irritant to the tissues. Venous thrombosis may follow the intravenous administration of thiopental and is said to be more common after 5% thiopental than after the use of 2.5% solution. In addition, local irritation may follow the accidental perivenous injection of thiopental, sequelae varying from slight pain to extensive tissue sloughing and necrosis. However, the most serious local complication is the intraarterial injection of thiopental, which can lead to serious damage to the blood supply of the affected limb. The injection causes severe burning pain that typically shoots down the forearm and into the hands and fingers. The intense arterial spasm that follows causes loss of the radial pulse and blanching of the arm. If the arterial supply continues to be compromised, cyanosis of the affected arm develops, followed by a deep purple discoloration which is finally followed by gangrene.

Many theories have been advanced to explain these changes. The intraarterial injection of thiopental releases norepinephrine from the vessel wall which may be the cause of the intense vascular spasm that immediately follows this accident. However, this spasm would be expected to be transitory, and other factors must be involved. Thrombosis has nearly always been demonstrated in cases where permanent damage has occured. The incidence of intraarterial injection is unknown, but no permanent complications have been reported following the use of a 2.5% solution of thiopental.

Treatment should be instituted immediately. A brachial plexus or stellate ganglion block should be performed to improve the blood supply to the affected limb. Papaverine, procaine, or tolazoline may be administered to cause local vasodilation. As thrombosis often occurs later, anticoagulant therapy should be commenced immediately with heparin. Operative removal of a thrombus may be required.

Pharmacokinetics. In the previous section, the distribution and elimination of thiopental were conceptualized using a physiologically based perfusion model in which anatomical and physiological comparisons of average organ size, average organ blood flow, and mean blood:tissue drug partition coefficients were made in a similar manner to that used to explain the uptake and distribution of the inhalational anesthetics. However, pharmacokinetic models examining the fate of intravenous thiopental using blood thiopental concentrations measured over a time period, more readily allow the prediction of an individual patient's rate of thiopental distribution and elimination.

When thiopental is administered intravenously in clinical doses, the initial decay is very rapid (producing the fast onset of sleep with rapid awakening) followed by a prolonged terminal elimination half-life. Thus, the decline in plasma concentration follows a multicompartmental model with fast and slow distribution half-lives of about 3 to 8 and 50 to 60 minutes, respectively, while the terminal elimination half-life is about 10 to 12 hours (Table 8.3). The volume of distribution at steady state is 2.5 L/kg, and the clearance is about 3.5 ml/kg/min. Elimination of thiopental is due in large part to hepatic metabolism, and very little thiopental is excreted unchanged in the urine. Thiopental has a low hepatic extraction ratio and, therefore, the extent of protein binding should limit its clearance and not hepatic blood flow (see Chapter 1, page 24). Thus, thiopental has a low clearance and relatively large volume of distribution, which results in a long elimination half-life. The plasma decay curves after intravenous administration of thiopental at clinical dosage levels exhibit first order kinetics (see Chapter 1). Plasma levels of thiopental necessary for the production of surgical anesthesia are in the region of 40 μg/ml.

Thiopental has been advocated for the treatment of cerebral ischemic injury when it may be administered in large doses by continuous intravenous infusion over a prolonged period. Recent evidence suggests that, as the dose of thiopental is increased, the pharmacokinetic behavior of thiopental changes from first-order with low doses to zero-order kinetics with high doses (see Fig. 1.8). In low doses (e.g, 5 mg/kg), thiopental exhibits

Table 8.3.
Pharmacokinetic Parameters of the Intravenous Barbiturate Anesthetics

		Distribution half-life (min)	Elimination half-life (hr)	Clearance (ml/kg/min)	Volume of distribution (L/kg)
Thiopental	Fast	2.5–8.5	5.1–11.6	3.4–3.6	1.53–2.5
	Slow	46.4–62.7			
Methohexital	Fast	5.6–6.2	1.6–3.9	10.9–12.1	1.13–2.2
	Slow	58.3			

Data from Hudson RJ, Stanski DR, Burch PG: Pharmacokinetics of methohexital and thiopental in surgical patients. *Anesthesiology* 59:215–219, 1983; Ghoneim MM, VanHamme MJ: Pharmacokinetics of thiopentone: effects of enflurane and nitrous oxide anaesthesia and surgery. *Br J Anaesth* 50:1237-1241, 1978; and Breimer DD: Pharmacokinetics of methohexitone following intravenous infusion in humans. *Br J Anaesth* 48:643-649, 1976.

first-order kinetics, whereby a constant fraction of drug is eliminated from the body in unit time and the rate of elimination and half-life is independent of plasma concentration. However, at high doses of thiopental (300 to 600 mg/kg), zero-order elimination kinetics results and, in these circumstances, a constant mass of drug is cleared from the body in unit time, so that the rate of elimination changes with plasma concentration and a rapid rise in plasma concentration will result with increased administration. This has clinical implications, because as the dose of thiopental is increased, the clearance falls so that it is important to monitor plasma concentrations of thiopental if this drug is to be administered by intravenous infusion over an extended period of time to ensure that dangerously high thiopental concentrations do not occur.

Table 8.3 summarizes the pharmacokinetic parameters of thiopental. When an anesthesiologist administers an intravenous anesthetic agent, the drug is usually titrated to a desired therapeutic end point or effect. In the clinical situation, it is very difficult to precisely define effect or pharmacodynamic response, although attempts have been made to correlate plasma concentrations with clinical end points, such as loss of corneal reflexes or response to skin incision. Recently, the electroencephalogram (EEG) has been used to model the pharmacokinetic-pharmacodynamic relationships of the intravenous anesthetics. Changes in EEG frequency and voltage are distilled using power spectral analysis to produce a spectral edge, which can then be used as a measure of effect (Fig. 8.7). Spectral edge is then related to thiopental concentrations using an inhibitory E_{max} sigmoid model. Thus, the thiopental concentration (IC_{50}) producing one-half of the maximum spectral edge shift is an index of brain sensitivity to thiopental. This technique has been used to describe the pharmacokinetic-dynamic relationships of not only the induction agents but narcotics, such as fentanyl and alfentanil, under various conditions.

Liver disease does not affect the phar-

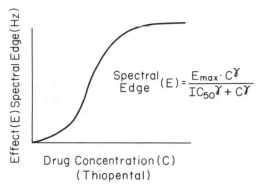

Figure 8.7. Pharmacodynamic model relating plasma concentration (*C*) to drug effect (*E*). E_{max} is the maximum effect due to the drug, i.e., the maximal decrease of the spectral edge induced by thiopental, *E* is the spectral edge, *C* is the plasma thiopental concentration, and IC_{50} is the concentration producing 50% of E_{max}, i.e., the thiopental concentration producing one-half the maximum spectral edge shift. IC_{50} is a measure of brain "sensitivity" to thiopental. γ is a power function describing the sigmoidicity or slope of the sigmoid concentration-response curve.

macokinetics of thiopental to any great extent, although plasma protein binding is markedly reduced in cirrhosis, probably as a result of the fall in albumin concentrations, which occurs in cirrhosis. Plasma binding is also reduced in renal disease, and the free fraction of thiopental in plasma is increased from 15.7% in normal individuals to 28% in patients with renal failure. This results in more drug being available for tissue distribution and an increased volume of distribution at steady state. Since total plasma clearance is also increased, elimination half-life is unchanged (see Fig. 1.21). However, when kinetic parameters are calculated on the basis of unbound (free) drug concentrations, there is very little difference between normal patients and those with renal failure. Although it is important to reduce the rate of administration of thiopental in patients with chronic renal failure to avoid unnecessarily high free concentrations, no reduction in total dose is required. The volume of distribution of such a highly lipid-soluble drug as thiopental is increased in obesity, probably because the drug so readily distributes into adipose tissue, leading to a prolonged elimination half-life and an unchanged clearance value.

Elderly patients have lower thiopental dose requirements for both induction and maintenance of anesthesia. The explanation for this clinical finding lies in the fact that, although brain sensitivity to thiopental (IC_{50})does not change with age, the initial volume of distribution of the central compartment (V_c or V_1) is smaller in elderly patients, resulting in higher plasma concentrations (Fig. 8.8) and, therefore, increased pharmacological effect. More recent work suggests that the pharmacokinetic changes seen in thiopental distribution may be more complicated than was first thought. The early blood samples obtained after thiopental administration which were used to calculate V_1 (Fig. 8.8) were probably obtained before complete intravascular mixing in the central compartment had occurred. In addition, some of the pa-

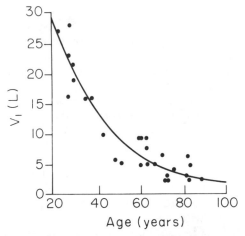

Figure 8.8.   Relationship of the initial volume of distribution (V_1) of thiopental to age. The dose of thiopental required to reach burst suppression on the EEG decreases with age. This decrease in dose requirement is not due to a change in brain sensitivity (IC_{50}) but due to a decrease in V_1 with increase in age. (With permission from Homer T, Stanski D: The effect of increasing age on thiopental disposition and anesthetic requirement. *Anesthesiology* 62:714–724, 1985.)

tients whose data is shown in Figure 8.8 received a bolus injection while others received a rapid thiopental infusion. The decrease in required dose of thiopental for induction of anesthesia in elderly patients might also be due to decreased rate of thiopental distribution from the central compartment to a second compartment which equilibrates rapidly with the central compartment. Although the plasma clearance of thiopental is relatively unaffected in older age groups, in some studies changes in protein binding in the elderly for thiopental have been shown to result in changes in volume of distribution and elimination half-life.

In contrast to the elderly, larger doses of thiopental are often recommended for anesthetic induction in young children. It is interesting that, although the dose of thiopental required to produce loss of lid and corneal reflexes is similar in pediatric patients and adults, the dose of thiopental required to produce loss of the trapezius reflex is larger in pediatric patients than in adults. Thus, if the trapezius reflex can be considered analogous to the stimulus of laryngoscopy and tracheal intubation, the dose of thiopental expected to prevent a response to this simulus is larger in young children. However, there is no difference between the rapid distribution half-life ($t_{1/2}\alpha$ or volume of distribution of the central compartment (V_c) in pediatric and adult patients. The terminal elimination half-life in children is about half that in adults accompanied by a thiopental clearance twice as great in infants and children as in adults. Thus, recovery may be more rapid for children if large or repeated doses of thiopental are given.

Suggested Dosage and Administration. Although it is possible to conduct all types of surgery under thiopental anesthesia, cardiovascular and respiratory depression and the prolonged recovery time associated with the use of large doses have led to the use of thiopental principally for the induction of general anesthesia. Rectal thiopental is still occasionally used to produce basal narcosis in children for short diagnostic procedures. However, thiopental has been superseded by drugs such as diazepam and midazolam for the production of sedation during short surgical operations, diagnostic procedures, or regional anesthesia.

Thiopental is usually administered as a 2.5% solution intravenously, the dose varying according to the age and physical status of the patient. A sleep induction dose may vary from 25 to 500 mg for the adult patient, but the generally accepted induction dose is 3 to 5 mg/kg. It should be given through a freely running intravenous line, so that there is direct access to the circulation should complications develop.

Toxicity, Precautions and Contraindications. *Complications.* 1. CARDIOVASCULAR. Knowledge of the cardiovascular depressant effects of thiopental requires that the administration of thiopental to patients suffering from cardiac disease or shock be undertaken with great caution. In particular, care should be exercised in the presence of constrictive pericarditis, coronary artery disease with poor left ventricular function, and mitral and aortic valvular disease where the patient may not be capable of withstanding the impairment of cardiovascular function induced by thiopental. Cardiovascular collapse and cardiac arrest have been reported following thiopental administration. If thiopental is to be administered to a patient with heart disease, it should be given slowly to allow sufficient time for the cardiovascular reflexes to compensate for the fall in cardiac output. A very rapid injection of a large dose may cause profound hypotension, a large decrease in systemic vascular resistance and, in addition, a fall in cornary artery perfusion pressure which may be especially hazardous in aortic valvular disease. The degree of hypotension following thiopental is said to be increased by opiate premedication.

2. RESPIRATORY. Respiratory complications include apnea, respiratory obstruction, laryngeal spasm, and bronchospasm. Laryngeal spasm may be triggered by a variety of stimuli, such as surgical stimulation, the premature insertion of the laryngoscope blade or airway, and pharyngeal secretions. Respiratory obstruction and an inadequate airway prior to induction are contraindications to

thiopental anesthesia. Facilities for intubation and ventilation should always be at hand when thiopental is administered.

3. LOCAL EFFECTS. Complications due to the local effects of thiopental, such as extravascular and intraarterial injection, have been discussed earlier in this chapter. However, it should be noted that pain on injection is low (9%) when compared to some of the new intravenous anesthetic induction agents.

4. ABNORMAL REACTIONS. Abnormal reactions, such as anaphylaxis, have been described but are extremely rare. Histamine release does occur, and a transient uticarial or blotchy, patchy red rash is sometimes seen.

5. EXCITATORY PHENOMENA. Excitatory phenomena, such as spontaneous involuntary muscle movement, sometimes occur, but are less frequent than following methohexital administration. The incidence of excitatory phenomena is said to be reduced by opiates, while the incidence of respiratory problems, such as cough and hiccough, is reduced by the preoperative use of atropine and hyoscine.

Contraindications. ABSOLUTE CONTRAINDICATIONS.

1. Respiratory obstruction or an inadequate airway before induction; a situation where it would not be possible to maintain an airway once general anesthesia was established.
2. Severe cardiovascular collapse or shock.
3. Unavailability of equipment to conduct a general anesthetic, and to perform intubation and ventilation.
4. Unavailability of an intravenous infusion for the administration of drugs and fluids.
5. Status asthmaticus, a situation where laryngeal spasm and respiratory depression are especially dangerous.
6. Porphyria

Porphyria is an inborn error of metabolism associated with disturbances in porphyrin metabolism. Porphyrins are pigments that possess a basic structure of four pyrrole rings linked by methane (—CH—) bridges and are found in chlorophyll, hemoglobin, and some of the cytochrome and peroxidase enzymes. They are formed from the precursors, aminolevulinic acid (ALA) and porphobilinogen. In the liver, ALA synthetase catalyzes the rate-limiting reaction for heme production (the formation of ALA from succinate and glycine within the mitochondria) and, therefore, controls the rate of synthesis of heme and porphyrin. ALA synthetase is increased in some types of porphyria.

The main clinical manifestations are intermittent attacks of nervous system dysfunction, abdominal pain, and sensitivity of the skin to sunlight. Exacerbations in patients who are normally asymptomatic may be precipitated by drugs, hormones, and liver disease. Clinical and biochemical manifestations may be induced by barbiturates, anticonvulsants, estrogens, contraceptives, and alcohol. Therefore, thiopental is contraindicated in porphyria. Some of the drugs that precipitate attacks of acute intermittent porphyria increase hepatic ALA synthetase activity, thus compounding the biochemical defects.

Drugs that are considered to be safe in porphyria include salicylates, morphine, meperidine, penicillins, phenothiazines, diphenhydramine, guanethidine, propranolol, atropine, neostigmine, propanidid, procaine, succinylcholine, and the inhalational anesthetics.

RELATIVE CONTRAINDICATIONS. If thiopental is used in the following situations, caution should be exercised as regards dose and rate of administration. The smallest effective dose should be used and given slowly because the arm-brain circulation time may be prolonged.

1. Cardiovascular disease, ischemic heart disease, hypertension, valvular heart disease.
2. Hypovolemia, hemorrhage, burns, fluid depletion, and dehydration.
3. Uremia.
4. Acute adrenocortical insufficiency.
5. Severe septicemia.

METHOHEXITAL

Methohexital is a barbiturate intravenous anesthetic agent that was developed during the search for an induction agent with a more rapid recovery than thiopental. It is a methylated oxybarbiturate, and its chemical structure is shown in Fig.

8.5. Methohexital has two asymmetric carbon atoms, so four isomers are possible. These have been divided into two pairs: α-dl and β-dl. The mixture of all four isomers was found to be a potent short-acting intravenous induction agent, but unfortunately produced excessive skeletal muscle activity and convulsions. Methohexital is the α-dl pair and produces hypnosis and sleep without the excessive motor phenomenon associated with the β isomer. It is 3 times as potent on a weight basis as thiopental, and recovery from anesthesia is shorter than after thiopental.

Pharmacological Effects. Many of the pharmacological effects of methohexital are similar to those described for thiopental, such as respiratory and cardiovascular depression. However, compared with thiopental, induction of anesthesia is associated with an increased incidence of excitatory phenomena. The incidence of tremor and involuntary muscle movements is reduced by narcotic premedication, while the incidence of cough and hiccough is diminished by atropine and hyoscine. Excitatory phenomena increase with larger doses.

Pharmacokinetics. Methohexital is 61% ionized at pH 7.4, and its plasma protein binding is similar to thiopental. Recovery of consciousness is due to redistribution of the drug from the central nervous system to muscle and fat. The pharmacokinetics of methohexital has been studied using a 60-minute zero-order infusion (rate = 0.05 mg/kg/min; dose, 3.0 mg/kg) in human volunteers, when the decrease in plasma concentration was best described by a two-compartmental kinetic model. There was a short distribution half-life (6.2 minutes), indicating that distribution from plasma to the tissues takes place very rapidly; the terminal elimination half-life was shorter (97 minutes) than that of thiopental due to the high metabolic clearance rate (12.1 ml/kg/min). The volume of distribution at steady state was 1.13 L/kg. The disposition of methohexital (2 to 3 mg/kg i.v. bolus) during halothane anesthesia in surgical patients also shows a high clearance (10.9 ml/kg/min), resulting in a shorter elimination half-life (3.9 hours) than that of thiopental (10 to 12 hours). Volume of distribution at steady state under these conditions was 2.2 L/kg, a value similar to that for thiopental. There is a short early distribution half-life of 5.6 minutes followed by a slow distribution half-life of 58.3 minutes. Therefore, the clearance of methohexital is about 4 times higher than that of thiopental, and the elimination half-life of methohexital is shorter than that of thiopental, reflecting the more rapid clinical recovery from methohexital administration, especially with large or repeated doses. Depsite the greater clearance of methohexital, it is important to recognize that redistribution still remains the major mechanism for terminating the effect of a single dose, reflecting the short early distribution half-life.

Table 8.3 describes the pharmacokinetic parameters of methohexital.

Suggested Dose and Administration. Methohexital is available for use as methohexital sodium for injection, and the pH of its aqueous solution is 11. It is usually given as a 1% solution. The recommended dose for a healthy patient is 1.0 to 1.5 mg/kg. It has been recommended for short procedures where rapid, complete recovery is desired.

Toxicity, Precautions, and Contraindications. Methohexital should be used with the same precautions as previously described for thiopental.

NONBARBITURATE INTRAVENOUS ANESTHETICS

Despite the current popularity of thiopental, intensive research is still ongoing for a nonbarbiturate intravenous anesthetic agent which possesses minimal respiratory and cardiovascular depression and in which rapid recovery from anesthesia is due to metabolism and excretion rather than just redistribution.

Dissociative Anesthetics

KETAMINE

Ketamine is an intravenous nonbarbiturate anesthetic agent which produces the clinical state of "dissociative anesthesia." It is relatively rapid acting, but

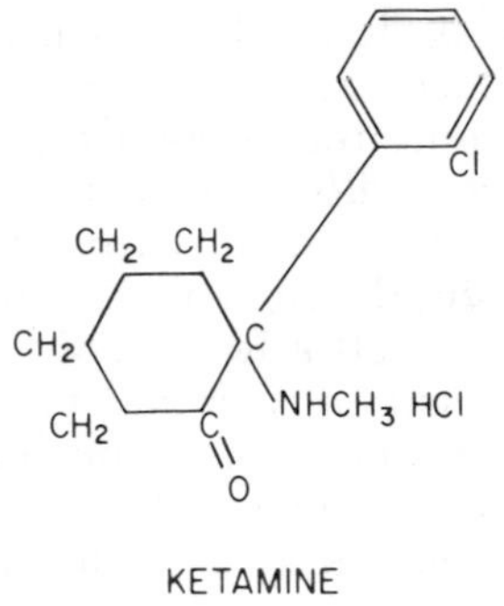

KETAMINE

Figure 8.9. Structural formula of ketamine hydrochloride.

its rate of onset is slower than that of thiopental. Although consciousness returns within 10 to 15 minutes of 2 mg/kg of ketamine intravenously, complete recovery is slow and protracted.

Chemical Structure. Ketamine is chemically related to phencyclidine and cyclohexamine. Its structural formula is given in Fig. 8.9. Since it contains an asymmetric carbon atom, ketamine exists as two isomers, the $(-)$ and the $(+)$ form, with the $(+)$ isomer being the more potent. The parenteral solution is a racemic mixture of ketamine, containing equal amounts of the two isomers. Infusions of the racemic mixture of the $(+)$-ketamine and $(-)$-ketamine isomers have been administered to volunteers when the isomer potency ratio for $(-)$:$(+)$ was found to be 1:3–5.

Pharmacological Effects

Central Nervous System. Ketamine produces an unusual trance-like cataleptic state, whereby the patient appears to be "dissociated" from his environment but not necessarily asleep. The patient may be awake with his eyes open or unconscious, and there is profound analgesia. This state has been called "dissociative" anesthesia. Spontaneous involuntary movements, nystagamus, and hypertonus may occur. Unlike the other intravenous anesthetic agents, ketamine can be given by both the intravenous and the intramuscular routes. The onset of action when given intravenously is 30 to 60 seconds and 3 to 8 minutes when administered intramuscularly. Analgesia associated with ketamine administration outlasts the period of anesthesia, and analgesia also occurs at subanesthetic doses of ketamine. Ketamine increases cerebral blood flow, cerebrospinal fluid pressure, and intracranial pressure and, therefore, should be avoided during neurosurgical anesthesia and in patients with increased intracranial pressure. In addition, cerebral oxygen consumption is not reduced as it is with thiopental.

Cardiovascular System. When ketamine was first introduced into clinical practice, it was quickly recognized that its lack of cardiovascular depression was an outstanding advantage. Ketamine possesses a cardiovascular stimulating effect, producing an increase in mean aortic pressure, pulmonary artery pressure, central venous pressure, heart rate, and cardiac index. The effect on peripheral resistance is variable. These cardiovascular changes are accompanied by striking elevations in circulating epinephrine and norepinephrine concentrations. The mechanism by which ketamine produces cardiovascular stimulation is unknown, but it is probably due to either central sympathetic stimulation or inhibition of the peripheral neuronal reuptake of catecholamines.

These features make ketamine a valuable induction agent for the poor-risk and hypovolemic patient, but the positve chronotropic and inotropic effects of ketamine are undesirable in patients with ischemic or valvular heart disease, because myocardial oxygen demand will be elevated by the increase in the stroke-work index and the rate-pressure product. Ketamine has been shown to increase pulmonary artery pressure in adults.

The use of ketamine in children with cyanotic heart disease is controversial. An increase in pulmonary vascular resistance adversely affects the degree or direction of shunting, while sympathetic stimulation might precipitate a hypercyanotic spell. However, recent clinical studies suggest that ketamine produces relatively minor increases in pulmonary and systemic arterial pressures in well-sedated children.

A direct short-lived myocardial depressant effect has been demonstrated in humans; the mean ejection fraction is reduced after 2.2 mg/kg of ketamine intravenously. In healthy patients, baroreceptor reflex function is well maintained during ketamine anesthesia. Cardiac arrhythmias are uncommon.

Respiratory System. The pharyngeal and laryngeal reflexes remain active during ketamine anesthesia, and aspiration is less likely to occur during this mode of anesthesia than with inhalational agents or the intravenous barbiturates. However, it is important to recognize that this protection is not absolute and that aspiration can still occur during ketamine anesthesia. Preservation of these protective reflexes may provoke laryngospasm and coughing secondary to secretions, blood, or manipulation of the mouth as in an attempted intubation or endoscopy. In addition, ketamine causes a marked increase in pharyngeal secretions and, therefore, an anticholinergic agent should be administered prior to ketamine. After the intravenous administration of 2 mg/kg of ketamine, there may be transient apnea followed by a reduction in respiratory rate and tidal volume. The bronchodilation produced by ketamine makes it a desirable agent in the treatment of a patient with asthma or obstructive airway disease.

Other Effects. Ketamine raises intraocular pressure and may cause postoperative nausea and vomiting. Patients have reported distressing psychic side effects such as hallucinations, alterations in perception of body image, and unpleasant dreams. Ketamine increases muscle tone and causes sudden jerky movements which may interfere with surgery and require sedation with diazepam.

Pharmacokinetics. After the intravenous administration of 2.2 mg/kg of ketamine, plasma ketamine concentration of 30,000 ng/ml at 30 seconds are produced, falling to around 1000 ng/ml at 10 minutes. The plasma ketamine concentration associated with analgesia is about 150 ng/ml, whereas concentrations at which awakening from anesthesia occurs range from around 600 to 1100 ng/ml. Thus, ketamine exhibits a range of concentrations where analgesia occurs without the loss of consciousness.

The distribution half-life $(t_{1/2\alpha})$ is about 11 to 17 minutes, while the elimination half-life $(t_{1/2\beta})$ is 2.5 to 3.1 hours, indicating that the recovery from the anesthetic action of ketamine is due to redistribution from brain to peripheral tissues. The final elimination is due predominantly to drug metabolism which proceeds relatively slowly. Plasma clearance is 17.5 to 19.1 ml/kg/min.

It is important to understand that, when surgical anesthesia is terminated, 50 to 60% of the drug still remains in the body in the active form, producing significant plasma levels (even though they are below those producing surgical anesthesia) which may make for a protracted emergence from anesthesia in the recovery room.

The pharmacokinetic profiles of the individual isomers are similar to the racemic mixtures. Ketamine serum concentrations have been related to EEG changes using the inhibitory sigmoid E_{max} model and the pharmacokinetic-pharmacodynamic relationships derived for both the ketamine enantiomers and the racemic mixture. It was found that the E_{max} value for the $(-)$-isomer is different from that of the $(+)$-isomer and the racemic mixture; a potency index defined as $IC_{50}/0.5E_{max}$ revealed a potency ratio of 1:1.7:5.6 for $(-)$-ketamine, racemic ketamine, and $(+)$-ketamine, respectively, indicating that the $(-)$-isomer partially antagonizes the EEG effects of the $(+)$-isomer when administered as a racemic mixture. Recovery of psychomotor skills was more rapid after either isomer compared with the racemic mixture. The degree of cardiovascular stimulation and psychomimetic activity appeared to be the same for both isomers.

Ketamine is extensively metabolized in the liver by hydroxylation and N-demethylation of the cyclohexylamine ring to form metabolites which are then conjugated and excreted in the urine. A major route of metabolism involves N-demethylation of ketamine to form norketamine, which appears to be one-fifth to one-third as potent as ketamine and may possess analgesic activity in humans. Norketamine can then be hydroxylated to form hydroxy-norketamine compounds, which in turn are then conjugated to form water-soluble compounds that are excreted in the urine. Very little unchanged ketamine appears in the urine. Some of the metabolites are pharmacologically active and may be important in the production of postoperative dreams and hallucinations. The disposition of ketamine in children is similar to that found in the adult, although children appear to produce more of the metabolite, norketamine.

Suggested Dosage and Administration. Ketamine may be used as an induction agent, a sole anesthetic agent for short diagnostic and surgical procedures, to provide pain relief outside the operating room for painful procedures such as dressing changes, and as a supplement to provide maintenance of anesthesia with nitrous oxide and muscle relaxants. Ketamine hydrochloride is available in vials containing 10 or 50 mg of ketamine per ml, respectively. An intravenous dose of 1.0 to 2.0 mg/kg is recommended for the induction of anesthesia, and unconsciousness usually lasts 5 to 15 minutes. If a longer effect is required, additional incremental doses may be given. Intramuscular doses, used mainly in children, are in the range of 5 to 10 mg/kg and usually produce surgical anesthesia with 3 to 5 minutes with a duration of action of 10 to 30 minutes. Lower doses of ketamine, e.g., 0.4 mg/kg, given by the intramuscular route produce analgesia lasting aporoximately 90 minutes. The continuous intravenous infusion of ketamine has been recommended for the production of analgesia without loss of consciousness for certain types of surgery, e.g., 5 to 20 μ/kg/min preceded by ketamine, 0.2 to 0.75 mg/kg i.v. bolus, or 2 to 4 mg/kg i.m. Ketamine, 15 to 30 μ/kg/min, as a continuous infusion has been administered to produce sleep and analgesia in combination with nitrous oxide/oxygen anesthesia and neuromuscular relaxants. Muscle relaxants may be necessary if ketamine is used to provide maintenance of anesthesia, since ketamine increases muscle tone. Diazepam reduces the incidence of involuntary muscle movements, and an antisialogogue such as glycopyrrolate reduces the amount of profuse salivation that may occur with ketamine administration.

Specific areas where ketamine may be indicated include:

1. Poor-risk surgical patients;
2. Pediatric surgery, where the intravenous induction of anesthesia is difficult;
3. Debridement, painful dressings, and skin-grafting procedures in patients suffering from burns;
4. Short procedures—diagnostic or surgical;
5. Cardiac catheterization;
6. Relief of postoperative pain.

Toxicity, Precautions, and Contraindications. Disadvantages of ketamine include its slow onset of action, increased muscle tone, jerky spontaneous muscular movements that occur during induction and anesthesia, cardiovascular stimulation, its slow recovery which is sometimes accompanied by disturbing emergence sequelae, and postoperative nausea and vomiting. Emergence sequelae are an important problem; auditory and visual hallucinations, restlessness, disorientation, confused and irrational behavior, and vivid dreams have all been reported in the immediate postoperative period and even up to 24 hours after ketamine anesthesia. The incidence of emergence complications may be reduced by heavy premedication and by diazepam and droperidol. Stimulation of the patient should be avoided during the recovery period. The more potent (+)-isomer of ketamine is associated with a more rapid recovery of psychomotor skills and less emergence reaction than the currently available racemic mixture.

Ketamine is contraindicated in patients with a history of cerebrovascular disease, hypertension, or ischemic and valvular disease of the heart. It should not be given to patients with increased intracranial or intraocular pressure.

Benzodiazepines

The benzodiazepines are a group of drugs that possess powerful anticonvul-

Figure 8.10.   The 1,4-benzodiazepine nucleus and the chemical structures of diazepam, lorazepam and midazolam.

sant, muscle relaxant, hypnotic, sedative, and tranquilizing properties. There are many derivatives of the 1,4-benzodiazepine nucleus (Fig. 8.10), but the ones of clinical importance include chlordiazepoxide, diazepam, oxazepam, clorazepate, flurazepam, temazepam, prazepam, lorazepam, flunitrazepam, and the water-soluble benzodiazepine, midazolam. All these drugs have similar neuropharmacological properties.

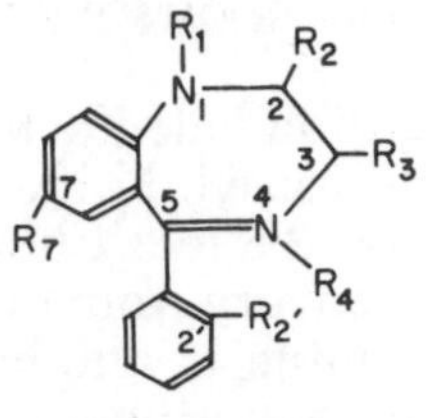

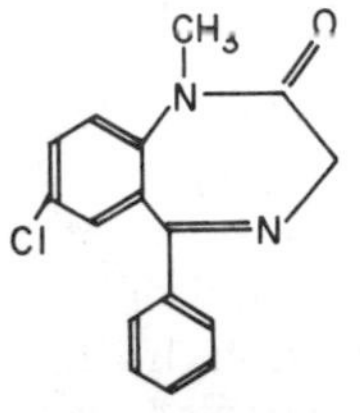

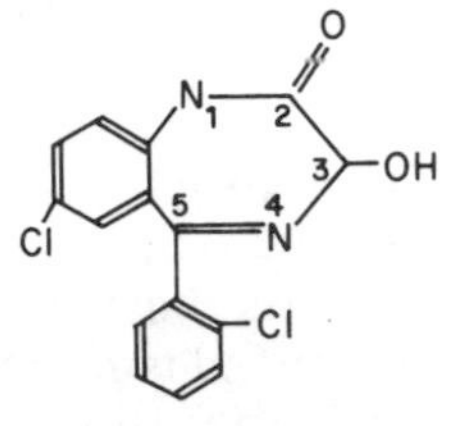

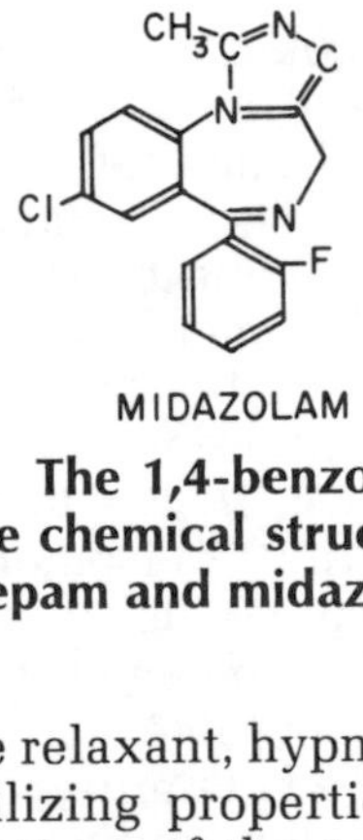

Over the last 10 years, great progress has been achieved in our understanding of the mechanism of action of the benzodiazepine group of drugs. An important inhibitory neurotransmitter in the brain is aminobutyric acid (GABA), while glycine is the major inhibitory neurotransmitter in the spinal cord and brainstem. The benzodiazepines, including diazepam and midazolam, augment or

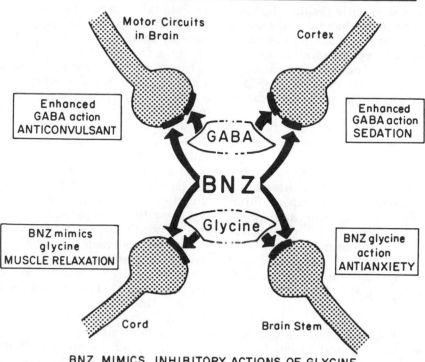

BNZ FACILITATES INHIBITORY ACTIONS OF GABA

Motor Circuits
in Brain

Cortex

Enhanced
GABA action
ANTICONVULSANT

Enhanced
GABA action
SEDATION

GABA

BNZ

Glycine

BNZ mimics
glycine
MUSCLE RELAXATION

BNZ glycine
action
ANTIANXIETY

Cord

Brain Stem

BNZ MIMICS INHIBITORY ACTIONS OF GLYCINE

Figure 8.11. Pharmacologic mechanisms for the benzodiazepine drugs.   The schematic diagram illustrates the actions of γ-aminobutyric acid *(GABA)* and glycine in presynaptic nerve terminals. The benzodiazepine drugs *(BNZ)* facilitate the inhibitory actions of GABA and mimic the inhibitory actions of glycine. (With permission from Richter JJ: Current theories about the mechanisms of benzodiazepines and neuroleptic drugs. *Anesthesiology* 54:66–72, 1981.)

facilitate GABA-ergic neurotransmission, producing sedation and anticonvulsant activity, while other central nervous system effects, such as anxiolysis and muscle relaxation, appear to be due to glycine-mimetic effects in the spinal cord and brainstem (Fig. 8.11).

Specific receptors for the benzodiazepines were first identified in the central nervous system in 1977. The highest concentration of receptors is found in the cerebral cortex, followed by the hypothalamus, cerebellum, corpus striatum and, finally, medulla. The identification of receptors or specific high-affinity binding sites for the benzodiazepines has led to the development of selective antagonists that bind to the benzodiazepine receptor and prevent benzodiazepine agonists from occupying the receptor site. The

benzodiazepine antagonist, flumazenil, is a specific benzodiazepine receptor antagonist and is described later in the chapter. The regional distribution of the benzodiazepine receptors parallels the distribution of GABA receptors, which suggests that, although benzodiazepines do not appear to bind to GABA receptor sites, they probably have some influence on GABA-containing neurons, since the overall effect of benzodiazepines binding to their receptors is to enhance the inhibitory effects of GABA.

The relative receptor binding affinities appear to correlate to some extent with the relative potencies of the individual benzodiazepines. The binding of diazepam, lorazepam, and midazolam has been studied in a receptor model in the rat cortex, when the rate of association with the benzodiazepine receptor for midazolam was slightly greater than for diazepam, but more than 30 fold greater than for lorazepam, indicating that midazolam and diazepam should have a more rapid onset of action. This has been showed to occur in clinical practice. Conversely, diazepam and midazolam dissociate from the receptor faster than lorazepam and, therefore, lorazepam has a longer duration of action than the other two benzodiazepines.

The benzodiazepines have been grouped depending on their elimination half-life as long acting (diazepam, flunitrazepam, and chlorazepate); intermediate acting (lorazepam and oxazepam); and short acting (midazolam and triazolam). The three benzodiazepines of most importance to anesthesiologists are midazolam, diazepam, and lorazepam.

DIAZEPAM

Diazepam is a benzodiazepine that is widely used by anesthesiologists for the induction of anesthesia, as a premedicant, to provide sedation during regional anesthetic techniques and as the sole anesthetic agent during short diagnostic or surgical procedures. Its chemical structure is given in Fig. 8.10. Diazepam is poorly soluble in water, and the solvent vehicle for parenteral diazepam contains several organic solvents (40% propylene glycol, 10% ethyl alcohol, 5% sodium benzoate, and 1.5% alcohol).

Central Nervous System. Both chlordiazepoxide and diazepam depress the limbic system; electrical discharge from the amygdaloid nuclei and amygdalohippocampal transmission are inhibited at low doses that do not depress other areas of the brain. In animal studies, diazepam was found to be a potent tranquilizer, muscle relaxant, and anticonvulsant agent. Aggression and hostility are reduced. In humans, diazepam possesses anxiety-reducing effects in doses that cause much less drowsiness than other tranquilizers.

Diazepam when administered intravenously causes drowsiness in about 30 seconds, although the patient is still responsive, while further administration causes unconsciousness. There is great individual variation in the dose required to produce sleep. Marked anterograde amnesia occurs, but retrograde amnesia is not a feature of diazepam when it is given as an induction agent. Analgesia is only sight, but there is no antanalgesia.

Diazepam has muscle relaxant activity, possibly due to several mechanisms, namely, facilitation of brainstem inhibitory interneurons and interference with interneuronal transmission at the spinal cord level. In addition, diazepam can directly depress motor nerve and muscle function in healthy adults and relax spastic muscles in patients with complete spinal cord transection.

The benzodiazepines have strong anticonvulsant activity and will prevent or stop generalized seizure activity produced by analeptic drugs or local anesthetics.

Diazepam reduces the minimum alveolar concentration (MAC) for halothane and, thus, anesthetic requirements are reduced following diazepam premedication.

Cardiovascular System. Diazepam is frequently used as an intravenous induction agent for patients with cardiac disease, because of its relative cardiovascular stability compared with the intravenous barbiturate anesthetic agents. Studies in humans indicate that, in clinical doses, diazepam does not exert a significant effect on the cardiovascular system, apart from a small fall in arterial blood pressure, comparable to that observed during sleep. Following the administration of 0.2 mg/kg intravenously to humans, minimal cardiovascular depressant effects are observed, although a small transient increase in heart rate may occur. In general, the hemodynamic effects of diazepam in patients who have valvular heart disease with either elevated filling pressures or poor ventricular function are small, and the relative cardiovascular stability of diazepam also makes diazepam a good induction agent for patients with ischemic heart disease. Diazepam, 0.5 mg/kg administered intravenously over 10 minutes to patients with coronary artery disease, causes a small decrease in systolic and mean arterial blood pressure, but heart rate, cardiac output, pulmonary arterial pressure, and systemic and vascular resistance are unchanged. However, diazepam is frequently combined with a narcotic analgesic, such as fentanyl, for anesthetic induction in patients with ischemic heart disease. In this situation, the combination of diazepam and fentanyl (50 μg/kg) decreases blood pressure, cardiac output, and systemic vascular resistance. In the laboratory, diazepam and fentanyl have been found to have additive dose-related negative inotropic effects. Although clinical doses of diazepam alone produce minimal cardiovascular effects, caution should be exercised when doses even as small as 0.125 mg/kg are combined with high-dose fentanyl anesthesia.

Diazepam can dilate coronary blood vessels and increase coronary blood flow in animals and humans; the clinical importance of this is uncertain at the present time. However, although coronary vasodilation may produce redistribution of myocardial flow to normal areas and, hence, increase regional ischemia (coronary steal syndrome), diazepam has not been reported to induce myocardial ischemia. Other studies have demonstrated that diazepam reduces myocardial oxygen demand and consumption. Dysrhythmias are uncommon.

Respiratory System. Following the administration of diazepam, 0.2 mg/kg intravenously, there is little clinically important effect on respiration in normal individuals. However, larger doses cause respiratory depression, and apnea has been reported especially in conjunction with opioid administration. Diazepam, 0.066 mg/kg intravenously, does not affect the respiratory response to carbon dioxide; however, premedication with large doses of diazepam (0.14 mg/kg) is associated with depression of the ventilatory response to carbon dioxide in some patients.

Pharmacokinetics. Diazepam is poorly absorbed when adminstered by the intramuscular route. However, after oral administration, diazepam is rapidly and completely absorbed, peak blood concen-

trations being achieved within 2 hours of administration.

When administered intravenously, there is relatively rapid initial distribution, followed by prolonged elimination. The metabolism of diazepam is slow, and elimination half-lives of 20 to 40 hours have been reported. Diazepam elimination is reduced in patients with cirrhosis. In the elderly patient, clearance is unchanged, but the half-life is prolonged due to an increase in volume of distribution. Diazepam is metabolized in the liver by N-demethylation to the major metabolic product desmethyldiazepam, C-3-hydroxylation of which yields oxazepam (Fig. 8.12). Direct C-3-hydroxylation of diazepam gives N-methyloxazepam. Oxazepam is then rapidly conjugated with glucuronide and excreted in the urine. Desmethyldiazepam has pharmacological activity and is metabolized even more slowly than diazepam. It accumulates in the plasma after repeated doses of diazepam because of its long half-life ($t\frac{1}{2}$ = 48 to 96 hours). After termination of chronic therapy, diazepam and desmethyldiazepam can be detected in the plasma for at least 1 week. Since diazepam has a long elimination half-life and because its metabolite has pharmacological activity, diazepam accumulates with repeated doses. Diazepam does not cause induction of the microsomal drug-metabolizing enzymes in the liver. Diazepam is extensively bound to plasma proteins (96 to 98%).

Diazepam readily crosses the placenta, and many studies have demonstrated higher total concentrations in the fetal circulation than in maternal blood.

Table 8.4 describes the pharmacokinetic parameters of diazepam and contrasts them with midazolam and lorazepam.

Suggested Dosage and Administration. Diazepam is available for oral and parenteral use. Intramuscular administration of diazepan is painful, and absorption from this site is often erratic and incomplete. Therefore, the oral or intravenous route is preferred. Thrombophlebitis is a frequent problem following intravenous injection, and diazepam should be given

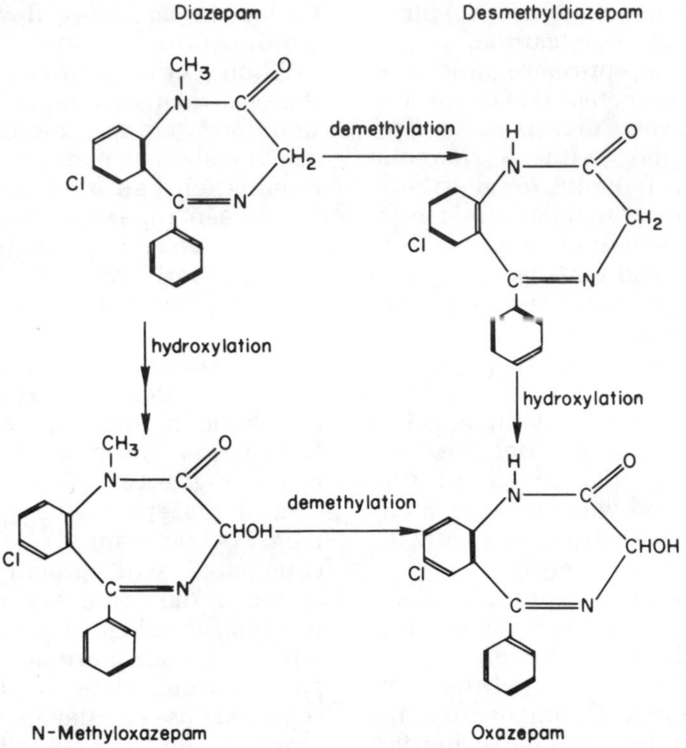

Figure 8.12.   Pathways for the biotransformation of diazepam to its major metabolites.

via a large vein. A cloudy suspension often forms in the intravenous line. Diazepam should not be mixed with other drugs. Midazolam is a rational alternative to diazepam when a parenteral benzodiazepine is required and pain on injection is a concern.

Diazepam is often given as a premedicant drug, because of its ability to allay

anxiety and apprehension in doses of 0.1 to 0.2 mg/kg orally, 1 to 2 hours before surgery. Diazepam is also a good induction agent for the aged, the poor-risk patient with cardiac disease, and the severely traumatized patient, when diazepam doses of 0.1 to 0.6 mg/kg intravenously may be required to induce unconsciousness. Rarely, diazepam may

Table 8.4.
Pharmacokinetic Parameters for the Benzodiazepines, Diazepam, Midazolam, and Lorazepam

Parameter	Diazepam	Midazolam	Lorazepam
V_d (L/kg)	0.7–1.7	1.1–2.5	1.1
Distribution $t_{1/2}$ (min)	30–40	6–30	2.7
Terminal $t_{1/2}$ (hr)	24–57	1.7–4.0	14.0
Clearance (ml/min/kg)	0.24–0.53	4.4–11.1	1.1
Protein bound (%)	98	94	91

Most of the data are taken from Reves JG, Fragen RJ, Vinik HR, Greenblatt DJ: Midazolam: pharmacology and uses. *Anesthesiology* 62:310-324,1985; Greenblatt DJ, Shader RI, Franke K, MacLaughlin DS, Harmatz JS, Allen MD, Werner A, Woo E: Pharmacokinetics and bioavailability of intravenous, intramuscular, and oral lorazepam in humans. *J Pharm Sci* 68:57-63, 1979; and Greenblatt DJ, Abernethy DR, Locniskar A, Harmatz JS, Limjuco RA, Shader RI: Effect of age, gender, and obesity on midazolam kinetics. *Anesthesiology* 61:27-35, 1984.

cause acute hypotension, and diazepam should be given slowly in 2.5-mg increments, the dose being titrated according to the clinical effect.

Other uses of diazepam in anesthesia and surgery include cardioversion, endoscopic procedures, dentistry, and minor surgical procedures. Diazepam has been used to provide sedation during labor and delivery, while large doses have been given as sedatives and anticonvulsants to eclamptic patients. However, in some cases diazepam given to the mother has caused lethargy, hypotonia, hypothermia, and respiratory depression in the neonate. Therefore, doses above 10 mg should be given with extreme caution during labor and delivery.

Toxicity, Precautions, and Contraindications. Unwanted effects that occur with diazepam administration include central nervous system depression, drowsiness, muscle weakness, ataxia, dysarthria, and respiratory depression. Tolerance and physical dependence may occur with chronic use. Pain and phlebitis at the injection site have been previously mentioned. The elimination half-life is increased in patients with liver disease and the elderly, and the dose should be reduced for these patients. Drug interactions are infrequent, but an important cause of side effects due to the use of benzodiazepines is the interaction with alcohol. Patients receiving diazepam on an outpatient basis should also be cautioned against taking other central nervous system depressants. Cimetidine reduces the clearance and prolongs the elimination half-life of both diazepam and its active metabolite, desmethyldiazepam. The degree of sedation is increased when diazepam is administered with cimetidine compared to when diazepam is given alone, reflecting the higher plasma concentrations of both parent drug and metabolite (see Chapter 23).

MIDAZOLAM

Midazolam is a water-soluble benzodiazepine with a low incidence of injection pain and postinjection phlebitis and thrombosis. It is a useful agent for premedication, sedation, and the induction of anesthesia.

Chemical Structure. Figure 8.10 gives the chemical structure of midazolam, which is a benzodiazepine with an imidazole ring structure. This drug exhibits a pH-dependent ring-opening phenomenon, whereby the benzodiazepine ring closes at pH values greater than 4.0 but opens reversibly at pH values less than 4.0. Physiological pH of 7.4 maintains the closed ring structure and may enhance lipid solubility. In an acidic aqueous solution, midazolam is water soluble (pK_a of midazolam is 6.5) and the parenteral formulation therefore does not contain organic solvents, such as propylene glycol, and is buffered to an acidic pH of 3.5. Once midazolam enters the body, the pH rapidly increases to 7.4, and the solubility properties of the drug change. At physiological pH, midazolam becomes highly lipid soluble; the partition coefficient between n-octanol and phosphate buffer at pH 3 is 34, but increases to 475 at pH 7.5. This increases the rate at which it enters the brain and increases the rate of onset of activity following intravenous administration. Midazolam is the most lipid-soluble benzodiazepine currently available, followed next by diazepam. Lorazepam is much less lipophilic.

The water solubility of midazolam results in a low incidence of injection pain and venous thrombosis when compared with diazepam, which is formulated in organic solvents.

Central Nervous System. Midazolam possesses anxiolytic, hypnotic, anticonvulsant, muscle relaxant, and anterograde amnestic properties, characteristic of the benzodiazepine class of drugs. It reduces cerebral metabolic rate and cerebral blood flow. However, cerebral perfusion pressure (which is equal to mean arterial pressure minus intracranial pressure) may be slightly decreased following midazolam administration, due to a tendency for systemic blood pressure to fall more than intracranial pressure. Intracranial pressure is not altered when midazolam, 0.27 mg/kg, is used for the induction of anesthesia in patients with intracranial lesions and, therefore, midazolam is a safe anesthetic agent for neurosurgical patients with intracranial pathology. Midazolam causes profound anterograde amnesia, which is more intense than diazepam, but of shorter duration than lorazepam. Emergence from induction is more rapid with midazolam than diazepam, but not when compared with thiopental. Thus, recovery times tend to be more prolonged following midazolam administration compared to thiopental; this may be important in an outpatient setting. Like diazepam, midazolam reduces the anesthetic requirements (MAC) for halothane in healthy patients.

Cardiovascular System. In healthy patients, midazolam, 0.15 mg/kg, causes a moderate reduction in systolic and diastolic blood pressure and an increase in heart rate. Systemic vascular resistance may decrease. Midazolam has also been administered to patients with ischemic heart disease, when the anesthetic agent in doses of 0.2 to 0.3 mg/kg caused similar hemodynamic changes. It is important to recognize that the cardiovascular effects produced by midazolam (0.3 mg/kg) are similar to those produced by thiopental when the barbiturate is administered in hypnotic doses of 3 to 4 mg/kg. However, when compared with diazepam (0.5 mg/kg) in the setting of ischemic heart disease, midazolam (0.2 mg/kg) has been shown to produce a greater decrease in blood pressure and increase in heart rate accompanied by a slightly greater decrease in systemic vascular resistance. Midazolam does not abolish the hemodynamic response to tracheal intubation, but smaller increases in heart rate and blood pressure appear to accompany induction by midazolam then diazepam.

The cardiovascular effects of midazolam can be explained by an understanding of the direct acute hemodynamic effects and the compensatory indirect homeostatic reflex changes which follow. Midazolam decreases myocardial contractility, decreases systemic vascular resistance, and causes venodilation, all of which result in a fall in arterial blood pressure. The decrease in systemic vascular resistance and venodilation reduce

cardiac filling pressure which further reduces cardiac output. The resultant hypotension activates the baroreceptor reflex arc, catecholamine stimulation occurs, and there is thus an increase in heart rate and myocardial contractility.

Midazolam administration to patients with stable coronary artery disease produces moderate decreases in coronary sinus blood flow and myocardial oxygen consumption, but no change in coronary vascular resistance. In contrast, diazepam and flunitrazepam have both been reported to decrease coronary vascular resistance. Coronary vasodilation or loss of autoregulation has been implicated in producing redistribution of myocardial blood flow to normal areas, thereby inducing regional ischemia (coronary steal syndrome). However, diazepam, flunitrazepam, and midazolam have not been reported to induce regional myocardial ischemia. Midazolam (0.2 mg/kg) has been successfully administered to patients with valvular heart disease, when the induction of anesthesia was associated with relative hemodynamic stability; there was a small decrease in mean arterial pressure and systemic vascular resistance, and the cardiac index was unchanged.

Respiratory System. In common with other intravenous anesthetic induction agents, midazolam causes dose-dependent respiratory depression. When midazolam is administered for the induction of anesthesia, apnea may occur, but the incidence and duration of apnea are greater with thiopental than midazolam. Equipotent doses of midazolam (0.15 mg/kg) and diazepam (0.3 mg/kg) equally depress the respiratory response to carbon dioxide. Small intravenous doses of midazolam (0.075 mg/kg) do not affect the ventilatory response to carbon dioxide, so that doses of midazolam used for premedication and sedation are not associated with clinically important respiratory depression in healthy individuals. Midazolam does not appear to cause bronchoconstriction. In patients with chronic obstructive pulmonary disease, the respiratory depressant effects of midazolam may be greater and more prolonged than those associated with normal healthy patients.

Other Effects. Adrenal steroidogenesis is not suppressed by the continuous intravenous administration of midazolam in the intensive care unit, in contrast to the suppression of adrenal steroidogenesis produced by etomidate (see page 209).

Pharmacokinetics. Midazolam is metabolized in the liver by hydroxylation to the major metabolite, 1-hydroxy midazolam, and a secondary metabolite, 4-hydroxy midazolam. Both 1- and 4-hydroxy midazolam metabolites are conjugated and then excreted in the urine as glucuronides. Although the metabolites have pharmacological activity, they are probably of little clinical importance. Very little unchanged midazolam (less than 1%) is excreted in the urine.

Midazolam is highly lipid soluble and, therefore, rapidly crosses the blood-brain barrier to gain access to benzodiazepine receptors in the central nervous system. It, therefore, has a rapid onset of clinical effect. Following intravenous administration (5.0 mg), midazolam concentrations decline biexponentially, with a distribution half-life of 6 to 30 minutes and an elimination half-life that may range from 1 to 4 hours (Table 8.4). The volume of distribution generally averages between 1 and 2.5 L/kg. The total clearance approximates 50% of hepatic blood flow and is in the region of 7 to 9 ml/min/kg. Orally administered midazolam undergoes substantial first-pass hepatic extraction, so that about 50% of the drug does not reach the systemic circulation. Midazolam is highly protein bound (94 to 96%).

Midazolam has a relatively large volume of distribution, short elimination half-life, and high clearance (Table 8.4), giving the drug a short duration of action and rapid recovery after single-dose intravenous administration. In contrast, diazepam has a high volume of distribution due to its high lipid solubility but possesses a low clearance and long elimination half-life so that recovery may be prolonged. Accumulation is thus much less likely to occur following repeated doses of midazolam than following diazepam

repeat-dose administration. Lorazepam has a low clearance (Table 8.4) and, therefore, its duration of action is longer than that of midazolam, and accumulation results with repeated doses.

The pharmacokinetic parameters of midazolam are altered in the elderly and obese; midazolam elimination half-life is increased and clearance reduced in elderly males. Midazolam volume of distribution is increased in obesity, leading to a prolonged elimination half-life with no change in clearance. Thus, continuous intravenous infusion rates should be reduced in both of these groups of patients.

There is minimal alteration of midazolam clearance in chronic renal disease. Plasma protein binding of midazolam is reduced in renal disease, but chronic renal failure does not alter the pharmacokinetics of unbound midazolam.

Suggested Dosage and Administration. Midazolam is available as a parenteral formulation (5 mg/ml and 1.0 mg/ml) for intravenous and intramuscular use. Midazolam may be given as a premedicant drug in doses of 0.07 to 0.08 mg/kg i.m. (i.e., 5.0 mg for an average adult) in which situation it has excellent anxiolytic and hypnotic properties. There is rapid and reliable absorption of midazolam from intramuscular sites, and intramuscular administration is not accompanied by pain or local irritation. It should be given intramuscularly 30 to 60 minutes before surgery, since peak effects occur 30 to 45 minutes after intramuscular injection.

Midazolam may be used intravenously for the induction of anesthesia in doses that range from 0.1 to 0.35 mg/kg depending on age, premedication, and patient physical status. It is extremely important to titrate the dose slowly according to clinical effect; increments as small as 1.0 mg should be cautiously administered until loss of consciousness is produced. The intravenous induction dose should be reduced in the presence of narcotic premedication, in patients with severe systemic disease, and in the elderly age group.

Midazolam is a logical agent to use as a hypnotic-amnesic drug during the maintenance of anesthesia. Incremental doses of 0.1 mg/kg have been administered with supplementation with fentanyl and nitrous oxide. The pharmacokinetic parameters of midazolam indicate that this drug may be administered by continuous intravenous infusion since it is likely that cumulation will be rare, and rapid recovery should result following discontinuation of the infusion. In addition, the metabolites are pharmaologically inactive. Prolonged infusions of 0.025 mg/kg/hour preceded by a bolus of 0.05 mg/kg have been administered to volunteers for over 26 hours when steady-state concentrations of around 34 to 48 ng/ml were rapidly achieved, and only a small and clinically unimportant (4 to 16%) fluctuation in individual steady-state concentrations was observed. Sedation occurs at plasma concentrations of 35 to 55 ng/ml, while sleep and deep hypnosis occur at plasma concentrations greater than 300 ng/ml. Concentrations that produce satisfactory sedation in the intensive care unit appear to be in the range of 145 to 250 ng/ml. Midazolam has been administered by continuous infusion for prolonged sedation of critical adult patients in the intensive care unit; the loading dose ranged from 0.15 to 0.5 mg/kg followed by a maintenance infusion rate of 0.1 to 20.0 μg/kg/min, depending on the degree of sedation produced. Midazolam has also been administered as an infusion of 2 to 6 μg/kg/min, preceded by a bolus of 0.2 mg/kg to provide sedation in a pediatric intensive care unit. Thus, as a general guide for midazolam administration by intravenous infusion, a satisfactory starting regimen appears to be 0.1 to 0.2 mg/kg as a loading dose followed by an infusion of 1.5 to 3.0 μg/kg/min (or 0.1 to 0.2 mg/kg/hour) titrated to clinical effect.

Midazolam is an ideal agent to provide intravenous sedation for cardioversion, endoscopic procedures, and during regional anesthetic procedures. Midazolam, 0.1 mg/kg, is generally administered for intravenous sedation in these circumstances.

Toxicity, Precautions, and Contraindications. Midazolam is generally a well-tolerated drug when administered intra-

venously for sedation, anesthesia induction, or intramuscularly for preoperative medication. Midazolam has a low incidence of phlebitis, thrombosis, and thrombophlebitis following intravenous injection. Unwanted effects that occur with midazolam administration include central nervous system depression with drowsiness and ataxia and cardiorespiratory depression. Midazolam should be used cautiously in patients with chronic obstructive pulmonary disease and should be avoided in the presence of severe hypovolemia. Dosage adjustments should be made for the elderly and poor-risk patient. Midazolam affects psychomotor function for several hours following administration, and patients should not drive for at least 8 hours after receiving the drug.

The histamine H_2-receptor antagonists, cimetidine and ranitidine, are frequently administered as part of a premedicant regimen before anesthesia and surgery. However, both cimetidine and ranitidine have been shown to increase the bioavailability of orally administered midazolam. In addition, there is a more marked hypnotic effect of midazolam in patients pretreated with ranitidine. It is important to note that other workers have failed to observe an interaction of either cimetidine or ranitidine with both intravenous and oral midazolam administration. The effect of cimetidine and ranitidine in increasing the systemic availability of oral midazolam, if it exists, is most probably due to a reduction in hepatic clearance; caution should therefore be exercised in prescribing midazolam for patients already receiving treatment with cimetidine or rantidine.

The central nervous system depression associated with midazolam may be reversed with the benzodiazepine antagonist, flumazenil (see later in the chapter).

LORAZEPAM

The structural formula of lorazepam is given in Figure 8.10. Lorazepam possesses a 3-hydroxy substitution on the benzodiazepine nucleus. It is much less lipophilic than diazepam and midazolam and therefore has a slow onset of action (20 to 40 minutes) when given by the intravenous route, making the drug unacceptable for use as an intravenous induction agent. However, it is used by anesthesiologists for premedication and therefore is included in this section.

Pharmacological Effects. Lorazepam is a benzodiazepine with pharmacological actions that are similar to diazepam, but of longer duration. It causes profound anterograde amnesia, and an intravenous bolus injection of 4 mg may produce this effect for up to 24 hours. Cardiovascular and respiratory stability is good.

Pharmacokinetics. Lorazepam is well absorbed orally, peak plasma concentrations being achieved within 3 hours of an oral dose. Systemic availability after oral administration is good, 80 to 93% of the oral dose reaching the systemic circulation. Lorazepam is extensively bound to plasma protein, with a free unbound fraction of 8 to 12%. The elimination half-life of lorazepam is about 10 to 14 hours (Table 8.4). Lorazepam is conjugated in the liver to the pharmacologically inactive glucuronide, which is then excreted in the urine.

The clinical implications of benzodiazepine oxidation versus conjugation are important. Essentially all benzodiazepines are metabolized in the liver by either microsomal oxidation as for diazepam or glucuronide conjugation as for lorazepam. Drug oxidation is depessed by many factors such as old age, disease states (e.g., hepatic cirrhosis), and concomitant drug administration (e.g., cimetidine). Conjugation, however, tends to be less impaired by the same factors. Thus, the elimination half-life of diazepam and chlordiazepoxide is increased in cirrhosis, but the elimination half-life of lorazepam, a conjugated benzodiazepine, is unaffected by cirrhosis. Similarly, cimetidine inhibits the metabolism of diazepam, but not lorazepam (see page 616).

Although intramuscular lorazepam is painful, it is rapidly and nearly completely absorbed from the injection site, in contrast to diazepam which is poorly absorbed when administered by this route.

Suggested Dosage and Administration. Lorazepam can be administered orally, in-

tramuscularly, or intravenously in doses of 1 to 5 mg to the adult patient. At the present time, it is used mainly by anesthesiologists in preanesthetic medication because of its profound amnesic, tranquilizing, and "anxiolytic" effects. Many patients do not recall events of the operative day after lorazepam premedication.

Flunitrazepam is a new benzodiazepine intravenous anesthetic 10 times more potent than diazepam. It is insoluble in water and is characterized by a slow onset, prolonged recovery time, and marked interindividual variability. Cardiovascular, amnesic, and sedative-hypnotic effects of flunitrazepam are similar to diazepam.

BENZODIAZEPINE ANTAGONISTS

A new class of specific benzodiazepine receptor antagonists has recently been described. The class consists of imidazobenzodiazepine derivatives which selectively inhibit the central nervous system effects of the classic benzodiazepine group of drugs by acting as antagonists at benzodiazepine receptors. Flumazenil is an example of a specific benzodiazepine receptor antagonist.

Flumazenil. Flumazenil, an imidazobenzodiazepine derivative structurally related to midazolam, is a new benzodiazepine antagonist. Flumazenil blocks the central nervous system effects of benzodiazepines and, thus, reverses the sedation and amnesia produced by midazolam and diazepam. It antagonizes the anxiolytic, muscle-relaxant, ataxic, anticonvulsant, sedative, and amnestic properties of the benzodiazepines, but is specific for the benzodiazepine receptor and therefore does not antagonize the effects of barbiturates, opiates, or ethanol. In very high doses, flumazenil has weak benzodiazepine-like agonist activity in animals, but so far, flumazenil does not appear to produce any clinically important agonist effects at therapeutic doses. Following intravenous administration, the onset of action is very rapid (within 5 minutes), but the duration of effect is relatively short, about 1 to 3.5 hours in keeping with an elimination half-life of about 60 minutes. Flumazenil appears to possess minimal cardiorespiratory effects, and early studies indicate that reversal of diazepam sedation in patients with coronary artery disease with flumazenil does not appear to be associated with any important changes in cardiovascular parameters. Flumazenil should prove useful in the reversal of the benzodiazepine effects of midazolam and diazepam, both following surgical anesthesia and in the intensive care unit. The dose required to reverse benzodiazepine-induced sedation is approximately 0.4 mg intravenously, with an initial starting dose of 0.1 mg; further 0.1-mg increments may be given up to a maximum of 1.0 mg.

Neuroleptanesthetics

The state of neuroleptanalgesia or neuroleptanesthesia is produced by the combination of the neuroleptic properties of the butyrophenone group of drugs with the profound analgesia induced with potent short-acting narcotics such as fentanyl. Neurolepsis was first described by Delay (1959) as a characteristic drug-induced behavioral syndrome in animals and humans. This syndrome is manifest in animals as inhibition of purposeful movements and learned conditioned behavior, inhibition of amphetamine-induced arousal, an increased tendency to maintain an induced posture (cataleptic immobility), and marked inhibition of apomorphine-induced vomiting. Drugs with neuroleptic properties may also exhibit other side effects, such as α-adrenergic blockade, hypotension, hypothermia, sedation, extrapyramidal effects, and anticholinergic properties. A neuroleptic state can be induced by a wide variety of drugs, but those of interest to the anesthesiologist fall into two classes:

1. Phenothiazines—of which chlorpromazine is the prototype;
2. Butyrophenones—typified by droperidol and haloperidol.

The mode of action of the neuroleptic drugs is thought to be due to competitive antagonism at dopaminergic receptors in the brain. The neuroleptic drugs have a predilection for areas in the brain rich in dopaminergic receptors, especially the chemoreceptor trigger zone (CTZ) and the extrapyramidal nigrostriatum.

The analgesic drugs that are used as part of this technique are described in Chapter 7, and only the butyrophenones will be discussed here.

BUTYROPHENONES

The butyrophenones induce a state of cataleptic immobility in humans where the patient appears to be in a tranquil trance-like state, free from pain and dissociated from his surroundings. However, many patients describe a state of mental restlessness and agitation not apparent to the observer. Hallucinations, loss of bodily image, and extrapyramidal side effects may also occur. In addition, the butyrophenones are potent inhibitors of chemoreceptor trigger zone-mediated vomiting. These drugs possess minimal cardiovascular and respiratory side effects.

DROPERIDOL

Droperidol, first synthesized by Janssen, is a butyrophenone derivative whose structural formula is given in Figure 8.13. It is frequently administered in combination with fentanyl as part of a neurolept technique. Although it has a faster onset and shorter duration of action than haloperidol, it does have a relatively long half-life (2 to 3 hours), and thus the pharmacological effects of droperidol often outlast those of the simultaneously administered fentanyl. It is a

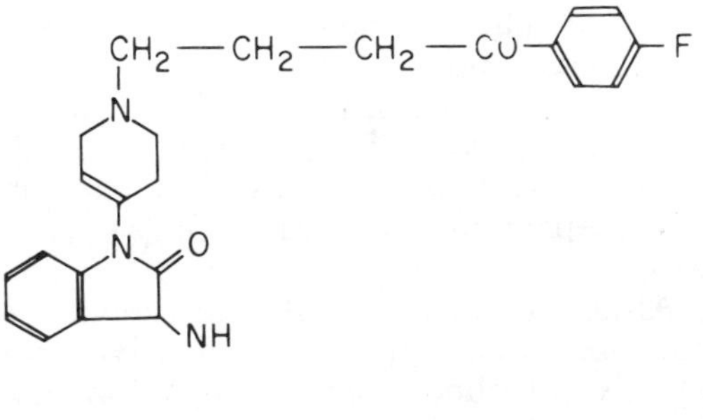

DROPERIDOL

Figure   8.13.   Structural   formula   of droperidol.

powerful antiemetic and is effective against opiate-induced vomiting. In addition, it has extrapyramidal side effects. In general, droperidol produces small hemodynamic changes, but it can inconsistently cause hypotension due to central nervous system and α-adrenergic blocking effects. Although the effect of droperidol on peripheral vascular resistance is small, there may be a pronounced fall in blood pressure following the use of droperidol in patients who are already receiving other vasodilator therapy, or who are hypovolemic. Arrhythmias are infrequent. Respiratory side effects are minimal. It has no analgesic effect. In humans, the combination of fentanyl and droperidol has little effect on or reduces cerebral blood flow.

Suggested Dosage and Administration. Droperidol is available for parenteral use: 2.5 mg/ml or as a fixed-dose mixture, "Innovar," where each ml contains 0.05 mg of fentanyl and 2.5 mg of droperidol. For premedication, 5 to 10 mg intramuscularly may be given to the adult (0.1 to 0.2 mg/kg) 1 hour before surgery. The intramuscular injection of droperidol alone has proven an unsatisfactory preoperative sedative, being associated with poor sedation, inner mental anxiety, and even refusal of surgery. Droperidol may also be administered intravenously for the induction of anesthesia in incremental doses of up to 10 mg alone or in combination with fentanyl. A typical procedure for the induction of anesthesia using the droperidol and fentanyl combination would be the slow intravenous administration of fentanyl, 0.004 mg/kg, and droperidol, 0.2 mg/kg, in small increments until the patient is asleep. This can then be followed by the administration of a muscle relaxant, intubation, and "neuroleptanesthesia" using nitrous oxide and oxygen. Unless the total dose of narcotics used is very low, it is important that the patient's ventilation be controlled during this type of anesthesia as respiration is invariably depressed. Neuroleptanalgesia and anesthesia have a wide variety of clinical applications including premedication, neuroradiological and neurosurgical procedures, aug-menting regional anesthetics, endoscopic procedures, repeat burns dressings, cardiovascular surgery, and as a supplement to nitrous oxide/muscle relaxant anesthesia.

Toxicity, Precautions, and Contraindications. Droperidol should be avoided in patients with Parkinsonism.

HALOPERIDOL

Haloperidol is a butyrophenone that is not often used by anesthesiologists because it has such a long duration of action. However, this property makes it useful for the drug treatment of psychoses, such as acute mania and schizophrenia. Haloperidol produces a high incidence of extrapyramidal reactions.

Imidazole Derivatives: Etomidate

Etomidate is a carboxylated imidazole derivative (Fig. 8.14) and possesses a high therapeutic index. Although water soluble, etomidate is formulated in 35% propylene glycol.

Central Nervous System. An induction dose of 0.1 to 0.4 mg/kg produces the rapid onset of sleep in one arm-brain circulation time, with the patient usually awakening within 7 to 14 minutes. Etomidate has a high incidence of excitatory phenomena, such as spontaneous involuntary muscle movement and tremor. Myoclonic movements occur in 10 to 35% of patients, but are not associated

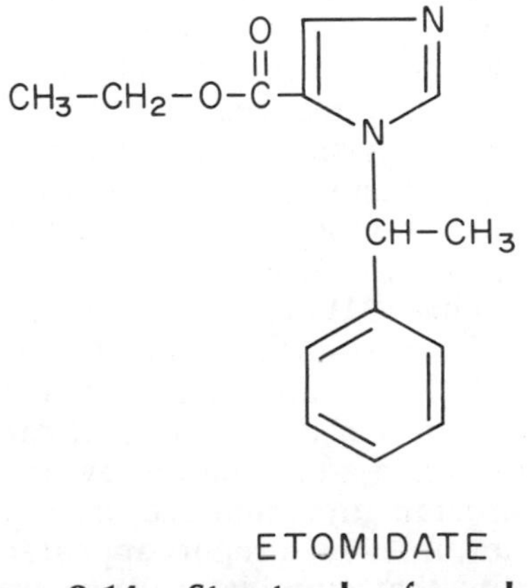

ETOMIDATE

Figure 8.14. Structural formula of etomidate.

with EEG changes. Opiate premedication reduces the severity and incidence of these side effects. Etomidate reduces both intracranial pressure and intraocular pressure and therefore is safe to use in patients with intracranial pathology. Cerebral metabolic rate, cerebral oxygen consumption, and cerebral blood flow are reduced. Since etomidate does not decrease systemic arterial pressure, cerebral perfusion pressure is maintained.

Cardiovascular System. When etomidate is compared to other currently available intravenous anesthetic agents, it is seen to cause the least hemodynamic effects; the lack of cardiovascular depression is an important consideration for patients with hypovolemia, cardiac tamponade, or low cardiac output in emergency situations in which rapid anesthesia induction is required. In healthy patients or patients with compensated ischemic heart disease, etomidate, 0.3 mg/kg, causes little change in heart rate, pulmonary artery pressure, cardiac index, systemic vascular resistance, or systemic arterial blood pressure. However, patients with valvular heart disease may exhibit a fall in systemic arterial blood pressure and a decrease in pulmonary artery pressure and cardiac index in some instances. Arrhythmias are uncommon.

Respiratory System. Etomidate reduces tidal volume and respiratory rate and may cause apnea, depending on dose and speed of injection. These decreases are less than those changes associated with thiopental administration. Etomidate does not appear to cause histamine release. Etomidate, 0.3 mg/kg, depresses the ventilatory response to carbon dioxide. Laryngospasm, cough, and hiccough may occur during induction with etomidate; the frequency may be reduced with opiate premedication.

Other Effects. When etomidate was introduced into anesthetic practice in Europe in 1973, it rapidly gained wide acceptance as a sedative for critically ill patients when administered by continuous infusion in intensive care units. However, in 1983, a report appeared that suggested that etomidate was associated with an increase in mortality in critically ill, multiple-trauma patients, due to adrenocortical hypofunction, since plasma cortisol levels were decreased in these patients. Etomidate has since been shown to be an even more potent inhibitor of steroid synthesis in vitro than metyrapone. Patients who receive etomidate infusions have marked adrenocortical suppression, which may still be present as long as 4 days after discontinuation of the infusion. Prolonged infusions of etomidate are associated with depressed cortisol production, decreases in plasma cortisol concentrations, and a flat or blunted endocrine response to exogenous adrenocorticotropic hormone (ACTH) administration. The effect of etomidate on adrenal function is present in patients receiving etomidate for induction followed by a short infusion or even as a single dose (0.4 mg/kg) for anesthesia induction. Etomidate when given as a single induction dose suppresses adrenal function for approximately 5 to 8 hours. The absence of adrenocortical response after etomidate administration is now known to be a result of adrenocortical enzyme inhibition, and the site of action has been identified as a concentration-dependent inhibition of the cytochrome P-450-dependent mitochondrial enzymes, 17-α- and 11-β-hydroxylase enzymes (Fig. 8.15). Thus, etomidate adminisration causes a decrease in cortisol, 17-α-hydroxyprogesterone, aldosterone, and corticosterone production (Fig. 8.16). Although etomidate may still be cautiously used for anesthesia induction as a single dose and may even have advantages in special situations, it should no longer be administered by continuous intravenous infusion.

Pharmacokinetics. Etomidate is probably primarily metabolized by ester hydrolysis or N-dealkylation in the liver. Etomidate is not hydrolyzed by human plasma cholinesterase. Following intravenous administration, etomidate produces a very short duration of hypnosis, due to rapid distribution and uptake into peripheral tissues, with an initial distribution half-life ($t_{1/2\alpha}$) of 2.6 to 3.9 minutes. The volume of distribution is about 2.3 to 4.5 L/kg, while the terminal elimination

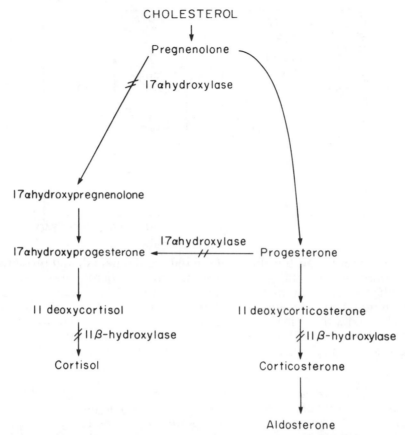

CHOLESTEROL
↓
Pregnenolone

17αhydroxylase

17αhydroxypregnenolone

17αhydroxyprogesterone ◄—— 17αhydroxylase —— Progesterone

11 deoxycortisol   11 deoxycorticosterone

11β-hydroxylase   11β-hydroxylase

Cortisol   Corticosterone

Aldosterone

Figure 8.15.   Inhibition of adrenal steroidogenesis by etomidate: the biosynthetic pathways for cortisol and aldosterone.   Etomidate inhibits the enzymes 17α-hydroxylase and 11 β-hydroxylase at the sites of action marked #. Thus, cortisol and aldosterone concentrations are reduced.

half-life has been reported to range from 70 to 275 minutes. Plasma clearance is between 11.5 and 25 ml/kg/min. Etomidate has an intermediate hepatic extraction ratio of 0.67. Etomidate is 75% bound to plasma proteins, and the unbound fraction is increased in renal and hepatic disease, probably due to lower albumin levels present in both these disease states. The disposition of etomidate is altered in elderly patients in a similar manner to that shown for thiopental (see page 190). The dose required for anesthesia induction is reduced in elderly patients, but using an inhibitory sigmoid E_{max} pharmacodynamic model similar to that described for thiopental, "sensitivity" (IC_{50}) to etomidate (i.e., the plasma concentration required to produce a given ef-

fect) has been shown to be unaltered with aging. However, the volume of distribution of the central compartment is reduced in the elderly, with resultant elevation in plasma etomidate concentrations. In addition, the clearance of etomidate is reduced in the aged.

Etomidate and fentanyl have been shown to interact in an interesting manner. During infusion of fentanyl, the clearance and volume of distribution of etomidate are reduced so that there may be prolongation of recovery after fentanyl-etomidate anesthesia. The mechanism for this drug interaction remains to be determined.

Like cimetidine, another substituted imidazole derivative, etomidate, has been shown to inhibit drug metabolism

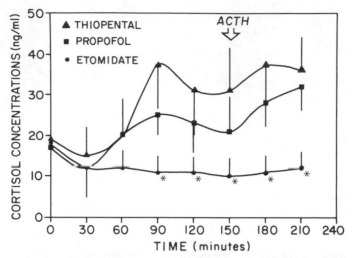

Figure 8.16. Comparison of the effects of etomidate, thiopental, and propofol on adrenocortical steroidogenesis. Blood cortisol concentrations before and after induction of anesthesia with thiopental, etomidate, or propofol. The ACTH stimulation test was performed 150 minutes post induction. *, $P < 0.05$ between blood cortisol concentrations for etomidate compared with those for thiopental and propofol. (With permission from Fragen RT, Weiss HW, Molteni A: The effect of propofol on adrenocortical steroidogenesis: a comparative study with etomidate and thiopental. *Anesthesiology* 66:839–842, 1987.)

both in vitro and in vivo in animals and humans. However, the effect is small, and clinically important adverse drug interactions are unlikely to occur. Although there has been speculation that the solvent for etomidate, propylene glycol, might be responsible for the inhibition of liver metabolism, propylene glycol has not been shown to have any significant effect on antipyrine clearance in humans.

Suggested Dose and Administration. Etomidate is available for intravenous administration as a 2-mg/ml solution. The dose for induction of anesthesia is 0.2 to 0.6 mg/kg and should be titrated to clinical effect in each patient; the average dose is usually 0.3 mg/kg injected over 30 to 60 seconds. Although etomidate has been administered by continuous infusion, its use by this route is now no longer recommended. The relative cardiovascular stability of etomidate makes it a useful agent in the presence of hypovolemia or low cardiac output.

Toxicity, Precautions, and Contraindications. Etomidate causes pain on injection when formulated in water; the incidence

of pain has been reported to range from 15 to 50%. The new formulation of etomidate in propylene glycol appears to have reduced the incidence of pain on injection to about 10%. Pain on injection and spontaneous involuntary movements can be decreased by narcotic and benzodiazepine premedication. The use of etomidate for anesthesia induction is associated with a relatively high incidence of postoperative nausea and vomiting.

Since etomidate inhibits adrenal steroidogenesis as discussed above, the clinical use of etomidate by continuous intravenous infusion is no longer justified, although it is still considered a useful agent for the induction of anesthesia.

The Hindered Phenols: Propofol

Propofol or 2,6-diisopropyl phenol represents a new class of intravenous anesthetic induction agents (Fig. 8.17). Propofol is insoluble in aqueous solution. It was first introduced into anesthetic practice in 1977 as a 1.0% solution solubilized in cremophor EL. This formulation was associated with hypersensitivity reac-

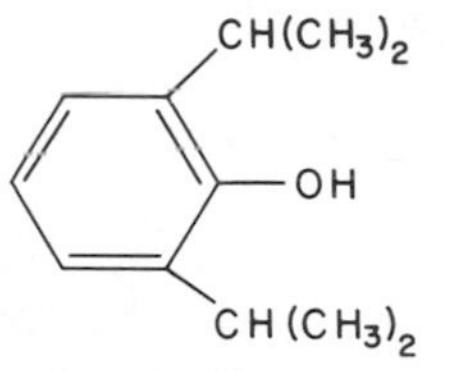

PROPOFOL

Figure 8.17. Structural formula of propofol.

tions in susceptible individuals. Because of the well-recognized concerns regarding anaphylactoid reactions in patients who receive anesthetic agents solubilized in cremophor EL, propofol is now formulated as a 1.0% egg lecithin emulsion which consists of 10% soybean oil, 2.25% glycerol, and 1.2% egg phosphatide. The new formulation does not cause histamine release and does not appear to produce serious hypersensitivity reactions. Induction of anesthesia is rapid with propofol (comparable to thiopental), and maintenance of anesthesia can be achieved with either continuous intravenous infusion or intermittent bolus injections. Nitrous oxide or opioids are often administered to provide analgesia.

Central Nervous System. Propofol produces the fast onset (less than 1 minute) of unconsciousness with rapid recovery; propofol, 2.0 mg/kg, produces a duration of anesthesia of about 4 minutes. It produces dose-dependent depression of central nervous system function. At low doses, propofol causes sedation and drowsiness, and as the dose is increased, loss of consciousness and anesthesia ensue. Propofol reduces intraocular pressure. The incidence of excitatory phenomena such as spontaneous involuntary movement is low, while myoclonic movements are not as frequent or severe as those associated with etomidate administration. Although recovery after propofol induction in the setting of inhalational anesthesia is not more rapid than that of thiopental, patients on awakening from anesthesia appear to have less postoperative sedation, are alert, and show no "hang over" effect. Some studies have shown that recovery from propofol when administered by continuous infusion is faster than that following inhalational isoflurane anesthesia, but the difference in recovery is usually small (under 10 minutes). Extensive studies of psychomotor function following propofol anesthesia have shown that impairment is minimal and that recovery is rapid and is at least as good or better than methohexital and isoflurane. Complete recovery may take up to 3.0 hours. Propofol anesthesia produces characteristic changes in the EEG (EEG frequency decreases on induction with a proportional increase in β activity), and blood concentrations of propofol negatively correlate with EEG frequency. Propofol provides a low incidence of nausea, vomiting, and headache.

Respiratory System. Propofol produces dose-dependent respiratory depression and, in some patients, may cause apnea. The incidence of apnea is greater after propofol than thiopental and may approach 100% if given in conjunction with a premedicant. A reduction in tidal volume and increase in respiratory rate precede the apneic period. Propofol decreases the slope of the ventilatory response to rebreathing carbon dioxide curve by about 40 to 60%. Laryngospasn, cough, and hiccough occasionally occur.

Cardiovascular Effects. Propofol produces dose-related cardiovascular depression similar in magnitude to or greater than that produced by thiopental in healthy patients. After induction of anesthesia, there is a decrease in arterial blood pressure and systemic vascular resistance accompanied by a compensatory increase in heart rate. Propofol has been administered to patients with ischemic heart disease, when an induction dose of 2.0 mg/kg produced a decrease in arterial blood pressure, peripheral vascular resistance, and a fall in stroke volume while cardiac output remained unchanged, but heart rate increased. On the other hand, in patients with valvular heart disease, propofol lowered mean arterial blood pressure, but heart rate decreased. These changes were associated with no change in cardiac index or stroke volume index.

Infusions of propofol for anesthesia maintenance for patients with coronary artery or peripheral vascular disease produce decreases in mean arterial pressure and systemic vascular resistance, which are associated with a decrease in cardiac output of up to about 30% in some studies.

Propofol has been used effectively in patients with good left ventricular function undergoing coronary artery bypass surgery. However, if fentanyl is added to the regimen, there is the possibility of pronounced hemodynamic depression. Left ventricular function has been assessed by radionuclide ventriculography and invasive monitoring in patients with coronary artery disease who received a propofol infusion with the addition of fentanyl, when it was shown that, in this setting, a propofol infusion for mainte-

nance of anesthesia produced a 15% decrease in arterial pressure associated with a decrease in cardiac index, but no decrease in systemic vascular resistance and no change in heart rate. The addition of fentanyl (5μg/kg) to the regimen produced a further decrease in blood pressure (35%), cardiac index, systemic vascular resistance, and heart rate. However, global ejection fraction and end systolic volume did not change, indicating that propofol alone or in combination with fentanyl did not alter left ventricular performance. However, the large fall in blood pressure might have deleterious effects on coronary perfusion in ischemic heart disease. Propofol should therefore be administered cautiously to patients with limited cardiac reserve or hypovolemia in whom a fall in peripheral vascular resistance or cardiac output might be disadvantageous. Cardiac dysrhythmias are uncommon.

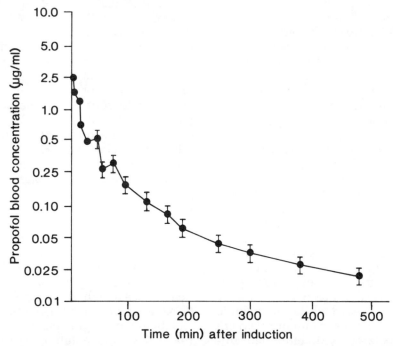

Figure 8.18.   Propofol blood concentrations following a single bolus dose (2.5 mg/ kg).   Note the rapid decline in the blood propofol concentrations as propofol rapidly distributes from the circulation to the tissues and that the data are best described as an open 3-compartment model with three different rate constants. (With permission from Cockshott ID: Propofol (Diprivan) pharmacokinetics and metabolism—an overview. *Post Grad Med J* 61 (Suppl 3):45–50, 1985.)

Other Effects. Propofol does not cause suppression of adrenal steroidogenesis (Fig. 8.16). Propofol interacts with the neuromuscular blocking agents; when it is administered during steady-state infusions of atracurium and vecuronium, the depth of neuromuscular blockade is increased, athough there is no effect on the duration of action of atracurium or vecuronium. The mechanism of this drug interaction is not known. Propofol does not cause histamine release.

Pharmacokinetics. The intravenous administration of a single bolus induction dose of propofol to surgical patients is followed by a rapid decline in propofol concentrations due to extensive distribution and elimination. A large number of pharmacokinetic studies have been performed, and some studies are best described as a two-compartment model, while others as a three-compartment model (Fig. 8.18). Propofol distributes very rapidly from the circulation to the

tissues, and the distribution half-life $(t_{1/2\alpha})$ has been reported to range from about 2.0 to 8.0 minutes. During the distribution phase, propofol blood concentrations rapidly decrease, and patients awaken from anesthesia when propofol concentrations are about 1.0 μg/ml (see next section). Volumes of distribution are high; the volume of distibution of the central compartment (V_1 or V_c) ranges from 13 to 70 L, the volume of distribution at steady state (Vd_{ss}) is reported to vary from 171 to 349 L, while the volume of distribution during elimination appears to range from 209 to 1008 L, reflecting the extensive tissue distribution of propofol. The plasma protein binding of propofol is approximately 98%.

In those studies where a two-compartment model was used, the terminal elimination half-life ranged from 1.0 to 3.0 hours, but when a three-compartment model was used, propofol elimination was biphasic with two elimination half-

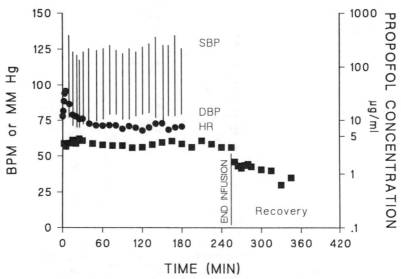

Figure 8.19. Propofol blood concentrations during intravenous infusion. Propofol induction was with 2 mg/kg followed by exponentially decreasing infusion rates of 0.2 mg/kg/min for 15 minutes, 0.15 mg/kg/min for 15 minutes, and 0.10 mg/kg/min thereafter to achieve constant "plateau" concentrations of about 3.0 μg/ml (■). Nitrous oxide (70%) was also administered. Note the short-lived increase in heart rate *(HR)* (•) at induction accompanied by a decrease in systolic *(SBP)* and diastolic *(DBP)* blood pressure. (With permission from Perry SM, Smith D, Wood M: Propofol for induction and maintenance of anesthesia: recovery characteristics. *Proceedings of the World Congress of Anaesthesiologists,* Washington, DC, 1988.)

lives: $t_{1/2\beta}$ of 34 to 64 minutes; and a $t_{1/2\gamma}$ for the terminal elimination phase, which was longer and ranged from 3 to 6.0 hours. Total-body clearance is high and has been reported to range from approximately 24 to 33 ml/kg/min. Since clearance exceeds hepatic blood flow, there must be other sites in addition to the liver that contribute to the elimination of propofol, and it has been suggested that propofol is perhaps metabolized by nonspecific esterases. Propofol total-body clearance following an infusion (total dose, 915 mg) for approximately 2 hours was about 2.0 L/min, volume of distribution at steady state was 160 L, and the elimination half-life was 116 minutes using a two-compartment

model. Propofol is metabolized in the liver by glucuronidation and sulfation to glucuronides and sulfate conjugates that are then excreted in the urine. Less than 0.3% of the administered dose is excreted unchanged in the urine, while approximately 40% is excreted in the urine as propofol glucuronide.

Pharmacodynamics. Propofol concentrations produced by a continuous infusion for general anesthesia at a rate of 0.15 mg/kg/min are shown in Figure. 8.19; "plateau" concentrations are about 3.0 μg/ml. In general, patients who are adequately anesthetized for major surgery require higher blood concentrations (around 4 μg/ml) than those for nonmajor surgery (around 3 μg/ml) (Fig.

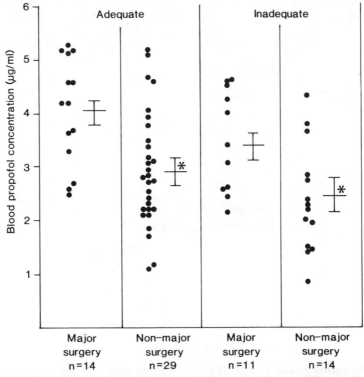

Figure 8.20. Blood concentrations of propofol required to produce adequate surgical anesthesia. Blood propofol concentrations (μg/ml) in relation to type of surgical procedure (major or nonmajor) at times of absence of autonomic responses (*adequate*) or presence of autonomic responses (*inadequate*) to surgical stimulation. Points individual patient values, *bars,* SEM. Significant differences between groups (major versus nonmajor surgery, $P < 0.05$, *). (With permission from Shafer A, Doze VA, Shafer SL, White PF: Pharmacokinetics and pharmacodynamics of propofol infusions during general anesthesia. *Anesthesiology* 69:348–356, 1988.)

8.20). Blood propofol concentrations at which 50% of patients are awake and oriented after surgery are 1.07 and 0.95 μg/ml, respectively (Fig. 8.21). Psychomotor performance appears to return to preoperative levels at concentrations of 0.38 to 0.43 μg/ml.

Factors Affecting Pharmacokinetics and Pharmacodynamics. The pharmacokinetic parameters of propofol are not affected by hepatic cirrhosis or renal failure. Anesthetic agents and anesthetic regimens may alter the disposition of propofol. Halothane has been shown to reduce the volume of distribution of propofol (both V_1 and V_d) and also reduce the elimination half-life ($t_{1/2\beta}$ and $t_{1/2\gamma}$). Fentanyl, which has previously been shown to alter the pharmacokinetics of etomidate,

has similar effects; V_1 and V_d are decreased and $t_{1/2\beta}$ and $t_{1/2\gamma}$ reduced. Propofol concentrations may therefore be higher when fentanyl is concomitantly administered. The elderly require dosage reductions; propofol clearance is reduced and the initial volume of distirbution (V_1) is reduced, leading to higher blood propofol concentrations and therefore increased drug effect. Half-life is unchanged.

Suggested Dose and Administration. The recommended dose for anesthesia induction is about 2.0 to 2.5 mg/kg. The dose should be reduced in elderly patients and in patients with cardiac disease or hypovolemia. The short duration of action and pharmacokinetic parameters described previously (i.e., a short $t_{1/2\beta}$ and high

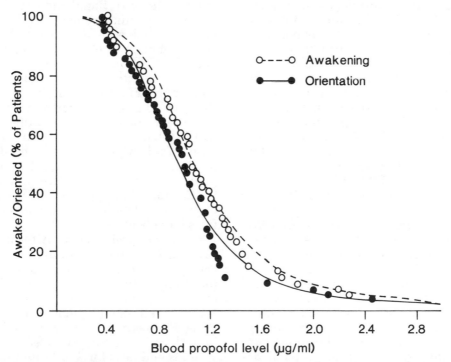

Figure 8.21. Propofol concentration-response curves for recovery from anesthesia. Concentration-response curves demonstrating the correlation between emergence from anesthesia (awakening and orientation) and propofol blood concentrations (μg/ml). The cumulative percentage of patients who were awake (o) or were oriented (•) at various blood propofol levels is shown. Note that blood propofol concentrations at which 50% of patients were awake (EC_{50}) and oriented after surgery were 1.07 and 0.95 μg/ml, respectively. (With permission from Shafer A, Doze VA, Shafer SL, White PF: Pharmacokinetics and pharmacodynamics of propofol infusions during general anesthesia. *Anesthesiology* 69:348–356, 1988.)

plasma clearance) make propofol an ideal agent for continuous intravenous infusion techniques for both anesthesia maintenance and sedation. However, in those studies where a 3-compartment model was used, the elimination is triphasic with a longer terminal elimination half-life $(t_{1/2\gamma})$ of 3 to 6 hours following a single bolus, suggesting that propofol might accumulate when administered for a very prolonged period of time with possible delayed recovery. However, when propofol has been given by continuous intravenous infusion for 4 hours, no delayed recovery has been observed. Propofol can be used for maintenance of anesthesia, when it can be administered by either continuous infusion or intermittent injection. Propofol has been administered as an adjuvant to anesthesia in conjunction with nitrous oxide at a rate of 50 to 55 μg/kg/min and without nitrous oxide as a total intravenous anesthetic technique at rates of 100 to 200 μg/ kg/min (0.1 to 0.2 mg/kg/min or 6 to 12 mg/kg/hour). Propofol has also been administered as a continuous intravenous infusion at a rate of 70 μg/kg/min during regional anesthesia to provide deep sedation. When propofol is used for anesthesia maintenance by an intermittent bolus technique, generally increments of about 25 to 50% of the induction dose are administered, with dose being titrated to clinical effect.

Toxicity, Precautions, and Contraindications. As for all intravenous anesthetic induction agents that cause cardiorespiratory depression, propofol should be used cautiously in patients with compromised cardiac disease or hypovolemic shock. Respiratory complications include apnea and respiratory depression. Excitatory effects are minimal. Pain or burning on injection may occur during propofol administration into a small vein, with an incidence as high as 30 to 40%. However, pain on injection may be reduced by injection into large veins of the antecubital fossa or forearm, when the incidence is reduced to 8 to 12%.

Steroid Anesthesia

The hypnotic properties of the steroids have been known for many years, and in

the 1950s Viadril (hydroxydione sodium succinate) was briefly used, but was abandoned due to its slow onset of action and tendency to cause thrombophlebitis. In 1971 Althesin, a mixture of two steroids, was introduced into clinical practice in Europe.

ALTHESIN (ALPHAXALONE AND ALPHADOLONE)

Althesin is a mixture of the two steroids: alphaxalone (3α-hydroxy-5α-pregnane-11,20-dione) and alphadolone acetate (21-acetoxy-3α-hydroxy-5α-pregnane-11,20-dione).

Althesin is a clear, colorless, viscid solution, containing 9 mg of alphaxalone and 3 mg of alphadolone acetate per ml. The solution also contains the solubilizing agent cremophor EL (polyoxyethylated castor oil). Rapid induction of anesthesia and high potency are known to be associated with the free 3α-hydroxy group on the steroid molecule, e.g., alphaxalone, but unfortunately these compounds are extremely insoluble, even in cremophor EL. However, it was found that the addition of another steroid, alphadolone acetate, increased the solubility of alphaxalone in cremophor EL more than 3-fold. Alphadolone is only-half as potent as alphaxalone. The mixture of alphaxalone and alphadolone is known as "Althesin." Although Althesin consists of two steroid molecules, no endocrine effects have been reported.

Pharmacological Effects. Althesin possesses a high therapeutic index (ratio of therapeutic to toxic dose), and in mice the therapeutic index of Althesin is 30.6 compared to values of 6.9 for thiopental, 7.4 for methohexital, and 8.5 for ketamine. Following intravenous administration, sleep is usually produced within 30 seconds and lasts for 7 to 11 minutes, depending on the dose administered. Excitatory side effects such as muscle tremors often occur and may be reduced by opiate premedication. The cardiovascular effects are similar to those produced by equivalent doses of thiopental and methohexital. Respiratory depression follows the intravenous injection of Althesin, and there may be a short period of apnea followed by rapid shallow breathing.

Coughing, hiccough, and laryngospasm have also been reported.

The most serious limitation to its clinical use is the hypersensitivity reactions that occur, which may be manifest as severe circulatory collapse, bronchospasm, edema, and a generalized erythematous reaction. One possible cause of these severe hypersensitivity reactions is histamine release. Estimates of the incidence vary from 1 in 10,000 to 1 in 1,000. Predisposing factors include a history of atopy, such as asthma or eczema, or previous exposure to Althesin. As similar reactions have been observed following propanidid (an intravenous induction agent discussed later in this chapter), it has been suggested that these reactions may be due to the solubilizing agent cremophor EL, which is common to both these drugs. The hypersensitivity reactions are potentially so serious in susceptible individuals that Althesin is now no longer manufactured. It has never been available in the United States.

The Eugenols: Propanidid

Propanidid has been in clinical use in Europe for many years and is included because its pharmacology and, in particular, metabolism are of special interest. Like Althesin, propanidid is no longer manufactured and has never been available in the United States. Propanidid is a nonbarbiturate ultrashort-acting anesthetic agent which is a derivative of eugenol. It is a pale yellow oil which is only slightly soluble in water. However, a 5% solution can be obtained by the use of a solubilizing agent, cremophor EL.

Pharmacological Effects. Propanidid produces sleep of a short duration when administered intravenously. Propanidid produces excitatory side effects, such as tremor or muscle movements, in about 11% of patients compared with 9% with equipotent doses of thiopental and 24% with methohexital. Hypotension and tachycardia also occur with propanidid. Respiratory effects are striking with marked hyperventilation being followed by a short period of apnea. Hypersensitivity reactions have been reported, including acute anaphylaxis.

Pharmacokinetics. The main advantage of propanidid is its rapid onset of action and fast recovery which are due to metabolism rather than to redistribution. Propanidid is broken down by pseudocholinesterase in plasma to its principal metabolite (98%) phenylacetic acid and to 4-carboxymethoxy phenylacetic acid (2%). Excretion is rapid, and 75 to 90% of the injected dose is eliminated as metabolites within 2 hours of administration. Propanidid may therefore prolong the effects of succinylcholine because both these drugs are metabolized by pseudocholinesterase.

BIBLIOGRAPHY

General

Clarke RSJ: New drugs—boon or bane? Premedication and intravenous induction agents. *Can Anaesth Soc J* 30:166–173, 1983.

Clarke RSJ, Dundee JW: Clinical studies of induction agents XV. A comparison of the cumulative effects of thiopentone, methohexitone, and propanidid. *Br J Anaesth* 38:401–405, 1966.

Clarke RSJ, Dundee JW, Garrett RT, McArdle GK, Sutton JA: Adverse reactions to intravenous anaesthetics. *Br J Anaesth* 47:575–585, 1975.

Davis PJ, Cook DR: Clinical pharmacokinetics of the newer intravenous anaesthetic agents. *Clin Pharmacokinet* 11:18–35, 1986.

Dhadphale PR, Jackson APF, Alseri S: Comparison of anesthesia with diazepam and ketamine vs morphine in patients undergoing heart-valve replacement. *Anesthesiology* 51:200–203, 1979.

Dundee JW: New IV anesthetics. *Br J Anaesth* 51:641–648, 1979.

Dundee JW, Wyant GM (ed): *Intravenous Anaesthesia*. Edinburgh, Churchill-Livingstone, 2nd edition 1988.

Duvaldestin P: Pharmacokinetics in intravenous anaesthetic practice. *Clin Pharmacokinet* 6:61–82, 1981.

Ghoneim MM, Korttila K: Pharmacokinetics of intravenous anesthetics: implications for clinical use. *Clin Pharmacokinet* 2:344–372, 1977.

Reilly CS, Nimmo WS: New intravenous anaesthetics and neuromuscular blocking drugs. *Drugs* 34:98–135, 1987.

Sear JW (ed): Intravenous anaesthesiology. *Clinics in Anaesthesiology*. London, WB Saunders, 2:1, 1984.

Sear JW: Toxicity of IV anaesthetics. *BR J Anaesth* 59:24–45, 1987.

Swerdlow BN, Holley FO: Intravenous anaesthetic agents: pharmacokinetic-pharmacodynamic relationships. *Clin Pharmacokinet* 12:79–110, 1987.

Watkins J, Clarke RSJ: Report of a symposium: adverse responses to intravenous agents. *Br J Anaesth* 50:1159–1163, 1978.

Whitwam JG: Intravenous induction agents in adverse reactions. In *Clinics in Anaesthesiology*. London, WB Saunders, 1984, vol 2, chap 4, p 30.

Barbiturates

Brodie BB: Physiological disposition and chemical fate of thiobarbiturates in the body. *Fed Proc* 11:632–639, 1952.

Brown SS, Lyons SM, Dundee JW: Intra-arterial barbiturates: study of some factors leading to intravascular thrombosis. *Br J Anaesth* 40:13–19, 1968.

Laiwah ACY, McColl KEL: Management of attacks of acute porphyria. *Drugs* 34:604–616, 1987.

Saidman LJ: Uptake, distribution, and elimination of barbiturates. In Eger EI II, (ed): *Anesthetic Uptake and Action.* Baltimore, Williams & Wilkins, 1974, chap 17.

Thiopental

Becker KE: Plasma levels of thiopental necessary for anesthesia. *Anesthesiology* 49:192–196, 1978.

Becker KE, Tonnesen AS: Cardiovascular effects of plasma levels of thiopental necessary for anesthesia. *Anesthesiology* 49:197–200, 1978.

Bischoff KB, Dedrick RL: Thiopental pharmacokinetics. *J Pharm Sci* 57:1346–1351, 1968.

Brett CM, Fisher DM: Thiopental, dose-response relations in unpremedicated infants, children, and adults. *Anesth Analg* 66:1024–1027, 1987.

Burch PG, Stanski DR: Decreased protein binding and thiopental kinetics. *Clin Pharmacol Ther* 32:212–217, 1982.

Carlon GC, Kahn RC, Goldiner PI, Howland WS, Turnbull A: Long-term infusion of sodium thiopental: hemodynamic and respiratory effects. *Crit Care Med* 6:311–316, 1978.

Chamberlain JH, Seed RGFL, Chung DC: Effect of thiopental on myocardial function. *Br J Anaesth* 49:865–870, 1977.

Christensen JH, Andreasen F, Jansen JA: The influence of age and sex on the pharmacokinetics of thiopentone. *Br J Anaesth* 53:1189–1195, 1981.

Couderc E, Ferrier C, Haberer JP, Henzel D, Duvaldestin P: Thiopentone pharmacokinetics in patients with chronic alcoholism. *Br J Anaesth* 56:1393–1397, 1984.

Crankshaw DP, Edwards NE, Blackman GL, Boyd MD, Chan HNJ, Morgan DJ: Evaluation of infusion regimens for thiopentone as a primary anesthetic agent. *Eur J Clin Pharmacol* 28:543–552, 1985.

Dundee JW: Editorial: fifty years of thiopentone. *Br J Anaesth* 56:211–213, 1984.

Eckstein JW, Hamilton WK, McCammond JM: The effect of thiopental on peripheral venous tone. *Anesthesiology* 22:525–528, 1961.

Fieldman EJ, Ridley RW, Wood EH: Hemodynamic studies during thiopental sodium and nitrous oxide anesthesia in humans. *Anesthesiology* 16:473–489, 1955.

Ghoneim MM, VanHamme MJ: Pharmacokinetics of thiopentone: effects of enflurane and nitrous oxide anaesthesia and surgery. *Br J Anaesth* 50:1237–1241, 1978.

Homer TD, Stanski DR: The effect of increasing age on thiopental disposition and anesthetic requirement. *Anesthesiology* 62:714–724, 1985.

Hudson RJ, Stanski DR, Burch PG: Pharmacokinetics of methohexitol and thiopental in surgical patients. *Anesthesiology* 59:215–219, 1983.

Jung D, Mayersohn M, Perrier D, Calkins J, Saunders R: Thiopental disposition as a function of age in female patients undergoing surgery. *Anesthesiology* 56:263–268, 1982.

Jung D, Mayersohn M, Perrier D, Calkins J, Saunders R: Thiopental disposition in lean and obese patients undergoing surgery. *Anesthesiology* 56:269–274, 1982.

Michenfelder JD, Theye RA: Cerebral protection by thiopental during hypoxia. *Anesthesiology* 39:510–517, 1973.

Pandele G, Chaux F, Salvadori C, Farinotti M, Duvaldestin P: Thiopental pharmacokinetics in patients with cirrhosis. *Anesthesiology* 59:123–126, 1985.

Pierce EC, Lambertsen CJ, Deutsch S, Chase PE, Linde HW, Dripps RD, Price HL: Cerebral circulation and metabolism during thiopental anesthesia and hyperventilation in man. *J Clin Invest* 41:1664–1671, 1962.

Price HL: A dynamic concept of the distribution of thiopental in the human body. *Anesthesiology* 21:40–45, 1960.

Price HL, Kovnat PJ, Safer JN, Coner EH, Price ML: The uptake of thiopental by body tissues and its relation to the duration of narcosis. *Clin Pharmacol Ther* 1:16–22, 1960.

Saidman LJ, Eger EI II: The effect of thiopental metabolism on duration of anesthesia. *Anesthesiology* 27:118–126, 1966.

Sonntag H, Hellberg K, Schenk HD, Donath U, Regensburger D, Kettler D, Duchanova H, Larsen R: Effects of thiopental (Trapanal) on coronary blood flow and myocardial metabolism in man. *Acta Anaesthesiol Scand* 19:69–78, 1975.

Sorbo S, Hudson RJ, Loomis JC: The pharmacokinetics of thiopental in pediatric surgical patients. *Anesthesiology* 61:666–670, 1984.

Stanski DR: Pharmacokinetic modelling of thiopental. *Anesthesiology* 54:446–448, 1981.

Stanski, DR, Mihm FG, Rosenthal MH, Kalman SM: Pharmacokinetics of high-dose thiopental used in cerebral resuscitation. *Anesthesiology* 53:169–171, 1980.

Stone HH, Donnelly CC: The accidental intra-arterial injection of thiopental. *Anesthesiology* 22:995–1006, 1961.

Turcant A, Delhumeau A, Premel-Cabic A, Granry JC, Cottineau C, Six P, Allain P: Thiopental pharmacokinetics under conditions of long-term infusion. *Anesthesiology* 63:50–54, 1985.

Methohexital

Breimer DD: Pharmacokinetics of methohexitone following intravenous infusion in humans. *Br J Anaesth* 48:643–649, 1976.

Ketamine

Bovill JG, Coppel DL, Dundee JW, Moore J: Current status of ketamine anaesthesia. *Lancet* 1:1285–1288, 1971.

Clements JA, Nimmo WS: Pharmacokinetics and analgesic effect of ketamine in man. *Br J Anaesth* 53:27–30, 1981.

Domino EF, Domino SE, Smith RE, Domino LE, Goulet JR, Domino KE, Zsigmond EK: Ketamine kinetics in unmedicated and diazepam-premedicated subjects. *Clin Pharmacol Ther* 36:645–653, 1984.

Grant IS, Nimmo WS, Clements JA: Pharmacokinetics and analgesic effect of IM and oral ketamine. *Br J Anaesth* 53:805–810, 1981.

Grant IS, Nimmo WS, McNicol LR, Clements JA: Ketamine disposition in children and adults. *Br J Anaesth* 55:1107–1111, 1983.

Hickey PR, Hansen DD, Cramolini GM, Vincent RN, Lang P: Pulmonary and systemic hemodynamic responses to ketamine in infants with normal and elevated pulmonary vascular resistance. *Anesthesiology* 62:287–293, 1985.

Morray JP, Lynn AM, Stamm SJ, Herndon PS, Kawabori I, Stevenson JG: Hemodynamic effects of ketamine in children with congenital heart disease. *Anesth Analg* 63:895–899, 1984.

Takeshita H, Okuda Y, Sari A: The effects of ketamine on cerebral circulation and metabolism in man. *Anesthesiology* 36:69–75, 1972.

White PF: Use of continuous infusion versus intermittent bolus administration of fentanyl or ketamine during outpatient anesthesia. *Anesthesiology* 59:294–300, 1983.

White PF, Ham J, Way WL, Trevor AJ: Pharmacology of ketamine isomers in surgical patients. *Anesthesiology* 52:231–239, 1980.

White PF, Schuttler J, Shafer A, Stanski DR, Horai Y, Trevor AJ: Comparative pharmacology of the ketamine isomers. *Br J Anaesth* 57:197–203, 1985.

White PF, Way WL, Trevor AJ: Ketamine—its pharmacology and therapeutic uses. *Anesthesiology* 56:119–136, 1982.

Wieber J, Gugler R, Hengstmann JH, Dengler HJ: Pharmacokinetics of ketamine in man. *Anaesthesist* 24:260–263, 1975.

Zsigmond EK, Domino EF: Ketamine: clinical pharmacology, pharmacokinetics, and current clinical uses. *Anesth Rev* 7:13–33, 1980.

Benzodiazepines

Bellantuono V, Reggi V, Tognoni G, Grattini S: Benzodiazepines: clinical pharmacology and therapeutic use. *Drugs* 19:195–219, 1980.

Colburn WA, Jack ML: Relationships between CSF drug concentrations, receptor binding characteristics, and pharmacokinetic and pharmacodynamic properties of selected 1,4-substituted benzodiazepines. *Clin Pharmacokinet* 13:179–190, 1987.

Dundee JW, Haslett WHK: The benzodiazepines—a review of their actions and uses relative to anesthetic practice. *Br J Anaesth* 42:217–234, 1970.

Greenblatt DJ, Arendt RM, Abernethy DR, Giles HG, Sellers EM, Shader RI: In vitro quantitation of benzodiazepine lipophilicity: relation to in vivo distribution. *Br J Anaesth* 55:985–989, 1983.

Greenblatt DJ, Shader RI: Benzodiazepines (two parts). *N Engl J Med* 291:1011–1015, 1974; *N Engl J Med* 291:1239–1243, 1974.

Greenblatt DJ, Shader RI, Abernethy DR: Current status of benzodiazepines (two parts). *N Engl J Med* 309:354–358, 1983; *N Engl J Med* 309:410–416, 1983.

Richter JJ: Current theories about the mechanisms of benzodiazepines and neuroleptic drugs. *Anesthesiology* 54:66–72, 1981.

Squires RF, Braestrup C: Benzodiazepine receptors in rat brain. *Nature* 266:732–734, 1977.

Whitwam JG: Editorial: benzodiazepine receptors. *Anaesthesia* 38:93–95, 1983.

Diazepam

Catchlove RFH, Kafer ER: The effects of diazepam on the ventilatory response to carbon dioxide and on steady-state gas exchange. *Anesthesiology* 34:9–13, 1971.

Cote P, Campeau L, Bournassa MG: Therapeutic implications of diazepam in patients with elevated left ventricular filling pressure. *Am Heart J* 91:747–751, 1976.

Ikram H, Rubin AP, Jewkes RF: Effect of diazepam on myocardial blood flow of patients with and without coronary artery disease. *Br Heart J* 35:626–630, 1973.

Kawar P, Carson IW, Clarke RSJ, Dundee JW, Lyons SM: Haemodynamic changes during induction of anaesthesia with midazolam and diazepam (Valium) in patients undergoing coronary artery bypass surgery. *Anaesthesia* 40:767–771, 1985.

Klotz U, Avant GR, Hoyumpa A, Schenker S, Wilkinson GR: The effects of age and liver disease on the disposition and elimination of diazepam in adult man. *J Clin Invest* 55:347–359, 1975.

Lowry KG, Dundee JW, McClean E, Lyons SM, Carson IW, Orr IA: Pharmacokinetics of diazepam and midazolam when used for sedation following cardiopulmonary bypass. *Br J Anaesth* 57:883–885, 1985.

Mandelli M, Gognoni G, Garattini S: Clinical pharmacokinetics of diazepam. *Clin Pharmacokinet* 3:72–91, 1978.

McCammon RL, Hilgenberg JC, Stoelting RK: Hemodynamic effects of diazepam and diazepam-nitrous oxide in patients with coronary artery disease. *Anesth Analg* 59:438–441, 1980.

Power SJ, Morgan M, Chakrabarti MK: Carbon dioxide response curves following midazolam and diazepam. *Br J Anaesth* 55:837–841, 1983.

Rao S, Sherbaniuk JW, Prasad K, Lee SJK, Sproule BJ: Cardiopulmonary effects of diazepam. *Clin Pharmacol Ther* 14:182–189, 1973.

Reves JG, Corssen G, Holcomb G: Comparison of two benzodiazepines for anaesthesia induction: midazolam and diazepam. *Can Anaesth Soc J* 25:211–214, 1978.

Reves JG, Kissin I, Fournier SE, Smith LR: Additive negative inotropic effect of a combination of diazepam and fentanyl. *Anesth Analg* 63:97–100, 1984.

Samuelson PN, Reves JG, Kouchoukos NT, Smith LR, Dole KM: Hemodynamic responses to anesthetic induction with midazolam or diazepam in patients with ischemic heart disease. *Anesth Analg* 60:802–809, 1981.

Tomicheck RC, Rosow CE, Philbin DM, Moss J, Teplick RS, Schneider RC: Diazepam-fentanyl interaction—hemodynamic and hormonal effects in coronary artery surgery. *Anesth Analg* 62:861–864, 1983.

Midazolam

Al-Khudhairi D, Whitwam JG, Chakrabarti MK, Askitopoulou H, Grundy EM, Powrie S: Haemodynamic effects of midazolam and thiopentone during induction of anaesthesia for coronary artery surgery. *Br J Anaesth* 54:831–835, 1982.

Allonen H, Ziegler G, Klotz U: Midazolam kinetics. *Clin Pharmacol Ther* 30:653–661, 1981.

Booker PD, Beechey A, Lloyd-Thomas AR: Sedation of children requiring artifical ventilation using an infusion of midazolam. *Br J Anaesth* 58:1104–1108, 1986.

Dundee JW, Halliday NJ, Harper KW, Brogden RN: Midazolam: a review of its pharmacological properties and therapeutic use. *Drugs* 28:519–543, 1984.

Fee JPH, Collier PS, Howard PJ, Dundee JW: Cimetidine and ranitidine increase midazolam bioavailability. *Clin Pharmacol Ther* 41:80–84, 1987.

Forster A, Gardaz JP, Suter PM, Gemperle M: Respiratory depression by midazolam and diazepam. *Anesthesiology* 53:494–497, 1980.

Forster A, Juge O, Morel D: Effects of midazolam on cerebral blood flow in human volunteers. *Anesthesiology* 56:453–455, 1982.

Fragen RJ, Gahl F, Caldwell N: A water-soluble benzodiazepine, R1 21-3981, for induction of anesthesia. *Anesthesiology* 49:41–43, 1978.

Gelman S, Reves JG, Harris D: Circulatory responses to midazolam anesthesia: emphasis on canine splanchnic circulation. *Anesth Analg* 62:135–139, 1983.

Greenblatt DJ, Abernethy DR, Locniskar A, Harmatz JS, Limjuco RA, Shader RI: Effect of age, gender, and obesity on midazolam kinetics. *Anesthesiology* 61:27–35, 1984.

Greenblatt DJ, Locniskar A, Scavone JM, Blyden GT, Ochs HR, Harmatz JS, Shader RI: Absence of interaction of cimetidine and ranitidine with intravenous and oral midazolam. *Anesth Analg* 65:176–180, 1986.

Heizman P, Eckert M, Ziegler WH: Pharmacokinetics and bioavailability of midazolam in man. *Br J Clin Pharmacol* 16:43S–49S, 1983.

Hoffman WE, Miletich DJ, Albrecht RE: The effects of midazolam on cerebral blood flow and oxygen consumption and its interaction with nitrous oxide. *Anesth Analg* 65:729–733, 1986.

Klotz U, Reimann TW: Chronopharmacokinetic study with prolonged infusion of midazolam. *Clin Pharmacokine* 9:469–474, 1984.

Lebowitz PW, Cote ME, Daniels AL, Bonventre JV: Comparative renal effects of midazolam and thiopental in humans. *Anesthesiology* 59:381–384, 1983.

Lebowitz PW, Cote ME, Daniels AL, Ramsey FM, Martyn JAJ, Teplick RS, Davison JK: Comparative cardiovascular effects of midazolam and thiopental in healthy patients. *Anesth Analg* 61:771–775, 1982.

Lloyd-Thomas AR, Booker PD: Infusion of midazolam in paediatric patients after cardiac surgery. *Br J Anaesth* 58:1109–1115, 1986.

Marty J, Nitenberg A, Blanchet F, Zouioueche S, Desmonts JM: Effect of midazolam on the coronary circulation in patients with coronary artery disease. *Anesthesiology* 64:206–210, 1986.

Melvin MA, Johnson BH, Quasha AL, Eger EI II: Induction of anesthesia with midazolam decreases halothane MAC in humans. *Anesthesiology* 57:238–241, 1982.

Persson P, Nilsson A, Hartvig P, Tamsen A: Pharmacokinetics of midazolam in total IV anaesthesia. *Br J Anaesth* 59:549–556, 1987.

Reitan JA, Porter W, Braunstein M: Comparison of psychomotor skills and amnesia after induction of anesthesia with midazolam or thiopental. *Anesth Analg* 65:933–937, 1986.

Reves JG, Fragen RJ, Vinik HR, Greenblatt DJ: Midazolam pharmacology and uses. *Anesthesiology* 62:310–324, 1985.

Reves JG, Vinik R, Hirschfield AM, Holcomb C, Strong S: Midazolam compared with thiopentone as a hypnotic component in balanced anaesthesia: a randomized, double-blind study. *Can Anaesth Soc J* 26:42–49, 1979.

Schulte-Sasse U, Hess W, Tarnow J: Haemodynamic responses to induction of anaesthesia using midazolam in cardiac surgical patients. *Br J Anaesth* 54:1053–1058, 1982.

Shapiro JM, Westphal LM, White PF, Sladen RN, Rosenthal MH: Midazolam infusion for sedation in the intensive care unit: effect on adrenal function. *Anesthesiology* 64:394–398, 1986

Lorazepam

Gate G, Galloon S: Lorazepam as a premedication. *Can Anaesth Soc J* 23:22–29, 1976

Greenblatt DJ: Clinical pharmacokinetics of oxazepam and lorazepam. *Clin Pharmacokinet* 6:89–105, 1981.

Greenblatt DJ, Shader RI: Prazepam and lorazepam, two new benzodiazepines. *N Engl J Med* 229:1342–1344, 1978.

Greenblatt DJ, Shader RI, Franke K, MacLaughlin DS, Harmatz JS, Allen MD, Werner A, Woo E: Pharmacokinetics and bioavailability of intravenous, intramuscular, and oral lorazepam in humans. *J Pharm Sci* 68:57–63, 1979.

Kothary SP, Brown ACD, Pandit UA, Samra SK, Pandit SK: Time course of antirecall effect of diazepam and lorazepam following oral administration. *Anesthesiology* 55:641–644, 1981.

Flumazenil

Barrett IE, Brady LS, Witkin JM: Behavioral studies with anxiolytic drugs. I. Interactions of the benzodiazepine antagonist R1 15-1788 with chlordiazepoxide, pentobarbital, and ethanol. *J Pharmacol Exp Ther* 233:554–559, 1985.

Brogden RN, Goa KL: Flumazenil: a preliminary review of its benzodiazepine antagonist properties, intrinsic activity, and therapeutic use. *Drugs* 35:448–467, 1988.

File SE, Pellow S: Intrinsic actions of the benzodiazepine receptor antagonist Ro 15-1788. *Psychopharmacology* 88:1–11, 1986.

Hunkeler W, Mohler H, Pieri L, Pole P, Bonetti EP, Cumin R, Schaffner R, Haefely W: Selective antagonists of benzodiazepines. *Nature* 290:514–516, 1981.

Klotz U, Kanto J: Pharmacokinetics and clinical use of flumazenil (Ro 15-1788). *Clin Pharmacokinet* 14:1–12, 1988.

Klotz U, Ziegler G, Ludwig L, Reimann IW: Pharmacodynamic interaction between midazolam and a specific benzodiazepine antagonist in humans. *J Clin Pharmacol* 25:400–406, 1985.

Lauven PM, Schwilden H, Stoeckel H, Greenblatt DJ: The effects of a benzodiazepine antagonist R1 15-1788 in the presence of stable concentrations of midazolam. *Anesthesiology* 63:61–64, 1985.

Ricou B, Forster A, Bruckner A, Chastonay P, Gemperle M: Clinical evaluation of a specific benzodiazepine antagonist (Ro 15-1788). *Br J Anaesth* 58:1005–1011, 1986.

Roncari G, Ziegler WH, Guentert TW: Pharmacokinetics of the new benzodiazepine antagonist Ro 15-1788 in man following intravenous and oral administration. *Br J Clin Pharmacol* 22:421–428, 1986.

Wolff J, Carl P, Clausen TG, Mikkelsen BO: Ro 15-1788 for postoperative recovery. *Anaesthesia* 41:1001–1006, 1986

Neuroleptanesthesia

Edmonds-Seal J, Prys-Roberts C: Pharmacology of drugs used in neuroleptanalgesia. *Br J Anaesth* 42:207–215, 1970

Prys-Roberts C, Kelman GR: The influence of drugs used in neuroleptanalgesia on cardiovascular and ventilatory function. *Br J Anaesth* 39:134–145, 1967

Etomidate

Arden JR, Holley FO, Stanski DR: Increased sensitivity to etomidate in the elderly: initial distribution versus altered brain response. *Anesthesiology* 65:19–27, 1986.

Arendt RM, Greenblatt DJ, deJong RH, Bonin JD, Abernethy CR, Ehrenberg BL, Giles HG, Sellers EM, Shader RI: In vitro correlates of benzodiazepine cerebrospinal fluid uptake, pharmacodynamic action, and peripheral distribution. *J Pharmacol Exp Ther* 227:98–106, 1983.

Atiba JO, Horai Y, White PF, Trevor AJ, Blaschke TF, Sung M-L: Effect of etomidate on hepatic drug metabolism in humans. *Anesthesiology* 68:920–924, 1988.

Bruckner JB, Gethmann JW, Patschke D, Tarnow J, Weymar A: Investigations into the effect of etomidate on the human circulation. *Anaesthesist* 23:322–330, 1974.

Carlos R, Calvo R, Erill S: Plasma protein binding of etomidate in patients with renal failure or hepatic cirrhosis. *Clin Pharmacokinet* 4:144–148, 1979.

Choi SD, Spaulding BC, Gross JB, Apfelbaum JL: Comparison of the ventilatory effects of etomidate and methohexitol. *Anesthesiology* 62:442–447, 1985.

Cold GE, Eskesen V, Eriksen H, Amtoft O, Madsen JB: CBF and CMRO2 during continuous etomidate infusion supplemented with N_2O and fentanyl in patients with supratentorial cerebral tumor. A dose response study. *Acta Anaesthesiol Scand* 29:490–494, 1985.

Daehlin L, Gran L: Etomidate and thiopentone: a comparative study of their respiratory effects. *Curr Ther Res* 27:706–713, 1980.

deRuiter G, Popescu DT, deBoer AG, Smeekens JB, Breimer DD: Pharmacokinetics of etomidate in surgical patients. *Arch Int Pharmacodyn Ther* 249:180–188, 1981.

Duthie DJR, Fraser R, Nimmo WS: Effect of induction of anaesthesia with etomidate on corticosteroid synthesis in man. *Br J Anaesth* 57:156–159, 1985.

Fish KJ, Rice SA, Margary J: Contrasting effects of etomidate and propylene glycol upon enflurane metabolism and adrenal steroidogenesis in Fischer 344 rats. *Anesthesiology* 68:189–193, 1988.

Fragen RJ, Weiss HW, Molteni A: The effect of propofol on adrenocortical steroidogenesis: a comparative study with etomidate and thiopental. *Anesthesiology* 66:839–842, 1987.

Ghoneim MM, VanHamme MJ: Hydrolysis of etomidate. *Anesthesiology* 50:227–229, 1979.

Giese JL, Stockham RJ, Stanley TH, Pace NL, Nelissen RH: Etomidate versus thiopental for induction of anesthesia. *Anesth Analg* 64:871–876, 1985.

Gooding JM, Weng JT, Smith RA, Berninger GT, Kirby RR: Cardiovascular and pulmonary responses following etomidate induction of anesthesia in patients with demonstrated cardiac disease. *Anesth Analg* 58:40–41, 1979.

Hebron BS, Edbrooke DL, Newby DM, Mather SJ: Pharmacokinetics of etomidate associated with prolonged IV infusion. *Br J Anaesth* 55:281–287, 1983.

Kenyon CJ, McNeil LM, Fraser R: Comparison of the effects of etomidate, thiopentone, and propofol on cortisol synthesis. *Br J Anaesth* 57:509–511, 1985.

Lambert A, Mitchell R, Robertson WR: Effect of propofol, thiopentone, and etomidate on adrenal steroidogenesis in vitro. *Br J Anaesth* 57:505–508, 1985.

Ledingham I McA, Watt I: Influence of sedation on mortality in critically ill multiple trauma patients. *Lancet* 1:1270, 1983.

Milde LN, Milde JH, Michenfelder JD: Cerebral functional, metabolic, and hemodynamic effects of etomidate in dogs. *Anesthesiology* 63:371–377, 1985.

Morgan M, Lumley J, Whitwam JG: Respiratory effects of etomidate. *Br J Anaesth* 49:233–236, 1977.

Moss E, Powell D, Gibson RM, McDowall DG: Effect of etomidate on intracranial pressure and cerebral perfusion pressure. *Br J Anaesth* 51:347–352, 1979.

Nelson EB, Egan JM, Abernethy DR: The effect of propylene glycol on antipyrine clearance in humans. *Clin Pharmacol Ther* 41:571–573, 1987.

Owen H, Spence AA: Editorial: etomidate. *Br J Anaesth* 56:555–557, 1984.

Renou AM, Vernheit J, Macrez P, Constant P, Billerey J, Khaderoo MY, Caille JM: Cerebral blood flow and metabolism during etomidate anaesthesia in man. *Br J Anaesth* 50:1047–1051, 1978.

Schuttler J, Wilms M, Stoeckel H, Schwinlden H, Lauven PM: Pharmacokinetic interaction of etomidate and fentanyl. *Anesthesiology* 59:A247, 1983.

Tarnow J, Hess W, Klein W: Etomidate, alfathesin, and thiopentone as induction agents for coronary artery surgery. *Can Anaesth Soc J* 27:338–344, 1980.

VanHamme MJ, Ghoneim MM, Ambere JJ: Pharmacokinetics of etomidate, a new intravenous anesthetic. *Anesthesiology* 49:274–277, 1978.

Wagner RL, White PP, Kan PB, Rosenthal RH, Feldman D: Inhibition of adrenal steroidogenesis by the anesthetic etomidate. *N Engl J Med* 310:1415–1421, 1984.

Wauquier A: Profile of etomidate: a hypnotic, anticonvulsant, and brain protective compound. Anaesthesia 38:26–33, 1983

Propofol

Adam HK, Briggs LP, Bahar M, Douglas EJ, Dundee JW: Pharmacokinetic evaluation of ICI 35 868 in man. Br J Anaesth 55:97–103, 1983.

Adam HK, Kay B, Douglas EJ: Blood disoprofol levels in anaesthetised patients. Anaesthesia 37:536–540, 1982.

Al-Khudhairi D, Gordon G, Morgan M, Whitwam JG: Acute cardiovascular changes following disoprofol: effects in heavily sedated patients with coronary artery disease. Anesthesia 37:1007–1010, 1982.

Aun C, Major E: The cardiorespiratory effects of ICI 35 868 in patients with valvular heart disease. Anaesthesia 39:1096–1100, 1984.

Baraka A: Severe bradycardia following propofol-suxamethonium sequence. Br J Anaesth 61:482–483, 1988.

Beller JP, Pottecher T, Lugnier A, Mangin P, Otteni JC: Prolonged sedation with propofol in ICU patients: recovery and blood concentration changes during periodic interruptions in infusions. Br J Anaesth 61:583–488, 1988.

Carlton JK, Bradbury WC: Chromatographic study of stearic hindrance in ortho-substituted alkyl phenols. J Am Chem Soc 78:1069–1070, 1956.

Coates DP, Monk CR, Prys-Roberts C, Turtle M: Hemodynamic effects of infusions of the emulsion formulation of propofol during nitrous oxide anesthesia in humans. Anesth Analg 66:64–70, 1987.

Cockshott ID, Briggs LP, Douglas EJ, White M: Pharmacokinetics of propofol in female patients. Br J Anaesth 59:1103–1110, 1987.

Cullen PM, Turtle M, Prys-Roberts C, Way WL, Dye J: Effect of propofol anesthesia on baroreflex activity in humans. Anesth Analg 66:1115–1120, 1987.

Doze VA, Shafer A, White PF: Propofol-nitrous oxide versus thiopental-isoflurane-nitrous oxide for general anesthesia. Anesthesiology 69:63–71, 1988.

Editorial: New awakening in anaesthesia—at a price. Lancet 1:1469–1470, 1987.

Fragen RJ, deGrood PM, Robertson EN, Booij LHDJ, Crul JF: Effects of premedication on diprivan induction. Br J Anaesth 54:913–915, 1982.

Fragen RJ, Hanssen EHJH, Denissen PAF, Booij LHDJ, Crul JF: Disoprofol (ICI 35868) for total intravenous anaesthesia. Acta Anaesthesiol Scand 27:113–116, 1983.

Fragen RJ, Weiss HW, Molteni A: The effect of propofol on adrenocortical steroidogenesis: a comparative study with etomidate and thiopental. Anesthesiology 66:839–842, 1987.

Gepts E, Camu F, Cockshott ID, Douglas EJ: Disposition of propofol administered as constant rate intravenous infusions in humans. Anesth Analg 66:1256–1263, 1987.

Glen JB, Hunter SC: Pharmacology of an emulsion formulation of ICI 35 868. Br J Anaesth 56:617–625, 1984.

Gold MI, Abraham EC, Herrington C: A controlled investigation of propofol, thiopentone, and methohexitone. Can J Anaesth 34:478–483, 1987.

Grounds RM, Twigley AJ, Carli F, Whitwam JG, Morgan M: The haemodynamic effects of intravenous induction: comparison of the effects of thiopentone and propofol. Anaesthesia 40:735–740, 1985.

Jessop E, Grounds RM, Morgan M, Lumley J: Comparison of infusions of propofol and methohexitone to provide light general anaesthesia during surgery with regional blockade. Br J Anaesth 57:1173–1177, 1985.

Johnston R, Noseworthy T, Anderson B, Konopad E, Grace M: Propofol versus thiopental for outpatient anesthesia. Anesthesiology 67:431–433, 1987.

Kay NH, Sear JW, Uppington J, Cockshott ID, Douglas EJ: Disposition of propofol in patients undergoing surgery. Br J Anaesth 58:1075–1079, 1986.

Kay NH, Uppington J, Sear JW, Allen MC: Use of an emulsion of ICI 35868 (propofol) for the induction and maintenance of anaesthesia. Br J Anaesth 57:736–742, 1985.

Kirkpatrick T, Cockshott ID, Douglas EJ, Nimmo WS: Pharmacokinetics of propofol (Diprivan) in elderly patients. Br J Anaesth 60:146–150, 1988.

Langley MS, Heel RC: Propofol. A review of its pharmacodynamic and pharmacokinetic properties and use of an intravenous anesthetic agent. Drugs 35:334–372, 1988.

Lepage J-Y, Pinaud ML, Hélias JH, Juge CM, Cozian AY, Farinotti R, Souron RJ: Left ventricular function during propofol and fentanyl anesthesia in patients with coronary artery disease: assessment with a radionuclide approach. Anesth Analg 67:949–955, 1988.

MacKenzie N, Grant IS: Comparison of the new emulsion formulation of propofol with methohexitone and thiopentone for induction of anaesthesia in day cases. Br J Anaesth 57:725–731, 1985.

MacKenzie N, Grant IS: Comparison of propofol with methohexitone in the provision of anaesthesia for surgery under regional blockade. Br J Anaesth 57:1167–1172, 1985.

MacKenzie N, Grant IS: Propofol for intravenous sedation. Anaesthesia 42:3–6, 1987.

Major E, Verniquet AJW, Yate PM, Waddell TK: Disoprofol and fentanyl for total intravenous anaesthesia. Anaesthesia 37:541–547, 1982.

Mirakhur RK, Shepherd WFI, Darrah WC: Propofol or thiopentone: effects on intraocular pressure associated with induction of anaesthesia and tracheal intubation (facilitated with suxamethonium). Br J Anaesth 59:431–436, 1987.

Monk CR, Coates DP, Prys-Roberts C, Turtle MJ, Spelina K: Haemodynamic effects of a prolonged infusion of propofol as a supplement to nitrous oxide anaesthesia. Br J Anaesth 59:954–960, 1987.

Mouton SM, Bullington J, Davis L, Fisher K, Ramsay S, Wood M: A comparison of propofol with the new emulsion formulation and thiopental for the induction of anesthesia. South Med J 81:611–615, 1988.

Newman LH, McDonald JC, Wallace PGM, Ledingham IMcA: Propofol infusion for sedation in intensive care. Anaesthesia 42:929–937, 1987.

O'Callaghan AC, Normandale JP, Grundy EM, Lumley J, Morgan M: Continuous intravenous infusion of disoprofol (ICI 35868, Diprivan). Anaesthesia 37:295–300, 1982.

Prys-Roberts C, Davies JR, Calverley RK, Goodman NW: Haemodynamic effects of infusions of diisopropyl phenol (ICI 35868) during nitrous oxide anaesthesia in man. *Br J Anaesth* 55:105–111, 1983.

Rampton AJ, Griffin RM, Stuart CS, Durcan JJ, Huddy NC, Abbott MA: Comparison of methohexital and propofol for electroconvulsive therapy: effects on hemodynamic responses and seizure duration. *Anesthesiology* 70:412–417, 1989.

Redfern N, Stafford MA, Hull CJ: Incremental propofol for short procedures. *Br J Anaesth* 57:1178–1182, 1985.

Robertson HN, Fragen RJ, Booij LHDJ, vanEdmond J, Crul JF: Some effects of diisopropyl phenol (ICI 35868) on the pharmacodynamics of atracurium and vecuronium in anaesthetized man. *Br J Anaesth* 55:723–728, 1983.

Rolly G, Versichelen L, Zubair NA: Use of ICI 35868 as an anesthetic induction agent. *Acta Anaesthesiol Belg* 31:241–247, 1980.

Schuttler J, Kloos S, Schwilden H, Stoeckel H: Total intravenous anaesthesia with propofol and alfentanil by computer assisted infusion. *Anaesthesia* 43 (suppl):2–7, 1988.

Schuttler J, Stoeckel M, Schwilden H: Clinical pharmacokinetics of Diprivan in volunteers and surgical patients. *Anesthesiology* 65:A555, 1986.

Shafer A, Doze VA, Shafer SL, White PF: Pharmacokinetics and pharmacodynamics of propofol infusions during general anesthesia. *Anesthesiology* 69:348–456, 1988.

Spelina KR, Coates DP, Monk CR, Prys-Roberts C, Norley I, Turtle MJ: Dose requirements of propofol by infusion during nitrous oxide anaesthesia in man. 1. Patients premedicated with morphine sulfate. *Br J Anaesth* 58:1080–1084, 1986.

Stephan H, Sonntag H, Schenk HD, Kettler D, Khambatta HJ: Effects of propofol on cardiovascular dynamics, myocardial blood flow, and myocardial metabolism in patients with coronary artery disease. *Br J Anaesth* 58:969–975, 1986.

Vanacker B, Dekegel D, Dionys J, Garcia R, Eeckhoutte LV, Dralants G, deWalle JV: Changes in intraocular pressure associated with the administration of propofol. *Br J Anaesth* 59:1514–1517, 1987.

Vermeyen KM, Erpels FA, Janssen LA, Beeckman CP, Hanegreefs GH: Propofol-fentanyl anaesthesia for coronary bypass surgery in patients with good left ventricular function. *Br J Anaesth* 59:1115–1120, 1987.

Wright PJ, Clarke RSJ, Dundee JW, Briggs LP, Greenfield AA: Infusion rates for anaesthesia with propofol. *Br J Anaesth* 56:613–616, 1984.

Steroid Anesthesia

Brogden RN, Speight TM, Avery GS: Alfathesin (Althesin-Glaxo): an independent report. *Drugs* 8:87–108, 1974.

9

Inhalational Anesthetic Agents

MARGARET WOOD

DEVELOPMENT OF THE INHALATIONAL ANESTHETIC AGENTS

In the late 1800s, the two anesthetic agents most commonly employed were chloroform and diethyl ether, and it was not until about 40 years ago that cyclopropane was introduced into clinical practice. Disadvantages of chloroform included hepatotoxicity, arrhythmias (ventricular fibrillation), and frequent nausea and vomiting, while diethyl ether was unpleasant to inhale and flammable, and its solubility resulted in a slow induction and recovery. Cyclopropane soon became popular due to the smooth, rapid induction of anesthesia and maintenance of arterial blood pressure that are associated with this anesthetic agent. However, the advent of cautery and diathermy equipment stimulated the search for nonflammable and nonexplosive compounds that could be more safely used in the operating room.

Volatile inhalational anesthetic agents can be divided into two groups: **halogenated hydrocarbons** or **ethers.** Examples of halogenated hydrocarbons include halothane, trichloroethylene, and chloroform. Hydrocarbons in which the hydrogen is replaced by fluorine are called fluorocarbons. Chlorine and bromine confer anesthetic potency to the hydrocarbon while fluorination produces stability. Halothane became available for clinical use in the 1950s and soon became the most widely used halogenated hydrocarbon anesthetic. However, it has become evident that halothane possesses undesirable effects, such as sensitization of the myocardium to catecholamines, cardiovascular depression, and hepatotoxicity. In addition, attention has centered on the possible risks of exposure to subanesthetic concentrations of inhalational agents in the operating room. These features have led to the development of more stable inhalational anesthetic agents—the new **halogenated ethers** of which enflurane and isoflurane are examples. Although the older members of the ether family are flammable, the new members of the series are not. In addition, generally ethers do not sensi-

tize the myocardium to circulating catecholamines. Thus, halogenated methylethyl ethers tend to be chemically stable and are not arrhythmogenic.

Isoflurane is now the most widely used potent volatile anesthetic in the United States. However, isoflurane has a pungent odor which makes it unpleasant to breathe and, although its cardiovascular effects suggest that it is less depressant to the circulation than enflurane or halothane, isoflurane causes a tachycardia. Isoflurane is a coronary artery vasodilator, and there is currently controversy as to whether isoflurane can produce myocardial ischemia by causing a coronary artery "steal" syndrome. Thus, new agents continue to be developed. Sevoflurane, for example, is an experimental fluorinated methyl-isopropyl ether whose solubility approaches that of nitrous oxide so that both induction and recovery are rapid. However, sevoflurane is not stable in soda lime and undergoes considerably more metabolism in vivo than isoflurane.

MINIMUM ALVEOLAR CONCENTRATION (MAC)

MAC is defined as the minimum alveolar concentration of anesthetic at one atmosphere that produces immobility in 50% of those patients or animals exposed to noxious stimulus. It is a measure of anesthetic potency. When MAC is determined in humans, the stimulus used is usually skin incision.

Anesthetic requirements (MAC) are reduced in hypothermia, pregnancy, and the elderly. Narcotic and diazepam premedication also reduce halothane MAC. Nitrous oxide, 70 to 75%, causes a marked reduction in halothane MAC of about 70%. In a study of 68 surgical patients, the minimum alveolar concentration of halothane in oxygen required to prevent movement in response to surgical incision was 0.74%, while addition of narcotic premedication decreased this value to 0.69%, and addition of nitrous oxide (without narcotic premedication) further decreased this value to 0.29%. Although hypocarbia does not appear to affect MAC, hypercarbia has "narcotic properties," and therefore anesthetic requirements are reduced. Metabolic acidosis and alkalosis have minimal effects on halothane MAC. Hypotension reduces anesthetic requirements, while chronic alcohol abuse produces a significant increase in MAC.

Drugs that affect central nervous system neurotransmitter release may alter anesthetic requirements. It is interesting that drugs such as reserpine and α-methyldopa which deplete central nervous system catecholamines decrease MAC, while d-amphetamine which releases catecholamines raises MAC, the significance of which is as yet undefined. Cocaine and ephedrine raise halothane MAC in dogs. Table 9.1 lists the MAC values for some of the inhalational anesthetic agents.

The dose of anesthetic that blocks the adrenergic (plasma norepinephrine concentration rise) and cardiovascular (increase in blood pressure and heart rate) response to skin incision in 50% of individuals has been termed MAC BAR and is 1.45 MAC for halothane, 1.6 MAC for enflurane, and 1.1 mg/kg for morphine when 60% nitrous oxide is also administered with each anesthetic.

PHARMACOKINETICS OF THE INHALATIONAL ANESTHETIC AGENTS

The aim of inhalational anesthesia is the development of an appropriate ten-sion or partial pressure of anesthetic agent within the brain. Knowledge of the factors affecting the uptake and distribution of the inhalational anesthetic agents provides vital information on the speed of induction, maintenance, and rate of recovery from a particular anesthetic agent.

The uptake and distribution of an inhalational anesthetic agent can be divided into four phases:

1. The introduction of a certain concentration of inhalational anesthetic agent from the anesthesia machine into the anesthetic circuit, i.e., the development of an inspired anesthetic concentration (C_i).
2. The uptake of anesthetic agent from the circuit into the lungs, i.e., the development of an alveolar anesthetic concentration (C_a).
3. The uptake of the anesthetic agent from the lungs to the arterial blood, i.e., the development of a blood anesthetic concentration (C_b).
4. Distribution of the anesthetic agent from the blood to the brain and other tissues.

There, thus, exists a series of partial pressure gradients between the partial pressure of the agent in the anesthetic circuit, the alveoli, arterial blood, and tissues. The rate of uptake of an inhalational anesthetic agent and, thus, the speed of induction are determined by the rate at which the alveolar concentration approaches the inspired anesthetic concentration. The uptake of anesthetic agent from the alveoli to blood is rapid

Table 9.1.
Physicochemical Properties of Some Inhalational Anesthetic Agents

Anesthetic	MAC* (% in oxygen)	MAC* (% in 70% N$_2$O)	Vapor pressure (mm Hg at 20°C)	Boiling point (°C at 760 mm Hg)
Nitrous oxide	105–110†		Gas	−88.5‡
Isoflurane	1.15	0.50	250	48.5
Enflurane	1.68	0.57	175	56.5
Halothane	0.75	0.29	243	50.2
Methoxyflurane	0.16	0.07	23	104.8

*MAC, minimum alveolar concentration (see text for definition). All values are expressed as percentages of one atmosphere.
†Hyperbaric nitrous oxide anesthesia would be required to attain 1 MAC.
‡At 50 atmospheres and 28°C.

initially as respiration brings anesthetic to the alveoli faster than it is removed by the blood. Uptake then slows down as the blood concentration rises until finally transfer from the inspired mixture to alveoli equals transfer from alveoli to blood (*point B*, Fig. 9.1). Uptake then continues at a slower rate until equilibrium is achieved in the tissues.

At equilibrium:

$$\frac{\text{Anesthetic blood concentration } (C_b)}{\text{Anesthetic alveolar concentration } (C_a)}$$
= Solubility of the anesthetic in blood (S)

Note that equilibrium means that the same anesthetic partial pressure exists in the blood and alveolar gas and does not mean equality of concentration in the two phases.

The **solubility** of a gas in a fluid is de-

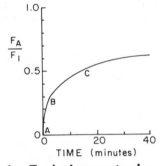

Figure 9.1. Typical curve to show the approach of the alveolar concentration to the inspired concentration. During the time *AB*, the first phase of the *curve,* there is a rapid rise in alveolar concentration as respiration brings anesthetic to the alveoli faster than it is removed by the blood. The *point B* on the *curve* represents the time when anesthetic uptake due to ventilation equals anesthetic uptake from the alveoli into the bloodstream. The second phase of the *curve,* the period *BC,* shows a relatively rapid rise in alveolar concentration resulting from equilibration of the anesthetic with tissues having a good blood supply— the vessel-rich group (VRG). The alveolar concentration subsequently rises more slowly, resulting in the third phase of the *curve,* as equilibrium occurs in muscle and fat.

$$\frac{F_A}{F_I} = \frac{\text{Alveolar concentration}}{\text{Inspired concentration}}$$

fined as the ratio of the concentration of dissolved gas to the concentration in the gas phase at equilibrium. This is referred to as the partition coefficient or the Ostwald solubility coefficient. Table 9.2 lists the partition coefficients of some of the inhalation anesthetics.

At equilibrium, the partial pressure of the inhalational anesthetic agent in blood and brain is approximately equal; and for each agent, there is a mean blood *concentration* at equilibrium which will produce surgical anesthesia. In addition, there is a precise relationship between anesthetic depth and blood and/or brain concentration. The more potent an agent, the lower the blood concentration required to produce anesthesia and, conversely, the less potent an anesthetic the higher the concentration required for surgical anesthesia.

In general, once equilibrium is achieved, arterial anesthetic partial pressure will approximate the alveolar anesthetic tension, and thus, the partial pressure of anesthetic agent within the alveoli closely governs the tension in the arterial blood and ultimately the tension of anesthetic agent within the brain.

The alveolar concentration depends on the balance between the factors affecting delivery of the anesthetic to the lungs and the factors affecting uptake from the lungs. Thus, alveolar concentration is determined by the *input* of the anesthetic minus the *loss* (uptake) of the anesthetic. Factors affecting the input or delivery of anesthetic agent to the lungs include (*a*) the inspired anesthetic concentration; and (*b*) the level of alveolar ventilation, while factors affecting uptake (loss) from the lungs include: (*a*) the solubility of the inhalational anesthetic agent in blood; (*b*) cardiac output; and (*c*) the difference between the level of agent in venous blood and the level in the alveolar gas.

LUNG "WASHIN"

Consider the introduction of an inhalational anesthetic agent into the lungs. The amount of anesthetic inhaled in the first breath is diluted in the lung volume, which at this time contains no anesthetic.

Table 9.2.
Partition Coefficients of Some Inhalational Anesthetic Agents at 37°C

Anesthetic	Blood/gas	Tissue/blood	Oil/gas
Cyclopropane	0.40 to 0.60	1.5 (brain-white) 1.16 (muscle) 1.16 (liver)	11.8
Nitrous oxide	0.47	1.13 (heart) 1.06 (brain) 1.00 (lung)	1.4
Isoflurane	1.40	2.6 (brain) 4.0 (muscle) 45.0 (fat)	98
Enflurane	1.91	1.45 (brain) 2.1 (liver) 1.7 (muscle) 36.2 (fat)	98
Halothane	2.3	2.6 (brain) 2.6 (liver) 1.6 (kidney) 3.5 (muscle) 60.0 (fat)	224
Methoxyflurane	13.0	2.34 (brain-white) 1.70 (brain-gray) 1.34 (muscle)	970

Most of the data are from Eger EI, Larson CP: Anesthetic solubility in blood and tissues: values and significance. *Br J Anaesth* 36:140–149, 1964; and Steward A, Allott PR, Cowles AL, Mapleson WW: Solubility coefficients for inhaled anesthetics for water, oil, and biological media. *Br J Anaesth* 45:282–293, 1973.

If

Alveolar ventilation = 0.3 L per breath

and

The effective lung volume into
which the anesthetic is diluted = 3.0 L,

let us consider the inhalation of an inspired gas mixture containing an anesthetic gas at a concentration of C_i (concentration/L), when C_a is the alveolar concentration in equilibrium with the required anesthetic blood concentration for surgical anesthesia (C_b).

The amount of anesthetic taken into the lungs at the first breath (0.3 C_i) is diluted immediately so that the alveolar concentration after the first breath is $(0.3/3)C_i$ or 0.1 C_i. Some of the anesthetic is then taken up by the blood perfusing the alveoli and carried away. If very little anesthetic is removed from the alveoli by the blood (low solubility), the alveolar concentration quickly rises towards the inspired concentration, C_i. If a large amount of the anesthetic is taken up by the blood (high solubility), the alveolar concentration rises more slowly toward the inspired concentration (Fig. 9.6). The repeated administration of a gas mixture carrying anesthetic at a concentration C_i to the total lung volume containing anesthetic at a lower concentration causes the anesthetic to accumulate within the alveoli. There comes a time when, during each inspiration, the amount of anes-

Table 9.3.
Anesthetic Concentrations and Partial Pressures for Surgical Anesthesia

Anesthetic	Solubility (S) in blood at 38°C	Blood concentration (C_b) (mM/L)	Alveolar concentration (C_a) (mM/L)	Partial pressure (mm Hg)
Ether	15.0	20.0	1.3	25.0
Halothane	2.3	1.0	0.43	8.3
Cyclopropane	0.47	4.1	8.7	170.0
Nitrous oxide	0.47	29.0	61.0	1200.0

Adapted with permission from Goldstein A, Aronow L, Kalman SM: *Principles of Drug Action: The Basis of Pharmacology,* ed 2. New York, John Wiley & Sons, 1974, p 339.

thetic agent taken up from the alveoli into the blood equals the amount of anesthetic taken up by the alveoli (*point B* of the curve in Fig. 9.1). In the case of an anesthetic of high solubility, the alveolar concentration would only be slightly higher than 0.1 C_i, since nearly all the anesthetic passes into the blood at each inspiration. However, for an anesthetic of low solubility, the alveolar concentration at point "B" would be almost C_i since very little is absorbed from the alveoli into the blood. In addition, anesthetics with low solubility (S) will have a high alveolar (C_a) than blood concentration (C_b) for surgical anesthesia, while anesthetics with a high solubility will have a higher blood than alveolar concentration for surgical anesthesia (Table 9.3). It is important to differentiate between the slow process of body saturation and the process of saturation of arterial blood concentration, to which the depth of anesthesia is closely related. The process whereby the alveolar anesthetic concentration completes the first phase of the curve (*point B*, Fig. 9.1) is called lung washin and is virtually complete within less than 2 minutes for most anesthetics.

FACTORS AFFECTING THE RATE OF DELIVERY OF ANESTHETIC TO THE LUNGS

The Inspired Anesthetic Concentration or Tension

The rate at which the alveolar tension rises and approaches the inspired anesthetic concentration is directly related to

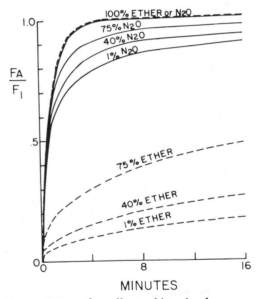

Figure 9.2.   The effect of inspired concentration on the rate of rise of alveolar anesthetic concentration. Increase in the inspired concentration of nitrous oxide and ether from 1 to 40 to 75 to 100% increases the rate of rise of the alveolar concentration of both nitrous oxide and ether. At 100% inspired concentration, the rate of rise of nitrous oxide and ether is the same and equals the washin rate of the lungs. F_A/F_I, alveolar/inspired concentration ratio. (With permission from Eger EI: Uptake of inhaled anesthetics: the concentration and second gas effects. In *Anesthetic Uptake and Action.* Baltimore, Williams & Wilkins, 1974, p 116.)

the inspired concentration (Fig. 9.2). The "concentration effect" states that the higher the inspired anesthetic concentration, the more rapid the rise in alveolar concentration. In theory, the rate of uptake of all inhalational anesthetic agents is equal when they are administered in 100% concentration, since when anesthetic uptake from the lungs occurs, the concentration, of anesthetic agent in the lungs remains at 100%. If however, we administer a lower inspired concentration and consider that the lung is filled with only 80% inhalational anesthetic agent and the other 20% is diluent gas that cannot be absorbed, then as the anesthetic agent is taken up by the lungs, the concentration of anesthetic agent within the lungs must fall and, thus, the rate at which the alveolar tension rises to

approach the inspired concentration is reduced. This is called the *concentration effect*—the effect which the inspired concentration of the anesthetic agent exerts on the speed with which that agent attains equilibrium.

The Second Gas Effect. The concentration effect is most noticeable with inhalational agents that can be administered over a wide range of inspired concentrations and which are taken up in large volumes, such as nitrous oxide. Such uptake results in (*a*) a concentrating effect and (*b*) a passive increase in the volume of gas inspired. When nitrous oxide and halothane (second gas) are administered concomitantly, the rate of increase of alveolar partial pressure of halothane is greater than if halothane is administered at the same inspired concentration with-

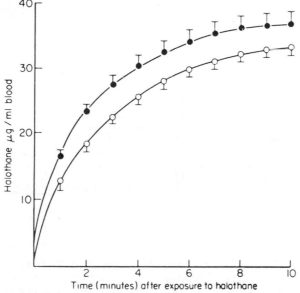

Figure 9.3.   The second gas effect. Mean blood halothane concentrations plotted against time for group A (O) and group B (●) patients. Group A received 0.4% halothane, 33% nitrous oxide, and 66% oxygen, while group B received 0.4% halothane, 66% nitrous oxide, and 33% oxygen. The increase in the rate of rise of arterial halothane concentration is demonstrated when halothane is administered with a higher concentration of nitrous oxide. Thus, the uptake of large volumes of a first gas (nitrous oxide) accelerates or augments the alveolar and, hence, arterial rate of rise of a second gas (halothane) administered concomitantly—the second gas effect. Note the rapid initial increase in blood concentration over the first 3 minutes, followed by a slower rate of increase to reach a steady-state concentration and the similarities between the shape of these curves and the one in Figure 9.1. (With permission from Tunstall ME, Hawksworth GM: Halothane uptake and nitrous oxide concentration. *Anaesthesia* 36:177–182, 1981.)

out nitrous oxide. The rapid uptake of a large volume of nitrous oxide causes a potential reduction of alveolar volume. This results in additional inflow of anesthetic gas from the machine to the alveolus and a net increase in alveolar ventilation. In addition, the uptake of a large volume of nitrous oxide causes an increased inflow of halothane and thus causes the alveolar partial pressure of halothane not to fall so much.

Figure 9.3 shows that the administration of halothane with a higher nitrous oxide concentration results in a secondary increase in the alveolar and arterial rate of rise of halothane, while Figure 9.4 illustrates the mechanisms for the production of the second gas effect. Similarly, the elimination of nitrous oxide accelerates that of halothane, by both alveolar dilution and an increased expired ventilation—"the reversed second gas effect."

Alveolar Ventilation

The greater the alveolar ventilation, the greater the rate of rise of alveolar anesthetic concentration (Fig. 9.5), when partial or nonrebreathing systems are employed. The more soluble the anesthetic agent, the greater the effect of increase in alveolar ventilation. Therefore, ether is most affected by changes in alveolar ventilation, and nitrous oxide is least affected.

FACTORS AFFECTING THE UPTAKE OF ANESTHETIC FROM THE LUNG

Solubility

The solubility of an inhalational anesthetic agent in blood is often expressed as the partition coefficient of the agent between blood and gas at body temperature, while the solubility of an agent in

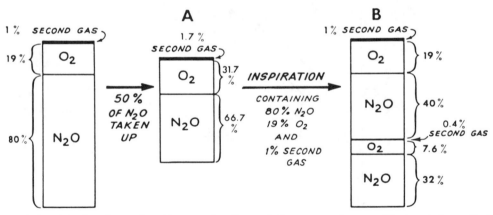

Figure 9.4. Mechanisms for the production of the second gas effect. A hypothetical lung, to illustrate the two proposed mechanisms in the production of the second gas effect. Part *A* is a diagrammatic illustration of how the second gas is concentrated in the lungs following the uptake of nitrous oxide. The hypothetical lung initially contains 80% nitrous oxide, 19% oxygen, and 1% second gas. If half the nitrous oxide is taken up, the remaining second gas now represents 1.7% (1 part in 60) of the total gas volume, while before it represented only 1% (1 part in 100). Consequently, the second gas has been concentrated in a smaller gas volume, and its alveolar concentration increases. Part *B* illustrates the effect of increased inspiratory ventilation on the concentrating effect. The inflowing gas contains the same proportions of nitrous oxide, oxygen, and second gas which were originally present. Though the absolute amount of second gas is increased (1 part to 1.4 parts), it represents a smaller proportion of the total gas volume, and its alveolar concentration falls from 1 part in 60 (1.7%) to 1.4 parts in 100 (1.4%). Therefore, the increased inspiratory ventilation dilutes the previously concentrated second gas and diminishes the magnitude of the second gas effect. (With permission from Stoelting RK, Eger EI: *Anesthesiology* 30:273–277, 1969.

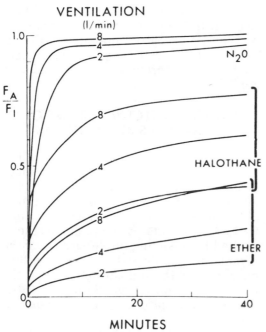

Figure 9.5. The effect of ventilation on the rate of rise of alveolar anesthetic concentration. If cardiac output and thus anesthetic uptake are held constant, then the rate of rise of alveolar concentration toward the inspired concentration (F_A/F_I) is accelerated by an increase in alveolar ventilation. (With permission from Eger EI: In *Anesthetic Uptake and Action.* Baltimore, Williams & Wilkins, 1974, p 123.)

tissues is expressed as the partition coefficient of the agent between blood and the tissue concerned at body temperature (see Table 9.2). Anesthetics are traditionally grouped as:

1. **Soluble** —methoxyflurane, diethyl ether
2. **Intermediate or moderately soluable** — halothane, enflurane, isoflurane
3. **Poorly soluable** —cyclopropane, nitrous oxide

Blood/gas solubility determines the rate of anesthetic induction, ease with which maintenance concentrations are changed, and speed of recovery.

Inhalational anesthetic agents with a high blood/gas partition coefficient, such as methoxyflurane, are highly soluble in blood and, thus, are removed in large quantities from the lungs by the pulmonary circulation, thereby lowering the al-

veolar anesthetic concentration or tension, resulting in a slow rise in alveolar concentrations, which are reflected in a slow rise in arterial and brain anesthetic tensions when the inspired concentration is maintained constant. Therefore, inhalational anesthetic agents with high blood/gas partition coefficients tend to be associated with the slow induction of anesthesia. In practice, this is overcome by raising the inspired anesthetic concentration to levels well above those required for the maintenance of anesthesia (overpressure). Insoluble anesthetic agents, such as nitrous oxide and cyclopropane, are removed in only small quantities from the alveoli, and the alveolar concentration soon equilibrates with the inspired concentration, resulting in the rapid induction of anesthesia. Figure 9.6 illustrates diagramatically the influence of solubility on the rate of rise of alveolar concentration. Oil/gas solubility (Table 9.2) parallels anesthetic potency; MAC times the oil/gas solubility coefficient results in a constant of 143 when all the commonly used inhalational anesthetic agents are averaged.

Cardiac Output

Cardiac output influences uptake by carrying away more or less inhalational anesthetic from the lungs. The greater the cardiac output, the greater the uptake of anesthetic agent from the alveoli by the blood and thus the slower the rate of

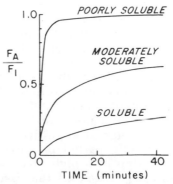

Figure 9.6. The influence of solubility on the rate of rise of alveolar concentration. F_A/F_I, alveolar/inspired concentration ratio.

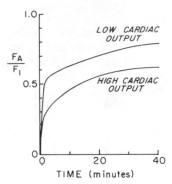

Figure 9.7. The effect of cardiac output on the rate of rise of alveolar anesthetic concentration. If ventilation is held constant, then the rate of increase of alveolar concentration will be slowed down by increases in cardiac output. This effect is greater with the more soluble anesthetics.

rise of alveolar concentration. When the cardiac output is reduced, less anesthetic is removed from the alveoli, and therefore the alveolar concentration approaches the inspired concentration more rapidly (Fig. 9.7).

The Alveolar to Mixed Venous Anesthetic Partial Pressure Difference

The third factor affecting the uptake of anesthetic agent from the lungs is the difference between the alveolar anesthetic partial pressure and the partial pressure of the agent in the venous blood returning to the lungs. The amount of anesthetic removed by the tissues will determine the alveolar to venous or arterial to venous anesthetic partial pressure difference, and depends on both the solubility of the agent in the tissues and the blood flow to the tissues. Thus, during the induction of anesthesia, the peripheral tissues remove a large proportion of the anesthetic brought to them, and the venous anesthetic partial pressure is very low. There is, therefore, a large alveolar to venous anesthetic partial pressure difference, resulting in a high level of anesthetic uptake. When all the tissues are equilibrated with the alveolar anesthetic partial pressure (this may take many hours or even days to occur), the anes-

thetic concentration in venous blood rises until there is no difference between the anesthetic partial pressure in the alveoli and the returning venous blood. Under these circumstances, uptake is zero.

FACTORS AFFECTING UPTAKE OF ANESTHETICS BY THE TISSUES

The total uptake of anesthetic at the tissues is equal to uptake from the lungs. When anesthetic is not removed by the tissues (as, for example, after saturation of the tissues), then the blood returning to the lungs contains as much anesthetic as the blood leaving the lungs. Thus, the alveolar to venous partial pressure difference is zero, there is no uptake, and the alveolar concentration closely approximates the inspired anesthetic concentration.

Factors affecting uptake of anesthetic by the tissues include tissue solubility, tissue blood flow, and the anesthetic partial pressure difference between arterial blood and the tissues (i.e., the concentration gradient). The capacity of the tissues to take up anesthetic depends on the size or volume of the tissue and the anesthetic's solubility in that tissue. Thus:

Tissue capacity
= Tissue volume × Tissue solubility

or

Tissue capacity = Tissue volume
× Tissue/blood partition coefficient

Tissue blood flow is also important and influences the *rate* at which tissue uptake proceeds. Fat has a large tissue capacity but small blood flow, so that the rate of rise of anesthetic partial pressure in fat is slow, but if the anesthetic were to be administered over a prolonged period of time, the eventual total uptake of anesthetic by fat would be great. However, in tissues with a large blood flow, the rate of rise is rapid, and tissue uptake soon ceases.

The body tissues have been divided into four groups according to their tissue capacity and level of perfusion (Table 9.4). The vessel-rich group (VRG), the

Table 9.4.
Tissue Group Characteristics

	VG (vessel rich)	MG (muscle)	FG (fat)	VPG (vessel poor)
Body Mass (%)	9	50	19	22
Volume (L) in a 70-kg man	6	33	14.5	12.5
Perfusion as % of cardiac output	75	18.1	5.4	1.5
Perfusion (L/min with a 6-L/min cardiac output)	4.5	1.09	0.32	0.08

Adapted with permission from Eger EI: *Anesthetic Uptake and Action.* Baltimore, Williams & Wilkins, 1974, p 88.

muscle group (MG), and the vessel-poor group (VPG) have similar tissue solubility but very different perfusion characteristics. The VRG is made up of tissues with a good blood supply and includes the brain, heart, kidney, splanchnic bed, and endocrine glands. Muscle and skin make up the MG, which has a moderately good blood supply, while the VPG consists of bone, ligaments, and cartilaginous tissue that has a very poor blood supply. Body fat (FG) has a poor blood supply, but a large tissue capacity. The VPG has little effect on uptake due to its extremely low perfusion. Figure 9.8 illustrates the uptake by the individual tissue groups for nitrous oxide and halothane. There is greatest uptake of anesthetic by the VRG in the first few minutes of anesthesia because this group of tissues receives the largest fraction of the cardiac output. Once equilibrium is established, tissue uptake by the vessel-rich group ceases; however, uptake by the muscle group and fat group continues and now contributes a greater proportion to total uptake. In 1 to 3 hours, equilibrium is established between the concentration in the arterial blood and muscle group, and uptake by fat then predominates and continues for many hours. It may theoretically take 5 days before halothane reaches equilibrium in fat.

The effect of tissue uptake on alveolar rate of rise is illustrated in Figure 9.9. The uptake of anesthetic by the tissues affects uptake at the lungs because, as uptake proceeds, the partial pressure difference between the alveolar gas and mixed venous blood falls. The anesthetic partial pressure in the VRG approaches the alveolar level more rapidly than tissue groups with poorer blood perfusion, MG and FG.

FACTORS AFFECTING RECOVERY FROM ANESTHESIA

The factors affecting the uptake and distribution of anesthetic agents during induction are also important during recovery from anesthesia. When the administration of an inhalational anesthetic agent is terminated, the factors that controlled the uptake of the anesthetic from the alveoli to blood also influence the effect of pulmonary ventilation on the rate of fall of alveolar anesthetic concentration; these are solubility, cardiac output, and the venous to alveolar anesthetic partial pressure difference. Therefore, recovery might be expected to be slow following anesthesia with highly soluble agents such as methoxyflurane, but rapid following anesthesia with poorly soluble agents such as nitrous oxide.

Metabolism of inhalational anesthetic agents is unimportant during anesthesia as complete inhibition or saturation of the metabolizing enzymes occurs. However, at low subanesthetic alveolar concentrations, hepatic metabolism becomes important for the elimination of halothane, but not for enflurane and isoflur-

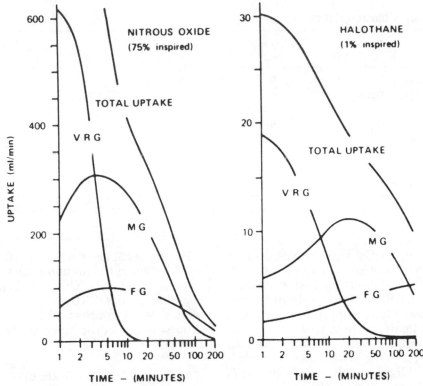

Figure 9.8.   Uptake of anesthetic by the tissues.   Total uptake is the sum of uptake by individual body tissues. The *uppermost curve* for each anesthetic is the sum of the three curves beneath it (with a slight time lag). The *curves* for nitrous oxide and halothane are identical in shape to those for all anesthetics. Uptake progressively decreases with duration of anesthesia and with saturation of the tissue depots. The order of saturation is always VRG first, then MG, and FG last. As noted in the illustration, the inspired concentration is constant at 75% nitrous oxide or 1% halothane. (With permission from Eger EI: Uptake of inhaled anesthetics: the alveolar to inspired anesthetic difference. In *Anesthetic Uptake and Action*. Baltimore, Williams & Wilkins, 1974, p 89.)

ane, since they undergo limited metabolism in comparison to halothane. As a result, alveolar concentrations of halothane fall below those of enflurane and isoflurane after about 1 and 3 hours, respectively, even though isoflurane and enflurane are less soluble than halothane. Figure 9.10 shows the comparative elimination of halothane, isoflurane, and enflurane over a 5-day period, indicating that the rate of elimination is similar for all three agents.

DIFFUSION HYPOXIA

The phenomenon of diffusion hypoxia was first described by Fink in 1955 and is

seen in the 10 minutes following discontinuation of anesthesia at the end of surgery. After nitrous oxide administration is terminated, the elimination of nitrous oxide into the lungs dilutes the oxygen within the alveoli and lowers the alveolar oxygen concentration. This is the reverse of the concentration effect. It can be prevented by the routine administration of oxygen when anesthesia is discontinued.

INDIVIDUAL INHALATIONAL ANESTHETIC AGENTS

Many of the traditional inhalational anesthetic agents such as cyclopropane and

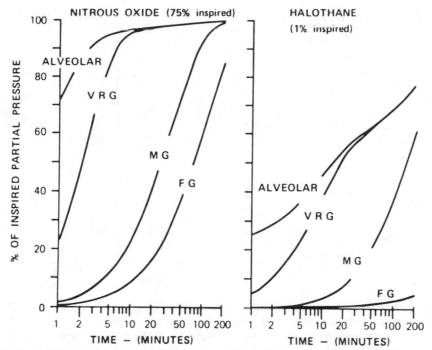

Figure 9.9.   Effect of tissue uptake on alveolar rate of rise.   Those tissue groups having a higher perfusion and lower solubility equilibrate sooner with the alveolar (i.e., arterial) anesthetic partial pressure. Thus, the VRG partial pressure rises more rapidly than that in the MG, and the MG partial pressure rises more rapidly than that in the FG. Tissue uptake may be obtained from these graphs as the alveolar/tissue partial pressure difference times the tissue perfusion. Peak uptake results from the peak difference between alveolar and tissue values and is therefore a function of both the alveolar and the tissue rate of rise. Note the logarithmic time scale. (With permission from Eger EI: Uptake of inhaled anesthetics: the alveolar to inspired anesthetic difference. In *Anesthetic Uptake and Action*. Baltimore, Williams & Wilkins, 1974, p 93.)

diethyl ether are now seldom used, and only the inhalational agents halothane, enflurane, isoflurane, and nitrous oxide will be discussed in detail in this chapter.

HALOGENATED HYDROCARBONS

Halothane

Halothane (2-bromo-2-chloro-1, 1, 1-trifluoroethane) is a fluorinated hydrocarbon. Its chemical structure is given in Figure 9.11.

PHYSICOCHEMICAL PROPERTIES

Halothane is a colorless liquid with a sweet nonirritating odor. Therefore, a rapid increase in inspired gas concentra-

tion is allowed, making halothane a suitable inhalational agent in children. It has a molecular weight of 197.39 and a specific gravity of 1.81 at 25°C. Table 9.1 lists some of its physicochemical properties. Because decomposition to HCL, HBr, free chlorine, bromine, and phosgene occurs when halothane is exposed to light, it is supplied in amber-colored bottles, to which 0.01% thymol is added to prevent the liberation of free bromine. Mixtures of halothane in air or oxygen are not explosive. Halothane is readily absorbed by rubber, but is less soluble in polyethylene.

The blood/gas partition coefficient of halothane at 37°C is 2.3 (Table 9.2) and, thus, it is considered moderately soluble,

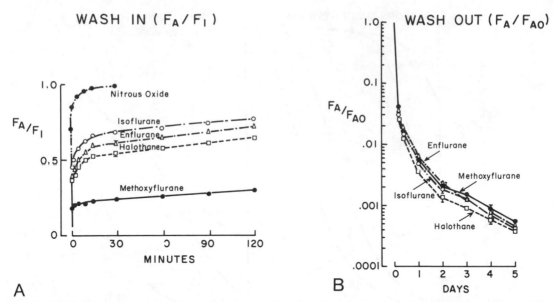

Figure 9.10. Recovery from anesthesia. The *left-hand panel* shows the rise in the ratio of alveolar to inspired concentration (F_A/F_I) for anesthetics of various blood-gas solubilities. The anesthetic vapors were delivered simultaneously at a concentration of 0.3 MAC. The *right-hand panel* shows the decline in alveolar concentration over 5 days expressed as the ratio of alveolar partial pressure (F_A) to the alveolar concentration immediately before discontinuation of anesthetic administration (F_{AO}). Note that F_A/F_{AO} is plotted on a logarithmic scale. The *curve* for wash-in (F_A/F_I) increased most rapidly with nitrous oxide and least rapidly with methoxyflurane, in accord with their respective solubilities in blood. However, for wash-out (F_A/F_{AO}), the curve for halothane fell below that for enflurane after about 70 minutes of wash-out and below that of isoflurane after 200 minutes. The more rapid decrease in halothane concentrations has been attributed to the elimination of halothane by the liver. Thus, metabolism can affect the rate of recovery from halothane anesthesia. It should be noted, however, that while uptake (wash-in) is as expected from anesthetic solubility data, the differences between the elimination curves are minimal.(With permission from Carpenter RL, Eger EI, Johnson BH, Unadkat JD, Sheiner LB: Pharmacokinetics of inhaled anesthetics in humans: measurements during and after the simultaneous administration of enflurane, halothane, isoflurane, methoxyflurane, and nitrous oxide. *Anesth Analg* 65:575–582, 1986.)

F   Br
| |
F – C – C – H
| |
F   Cl

HALOTHANE

F   F   F
| | |
H – C – C – O – C – H
| | |
Cl F   F

ENFLURANE

F   H   F
| | |
F – C – C – O – C – H
| | |
F   Cl   F

ISOFLURANE

Figure 9.11. Structural formulae of the inhalational anesthetic agents.

resulting in the fairly rapid induction and recovery from anesthesia.

CENTRAL NERVOUS SYSTEM

Halothane anesthesia causes depression of the central nervous system. Volatile anesthetics, in general, are cerebral vasodilators. Cerebral blood flow is increased and cerebral vascular resistance decreased during halothane anesthesia, provided that profound hypotension does not occur. This may lead to an increase in intracranial pressure, especially in the presence of a space-occupying intracranial lesion. Hyperventilation before the administration of halothane anesthesia is said to prevent or ameliorate the rise in intracranial pressure. Autoregulation of cerebral blood flow in response to changes in blood pressure is lost during halothane anesthesia.

The largest increase in cerebral blood flow occurs with halothane anesthesia, is intermediate with enflurane, and least with isoflurane. In addition, volatile anesthetics produce dose-dependent reductions in cerebral metabolic oxygen requirements.

Inhalational anesthetics cause dose-dependent depression of the amplitude and increase in the latency of the cortical component of median nerve somatosensory-evoked potentials; these changes are least with halothane, intermediate with isoflurane, and greatest with enflurane.

CARDIOVASCULAR SYSTEM

Volatile anesthetics have complex cardiovascular effects on both the myocardium and the peripheral circulation. All inhalational anesthetic agents depress myocardial function in a dose-related fashion. In addition to direct negative inotropic effects, indirect effects on the myocardium may occur due to secondary changes in cardiac preload or afterload or to reflex nervous system effects. It is generally accepted that the calcium ion is the most important mediator of acute changes in myocardial contractile activation, and inhalational anesthetics may produce their direct negative inotropic effects by interference with some of the steps involved in excitation-contraction coupling in the heart. Thus, anesthetics may act at a number of subcellular sites in myocardial muscle, such as the sarcolemma and sarcoplasmic reticulum, to decrease the level of intracellular ionized calcium and also to modify the sensitivity or responsiveness of the contractile proteins to activation by calcium. The possible mechanisms of anesthetic depression of myocardial contractility are extensively discussed in the review by Rusy and Komai.

In vitro studies performed in 1971 on the isolated papillary muscle of the cat

indicated that halothane depresses myocardial contractility and that, when enflurane, halothane, methoxyflurane, cyclopropane, and diethyl ether are administered at equal MAC, the order of depression of myocardial contractility is enflurane > halothane > methoxyflurane > cyclopropane > diethyl ether. Since that time, many studies have been carried out to determine the relative effects of the three most commonly used anesthetics, halothane, enflurane, and isoflurane, on myocardial contractility, often with conflicting results. More recent work using isolated ventricular myocardium has shown that isoflurane has a lesser direct inotropic effect than both halothane and enflurane at equipotent concentrations (Figure 9.12). Halothane and enflurane appear to be equipotent myocardial depressants.

Although clinical cardiovascular studies in humans are difficult to perform and in many cases the pharmacological effects of premedication, intravenous induction agents, and muscle relaxants need to be taken into account, myocardial contractility has been shown to be consistently impaired by halothane.

Filner and Karliner, using serial invasive and noninvasive measurements of left ventricular function in healthy volunteers, have demonstrated that halothane depresses left ventricular function at levels commonly employed for general anesthesia. They constructed composite ventricular function curves for the subjects at 1.25 and 1.75 MAC halothane administered in 100% oxygen (Figure 9.13); the curves showed displacement downward and to the right with increasing halothane concentration. Another study by Sonntag and coworkers also demonstrated that halothane has a direct depressant effect on left ventricular function. Their investigations of left ventricular function during halothane anesthesia using a Swan-Ganz catheter and direct left ventricular catheterization indicated that does-related decreases in left ventricular function are accompanied by increases in left ventricular filling pressures (Figure 9.14).

The administration of halothane dur-

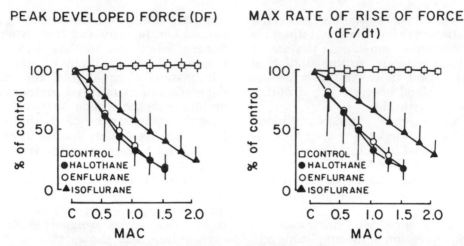

PEAK DEVELOPED FORCE (DF)   MAX RATE OF RISE OF FORCE
                                              (dF/dt)

Figure 9.12. Volatile anesthetics and myocardial contractility.   The effects of halothane, enflurane, and isoflurane on myocardial contractility in the isolated ventricular myocardium of the ferret. Isoflurane, enflurane, and halothane all caused a dose-dependent decrease in contractility, but the negative inotropic effect of isoflurane is less than that of halothane or enflurane. (With permission from Housmans PR, Murat I: Comparative effects of halothane, enflurane, and isoflurane at equipotent anesthetic concentrations on isolated ventricular myocardium of the ferret. I. Contractility. *Anesthesiology* 69:451–463, 1988.)

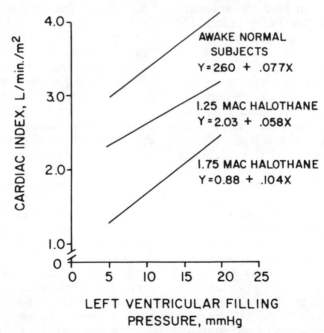

Figure 9.13. Left ventricular function and halothane anesthesia.   Composite left ventricular function curves at two levels of halothane anesthesia compared with a left ventricular function curve derived from data obtained in normal awake subjects. Left ventricular "filling" pressure for the awake subjects refers to left ventricular end diastolic pressure, and for the anesthetized subjects to mean pulmonary capillary ("wedge") pressure (PAW). (With permission from Filner BE, Karliner JS: Alterations of normal left ventricular performance by general anesthesia. *Anesthesiology* 45:610–621, 1976.)

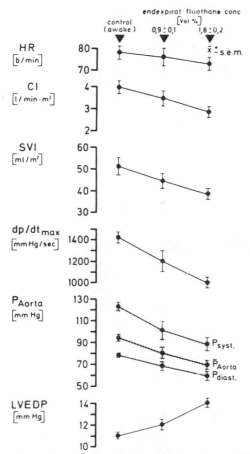

Figure 9.14. Effects of halothane on left ventricular function in humans. HR, heart rate; CI, cardiac index; SVI, stroke volume index; dp/dt_{max}, maximum rate of left ventricular pressure development; P_{syst}, systolic aortic pressure; P_{diast}, diastolic aortic pressure: P_{aorta}, mean aortic pressure; LVEDP, left ventricular end diastolic pressure. (With permission from Sonntag H, Donath U, Hillebrand W, Merin RG, Radke J: Left ventricular function in conscious man and during halothane anesthesia. *Anesthioloyg* 48:320–324, 1978.

ing controlled ventilation is accompanied by a dose-related reduction in systemic arterial blood pressure, cardiac output, and stroke volume. Mean right atrial pressure is increased. Total peripheral vascular resistance is unchanged, although at light anesthetic levels skin blood flow is increased. It is interesting

that prolonged anesthetia (5 hours) is associated with a gradual improvement of some cardiovascular parameters and that cardiac output, stroke volume, left ventricular work (stroke work), muscle blood flow, and mean right atrial pressure all return toward or above awake values. However, total peripheral vascular resistance falls and heart rate increases with prolonged duration of halothane anesthesia.

The cardiovascular effects of halothane are modified in the presence of spontaneous respiration and are shown in Figure 9.15. These changes have been attributed to (a) the effect of increased sympathetic activity due to elevated arterial carbon dioxide concentrations during spontaneous respiration and (b) the changes in intrathoracic pressure that occur during controlled ventilation.

The effects of halothane on heart rate and rhythm have been widely investigated. Some investigators have shown that halothane does not affect heart rate, while other workers have demonstrated that halothane anesthesia frequently slows cardiac rate. Halothane may cause direct depression of the S-A node and increase the refractory period of the A-V conduction system. Arrhythmias reported during halothane anesthesia include sinus bradycardia and nodal or junctional rhythms. Halothane also "sensitizes" the myocardium to the effects of endogenous and exogenous catecholamines (see Chapter 13 and Chapter 16), especially in the presence of hypercarbia. Bigeminy, multifocal ventricular ectopic beats, and even ventricular fibrillation may occur. While the arrhythmias which develop during halothane anesthesia are usually benign, they may not be in the presence of disease states (for example, ischemic heart disease), hypoxia, hypercarbia, or electrolyte abnormalites. The mechanism by which halothane sensitizes the myocardium to catecholamines is unknown, but since the threshold dose for epinephrine-induced arrhythmias is increased to a greater extent by α_1-blockade with prazosin than by relatively selective β_1-blockade with metropolol in dogs, it has been suggested that both α_1-

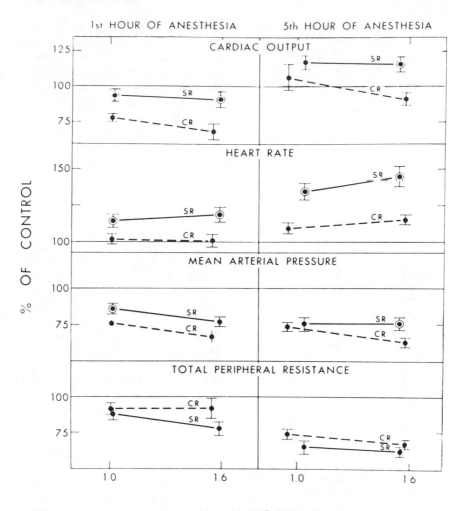

1st HOUR OF ANESTHESIA   5th HOUR OF ANESTHESIA

CARDIAC OUTPUT

HEART RATE

MEAN ARTERIAL PRESSURE

TOTAL PERIPHERAL RESISTANCE

% OF CONTROL

% HALOTHANE

Figure 9.15.   Cardiovascular effects of halothane during spontaneous and controlled respiration.   Values in the spontaneous respiration group and the controlled respiration group in the first and fifth hours of anesthesia. The percentage of control versus percentage of end tidal halothane is plotted for each variable. *Solid line SR,* spontaneous respiration; *dashed line CR,* controlled respiration. (With permission from Bahlman SH, Eger EI, Halsey MJ, Stevens WC, Shakespeare TF, Smith NT, Cromwell TH, Fourcade H: The cardiovascular effects of halothane in man during spontaneous ventilation. *Anesthesiology* 36:494–502, 1972.)

and β-receptors may be important in the production of epinephrine-induced arrhythmias. Other experiments have demonstrated a synergistic interaction between α_1 (phenylephrine) and β (isoproterenol) adrenoreceptor agonsts in the production of arrhythmias during halothane anesthesia. It has been further postulated that elevation in blood pressure (secondary to the α_1 effects of epinephrine, for example) may also contribute to the halothane-epinephrine-induced arrhythmias. Although recommendations of concentration and dose of epinephrine have been made for use during halothane anesthesia (See Chapter 13), it is wise to avoid the use of epinephrine during halothane whenever possible.

The effect of halothane on sympathetic nervous system activity may explain some of the observed hemodynamic changes that occur during halothane anesthesia. Plasma catecholamine concentrations are depressed in rats anesthetized by halothane and, in addition, halothane reduces stress-induced increases in levels of plasma total catecholamines and norepinephrine in rats. However, studies in humans have shown an increase in plasma norepinephrine concentrations during the induction of halothane anesthesia; this may have been related to the fall in blood pressure that occurred, since there was an inverse relationship between the rate-pressure product and plasma norepineprhine concentration.

RESPIRATORY SYSTEM

Increasing inspired concentrations of halothane lead to a progressive depression of the respiratory center, resulting in shallow and rapid respiration. Both tidal and minute volume are decreased. Potent inhalational agents are known to be bronchodilators, and bronchomotor tone is reduced in an animal model of antigen-induced asthma. The mechanism for the reduction in airway resistance produced by halothane is unclear; but it is possible that stimulation of bronchial β-adrenergic receptors is responsible (see Chapter 13). Halothane does not appear to exert a protective effect on the airway via inhibition of bronchoactive mediators, since plasma histamine levels remain elevated in laboratory animal studies. Whatever the mechanism, there is no clear evidence that halothane is beneficial in treating status asthmaticus that has failed to respond to conventional medical therapy.

There is suppression of both salivary and bronchial secretions even in subjects who have not received atropine. Halothane causes a dose-related reduction in the ventilatory response to carbon dioxide.

RENAL SYSTEM

Halothane (1 MAC) causes a reversible decrease in both glomerular filtration rate and renal blood flow and a dose-related decrease in urine output. Halothane does not alter autoregulation of renal blood flow.

MUSCLE

Halothane potentiates the neuromuscular relaxation produced by nondepolarizing skeletal muscle relaxants such as d-tubocurarine and pancuronium. The effect of inhalational anesthetic agents at the neuromuscular junction is discussed in Chapter 10.

REPRODUCTIVE SYSTEM

Halothane produces dose-dependent relaxation of uterine muscle in both pregnant and nonpregnant women. This relaxation may be due to stimulation of adrenergic β-receptors in the uterus. Inhibition of uterine contraction during labor and delivery by halothane may cause uterine atony accompanied by increased blood loss, and halothane should be avoided in these circumstances. Halothane is, however, valuable when uterine relaxation is required, for example, during the manual removal of a retained placenta.

LIVER

Factors affecting hepatic blood flow include sympathetic nervous system activity, surgery, hypoxia, hypercarbia, splanchnic reflexes, and exogenously administered drugs. Halothane (inspired concentration of approximately 1.5%) causes hepatic blood flow to fall by about 25 to 30%, which is unaccompanied by a change in splanchnic vascular resistance. It, therefore, appears that the fall in hepatic blood flow during halothane anesthesia is due to the fall in hepatic perfusion pressure, resulting from a reduction in arterial blood pressure. If the arterial carbon dioxide tension is allowed to rise during halothane anesthesia, splanchnic vascular resistance is reduced, and liver blood flow may be increased. Bromosulphthalein retention is increased following the administration of halothane. The association of halothane with postoperative hepatic dysfunction will be discussed later in this Chapter.

BIOTRANSFORMATION

Halothane is now known to be metabolized by the mixed-function oxidase system in the endoplasmic reticulum of the liver. Estimates of the extent of halothane metabolism vary and have been reported to be between 11 and 21% when approximately 1.0% halothane was administered. However, higher rates of halothane metabolism (41 to 55%) have been found when lower concentrations of halothane (0.11 to 0.43%) were employed. Thus, the importance of metabolism for halothane elimination may depend on the anesthetic concentration administered. It appears that a greater fraction of the halothane taken up at subanesthetic concentrations as opposed to anesthetizing concentrations is metabolized. This may be because at anesthetizing doses, hepatic enzyme systems are saturated, and anesthetic metabolism then plays a smaller role in the rate at which elimination occurs.

Halothane metabolism may proceed along two routes: **oxidative** and **reductive** (Figure 9.16). Trifluoroacetic acid and free bromide ion are metabolites that are produced via the oxidative pathway. Trifluoroacetic acid is detectable in the urine for many days after anesthesia. Cohen, using radiolabeled halothane in heart transplant donors, identified three major urinary metabolites of halothane: trifluoroacetic acid; N-trifluoroacetyl 1-2-aminoethanol; and N-acetyl-S-(2 bromo-2-chloro-1,1-difluoroethyl)-L-cysteine. Chloride and bromide ions are readily removed from halothane, but only a small amount of fluoride ion is liberated under normal circumstances since the bond energy for C-F is greater than that of C-Br and C-Cl. It is interesting that bromide is formed by both oxidative and reductive routes of biotransformation. Blood bromide concentrations might contribute to postoperative somnolence; levels as high as 3.0 mEq/L of plasma have been reported. Inhibition of oxidative metabolism of halothane is reported by cimetidine and possibly also by isoflurane.

Two volatile reductive metabolites, 2-chloro-1, 1, 1-trifluoroethane (CF_3CH_2C) and 2-chloro-1,1-difluoroethylene (CF_2CHCl) have been identified in humans and animals during halothane anesthesia. The volatile metabolite 2-

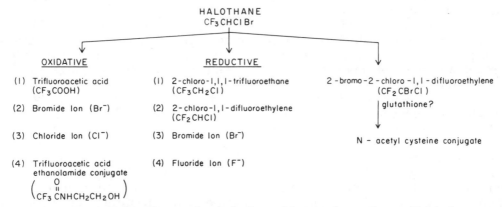

Figure 9.16.   Proposed pathways for halothane biotransformation.   *Oxidative* metabolism proceeds to produce trifluoroacetic acid and trifluoroacetic acid ethanolamide conjugate which have been isolated in the urine. Inorganic bromide is also produced. *Reductive* metabolism proceeds to form 2-chloro-1,1,1-trifluoroethane and 2-chloro-1,1-difluoroethylene, which are found in the breath. Inorganic bromide and fluoride are also metabolites formed by this route and are found in the urine. The volatile metabolite 2-bromo-2-chloro-1,1-difluoroethylene is found in the expired breath of patients under semiclosed or closed circuit conditions. It is produced by the passage of halothane through soda lime and is possibly excreted in the urine as the *N*-acetyl cysteine conjugate, described by Cohen (see text).

bromo-2-chloro-1,1-difluoroethylene (CF_2CBrCl) is due to a reaction of halothane with soda lime within the anesthetic circuit. The liberation of fluoride ion is thought to proceed by the reductive pathway. The various proposed pathways for halothane biotransformation are summarized in Figure 9.16.

Halothane has been shown to induce cytochrome P-450 in rats. However, it is a weak inducing agent (*cf.* phenobarbital, see Chapter 2), and long periods of exposure are required to produce this effect. In addition, halothane metabolism is inducible by phenobarbital. Exposure of anesthetists to measured trace concentrations of halothane for 10 days results in enzyme induction. A study in humans in which the drug-metabolizing ability of operating room personnel was compared with that of a group who did not work in the operating room showed increased drug-metabolizing ability in the operating room group (see page 50), possibly due to enzyme induction by inhalational anesthetic agents, such as halothane.

HALOTHANE HEPATOTOXICITY

Although halothane has been widely used as an inhalational anesthetic for over 30 years, the major reason for its decline in popularity is the association of halothane with liver damage—"halothane hepatitis." The first reports that halothane might be hepatotoxic appeared in 1958, and increasing concern led to the National Halothane Study (1966). This was a retrospective analysis of about 850,000 anesthetics between the years 1959 and 1962. This study, however, neither proved nor disproved a relationship between hepatic necrosis and halothane anesthesia, but did support the safety of halothane as an inhalational anesthetic agent. Laboratory experiments during this period failed to reveal a direct toxic action of halothane on the liver at clinical concentrations, and the existence of halothane hepatitis became the subject of considerable debate. Today, it is accepted that liver necrosis can follow the administration of halothane, but the mechanism is still unclear. A variety of causative mechanisms have been suggested including hypersensitivity, liver hypoxia, metabolism of halothane to destructive reactive intermediates via the reductive pathway, metabolism to a metabolite-protein hapten that possesses immunological properties, and finally that postoperative hepatic dysfunction is actually not a result of halothane administration, but of viral hepatitis. However, the two major mechanisms of halothane hepatoxicity investigated over the last 15 years are:

1. Biotransformation of halothane to toxic intermediate metabolites;
2. Sensitization to halothane or its metabolites, or to a new antigen induced by the reaction of a halothane metabolite with liver cell macromolecules.

Halothane hepatitis occurs about 2 to 5 days after anesthesia and surgery when typically fever, nausea, and vomiting develop followed by jaundice. A rash and eosinophilia may also occur. Estimates of the incidence of severe liver damage associated with halothane anesthesia vary between 1 in 6,000 and 1 in 35,000. The overall incidence of postoperative jaundice is not known, but may be in the region of 4 per 1,000 anesthetics. It should be stressed that the most common causes of postoperative hepatic dysfunction include viral hepatitis, the use of blood transfusions, or damage by known hepatotoxins. Two distinct forms of liver damage have now been defined:

1. A mild relatively common form (up to 20% of patients exposed to halothane) in which serum aminotransferases are raised during the first and second postoperative weeks after receiving halothane (type I, minor).
2. A rare form in which massive liver cell necrosis occurs leading to liver failure and even death (type II, major).

An increased incidence of liver damage has been reported after repeated exposure to halothane within a short period of time. This seems to suggest that halothane hepatitis might be due to an abnormal immune response. Supportive evidence for a hypersensitivity reaction includes fever, eosinophilia, arthralgia, and rash. In addition, it has been suggested that an immune-mediated response might be related to the binding of halothane intermediates to liver macromolecules, which then triggers the hypersensitivity response in susceptible individuals. Thus, sensitization is directed toward liver cells altered as a result of exposure to halothane or halothane metabolites.

It is now recognized that the biotransformation of halothane may play a major role in the production of halothane hepatotoxicity. Usually metabolism of drugs converts pharmacologically active lipid-soluble compounds to more polar pharmacologically inactive water-soluble products which are easily excreted. However, during the metabolism of some drugs, reactive unstable intermediaries are formed which bind to various cellular constituents. Because of the instability and reactivity of these intermediates, they are hard to detect in, for example, plasma samples and usually bind to tissues close to their site of production, which for many drugs is the microsomal mixed-function oxidase system of the liver. Such irreversible binding of halothane intermediate metabolites to liver macromolecules might be related to halothane hepatotoxicity.

Halothane undergoes both oxidative and reductive biotransformation (see previous section), and both routes are associated with the generation of reactive metabolites which covalently bind to hepatocellular macromolecules. In the last decade, animal experiments have suggested that the reductive pathway leads to the formation of reactive intermediates and subsequent hepatotoxicity, and that halothane metabolism under hypoxic conditions and enzyme induction (to promote metabolism along the reductive pathway) produces reactive metabolites that bind to cellular constituents and cause hepatic damage. *In vitro* covalent binding of halothane to liver lipids and protein is enhanced by an anerobic atmosphere, while the binding of radiolabeled halothane in isolated perfused rat livers is increased during conditions of hypoxia and enzyme induction.

Animal models for halothane hepato-toxicity have been developed. In one model, rats, pretreated with phenobarbital and anesthetized with halothane at low oxygen concentrations (7 to 14% oxygen), develop centrilobular hepatic necrosis and exhibit a 3-fold increase in the covalent binding of radiolabeled halothane metabolites to hepatic microsomal lipids. In addition, there is a significant elevation in the plasma fluoride concentration. The defluorination of halothane occurs via the reductive pathway (see previous section), and plasma fluoride concentrations correlate with toxicity in the hypoxic enzyme-induced model. In addition, two volatile metabolites of halothane, 1,1,1-trifluorochloroethane and 1,1-difluoro-2-chloroethylene, are also end products of reductive metabolism; their formation is enhanced by phenobarbital pretreatment and hypoxia. Thus, there is evidence that the reductive pathway for halothane biotransformation leads to hepatic damage in animals. Cimetidine, which inhibits the metabolism of halothane, is associated with a decreased incidence and severity of liver damage in the phenobarbital-hypoxia rat model, implicating halothane metabolism as an important etiological factor in halothane-induced liver injury. It is interesting to note that the same two volatile metabolites have been found in humans even at inspired oxygen concentrations of nearly 100%, but their relationship to toxicity in humans is not known.

Another animal model that was studied a number of years ago involves pretreatment with triiodothyronine. Halothane anesthesia (1%) for 2 hours in 21% oxygen causes centrilobular hepatic necrosis in rats. More recently, a guinea pig model has been developed, in which the animals develop liver damage after 4 hours of halothane anesthesia in 21% oxygen; enzyme induction is not required. Other animal experiments have suggested that hypoxia per se is important in the production of halothane hepatotoxicity.

It should be emphasized that the evidence linking the biotransformation of halothane to toxicity has been obtained in animals, and caution must be exercised before extrapolating these findings to humans.

Clinical studies have shown that patients with halothane hepatotoxicity have circulating antibodies reacting with altered liver cell membrane determinants. In contrast to the direct hepatotoxicity shown in animal experiments in which reactive metabolites are generated via the reductive route, the production of the halothane-altered determinant is associated with the oxidative route. A specific circulating antibody found in the sera of patients with hepatic failure following multiple halothane anesthetics reacts with an antigen present on the membrane of hepatocytes isolated from halothane-exposed rabbits—"the halothane antigen."

Thus, there are two possible mechanisms of halothane toxicity, both of which are related to halothane biotransformation; (a) a direct reaction via the reductive pathway; and (b) an immune-mediated reaction where the antigen is associated with the oxidative route (Figure 9.17). Neuberger and Davis have speculated that the mild reaction is due to toxic metabolites generated via the reductive pathway, while the rare severe reaction is due to an immune reaction in which the antigen is associated with the oxidative route and the patient possesses an antibody reacting with halothane-altered liver cells. Thus, the diagnosis of halothane hepatotoxicity can now be confirmed serologically by the presence of *in vitro* antibodies reacting with halothane-altered liver cell membrane antigens.

Pharmacogenetic factors have been suggested to play a role in the etiology of halothane hepatotoxicity, since it is known that species and strain differences exist for susceptibility to halothane hepatotoxicity in animals and that halothane hepatotoxicity has been demonstrated in three pairs of closely related women.

Although halothane metabolism may play a central role in the production of halothane hepatotoxicity, it is likely that the etiology of halothane-induced liver disease is multifactorial, and other factors such as reduced hepatic blood flow secondary to halothane-induced cardiovascular depression, surgical trauma, hypoxia, and genetic factors are also important (Figure 9.18).

SUGGESTED DOSAGE AND
ADMINISTRATION

Inspired concentrations of 2.0 to 3.0% may be necessary for the induction of anesthesia, while maintenance concentra-

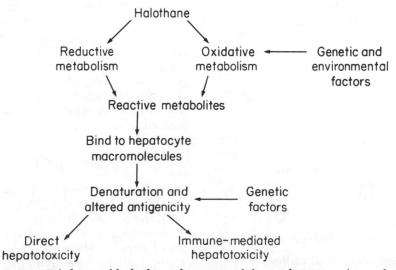

Figure 9.17. Etiology of halothane hepatotoxicity and routes of metabolism.

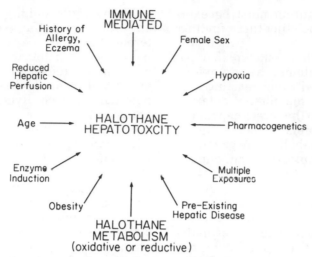

Figure 9.18.   Factors affecting halothane hepatotoxicity.

tions are in the region of 0.25 to 2.5%. Maintenance concentrations depend on many factors; these include the age and physical status of the patient, premedication, and the percentage concentration of nitrous oxide being administered.

Since repeat administrations of halothane have been associated with hepatotoxicity, and enflurane and isoflurane are readily available, there is now no indication for the repeated use of halothane within at least 6 months of previous administration.

PRESENT STATUS

For many years halothane was the most important volatile anesthetic agent in clinical practice, despite its arrhythmogenic effects and its potential to cause hepatotoxicity. However, when enflurane was released for clinical use in the early 1970s, it soon supplanted halothane as the most widely used inhalational anesthetic agent in the United States. Today, halothane continues to be used in children, because it is a more pleasant agent to breathe than either enflurane or isoflurane and because of the belief (perhaps not correct) that halothane hepatotoxicity is rare in this age group.

Chloroform and Trichloroethylene

Trichloroethylene and chloroform are no longer used today. Trichloroethylene is decomposed by alkali and heat to form the toxic flammable substance, dichloroacetylene, which may break down further to phosgene and carbon monoxide. The breakdown products are highly toxic, causing lesions of cranial nerves C5, and also C3, 7, and 8. Therefore, trichloroethylene should not be used in breathing circuits requiring soda lime. Trichloroethylene anesthesia is associated with bradycardia and tachypnea with shallow respiration, while deeper anesthesia causes cardiac dysrhythmias, especially in the presence of spontaneous ventilation. Trichloroethylene increases cerebral blood flow and intracranial pressure. The incidence of nausea and vomiting after trichloroethylene anesthesia is higher than after halothane anesthesia.

Chloroform is hepatotoxic and nephrotoxic. During chloroform anesthesia, the myocardium is sensitized to catecholamines, cardiac irritability occurs, and ventricular fibrillation may result.

ANESTHETIC ETHERS

Although diethyl ether was used by Crawford Long in 1841, it was Morton in 1846 who conducted the famous ether demonstration at the Massachusetts General Hospital. Since that time many anesthetic ethers have been introduced. Diethyl ether is flammable and explosive under certain circumstances, whereas the new ethers are nonflammable and nonexplosive. When halothane and methoxyflurane were introduced into anesthetic practice, it was thought that they did not undergo biotransformation and that they were eliminated from the body in the unchanged state. It is now known that significant metabolism does occur and that the metabolic products may exert toxic effects on the liver and kidney. The toxic effects of these agents stimulated the search for new inert volatile anesthetics with improved cardiovascular stability. The ethers are likely to be more useful than the hydrocarbons, and a new series of compounds, the fluorinated methyl ethers (of which enflurance and its isomer, isoflurane, are the most noted), have been developed.

Enflurane

Enflurane, 2-chloro-1,1,2-trifluoroethyl difluoromethyl ether, is a fluorinated methyl ethyl ether. Its chemical structure is given in Figure 9.11.

PHYSICOCHEMICAL PROPERTIES

Enflurane is a clear, colorless, nonflammable volatile liquid with a mild sweet odor. Enflurane is more stable than halothane and does not contain a preservative. It has a molecular weight of 184.5 and a specific gravity at 25°C of 1.52. Table 9.1 lists some of its physicochemical properties. Enflurane is nonflammable and nonexplosive at all concentrations in air or oxygen. The MAC of enflurane is 1.68 in pure oxygen (see Table 9.1) and, therefore, it is less potent than halothane.

The blood/gas partition coefficient of enflurane at 37°C is 1.91 (Table 9.2), producing a slightly more rapid induction of anesthesia with enflurane than with halothane.

CENTRAL NERVOUS SYSTEM

Soon after its introduction into clinical practice, it was noted that tonic-clonic twitching of the muscles of the face and limbs may develop during the administration of high concentrations of enflur-

ane, especially if there is associated hypocapnia. A characteristic EEG pattern occurs; a high voltage fast frequency pattern progresses to spike-dome complexes alternating with a period of silence or frank "seizure" activity. Tonic-clonic responses may be terminated by reducing the inspired concentration of enflurane and returning the arterial carbon dioxide tension to normal.

Although studies of enflurane anesthesia in patients suffering from various types of epilepsy do not show that seizure activity is provoked, it is recommended that enflurane not be administered to patients with a history of epilepsy.

Enflurane causes cerebral vasodilation and, provided arterial blood pressure is maintained, cerebral blood flow is increased. However, reductions in cerebral flow may follow profound decreases in arterial pressure. The effects of enflurane on intracranial pressure are variable; either no change or small and inconsistent increases in pressure have been reported in neurosurgical patients who are hyperventilated and receive low concentrations of enflurane.

CARDIOVASCULAR EFFECTS

The hemodynamic effects of enflurane are qualitatively similiar to those of halothane, but discussion has centered on the relative extent of cardiovascular depression that these two agents exert. Early clinical reports showed that, in the presence of hypocarbia, normocarbia, and hypercarbia, cardiac output and arterial pressure were well maintained. These early studies were interpreted to indicate that enflurane produces minimal cardiovascular depression in humans. Animal and human studies have since shown that enflurane causes dose-dependent cardiovascular depression similar to or greater than that of halothane. It is probable that the conflicting data obtained from clinical investigations in humans are due in part to the differing levels of enflurane anesthesia employed; levels above 1.5 MAC may cause pronounced cardiovascular depression, especially if administered over a prolonged period of time. Enflurane possesses a narrow margin of safety between concentrations required for surgical anesthesia and dangerous cardiovascular depressant levels.

In vitro studies of the inotropic effect of enflurane on cat papillary muscle have shown that enflurane produces dose related reversible depression of myocardial contractility. Merin and coworkers have demonstrated that in intact dogs with chronically implanted transducers, 3.6% enflurane depresses left ventricular function, myocardial blood flow, and metabolism. The cardiovascular effects of halothane (2.0 MAC) resembled those of enflurane (1.6 MAC), suggesting that enflurane depresses myocardial contractility more than halothane at equipotent doses.

Enflurane anesthesia depresses arterial blood pressure, stroke volume, and systemic vascular resistance. Calverly and colleagues found that, in human volunteers, 1.0 MAC enflurane during controlled ventilation depresses cardiac output, stroke volume, arterial blood pressure, and systemic vascular resistance, while 2.0 MAC enflurane produces unacceptable progressive and profound hypotension. These cardiovascular changes are more marked during normocarbia and controlled ventilation than during spontaneous respiration and hypercarbia. During prolonged enflurane anesthesia, myocardial function recovers partially at light but not deep levels of enflurane anesthesia. Arterial hypotension is thus a frequent occurrence during enflurane anesthesia, but the blood pressure tends to return toward preanesthetic levels with surgical stimulation. It appears that enflurane produces cardiovascular depression by both a direct negative inotropic effect on the heart and a decrease in peripheral vascular resistance. Heart rate tends to increase or remain constant, and bradycardia does not usually occur. Although enflurane sensitizes the myocardium to the effects of endogenous and exogenous catecholamines, a lower incidence of dysrhythmias is associated with the administration of epinephrine during enflurane

anesthesia than with halothane (see Chapter 16). Enflurane causes a dose-related inhibition of spontaneous catecholamine release, and plasma catecholamine concentrations do not rise during enflurane anesthesia.

Propranolol accentuates the hemodynamic effects of enflurane more than those of halothane in dogs. Enflurane also impairs the response to volume depletion following 20% withdrawal of blood volume in the presence of β-adrenergic blockade. The adverse hemodynamic effects of calcium antagonist administration are greater during enflurane anesthesia than during halothane anesthesia in animal studies (see Chapter 18).

RESPIRATORY SYSTEM

Enflurane produces dose-dependent depression of respiration, which is more pronounced than that of other inhalational anesthetics at comparable MAC levels of anesthesia. Tidal volume is diminished, while respiratory rate remains unchanged or slightly increased. A reduced ventilatory response to hypoxia and hypercarbia is observed in dogs anesthetized with 1.0 MAC enflurane. Enflurane is nonirritating to the respiratory tract and coughing, laryngospasm, and increases in secretions are uncommon. Bronchodilation occurs.

RENAL SYSTEM

The renal effects of enflurane in humans include a reduction in renal blood flow, glomerular filtration rate, and urinary flow rate. These reductions are of the same order as occur with other volatile anesthetic agents. Enflurane is metabolized in humans (see biotransformation below) with the production of inorganic fluoride. Maximum serum fluoride concentrations after enflurane anesthesia do not approach critical concentrations for renal toxicity, and it would be reasonable to assume that the danger of renal damage after enflurane anesthesia is slight in normal subjects. Peak serum concentrations below 20 μmol/L have been reported after enflurane anesthesia, while serum concentrations of about 50 μmol/L are usually necessary for the production of fluoride renal toxicity. The maximum serum fluoride concentrations following the administration of enflurane to anephric subjects and patients suffering from severe renal disease do not differ significantly from each other, nor from those patients with normal renal function. However, low fluoride concentrations (15 μmol/L) following enflurane anesthesia have been associated with a 25% reduction in maximum urine concentrating ability. The finding that even relatively low concentrations of fluoride may temporarily alter renal function suggests that enflurane anesthesia might be potentially harmful in patients with preexisting renal disease.

MUSCLE

Enflurane causes dose-related depression of neuromuscular transmission and thus provides good muscular relaxation, which may be sufficient for abdominal surgery. However, the administration of a nondepolarizing muscle relaxant allows the use of a lower concentration of enflurane. Enflurane potentiates the effects of the nondepolarizing muscle relaxants, and smaller doses of d-turocurarine and pancuronium are required during enflurane anesthesia than during the administration of equipotent (equal MAC) concentrations of halothane (see Chapter 10).

REPRODUCTIVE SYSTEM

Uterine muscle is relaxed by enflurane. The response of the uterus to oxytocin is maintained, provided that high inspired concentrations (over 2.5 to 3.0%) are not employed.

LIVER

Evidence of slight hepatic dysfunction has been reported during and after surgery with enflurane anesthesia (increase in standard liver function test values), while prolonged periods of enflurane anesthesia (9.0 MAC hours) in young volunteers cause only slight reversible changes in liver function. Nevertheless, there have been isolated case reports of hepatic damage in association with enflurane anesthesia. Enflurane administration under hypoxic conditions to phenobarbital-pretreated rats does not cause centrilobular necrosis (see Halothane Hepatotoxicity).

BIOTRANSFORMATION

The biotransformation of enflurane in humans is only about one-fifth that of halothane with only about 2.0 to 8.0% of the administered dose being metabolized, chiefly in the liver. Chase and co-workers have reported that 82.7% of administered enflurane is excreted unchanged by the lungs and 2.4% is excreted in the urine as nonvolatile fluorinated metabolites. The very low biodegradation of enflurane is attributed to its chemical stability and low-fat solubility, so that enflurane rapidly leaves fatty tissues when anesthesia is discontinued and thus is available for metabolism for only a short period of time.

Like methoxyflurane (another fluorinated ether), enflurane is metabolized to inorganic and organic fluoride via oxidative metabolism. The molecule is thus broken down to yield difluoromethyldifluoracetic acid and chloride and fluoride ions.

Enzyme induction by phenobarbital treatment increases methoxyflurane metabolism in rats and causes a parallel increase in renal toxicity, but there is no increase in urinary fluoride excretion when phenobarbital-pretreated rats are exposed to enflurane. However, enzyme induction increases the liberation of fluoride from enflurane in isolated liver microsomes in vitro. This difference in metabolism in vivo and in vitro is probably due to the low tissue solubility of enflurane, so that in vivo the availability of the substrate (enflurane) becomes the rate-limiting factor, whereas in vitro, the substrate concentration is controlled and the effect of enzyme induction leads to a significant increase in enflurane metabolism to fluoride. Figure 9.19 compares the in vitro metabolism of methoxyflurane, enflurane, and isoflurane. The ratio of inorganic fluoride released by the biotrans-

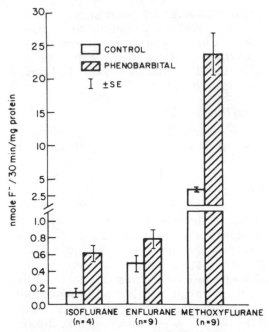

Figure 9.19.   Histograms showing the defluorination of isoflurane, enflurane, and methoxyflurane in hepatic microsomes from rats pretreated with phenobarbital and in control rats not treated with phenobarbital. (With permission from Greenstein LR, Hitt BA, Mazze RI: Metabolism *in vitro* of enflurane, isoflurane, and methoxyflurane. *Anesthesiology* 42:420–424, 1975.)

formation of methoxyflurane, enflurane, and isoflurane was 23:3:1 using hepatic microsomes from non-enzyme-induced (no phenobarbital pretreatment) rats and 39:1.3:1 using microsomes from rats pretreated with phenobarbital. The defluorination of enflurane in humans is not inducible with phenobarbital or the 3-methylcholanthrene group of inducing agents.

Although many cases of nephrotoxicity following methoxyflurane anesthesia have been reported, only a small number of cases have been associated with enflurane administration. In one case, the patient had a high peak serum fluoride concentration and was receiving the antituberculous drug, isoniazid. Animal studies have since shown that enflurane defluorination is enhanced following iso-

niazid treatment. Increased defluorination of enflurane has now been demonstrated in patients who are "fast acetylators" (see page 49) treated with the antituberculous drug, isoniazid. There is a bimodal distribution of enzyme induction following isoniazid treatment, with some (approximately 50%) patients having high and others normal fluoride concentrations. Isoniazid is metabolized to isonicotinic acid and acetylhydrazine. Acetylhydrazine is subsequently broken down to hydrazine and acetic acid. Rapid acetylators have higher hydrazine concentrations than slow acetylators, and it is hydrazine that induces increased formation of cytochrome P-451, leading to increased enflurane defluorination.

Suggested Dosage and Administration

Enflurane is a less potent anesthetic agent than halothane. The induction of anesthesia usually requires an inspired concentration of 3 to 4%, while the maintenance concentration is between 1.5 and 3%. Ventilation to maintain normocarbia is advisable to prevent central nervous system complications.

Isoflurane

PHYSICOCHEMICAL PROPERTIES

Isoflurane (1-chloro-2,2,2-trifluoroethyl difluoromethyl ether) is a halogenated methyl ethyl ether and is an isomer of enflurane; its structual formula is given in Figure 9.11. It is a clear colorless liquid which is nonflammable in air, nitrous oxide, and oxygen. Some of its physicochemical properties are listed in Table 9.1. The vapor pressures of halothane and isoflurane are nearly identical. Isoflurane does not require a preservative to prevent its decomposition.

As it is relatively insoluble in blood (blood/gas partition coefficient of 1.4) (Table 9.2), induction and recovery might be expected to be more rapid than with halothane anesthesia. However, the airway irritability of isoflurane often results in a slower than expected induction during clinical anesthesia.

CENTRAL NERVOUS SYSTEM

Isoflurane produces dose-related depression of the central nervous system. It causes progressive electroencephalographic (EEG) changes that generally are similar to those produced by other volatile anesthetics. At 1.0 MAC anesthesia, EEG frequency decreases and voltage increases. At 1.5 MAC, burst suppression occurs and the voltage begins to diminish, while at 2.0 MAC, the electroencephalogram becomes isoelectric. It does not produce convulsive electroencephalographic abnormalities, characteristic of enflurane, even at deep levels of anesthesia, with or without hypocapnia.

As discussed earlier in the chapter, volatile anesthetics are cerebral vasodilators (Fig. 9.20). No change in cerebral blood flow occurs when isoflurane is administered in concentrations of 0.6 or 1.1 MAC. Similar results are obtained at 0.6 MAC for halothane and enflurane, but at 1.1 MAC, cerebral blood flow increases 30 to 50% with enflurane and almost 200% with halothane. At 1.6 MAC, cerebral blood flow is increased 2-fold for enflurane and isoflurane and 4-fold for halothane. Cerebral vascular resistance is thus decreased during isoflurane anesthesia and may cause an increase in intracranial pressure. The cerebral vasodilating properties of isoflurane can be effectively attenuated by establishment

of hypocapnia. The limited changes in cerebral blood flow associated particularly with low concentrations of isoflurane as compared to halothane and enflurane mean it is less likely to increase intracranial pressure. Cerebral oxygen consumption is decreased by isoflurane. Autoregulation of cerebral blood flow in response to changes in blood pressure is maintained during isoflurane anesthesia.

Isoflurane has perhaps become the volatile anesthetic agent of choice in neurosurgical anesthetic practice for three reasons: effects on intracranial pressure; possible cerebral protective effects; and its metabolic effects during induced hypotension. Whether isoflurane provides cerebral protection has been the subject of debate over the last 5 years; evidence from laboratory studies that isoflurane may provide some degree of cerebral protection is conflicting and, although isoflurane may offer protective effects in regional cerebral ischemia, it does not appear to offer as great protection as that associated with thiopental. Although the potent volatile anesthetics may be associated with increases in intracranial pressure, isoflurane is less deleterious in this situation than halothane or enflurane. Isoflurane has also been administered to provide controlled hypotension, and it has been shown that cerebral oxygen balance is generally not disturbed. In animals, nitroprusside-induced hypotension produces far greater metabolic effects (ATP, lactate) than isoflurane-induced hypotension. The cerebral metabolic rate for oxygen was reduced more by isoflurane than nitroprusside. Clinical studies also show that controlled hypotension with isoflurane does not cause major disturbances in cerebral oxygen balance.

CARDIOVASCULAR SYSTEM

Like other inhalational anesthetics, isoflurane depresses the contractility of isolated myocardial muscle in vitro. Isoflurane decreases the mean maximal velocity of shortening, the mean maximal developed force, and other indices of myocardial contractility in a dose-depen-

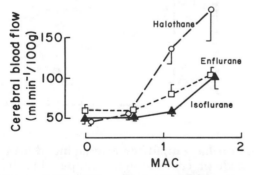

Figure 9.20. The effect of volatile anesthetics on cerebral blood flow. (With permission from Eger EI: The pharmacology of isoflurane. *Br J Anaesth* 56:71S–99S, 1984.)

dent manner. At equipotent doses, these effects of isoflurane are comparable to or less than those of halothane, but are greater than those of diethyl ether. However, in vivo, isoflurane may be less depressant to the myocardium and circulation than other volatile anesthetics. Cardiac output is maintained in human volunteers given 1.0 to 1.8 MAC isoflurane, while in contrast, enflurane and halothane produce a dose-related depression of cardiac output (Fig. 9.21). Volatile anesthetics produce dose-dependent reductions in blood pressure with isoflurane and enflurane producing greater decreases than halothane. The fall in blood pressure produced by halothane is probably due mainly to a decrease in myocardial contractility and cardiac output, while for isoflurane, the greater decrease in blood pressure is due not only to a decrease in myocardial contractility but more importantly to a profound decrease in peripheral vascular resistance (see later in section). The decrease in blood pressure produced by isoflurane is offset by an increase in heart rate so that cardiac output is unchanged.

In some patients, a significant tachycardia may occur, and heart rate generally is higher with isoflurane than with halothane. It has been suggested that the increase in heart rate is due to stimulation of baroreceptors secondary to a decrease in arterial blood pressure. Isoflurane, like halothane, has been shown to attenuate the carotid sinus baroreceptor reflex, but at comparable doses, isoflurane appears to be less depressant than halothane on baroreflex-induced changes in heart rate. Cardiac arrhythmias are uncommon. Isoflurane does not sensitize the myocardium to the arrhythmogenic effects of circulating catecholamines to the same extent as halothane (see Chapter 13 and Chapter 16).

Isoflurane decreases systemic vascular resistance in a dose-dependent fashion that is greater than that produced by enflurane. Halothane only produces mild changes in peripheral vascular resistance. Isoflurane thus decreases vascular

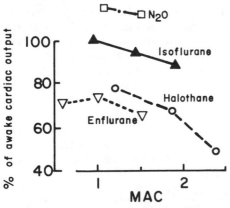

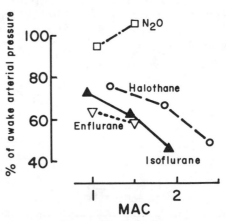

Figure 9.21.   The effect of volatile anesthetics on cardiac output and arterial blood pressure.   Note the effect of isoflurane and nitrous oxide on cardiac output compared to the decrease in cardiac output produced by halothane and enflurane *(left-hand panel).* Isoflurane, halothane, and enflurane, but not nitrous oxide, decrease arterial blood pressure in a dose-related fashion *(right-hand panel).* The maintenance of cardiac output by isoflurane despite a fall in arterial blood pressure is probably due to the compensatory increase in heart rate. (With permission from Eger EI: The pharmacology of isoflurane. *Br J Anaesth* 56:71S–99S, 1984.)

tone in many vascular beds, including skin, muscle, intestine, kidney, brain, and heart. Blood flow is increased to muscle and skin.

Volatile anesthetics exert little effect on the pulmonary circulation, and isoflurane anesthesia results in no change in pulmonary artery or occlusion pressure while pulmonary vascular resistance is unchanged. The effect of volatile anesthetics on hypoxic pulmonary vasoconstriction is controversial, and although it has been suggested that halothane, enflurane, and isoflurane depress hypoxic pulmonary vasoconstriction in the laboratory, Rogers and Benumof have shown in patients that halothane and isoflurane administration does not alter shunt fraction or decrease arterial oxygenation during "one-lung anesthesia."

The cardiovascular effects of isoflurane (1.0 to 2.0 MAC) have been studied in unpremedicated human volunteers when ventilation was controlled to maintain normal P_aCO_2; systemic arterial blood pressure and total peripheral resistance fell, but cardiac output was maintained, possibly due to an increase in heart rate. With increased duration of anesthesia (5 hours), there were only minor changes in cardiovascular function. Isoflurane is a potent respiratory depressant, and it might be predicted that spontaneous ventilation with consequent hypercarbia and the reflex sympathetic stimulation produced by CO_2 retention would alter the cardiovascular response to isoflurane. This has been shown to occur; during spontaneous respiration, cardiac output and heart rate are further increased. Cardiovascular responses to isoflurane (1.0 and 1.5 MAC) have also been examined in surgical patients; stroke volume fell but there was a significant increase in heart rate such that there was no change in cardiac output. Systemic vascular resistance decreased, and arterial blood pressure was well maintained. As with enflurane, surgical stimulation causes arterial blood pressure to rise.

The coronary circulation consists of large proximal coronary arteries (that are dilated, for example, by nitroglycerin) and smaller arteries and arterioles in the myocardium that contribute to the major part of the total coronary vascular resistance and dilate in response to adenosine and metabolic products to maintain a balance between oxygen supply and demand. Drugs that dilate coronary arterioles have the potential to divert the blood supply from ischemic to nonischemic areas—**coronary steal syndrome.**

Volatile anesthetics, including isoflurane, dilate coronary arteries in animals and humans. However, isoflurane is an extremely potent coronary artery vasodilator, and controversy currently exists as to the relative influence of halothane, enflurane, and isoflurane on myocardial ischemia. It has been suggested that isoflurane-induced coronary artery vasodilation produces a "steal" syndrome in patients with coronary artery disease; diseased portions of the coronary bed may be dilated maximally and unable to further dilate following isoflurane administration, while normal portions of the coronary artery dilate in response to isoflurane. Thus, it is hypothesized that normal beds "steal" blood from diseased beds, producing inadequate oxygenation and ischemia in diseased areas of the myocardium. Some workers (Reiz et al,) have observed a high incidence of ischemia (ST changes on the electrocardiogram and metabolic evidence) in patients with coronary artery disease anesthetized with isoflurane, while other clinical studies have failed to confirm these findings. Laboratory studies have shown coronary artery steal during isoflurane anesthesia in a dog model of chronic coronary occlusion. Other animal studies have shown that isoflurane is a potent coronary artery vasodilator and that at high concentrations severe myocardial depression occurs, leading to further decrease in arterial pressure and cardiac output, and the consequent reduced perfusion pressure causes a fall in coronary blood flow. It appears that isoflurane preferentially dilates small vessels, and it is interesting that other coronary vasodilators that also dilate small vessels such as adenosine and dipyridamole have been shown to cause "coronary steal." While the results of these laboratory studies in animals cannot be simply extrapolated to the clinical situation in which the production of myocardial ischemia depends on so many other factors, it would appear prudent to be cautious in the use of isoflurane in patients with ischemic heart disease and poor left ventricular function and to continue to control the factors that relate myocardial oxygen supply and demand when isoflurane is administered to these patients. It is thus especially important to maintain coronary perfusion pressure during isoflurane anesthesia in patients with coronary artery disease.

Hemodynamic interactions between the volatile anesthetics and the β-adrenergic blocking agents and calcium antagonists are important in clinical anesthetic practice (see Chapter 14 and Chapter 18). However, isoflurane appears to potentiate the cardiovascular effects of the β-blockers less than halothane, while the complex effects of concomitant administration of isoflurane and the calcium antagonists are discussed in Chapter 18, page 00.

RESPIRATORY SYSTEM

Isoflurane depresses respiration in a dose-related manner and produces a decrease in tidal volume without an increase in respiratory rate. Arterial carbon dioxide (P_aCO_2) increases in a dose-related fashion in volunteers given enflurane, isoflurane, and halothane (but not nitrous oxide), but the increase in P_aCO_2 is greater with isoflurane than halothane, but less than with enflurane, suggesting that isoflurane is a more potent respiratory depressant than halothane but less than enflurane. All volatile anesthetics decrease the ventilatory response to carbon dioxide, and isoflurane appears to depress the ventilatory response to carbon dioxide more than halothane. Isoflurane also depresses the ventilatory response to hypoxia, even at subanesthetic concentrations.

MUSCLE

Isoflurane directly depresses skeletal muscle contractility. Skeletal muscular relaxation is therefore good and like enflurane, isoflurane markedly potentiates the actions of the nondepolarizing muscle relaxants. Isoflurane produces greater skeletal muscle relaxation than halothane, when administered alone or in combination with the nondepolarizing muscle relaxants. The interaction of isoflurane and the neuromuscular blocking agents is further discussed in Chapter 10.

BIOTRANSFORMATION

Isoflurane is an extremely stable anesthetic agent and undergoes only limited metabolism. Holaday and colleagues have shown that 95% of an administered dose is recovered in exhaled air, while the postoperative increase in urinary excretion of fluoride accounts for less than 0.2% of fluorine administered as isoflurane. The major metabolites are trifluoroacetic acid and fluoride ion. The metabolism of isoflurane to inorganic fluoride is of insufficient magnitude to cause renal dysfunction in surgical patients. Reductive metabolism probably does not occur with isoflurane. Isoflurane may affect the metabolism of other anesthetics, and isoflurane has been shown to inhibit the oxidative metabolism of halothane. The concurrent administration of isoflurane and halothane to rats has been shown to decrease the appearance of nonvolatile halothane metabolites.

Since isoflurane is less soluble in blood and fat than halothane, this would tend to enhance its rate of elimination in relation to the more lipid-soluble halothane. However, halothane because of its greater metabolism is more rapidly removed from the body 1 to 2 hours after discontinuation of anesthesia.

TOXICITY

The resistance of isoflurane to biodegradation suggests that isoflurane should have limited potential to produce metabolite-induced organ toxicity. Isoflurane has not been shown to be mutagenic. A report by Corbett of increased incidence of hepatic neoplasms in mice undergoing repeated anesthetics with isoflurane delayed the clinical introduction of isoflurane. This was later disproved by Eger and coworkers, and isoflurane was introduced into clinical practice in 1980.

RENAL SYSTEM

Renal blood flow, glomerular filtration rate, and urinary flow rate decrease during isoflurane anesthesia. Isoflurane is not nephrotoxic.

LIVER

Isoflurane anesthesia does not result in postanesthetic increases in serum transaminases or increase in bromsulphthalein retention. There is no evidence that isoflurane is hepatotoxic in humans, although there is some evidence in animals to suggest that, when severe hypoxia is also present (10% inspired oxygen concentration), isoflurane, enflurane, thiopental, and fentanyl all produce centrilobular necrosis of the liver. This effect is probably due to hepatic hypoxia rather than isoflurane itself.

Isoflurane and halothane both reduce portal vein blood flow in animals, while hepatic arterial blood flow increases during isoflurane but remains unchanged during halothane administration, suggesting that hepatic oxygen supply is maintained to a greater extent during isoflurane than halothane anesthesia.

SUGGESTED DOSAGE AND ADMINISTRATION

Isoflurane concentrations for induction should be increased slowly to avoid breath-holding and coughing. After an initial increase in isoflurane to 0.5 to 1.0%, increases of 0.1 to 0.25% are taken every four breaths if tolerated. Approximate induction concentrations are around 2.5% while maintenance concentrations are in the range of 1.0 to 1.5%.

PRESENT STATUS

Isoflurane has become the most widely used volatile anesthetic in the United States today. Advantages of isoflurane include cardiovascular stability, lack of sensitization of the heart to circulating catecholamines, limited biodegradation resulting in reduction in hepatorenal tox-

icity, good neuromuscular relaxation, and no central nervous system excitatory effects. However, the status of isoflurane in patients with coronary artery disease remains ill defined.

Methoxyflurane

PHYSICOCHEMICAL PROPERTIES

The physicochemical constants of methoxyflurane are listed in Table 9.1. The vapor pressure of methoxyflurane is 22.5 mm Hg at 20°C (Table 9.1) so that the maximum inspired concentration that can be attained is approximately 3% (23/760 × 100 = 3%). Methoxyflurane is highly soluble in blood (Table 9.2) and, hence, the attainment of an anesthetic arterial concentration is slow. All these factors lead to a slow, prolonged induction. However, since MAC is 0.16% (Table 9.1), induction can be accomplished with inspired concentrations of 2 to 3%. Methoxyflurane is highly fat soluble (Table 9.2) and, therefore, recovery from anesthesia is also slow.

CENTRAL NERVOUS SYSTEM

As with all potent inhalational anesthetic agents, deep levels of anesthesia produce direct depression of the respiratory and vasomotor centers of the medulla. Methoxyflurane possesses good analgesic properties at subanesthetic concentrations and was at one time used for the production of analgesia during labor and delivery (see Chapter 12). Methoxyflurane causes vasodilatation of cerebral vessels resulting in increased cerebral blood flow and intracranial pressure. Cerebral oxygen consumption is decreased.

CARDIOVASCULAR SYSTEM

Although methoxyflurane is an anesthetic ether, its cardiovascular effects resemble those of halothane rather than diethyl ether. Methoxyflurane produces cardiovascular depression in a dose-related manner. Arterial blood pressure, cardiac output, stroke volume, and systemic vascular resistance are decreased while heart rate is usually increased slightly. Hypotension is probably due at least in part to a decrease in cardiac output as methoxyflurane has been shown to markedly depress left ventricular function. Methoxyflurane does not appear to stimulate the sympathetic nervous system, and concentrations of circulating catecholamines do not increase in dogs. Methoxyflurane has been shown to decrease adrenal medullary catecholamine secretion in rats, probably due to a direct effect of methoxyflurane on the chromaffin cell. Although some slowing of the heart may occur as the concentration of methoxyflurane is increased, generally heart rate and rhythm are stable.

RESPIRATORY SYSTEM

Methoxyflurane depresses respiration in a dose-dependent fashion. Tidal volume is reduced.

RENAL SYSTEM

Renal blood flow, glomerular filtration rate, and urine flow are reduced, as previously described for halothane. A serious disadvantage of methoxyflurane is its potential to cause vasopressin-resistant high output renal failure in some patients during the postoperative period. This nephropathy is manifest by polyuria, weight loss, hypernatremia, increased serum osmolarity, and elevated blood urea. Methoxyflurane undergoes biotransformation in the liver to inorganic fluoride (Fig. 9.19), and plasma and urine inorganic fluoride concentrations rise. When plasma fluoride concentrations exceed 40 to 50 μM/L, direct damage to the renal tubules may occur, possibly due to fluoride inhibition of the enzyme systems necessary for sodium transport in the ascending loop of Henle or early distal tubule. Animal studies have demonstrated that the severity of renal functional and pathological changes is directly proportional to the dose of methoxyflurane administered. The relationship of these changes in the kidney to the presence of inorganic fluoride has been confirmed by the injection of equivalent amounts of sodium fluoride in rats, sodium fluoride injections producing similar changes in renal function and

histology to those observed after methoxyflurane anesthesia. In addition, rats pretreated with phenobarbital (enzyme induced) and anesthetized with methoxyflurane exhibit increased renal toxicity associated with increased urinary excretion of inorganic fluoride. Patients anesthetized with methoxyflurane for 2.0 MAC hours* or less usually have plasma serum inorganic fluoride levels below 40 μM/L and do not develop nephrotoxicity. Subclinical toxicity may occur at a dosage of 2.5 to 3.0 MAC hours, when serum fluoride levels are in the range of 50 to 80 μM/L. These patients may exhibit a delayed return to maximum preoperative urine osmolality and are unresponsive to vasopressin administration. Mild clinical toxicity (no response to vasopressin administration, serum hyperosmolality, azotemia, hypernatremia, polyuria, low urine osmolality) develops when inorganic fluoride levels exceed 90 μM/L due to methoxyflurane administration at a dosage of 5.0 MAC hours. Serious clinical toxicity results when methoxyflurane is administered for greater than 7.0 MAC hours resulting in peak serum inorganic levels between 80 to 175 μM/L, unless care is taken to prevent dehydration by maintaining water and electrolyte balance. In this situation, serious serum and urine abnormalities may make postoperative management extremely difficult. The toxicity of methoxyflurane is increased by known nephrotoxic drugs such as gentamycin, kanamycin, and tetracycline and, in addition, enzyme inducing agents (phenobarbital) may also increase renal toxicity by increasing the biotransformation of methoxyflurane. The nephrotoxicity of methoxyflurane has resulted in a dramatic decline in its use. It has been suggested that, if methoxyflurane is to be used at all, it should be administered in low dosage for a short period of time, so that the maximum exposure is less than 2.0 to 2.5 MAC hours.

---

*MAC hours, methoxyflurane concentration in MAC units multipled by the duration of anesthetic administration in hours.

BIOTRANSFORMATION

Methoxyflurane undergoes extensive metabolism to carbon dioxide, oxalic acid, methoxydifluoroacetic acid, and inorganic chloride and fluoride ion. Some studies have shown that more than 30% of the absorbed anesthetic is metabolized in humans. Methoxyflurane can be biotransformed by two pathways: ether cleavage and dechlorination. Oxidative cleavage of the ether linkage, mediated by the microsomal cytochrome P-450 system, results in the release of inorganic fluoride. The second pathway, the dehalogenation of methoxyflurane, results in the formation of methoxydifluoroacetic acid and inorganic chloride. The production of inorganic fluoride is of great concern as renal toxicity has been related to serum fluoride concentration (see previous section). Phenobarbital pretreatment in rats stimulates metabolism and causes the production of greater amounts of inorganic fluoride and increased evidence of renal toxicity.

PRESENT STATUS

The biotransformation of methoxyflurane to inorganic fluoride with associated nephrotoxicity is a serious disadvantage to the clinical use of methoxyflurane, and the drug is no longer used today.

Diethyl Ether

Diethyl ether is rarely used today. It is highly flammable and explosive, particularly in an oxygen-enriched atmosphere. During diethyl ether anesthesia, arterial blood pressure and cardiac output are well maintained. There is evidence of increased sympathetic nervous system activity, and circulating concentrations of catecholamines are increased. Diethyl ether does not sensitize the myocardium to the effects of endogenous or exogenous catecholamines. Bronchial secretions are increased, and coughing, salivation, and laryngeal spasm may occur. Respiratory rate is markedly increased. There is a high incidence of postoperative nausea and vomiting.

ANESTHETIC GASES

DEFINITION OF GAS AND VAPOR

The *critical temperature* is defined as the temperature above which a substance cannot be liquefied by compression. Therefore, a substance is a *gas* when at a temperature above its critical value. Molecules are able to leave the surface of a liquid by evaporation at temperatures below the critical value and thus constitute a *vapor* above the liquid phase—that is, a vapor is the gaseous phase above the liquid phase at a temperature below the critical value. A *saturated vapor* is one in equilibrium with its own liquid so that the number of molecules leaving the liquid phase is the same as those reentering it. The pressure exerted by the molecules in the vapor phase at equilibrium is called the *saturated vapor* pressure at that temperature. Anesthetic gases, therefore, have a vapor pressure above ambient pressure at room temperature. The two most widely known anesthetic gases are nitrous oxide and cyclopropane. Cyclopropane is highly flammable, forms explosive mixtures in air, oxygen, and/or nitrous oxide, and therefore is rarely used today.

Nitrous Oxide

Nitrous oxide was first prepared by Priestley in 1772; Humphrey Davy suggested that it might have anesthetic and analgesic properties in 1779. It was first used in clinical practice by Cotton and Wells in the United States in 1844.

PHYSICOCHEMICAL PROPERTIES

Nitrous oxide (N_2O) is a colorless gas with a sweet smelling odor. It is stored in steel cylinders as a colorless liquid under pressure and in equilibrium with the gaseous phase (vapor). The critical temperature of nitrous oxide is 36.5°C, and the pressure required to liquefy it at just below this temperature is 74 atmospheres (the more a gas is cooled, the less the pressure required to liquefy it). The pressure inside a cylinder containing liquid nitrous oxide is 750 lb/in² or approximately 51 atmospheres at room temperature. The pressure of the vapor above liquid nitrous oxide varies with temperature. At 0°C, the vapor pressure is 31 atmospheres, at 20°C the vapor pressure is 51 atmospheres, while in hot climates, if the temperature is above the critical temperature of nitrous oxide (36.5°C), the contents of the cylinder will be wholly gaseous. Under normal operating room conditions (20°C), when the cylinder valve is opened, gaseous nitrous oxide escapes and is immediately replaced by further vapor from the liquid. When the cylinder is half empty, there is still liquid in the cylinder and, thus, the pressure in the cylinder is still 51 atmospheres. When all the liquid has evaporated, the pressure of the gas within the cylinder begins to fall. Thus, the pressure gauge does not give an accurate indication of the amount of nitrous oxide in the cylinder, and as long as liquid is present in the cylinder, the pressure remains at 51 atmospheres. Heat is required for the vaporization of nitrous oxide and, thus, if evaporation is rapid, the cylinder becomes cold and may even accumulate a deposit of frost due to freezing of the water vapor in the air immediately around the cylinder.

The molecular weight of nitrous oxide is 44.02, and the specific gravity at 25°C is 1.53. Other physicochemical constants are given in Table 9.1. Nitrous oxide is neither flammable nor explosive, but supports the combustion of flammable agents.

IMPURITIES OF NITROUS OXIDE

Nitrous oxide is prepared commercially by heating ammonium nitrate to temperatures between 245 and 270°C.

$$NH_4NO_3 \xrightarrow[245-270°C]{Heat} N_2O + 2H_2O$$

Ammonium nitrate → nitrous oxide + water

A strong solution of ammonium nitrate when heated produces nitrous oxide and in addition ammonia, nitric acid, nitrogen, and traces of nitric oxide (NO) and nitrogen dioxide (NO_2). Cooling of the emerging gases results in the conversion of ammonia and nitric acid to ammonium

nitrate which is then returned to the reactor. However, contamination of nitrous oxide with the higher oxides of nitrogen can have serious consequences. Inhalation of nitrogen dioxide and nitric oxide causes laryngospasm and cyanosis. The cyanosis is due in part to the formation of methemoglobin. Pulmonary edema develops followed by chemical pneumonitis, resulting in acute respiratory failure. Acute circulatory collapse also occurs due to profound peripheral vasodilation. Treatment includes oxygen therapy, positive pressure ventilation, steroids, antibiotics, bronchial lavage and suction, and methylene blue, 2 mg/kg, intravenously in order to reduce the methemoglobinemia. Fiberoptic bronchoscopy and suctioning may be beneficial.

PHARMACOKINETICS

Nitrous oxide is a potent analgesic but weak anesthetic agent (MAC is 105%; Table 9.1). The approach of the alveolar concentration to the inspired concentration, i.e., the rate of uptake, is relatively rapid due to the low blood gas partition coefficient (Table 9.2), and arterial blood saturation occurs quickly; the volume rate of uptake of nitrous oxide after inhalation of an 80% nitrous oxide-20% oxygen mixture at 1 minute is 1 L/min, at 5 minutes is 500 ml/min, and at 90 minutes is about 100 ml/min. The time taken to achieve 90% arterial saturation is in general about 20 minutes, while the time taken to reach full saturation including the tissues is about 5 hours. This large uptake of gas from the alveoli results in the *second gas* effect and the *concentration* effect (see previous section). The time required for elimination of nitrous oxide is similar to that required for uptake; the body tissues require about 5 hours to lose 90% of their nitrous oxide. Arterial blood loses 70% of its nitrous oxide in 3 minutes, 90% in 20 minutes. Recovery is therefore rapid. Hypoxia can occur during recovery from nitrous oxide if the patient is allowed to breathe room air. The rapid diffusion of nitrous oxide from the tissues and blood to the alveoli markedly reduces the alveolar concentration of oxygen, resulting in arterial hypoxemia. This has been described by Fink as "diffusional hypoxia" (see previous section). It can be prevented by oxygen administration during the period of nitrous oxide elimination in the early recovery period.

Although nitrous oxide is considered to have low blood solubility, it is very soluble in blood when compared with nitrogen; 100 ml of blood will carry about 46 ml of nitrous oxide. The blood/gas partition coefficient for nitrous oxide is 34 times that of nitrogen, with the result that during nitrous oxide anesthesia any closed gas-filled cavity in the body expands due to the slow exchange of nitrogen from the cavity for rapid exchange of large volumes of nitrous oxide from the blood. Examples of such closed cavities include pneumothorax, pneumopericardium, occluded middle ear, loops of intestine in intestinal obstruction, and lung or renal cysts. Large increases in pressure and volume occur within these cavities, and nitrous oxide should be avoided in these situations.

Nitrous oxide can produce surgical anesthesia in normal subjects only when administered under hyperbaric conditions; a 50:50 mixture of nitrous oxide and oxygen at 2 atmospheres pressure produces surgical anesthesia, while the same 50:50 mixture of nitrous oxide and oxygen at one atmosphere does not usually produce loss of consciousness, although it produces excellent analgesia. Unconsciousness is produced by nitrous oxide concentrations of 80 to 100% in healthy subjects, but the dangers of hypoxia make this an unacceptable technique; today, nitrous oxide is always used in combination with other agents.

Nitrous oxide is predominantly eliminated unchanged in the expired gas. It has recently become recognized that nitrous oxide might undergo biotransformation in animals.

CENTRAL NERVOUS SYSTEM

Nitrous oxide depresses the central nervous system and produces analgesia (and unconsciousness depending on the clinical status of the patient). Nitrous oxide increases cerebral blood flow and intracranial pressure, but cerebral blood flow remains responsive to carbon dioxide. The ability of nitrous oxide to elevate intracranial pressure is probably less than the volatile anesthetic agents, perhaps because of its sub-MAC dosage restriction. The use of a barbiturate induction—droperidol-fentanyl—relaxant anesthetic technique can cause a moderate decrease in intracranial pressure when used with nitrous oxide.

CARDIOVASCULAR SYSTEM

Since nitrous oxide is only a weak anesthetic agent, it has generally been considered in the past to have minimal effects on cardiovascular dynamics. However, it has become evident that the cardiovascular effects of nitrous oxide are complex and depend on whether nitrous oxide is administered alone or in combination with narcotic or inhalational anesthesia. Nitrous oxide has been shown to have a direct myocardial depressant effect during studies on isolated cat papillary muscle, while studies in human volunteers have demonstrated that the administration of 40% nitrous oxide in oxygen as compared with 40% nitrogen in oxygen produces small but potentially important depression in ventricular function. Cardiac output, heart rate, and contractility were reduced while systemic vascular resistance increased. Thus, there was no change in arterial blood pressure. In addition, there was a small rise in urinary catecholamines. These results suggest that nitrous oxide may produce weak sympathomimetic, α-adrenergic effects.

The cardiovascular effects of the addition of nitrous oxide to other anesthetic agents have also been studied in human volunteers. The addition of 70% nitrous oxide in oxygen to morphine anesthesia (2 mg/kg intravenously) results in a reduction in heart rate and cardiac output and a rise in peripheral resistance and central venous pressure. Blood pressure is unchanged. When nitrous oxide is added to inhalational anesthesia, the results have been conflicting in some instances. However, it appears that adding nitrous oxide to halothane-oxygen anesthesia results in less depression of the cardiovascular system than comparable levels of halothane-oxygen anesthesia; when nitrous oxide is added to halothane in healthy unpremedicated subjects, the mixture usually produces an α-adrenergic-like response; arterial blood pressure, systemic vascular resistance, and central venous pressure are increased while the heart rate and cardiac output are unchanged. However, the addition of nitrous oxide to enflurane anesthesia produces minimal changes, and there is no evidence of sympathetic stimulation.

The effects of nitrous oxide in combination with narcotic or inhalational anesthetic agents in surgical patients with heart disease are variable. During halothane anesthesia, the addition of nitrous oxide, 60%, causes no change in hemodynamic parameters compared with halothane alone in patients with valvular heart disease. Addition of nitrous oxide, 60%, to morphine-oxygen anesthesia (morphine, 1.0 mg/kg intravenously) in patients undergoing open heart surgery causes mean arterial pressure and cardiac index to fall and systemic vascular resistance to increase. Another study investigated the effects of ventricular function following the addition of 50% nitrous oxide to morphine-oxygen anesthesia during coronary artery surgery in patients with angiographically demonstrable coronary artery disease and normal ventricular contractility. Mean arterial pressure, cardiac index, stroke index, and other indices of left ventricular function decreased, while mean pulmonary artery pressure and left ventricular end diastolic pressure increased. Heart rate and systemic vascular resistance remained unchanged.

The effects of nitrous oxide on myocardial function in patients with coronary artery disease have also been investigated during cardiac catheterization. Nitrous oxide, 40%, decreased arterial blood pressure and myocardial contractility and increased left ventricular end diastolic pressure in patients with angiographically demonstrable occlusive coronary disease and evidence of previously impaired left ventricular function. Nitrous oxide had no significant cardiovascular effect in patients with angina, but no angiographically demonstrable coronary arterial disease.

RESPIRATORY SYSTEM

The effects of nitrous oxide on the respiratory system are small. The administration of 50% nitrous oxide does not affect the ventilatory response to carbon dioxide, and no change in bronchomotor tone occurs.

HEMATOLOGICAL SYSTEM

It became evident many years ago that the administration of nitrous oxide could depress hematopoietic function when it was shown that the prolonged use of nitrous oxide in the management of tetanus resulted in anemia, leucopenia, and thrombocytopenia. More recently, it has become apparent that nitrous oxide also causes megaloblastic anemia. Amess and coworkers have shown that 50% nitrous oxide administered to patients after cardiopulmonary bypass operations for 24 hours causes megaloblastic changes in the bone marrow that can be partially prevented by folinic acid or vitamin B_{12} administration. Vitamin B_{12}, a bound coenzyme of methionine synthase, has a tetrapyrrole ring with a monovalent cobalt at the center. Nitrous oxide will react chemically with vitamin B_{12}; Cob(I)alamin is oxidized to Cob(III) alamin which can no longer function as a methyl carrier so that there is a reduction in the activity of vitamin B_{12}. Thus, methionine synthase activity is inhibited by nitrous oxide. Methionine synthase is required for the conversion of homocysteine to methionine and for the demethylation of methyl tetrahydrofolate to tetrahydrofolate, which is essential for DNA synthesis. By inhibiting methionine synthase, nitrous oxide administration leads to interference in DNA synthesis, manifest by an abnormal deoxyuridine suppression test, a test used in vitamin B_{12} deficiency.

Megaloblastic changes in bone marrow have not only been found in patients who have been exposed to anesthetic concentrations of nitrous oxide for 24 hours, but also in critically ill patients who have been exposed to much shorter durations of about 2 to 6 hours. It has been estimated that a minimum of 5 hours of exposure to 50% nitrous oxide is required in healthy patients before evidence of bone marrow dysfunction becomes evident, while debilitated patients may be more susceptible. It is important to appreciate that the hematological effects of nitrous oxide are reversible on withdrawal of nitrous oxide in healthy patients. Dentists and other health care workers who chronically abuse nitrous oxide have been shown to exhibit signs and symptoms of neurologic disease which tend to improve when abuse is discontinued.

REPRODUCTIVE SYSTEM

Nitrous oxide does not alter uterine tone and contractility during labor and delivery. However, nitrous oxide has been shown to be teratogenic when administered in anesthetic concentrations to animals during early pregnancy. It has been shown, for example, that nitrous oxide and halothane anesthesia for 3 hours causes fetal resorption in pregnant hamsters and that 50% (but not 35%) nitrous oxide for 24 hours produces teratogenic effects in rats. Nitrous oxide inhibits rat fetal methionine synthase activity (but not human placental methionine synthase activity), and thus it has been suggested that the teratogenic effects of nitrous oxide are due to interference with DNA synthesis by altered folate metabolism, since nitrous oxide irreversibly oxidizes vitamin B_{12}, making it inactive as a coenzyme (see previous section). This results in two effects. There is (a) decreased conversion of deoxyuridine (dUrd) to thymidine and (b) decreased conversion of homocysteine to methionine, reactions that are catalyzed by the enzymes thymidylate synthetase and methionine synthase, respectively. It is speculated that nitrous oxide administration might lead to decreased DNA synthesis in the embryo. Indeed, exposure of pregnant rats to nitrous oxide has been shown to decrease DNA synthesis and content in rat embryos. Folinic acid administration protects against nitrous oxide teratogenicity in the rat.

These laboratory studies have led some workers to recommend that nitrous oxide should not be used in the first and second trimesters of pregnancy. However, a small but detailed study of about 400 births by Crawford and Lewis found no evidence of nitrous oxide teratogenicity in early human pregnancy. At the present time, there is no definitive evidence to suggest that the brief use of nitrous oxide has proven harmful to adults or the fetus.

Cyclopropane

Cyclopropane is a colorless, highly flammable, explosive gas that is little used today. Cyclopropane is a rapidly acting anesthetic due to its low blood/gas partition coefficient, and it is, therefore, easy to achieve dangerous levels of anesthesia quickly. It causes stimulation of the sympathetic nervous system; cardiac output, arterial blood pressure, and peripheral vascular resistance are increased. There is increased myocardial irritability, and dysrhythmias are not uncommon in the presence of an elevated arterial carbon dioxide tension. Cyclopropane is a marked respiratory depressent, and laryngospasm and bronchospasm may occur. Postoperative nausea and vomiting are common.

BIBLIOGRAPHY

General

Brown BR, Crout JR: A comparative study of the effects of five general anesthetics on myocardial contractility. 1. Isometric conditions. *Anesthesiology* 34:236–245, 1971.

Brown BR, Gandolfi AJ: Adverse effects of volatile anaesthetics. *Br J Anaesth* 59:14–23, 1987.

Burnie JP: Molecular mechanisms of general anaesthesia. *Anaesthesia* 36:1027–1039, 1981.

Cahalan M, Johnson BH, Eger EI: Relationship of concentrations of halothane and enflurane to their metabolism and elimination in man. *Anesthesiology* 54:3–8, 1981.

Carpenter RL, Eger EI, Johnson BH, Unadkat JD, Sheiner LB: Does the duration of anesthetic administration affect the pharmacokinetics or metabolism of inhaled anesthetics in humans? *Anesth Analg* 66:1–8, 1987.

Cohen EN, Bellville JW, Brown BW: Anesthesia, pregnancy, and miscarriage: a study of operating room nurses and anesthetists. *Anesthesiology* 35:343–347, 1971.

Dale O, Brown BR: Clinical pharmacokinetics of

the inhalational anaesthetics. *Clin Pharmacokinet* 12:145–167, 1987.

Duvaldestine P, Mazze RI, Nivoche Y, Desmonts JM: Occupational exposure to halothane results in enzyme induction in anesthetists. *Anesthesiology* 54:57–60, 1981.

Editorial: Molecular mechanisms of general anesthesia. *Lancet* 2:455–456, 1981.

Eger EI: Respiratory and circulatory factors in uptake and distribution of volatile anaesthetic agents. *Br. J Anaesth* 36:155–171, 1964.

Eger EI: *Anesthetic Uptake and Action.* Baltimore, Williams & Williams, 1974.

Eger EI, Larson CP Jr: Anaesthetic solubility in blood and tissues: values and significance. *Br J Anaesth* 36:140–149, 1964.

Epstein RM, Rackow H, Salanitre E, Wolf GL: Influence of the concentration effect on the uptake of anesthetic mixtures: the second gas effect. *Anesthesiology* 25:364–371, 1964.

Featherstone RM, Schoenborn BP: Protein and lipid binding of volatile anaesthetic agents. *Br. J. Anaesth* 36:150–154, 1964.

Filner BE, Karliner JS: Alterations of normal left ventricular performance by general anesthesia. *Anesthesiology* 45:610–621, 1976.

Fineberg HV, Pearlman LA, Gabel RA: The case for abandonment of explosive anesthetic agents. *N Engl J Med* 303:613–617, 1980.

Fink BR, Cullen BF: Anesthetic pollution: what is happening to us? *Anesthesiology* 45:79–83, 1976.

Frumin MJ, Edelist G: Diffusion anoxia: a critical reappraisal. *Anesthesiology* 31:243–249, 1969.

Greenstein LR, Hitt BA, Mazze RI: Metabolism in vitro of enflurane, isoflurane, and methoxyflurane. *Anesthesiology* 42:420–424, 1975.

Halsey MJ: A reassessment of the molecular structure-functional relationships of the inhaled general anaesthetics. *Br J Anaesth* 56:9S–25S, 1984.

Himmelstein KJ, Lutz RJ: A review of the applications of physiologically based pharmacokinetic modeling. *J Pharmacokinet Biopharmacol* 7:127–145, 1979.

Housmans PR, Murat I: Comparative effects of halothane, enflurane, and isoflurane at equipotent anesthetic concentrations on isolated ventricular myocardium of the ferret. I. Contractility. *Anesthesiology* 69:451–463, 1988.

Housmans PR, Murat I: Comparative effects of halothane, enflurane, and isoflurane at equipotent anesthetic concentrations on isolated ventricular myocardium of the ferret. II. Relaxation. *Anesthesiology* 69:464–471, 1988.

Johnston RR, Eger EI, Wilson CA: Comparative interaction of epinephrine with enflurane, isoflurane, and halothane in man. *Anesth Analg* 55:709–712, 1986.

Jones RM: Clinical comparison of inhalation anesthetic agents. *Br J Anaesth* 56:57S–69S, 1984.

Knill-Jones RP, Moir DD, Rodrigues LV, Spence AA: Anaesthetic practice and pregnancy: controlled survey of women anaesthetists in the United Kingdom. *Lancet* 1:1326–1328, 1972.

Knill-Jones RP, Newman BJ, Spence AA: Anaesthetic practice and pregnancy: controlled survey of male anaesthetists in the United Kingdom. *Lancet* 2:807–809, 1975.

Larson CP, Eger EI, Severinghaus JW: Ostwald solubility coefficients for anesthetic gases in various fluids and tissues. *Anesthesiology* 23:686–689, 1962.

Larson CP, Mazze RI, Cooperman LH, Wollman H: Effects of anesthetics on cerebral, renal, and splanchnic circulations: recent developments. *Anesthesiology* 41:169–181, 1974.

Mapleson WW: Circulation-time models of the uptake of inhaled anaesthetics and data for quantifying them. *Br J Anaesth* 45:319–334, 1973.

Mazze RI: Metabolism of the inhaled anaesthetics: implications of enzyme induction. *Br J Anaesth* 56:27S–41S, 1984.

Miller RD, Way WL, Dolan WM, Stevens WC, Eger EI: Comparative neuromuscular effects of pancuronium, gallamine, and succinylcholine during Forane and Halothane anesthesia in man. *Anesthesiology* 35:509–514, 1971.

Munson ES, Eger EI: The effects of hyperthermia and hypothermia on the rate of induction of anesthesia: calculations using a mathematical model. *Anesthesiology* 33:515–519, 1970.

Munson ES, Embro WJ: Enflurane, isoflurane, and halothane and isolated human uterine muscle. *Anesthesiology* 46:11–14, 1977.

Palahniuk RJ, Shnider SM, Eger EI: Pregnancy decreases the requirement for inhaled anesthetic agents. *Anesthesiology* 41:82–83, 1974.

Perry LB, Van Dyke RA, Theye RA: Sympathoadrenal and hemodynamic effects of isoflurane, halothane, and cyclopropane in dogs. *Anesthesiology* 40:465–470, 1974.

Pope WDB, Halsey MJ, Landsown AGB, Simmonds A. Bateman PE: Fetotoxicity in rats following chronic exposure to halothane, nitrous oxide, or methoxyflurane. *Anesthesiology* 48:11–16, 1978.

Price ML, Price HL: Effects of general anesthetics on contractile response of rabbit aortic strips. *Anesthesiology* 23:16–20, 1962.

Quasha AL, Eger EI, Tinker JH: Determination and applications of MAC. *Anesthesiology* 53:315–334, 1980.

Report of an Ad Hoc Committee on the Effect of Trace Anesthetics on the Health of Operating Room Personnel. American Society of Anesthesiologists. Occupational disease among operating room personnel: a national study. *Anesthesiology* 41:321–340, 1974.

Rice SA, Sbordone L, Mazze RI: Metabolism by rat hepatic microsomes of fluorinated ether anesthetics following isoniazid administration. *Anesthesiology* 53:489–493, 1980.

Roizen MF, Horrigan RW, Frazer BM: Anesthetic doses blocking adrenergic (stress) and cardiovascular responses to incision—MAC BAR. *Anesthesiology* 54:390–398, 1981.

Rusy BF: Anesthetic action in heart muscle: further insights through the study of myocardial mechanics. *Anesthesiology* 69:445–447, 1988.

Rusy BF, Komai H: Anesthetic depression of myocardial contractility: a review of possible mechanisms. *Anesthesiology* 67:745–766, 1987.

Sakai T, Takaori M: Biodegradation of halothane, enflurane, and methoxyflurane. *Br J Anaesth* 50:785–791, 1978.

Spence AA, Cohen EN, Brown BW, Knill-Jones RP, Himmelberger DV: Occupational hazards for operating room based physicians. *JAMA* 238:955–959, 1977.

Steward A, Allott PR, Cowles AL, Mapleson WW: Solubility coefficients for inhaled anaesthetics for water, oil and biological media. *Br. J. Anaesth* 45:282–293, 1973.

Stoelting RK, Eger EI: An additional explanation for the second gas effect: a concentrating effect. *Anesthesiology* 30:273–277, 1969.

Stoelting RK, Longnecker DE: The effect of right-to-left shunt on the rate of increase of arterial anesthetic concentration. *Anesthesiology* 36:352–356, 1972.

Terrell RC: Physical and chemical properties of anaesthetic agents. *Br J Anaesth* 56:3S–7S, 1984.

Tunstall ME, Hawksworth GM: Halothane uptake and nitrous oxide concentration. Arterial levels during cesarean section. *Anaesthesia* 36:177–182, 1981.

Vitez TS, White PF, Eger EI: Effects of hypothermia on halothane MAC and isoflurane MAC in the rat. *Anesthesiology* 41:80–81, 1974.

Wahrenbrock EA, Eger EI, Laravuso RB, Maruschak G: Anesthetic uptake—of mice and men (and whales). *Anesthesiology* 40:19–23, 1974.

Walts LT, Forsythe AB, Moore JG: Occupational diseases among operating room personnel. *Anesthesiology* 42:608–611, 1975.

Wood M, Uetrecht J, Sweetman B, Shay S, Phythyon JM, Wood AJJ: The effect of cimetidine on anesthetic metabolism and toxocity. *Anesth Analg* 65:481–488, 1986.

Halothane

Allott PR, Steward A, Mapleson WW: Pharmacokinetics of halothane in the dog. *Br J Anaesth* 48:279–295, 1976.

Bahlman SH, Eger EI, Halsey MJ, Stevens WC, Shakespeare TF, Smith NT, Cromwell TH, Fourcade H: The cardiovascular effects of halothane in man during spontaneous ventilation. *Anesthesiology* 36:494–502, 1972.

Bahlman SH, Eger EI, Smith NT, Stevens WC, Shakespeare TF, Sawyer DC, Halsey MJ, Cromwell TH: The cardiovascular effects of nitrous oxide-halothane anesthesia in man. *Anesthesiology* 35:274–285, 1971.

Beneken Kolmer HH, Burm AG, Cramers CA, Ramakers JM, Vader JL: The uptake and elimination of halothane in dogs: a two or multicompartment system? *Br J Anaesth* 47:1169–1175, 1975.

Brody GL, Sweet RB: Halothane anesthesia as a possible cause of massive hepatic necrosis. *Anesthesiology* 24:29–37, 1963.

Brown BR: Pharmacogenetics and the halothane hepatitis mystery. *Anesthesiology* 55:93–94, 1981.

Brown BR, Sipes IG: Biotransformation and hepatotoxicity of halothane. *Biochem Pharmacol* 26:2091–2094, 1977.

Bunker JP, Blumenfeld CM: Liver necrosis after halothane anesthesia: cause or coincidence. *N Engl J Med* 268:531–534, 1963.

Carpenter RL, Eger EI, Johnston BH, Unadkat JD, Sheiner LB: The extent of metabolism of inhaled anesthetics in humans. *Anesthesiology* 65:210–205, 1986.

Cohen EN, Trudell JR, Edmunds HN, Watson E: Urinary metabolites of halothane in man. *Anesthesiology* 43:392–401, 1975.

Cousins MJ, Sharp JH, Gourley GK, Adams JF, Haynes WD, Whitehead R: Hepatotoxicity and halothane metabolism in an animal model with application for human toxicity. *Anaesth Intens Care* 7:9–24, 1979.

Editorial: Halothane-associated liver damage. *Lancet* 1:1251–1252, 1986.

Eger EI, Smith NT, Stoelting RK, Cullen DJ, Kadis LB, Whitcher CE: Cardiovascular effects of halothane in man. *Anesthesiology* 32:396–409, 1970.

Farrell G, Prendergast D, Murray M: Halothane hepatitis. Detection of a constitutional susceptibility factor. *N Engl J Med* 313:1310–1314, 1985.

Gelman S, Van Dyke R: Mechanism of halothane-induced hepatotoxicity: another step on a long path. *Anesthesiology* 68:479–482, 1988.

Gourlay GK, Adams JF, Cousins MJ, Hall P: Genetic differences in reductive metabolism and heptotoxicity of halothane in three rat strains. *Anesthesiology* 55:96–103, 1981.

Hayashi Y, Sumikawa K, Tashiro C, Yashiya I: Synergistic interaction of α_i- and β-adrenoceptor agonist induction arrhythmias during halothane anesthesia in dogs. *Anesthesiology* 68:902–907, 1988.

Hermens JM, Edelstein G, Hanifen JM, Woodward WR, Hirshman CA: Inhalational anesthesia and histamine release during bronchospasm. *Anesthesiology* 61:69–72, 1984.

Hickey RF, Graf PD, Nadee JA, Larson CP: The effects of halothane and cyclopropane on total pulmonary resistance in the dog. *Anesthesiology* 31:334–343, 1969.

Hirshman CA, Edelstein G, Peetz S, Wayne R, Downes H: Mechanism of action of inhalational anesthesia on airways. *Anesthesiology* 56:107–111, 1982.

Hoft RH, Bunker JP, Goodman HI, Gregory PB: Halothane hepatitis in three pairs of closely related women. *N Engl J Med* 304:1023–1024, 1981.

Hubbard AK, Roth TP, Gandolfi AJ, Brown BR, Webster NR, Nunn JF: Halothane hepatitis patients generate an antibody response toward a covalently bound metabolite of halothane. *Anesthesiology* 68:791–796, 1988.

Kenna JG, Neuberger J, Mieli-Vergani G, Mowat AP, Williams R: Halothane hepatitis in children. *Br Med J* 294:1209–1211, 1987.

Kenna JG, Neuberger J, Williams R: An enzyme-linked immunosorbent assay for detection of antibodies against halothane-altered hepatocyte antigens. *J Immunol Methods* 75:3–14, 1984.

Klatskin G, Kimberg DV: Recurrent hepatitis attributable to halothane sensitization in an anesthetist. *N Engl J Med* 280:515–522, 1969.

Larson CP, Eger EI, Severinghaus JW: The solubility of halothane in blood and tissue homogenates. *Anesthesiology* 23:349–355, 1962.

Lee RC, Sipes IG, Gandolfi AJ, Brown BR: Factors influencing halothane hepatotoxicity in the rat hypoxic model. *Toxic Appl Pharmacol* 52:267–277, 1980.

Lunam CA, Cousins MJ, Hall PM: Guinea-pig model of halothane-associated hepatotoxicity in the absence of enzyme induction and hypoxia. *J Pharmacol Exp Ther* 232:802–809, 1985.

Maiorino RM, Sipes IG, Gandolfi AJ, Brown BR, Lind RC: Factors affecting the formation of chloro-trifluoroethane and chlorodifluoroethylene from halothane. *Anesthesiology* 54:383–389, 1981.

Maze M, Smith CM: Identification of receptor mechanism mediating epinephrine-induced arrhythmias during halothane anesthesia in the dog. *Anesthesiology* 59:322–326, 1983.

Maze M, Smith CM, Baden JM: Halothane anesthesia does not exacerbate hepatic dysfunction in cirrhotic rats. *Anesthesiology* 62:1–5, 1985.

McDowell DG: Effects of clinical concentrations of halothane on the blood flow and oxygen uptake of the cerebral cortex. *Br J Anaesth* 39:186–196, 1967.

McLain GE, Sipes IG, Brown BR: An animal model of halothane hepatotoxicity: roles of enzyme induction and hypoxia. *Anesthesiology* 51:321–326, 1979.

Metz S, Maze M: Halothane concentration does not alter the threshold for epinephrine-induced arrhythmias in dogs. *Anesthesiology* 62:470–474, 1985.

Mukai S, Morio M, Fujii I, Hanaki C: Volatile metabolites of halothane in the rabbit. *Anesthesiology* 47:248–251, 1977.

Munson ES, Larson CP, Badad AA, Regan MJ, Buechel DR, Eger EI: The effects of halothane, fluroxene, and cyclopropane on ventilation: a comparative study in man. *Anesthesiology* 27:716–728, 1966.

National Halothane Study: Possible association between halothane anesthesia and post-operative hepatic necrosis. Report by Subcommittee on the National Halothane Study of the Committee on Anesthesia, National Academy of Science. *JAMA* 197:775–788, 1966.

Neuberger J, Gimson AES, Davis M, Williams R: Specific serological markers in the diagnosis of fulminant hepatic failure associated with halothane anesthesia. *Br J Anaesth* 55:15–19, 1983.

Neuberger J, Vergani D, Mieli-Vergani G, Davis M, Williams R: Hepatic damage after exposure to halothane in medical personnel. *Br J Anaesth* 53:1173–1177, 1981.

Pohl LR, Gillette JR: A perspective on halothane-induced hepatotoxicity. *Anesth Analg* 61:809–811, 1982.

Prys-Robert C, Gersh BJ, Baker B, Reuben SR: The effects of halothane on the interactions between myocardial contractility, aortic impedance, and left ventricular performance. *Br J Anaesth* 44:634–649, 1972.

Raventos J, Lemon PG: The impurities in fluothane: their biological properties. *Br J Anaesth* 37:716–737, 1965.

Roizen MF, Moss J, Henry DP, Kopin IJ: Effect of halothane on plasma catecholamines. *Anesthesiology* 41:432–439, 1974.

Roizen MR, Moss J, Henry DP, Wiese V, Kopin IJ: Effect of general anesthetics on handling and decapitation-induced increases in sympathoadrenal discharge. *J Pharmacol Exp Ther* 204:11–18, 1978.

Ross WT, Daggy BP, Cardell RR: Hepatic necrosis caused by halothane and hypoxia in phenobarbital-treated rats. *Anesthesiology* 51:327–333, 1979.

Saraiva RA, Willis BA, Steward A, Lunn JN, Mapleson WW: Halothane solubility in human blood. *Br J Anaesth* 49:115–119, 1977.

Schieble TM, Costa AK, Heffel DF, Trudell JR: Comparative toxicity of halothane, isoflurane, hypoxia, and phenobarbital induction in monolayer cultures of rat hepatocytes. *Anesthesiology* 68:485–494, 1988.

Seagard JL, Hopp FA, Bosnjak ZJ, Elegbe EO, Kampine JP: Extent and mechanism of halothane sensitization of the carotid sinus baroreceptors. *Anesthesiology* 58:432–437, 1983.

Sharp JH, Trudell JR, Cohen EN: Volatile metabolites and decomposition products of halothane in man. *Anesthesiology* 50:2–8, 1979.

Sonntag H, Donath U, Hillebrand W, Merin RG, Radke J: Left ventricular function in conscious man and during halothane anesthesia. *Anesthesiology* 48:320–324, 1978.

Stock JGL, Strunin L: Unexplained hepatitis following halothane. *Anesthesiology* 63:424–439, 1985.

Stoelting RK, Reis RR, Longnecker DE: Hemodynamic responses to nitrous oxide-halothane in patients with valvular heart disease. *Anesthesiology* 37:430–435, 1972.

Sumikawa K, Ishizaka N, Suzaki M: Arrhythmogenic plasma levels of epinephrine during halothane, enflurane, and pentobarbital anesthesia in the dog. *Anesthesiology* 58:322–325, 1983.

Uetrecht J, Wood AJJ, Phythyon JM, Wood M: Contrasting effects on halothane hepatotoxicity in the phenobarbital-hypoxia and triiodothyronine model: mechanistic implications. *Anesthesiology* 59:196–201, 1983.

Van Dyke RA, Gandolfi AJ: Anaerobic release of fluoride from halothane, relationship to the binding of halothane and metabolites to hepatic cellular constituents. *Drug Metab Dispos* 4:40–44, 1976.

Van Dyke RA, Wood CL: Binding of radioactivity from ^{14}C-labelled halothane in isolated perfused rat livers. *Anesthesiology* 38:328–332, 1973.

Vergani D, Meili-Vergani G, Alberti A, Neuberger J, Eddleston ALWF, Davis M, Williams R: Antibodies to the surface of halothane-altered rabbit hepatocytes in patients with severe halothane-associated hepatitis. *N Engl J Med* 303:66–71, 1980.

Widger LA, Gandolfi AJ, Van Dyke RA: Hypoxia and halothane metabolism in vivo: release of inorganic fluoride and halothane metabolite binding to cellular constituents. *Anesthesiology* 44:197–201, 1976.

Isoflurane

Adams RW, Cucchiara RF, Gronert GA, Messick JM, Michenfelder JD: Isoflurane and cerebrospinal fluid pressure in neurosurgical patients. *Anesthesiology* 54:97–99, 1981.

Artru AA: Relationship between cerebral blood volume and CSF pressure during anesthesia with isoflurane or fentanyl in dogs. *Anesthesiology* 60:575–579, 1984.

Becker LC: Is isoflurane dangerous for the patient with coronary artery disease? *Anesthesiology* 66:259–261, 1987.

Blaise G, Sill JC, Nugent M, Van Dyke RA, Vanhoutte PM: Isoflurane causes endothelium-dependent inhibition of contractile responses of canine coronary arteries. *Anesthesiology* 67:513–517, 1987.

Buffington CW, Romson JL, Levine A, Duttlinger NC, Huang AH: Isoflurane induces coronary steal in a canine model of chronic coronary occlusion. *Anesthesiology* 66:280–292, 1987.

Campkin TV: Isoflurane and cranial extradural pressure. *Br J Anaesth* 56:1083–1087, 1984.

Cromwell TH, Eger EI, Stevens WC, Dolan WM: Forane uptake, excretion, and blood solubility in man. *Anesthesiology* 35:401–408, 1971.

Cromwell TH, Stevens WC, Eger EI, Shakespeare TF, Halsey, MJ, Bahlman SH, Fourcade HE: The cardiovascular effects of compound 469 (Forane) during spontaneous ventilation and CO$_2$ challenge in man. *Anesthesiology* 35:17–25, 1971.

Cutfield GR, Francis CM, Foex P, Jones LA, Ryder WA: Isoflurane and large coronary artery haemodynamics. *Br J Anaesth* 60:784–790, 1988.

Eger EI: Isoflurane: a review. *Anesthesiology* 55:559–576, 1981.

Eger EI: The pharmacology of isoflurane. *Br J Anaesth* 56:71S–99S, 1984.

Eger EI, Stevens WC, Cromwell TH: The electroencephalogram in man anesthetized with Forane. *Anesthesiology* 35:504–508, 1971.

Eger EI, White AE, Brown CL, Biava CG, Corbett TH, Stevens WC: A test of the carcinogenicity of enflurane, isoflurane, halothane, methoxyflurane, and nitrous oxide in mice. *Anesth Analg* 57:678–694, 1978.

Fourcade HE, Stevens WC, Larson CP, Cromwell TH, Bahlman SH, Hickey RF, Halsey MJ, Eger EI: The ventilatory effects of Forane, a new inhaled anesthetic. *Anesthesiology* 35:26–31, 1971.

Graves CL, McDermitt RW, Bidwai A: Cardiovascular effects of isoflurane in surgical patients. *Anesthesiology* 41:486–489, 1974.

Grosslight K, Foster R, Colohan AR, Bedford RF: Isoflurane for neuroanesthesia: risk factors for increases in intracranial pressure. *Anesthesiology* 63:533–536, 1985.

Hitt BA, Mazze RI, Cousins MJ, Edmunds HN, Barr GA, Trudell JR: Metabolism of isoflurane in Fischer 344 rats and man. *Anesthesiology* 40:62–67, 1974.

Holaday DA, Fiserova-Bergerova V, Latto IP, Zumbiel MA: Resistance of isoflurane to biotransformation in man. *Anesthesiology* 43:325–332, 1975.

Mazze RI, Cousins MJ, Barr GA: Renal effects and metabolism of isoflurane in man. *Anesthesiology* 40:536–542, 1974.

Michenfelder JD: Does isoflurane aggravate regional cerebral ischemia? *Anesthesiology* 66:451–452, 1987.

Miller RD, Eger EI, Way WL, Stevens WC, Dolan WM: Comparative neuromuscular effects of Forane and halothane alone and in combination with d-tubocurarine in man. *Anesthesiology* 35:38–42, 1971.

Moffitt E, Barker RA, Glenn JJ, Imrie DD, DelCampo C, Landymore RW, Kinley CE, Murphy DA: Myocardial metabolism and hemodynamic responses with isoflurane anesthesia for coronary arterial surgery. *Anesth Analg* 65:53–61, 1986.

Nehls DG, Todd MM, Spetzler RF, Drummond JC, Thompson RA, Johnson PC: A comparison of the cerebral protective effects of isoflurane and barbiturates during temporary focal ischemia in primates. *Anesthesiology* 66:453–464, 1987.

Newberg LA, Milde JH, Michenfelder JD: Systemic and cerebral effects of isoflurane-induced hypotension in dogs. *Anesthesiology* 60:541–546, 1984.

Nunn JF: Isoflurane as a routine anesthetic in general surgical practice. *Br J Anaesth* 57:461–475, 1985.

O'Young J, Mastrocostopoulos G, Hilgenberg A, Palacios I, Kryitisis A, Lappas D: Myocardial circulatory and metabolic effects of isoflurane and sufentanil during coronary artery surgery. *Anesthesiology* 66:653–658, 1987.

Pollard JB, Hill RF, Lowe JE, Cummings RG, Simeone DM, Menius JA, Reves JG: Myocardial tolerance to total ischemia in the dog anesthetized with halothane or isoflurane. *Anesthesiology* 69:17–23, 1988.

Priebe HJ: Differential effects of isoflurane on regional right and left ventricular performances, and on coronary, systemic, and pulmonary hemodynamics in the dog. *Anesthesiology* 66:262–272, 1987.

Priebe HJ: Isoflurane causes more severe regional myocardial dysfunction than halothane in dogs with a critical coronary artery stenosis. *Anesthesiology* 69:72–83, 1988.

Priebe HJ, Foex P: Isoflurane causes regional myocardial dysfunction in dogs with critical coronary artery stenoses. *Anesthesiology* 66:293–300, 1987.

Reiz S, Balfors E, Sorensen MB, Ariola S, Friedman A, Truedsson H: Isoflurane—a powerful coronary vasodilator in patients with coronary artery disease. *Anesthesiology* 59:91–97, 1983.

Roberts SL, Gilbert M, Tinker JH: Isoflurane has a greater margin of safety than halothane in swine with and without major surgery or critical coronary stenosis. *Anesth Analg* 66:485–491, 1987.

Seagard JL, Elegbe EO, Hopp FA, Bosnjak ZJ, Van Colditz JH, Kalbfleisch JH, Kampine JP: Effects of isoflurane on the baroreceptor reflex. *Anesthesiology* 59:511–520, 1983.

Sill JC, Bove AA, Nugent M, Blaise GA, Dewey JD, Grabau C: Effects of isoflurane on coronary arteries and coronary arterioles in the intact dog. *Anesthesiology* 66:273–279, 1987.

Sprague DH, Yang JC, Hgai SH: Effects of isoflurane and halothane on contractility and the cyclic 3',5'-adenosine monophosphate system in the rat aorta. *Anesthesiology* 40:162–167, 1974.

Stevens WC, Cromwell TH, Halsey MJ, Eger EI, Shakespeare TF, Bahlman SH: The cardiovascular effects of a new inhalation anesthetic, Forane, in human volunteers at constant arterial carbon dioxide tension. *Anesthesiology* 35:8–16, 1971.

Takekawa S, Traber KB, Hantler CB, Tait AR, Gallagher KP, Knight PR: Effects of isoflurane on myocardial blood flow, function, and oxygen consumption in the presence of critical coronary stenosis in dogs. *Anesth Analg* 66:1073–1082, 1987.

Tarnow J, Markschies-Hornung A, Schulte-Sasse U: Isoflurane improves the tolerance to pacing-induced myocardial ischemia. *Anesthesiology* 64:147–156, 1986.

Todd MM, Drummond JC: A comparison of the

cerebrovascular and metabolic effects of halothane and isoflurane in the cat. *Anesthesiology* 60:276–282, 1984.

Enflurane

Black GW: Enflurane. *Br J Anaesth* 51:627–640, 1979.

Calverley RK, Smith NT, Jones CW, Prys-Roberts C, Eger EI: Ventilatory and cardiovascular effects of enflurane anesthesia during spontaneous ventilation in man. *Anesth Analg* 57:610–618, 1978.

Calverley RK, Smith NT, Prys-Roberts C, Eger EI, Jones CW: Cardiovascular effects of enflurane anesthesia during controlled ventilation in man. *Anesth Analg* 57:619–628, 1978.

Chase RE, Holaday DA, Fiserova-Bergerova V, Saidman LJ, Mack FE: The biotransofrmation of Ethrane in man. *Anesthesiology* 35:262–267, 1971.

Coleman AJ, Downing JW: Enflurane anesthesia for Cesarean section. *Anesthesiology* 43:354–357, 1975.

Cousins MJ, Greenstein LR, Hitt BA, Mazze RI: Metabolism and renal effects of enflurane in man. *Anesthesiology* 44:44–53, 1976.

Dooley JR, Mazze RI, Rice SA, Borel JD: Is enflurane defluorination inducible in man. *Anesthesiology* 50:213–217, 1979.

Dykes MHM: Is enflurane hepatotoxic? *Anesthesiology* 61:235–237, 1984.

Eger EI, Calverley RK, Smith NT: Changes in blood chemistries following prolonged enflurane anesthesia. *Anesth Analg* 55:547–549, 1976.

Fogdall RP, Miller RD: Neuromuscular effects of enflurane alone and combined with d-tubocurarine, pancuronium, and succinylcholine in man. *Anesthesiology* 42:173–178, 1975.

Gothert M, Wendt J: Inhibition of adrenal medullary catecholamine secretion by enflurane. 1. Investigations in vivo. *Anesthesiology* 46:400–403, 1977.

Horan BF, Prys-Roberts C, Hamilton WK, Roberts JG: Haemodynamic responses to enflurane anaesthesia and hypovolemia in the dog, and their modification by propranolol. *Br J Anaesth* 49:1189–1197, 1977.

Jensen BH, Ruhwald H, Berthlesen P, Brochner-Mortenssen J: Glomerular filtration rate during enflurane anaesthesia. *Acta Anaesth Scand* 21:13–15, 1978.

Kemmotsu O, Hashimoto Y, Shimosato S: The effects of fluroxene and enflurane on contractile performance of isolated papillary muscles from failing hearts. *Anesthesiology* 40:252–260, 1974.

Mazze RI, Calverley RK, Smith NT: Inorganic fluoride nephrotoxicity: prolonged enflurane and halothane anesthesia in volunteers. *Anesthesiology* 46:265–271, 1977.

Merin RG, Kumazawa T, Luka NL: Enflurane depresses myocardial function, perfusion and metabolism in the dog. *Anesthesiology* 45:501–507, 1976.

Moss E, Dearden NM, McDowall DG: Effects of 2% enflurane on intracranial pressure and cerebral perfusion pressure. *Br J Anaesth* 55:1083–1088, 1983.

Rydvall A, Haggmark S, Nyhman H, Reiz S: Effects of enflurane on coronary haemodynamics in patients with ischaemic heart disease. *Acta Anaesthesiol Scand* 28:690–695, 1984.

Wharton RS, Mazze RI, Wilson AI: Reproduction and fetal development in mice chronically exposed to enflurane. *Anesthesiology* 54:505–510, 1981.

Methoxyflurane

Bagwell EE, Woods EF: Cardiovascular effects of methoxyflurane. *Anesthesiology* 23:51–57, 1962.

Barr GA, Cousins MJ, Mazze RI, Hitt BA, Kosek JC: A comparison of the renal effects and metabolism of enflurane and methoxyflurane in Fischer 344 rats. *J Pharmacol Exp Ther* 188:257–264, 1974.

Black GW, McArdle L: The effects of methoxyflurane (Penthrane) on the peripheral circulation in man. *Br J Anaesth* 37:947–951, 1955.

Cousins MJ, Mazze RI, Kosek JC, Hitt BA, Love FV: The etiology of methoxyflurane nephrotoxicity. *J Pharmacol Exp Ther* 190:530–541, 1974.

Cousins MJ, Mazze RI: Methoxyflurane toxicity: a study of dose response in man. *JAMA* 255:1611–1616, 1973.

Mazze RI, Cousins MJ: Combined nephrotoxicity of gentamicin and methoxyflurane anesthesia in man. *Br J Anaesth* 45:394–398, 1973.

Mazze RI, Cousins MJ, Kosek JC: Dose-related methoxyflurane nephrotoxicity in rats: a biochemical and pathologic correlation. *Anesthesiology* 36:571–587, 1972.

Mazze RI, Shue GL, Jackson SH: Renal dysfunction associated with methoxyflurane anesthesia: a randomized, prospective clinical evaluation. *JAMA* 216:278–288, 1971.

Mazze RI, Trudell JR, Cousins MJ: Methoxyflurane metabolism and renal dysfunction: clinical correlation in man. *Anesthesiology* 35:247–252, 1971.

Walker JA, Eggers GWN, Allen CR: Cardiovascular effects of methoxyflurane anesthesia in man. *Anesthesiology* 23:639–642, 1962.

Nitrous Oxide

Amos RJ, Amess JAL, Nancekievill DG, Rees GM: Prevention of nitrous oxide-induced megaloblastic changes in bone marrow using folinic acid. *Br J Anaesth* 56:103–107, 1984.

Baden JM, Rice SA, Serra M, Kelley M, Mazze R: Thymidine and methionine syntheses in pregnant rats exposed to nitrous oxide. *Anesth Analg* 62:738–741, 1983.

Baden JM, Serra M, Mazze RI: Inhibition of fetal methionine synthase by nitrous oxide. *Br J Anaesth* 56:523–526, 1984.

Baden JM, Serra M, Mazze RI: Inhibition of rat fetal methionine synthase by nitrous oxide. *Br J Anaesth* 59:1040–1043, 1987.

Bennett GM, Loeser EA, Kawamura R, Stanley TH: Cardiovascular responses to nitrous oxide during enflurane and oxygen anesthesia. *Anesthesiology* 46:227–229, 1977.

Brodsky JB, Cohen EN, Brown BW, Wu ML, Whitcher CE: Exposure to nitrous oxide and neurologic disease among dental professionals. *Anesth Analg* 60:297–301, 1981.

Bussard DA, Stoelting RK, Peterson C, Ishaq M: Fetal changes in hamsters anesthetized with nitrous oxide and halothane. *Anesthesiology* 41:275–278, 1974.

Chapman WP, Arrowood JG, Beecher HK: The anesthetic effects of low concentrations of nitrous oxide compared in man with morphine sulfate. *J Clin Invest* 22:871–875, 1943.

Clutton-Brock J: Two cases of poisoning by contamination of nitrous oxide with higher oxides of nitrogen during anaesthesia. *Br J Anaesth* 39:388–392, 1967.

Crawford J, Lewis M: Nitrous oxide in early human pregnancy. *Anaesthesia* 41:900–905, 1986.

Dreyer C, Bischoff D, Gothert M: Effects of methoxyflurane anesthesia on adrenal medullary catecholamine secretion evoked by splanchnic-nerve stimulation. *Anesthesiology* 41:18–26, 1974.

Editorial: Oxides of nitrogen and health. *Lancet* 1:81–82, 1981.

Eger EI, Saidman LJ: Hazards of nitrous oxide anesthesia in bowel obstruction and pneumothorax. *Anesthesiology* 26:61–66, 1965.

Eisele JH, Reitan JA, Massumi RA, Zelis RF, Miller RR: Myocardial performance and N_2O analgesia in coronary-artery disease. *Anesthesiology* 44:16–20, 1976.

Eisele JH, Smith NT: Cardiovascular effects of 40 percent nitrous oxide in man. *Anesth Analg* 51:956–963, 1972.

Fink BR, Shepard TH, Blandau RJ: Teratogenic activity of nitrous oxide. *Nature* 214:146–148, 1967.

Fukunaga AF, Epstein RM: Sympathetic excitation during nitrous oxide-halothane anesthesia in the cat. *Anesthesiology* 39:23–36, 1973.

Gillman MA: Haematological changes caused by nitrous oxide. Cause for Concern? *Br J Anaesth* 59:143–147, 1987.

Goldberg AH, Sohn YZ, Phear WPC: Direct myocardial effects of nitrous oxide. *Anesthesiology* 37:373–380, 1972.

Hansen DK, Billings RE: Effects of nitrous oxide on macromolecular content and DNA synthesis in rat embryos. *J Pharmacol Exp Ther* 238:985–989, 1986.

Hornbein TF, Martin WE, Bonica JJ, Freund FG, Parmentier P: Nitrous oxide effects on the circulatory and ventilatory responses to halothane. *Anesthesiology* 31:250–260, 1969.

Johnson MC, Swartz HM, Donati RM: Hematologic alterations produced by nitrous oxide. *Anesthesiology* 34:42–49, 1971.

Keeling PA, Rocke DA, Nunn JF, Monk SJ, Lumb MJ, Halsey MJ: Folinic acid protection against nitrous oxide teratogenicity in the rat. *Br J Anaesth* 58:528–534, 1986.

Konieczko KM, Chapple JC, Nunn JF: Fetotoxic potential of general anaesthesia in relation to pregnancy. *Br J Anaesth* 59:449–454, 1987.

Kripke BJ, Talarico L, Shah NK, Kelman AD: Hematologic reaction to prolonged exposure to nitrous oxide. *Anesthesiology* 47:342–348, 1977.

Landon MJ, Toothill VJ: Effect of nitrous oxide on placental methionine synthase activity. *Br J Anaesth* 58:524–527, 1986.

Lappas DG, Buckley MJ, Laver MB, Daggett WM, Lowenstein E: Left ventricular performance and pulmonary circulation following addition of nitrous oxide to morphine during coronary artery surgery. *Anesthesiology* 43:61–69, 1975.

Masuda T, Ikeda K: Elimination of nitrous oxide accelerates elimination of halothane: reversed second gas effect. *Anesthesiology* 60:567–568, 1984.

Mazze RI: Nitrous oxide during pregnancy. *Anaesthesia* 41:897–899, 1986.

Mazze RI, Fujinaga M, Baden JM: Reproductive and teratogenic effects of nitrous oxide, fentanyl, and their combination in Sprague-Dawley rats. *Br J Anaesth* 59:1291–1297, 1987.

Mazze RI, Fujinaga M, Rice SA, Harris SB, Baden JM: Reproductive and teratogenic effects of nitrous oxide, halothane, isoflurane, and enflurane in Sprague-Dawley rats. *Anesthesiology* 64:339–344, 1986.

McDermott RW, Stanley TH: The cardiovascular effects of low concentrations of nitrous oxide during morphine anesthesia. *Anesthesiology* 44:89–91, 1974.

Munson ES: Transfer of nitrous oxide into body air cavities. *Br J Anaesth* 46:202–209, 1974.

Munson ES, Merrick HC: Effect of nitrous oxide on venous air embolism. *Anesthesiology* 27:783–787, 1966.

Nunn JF: Clinical aspects of the interaction between nitrous oxide and vitamin B_{12}. *Br J Anaesth* 59:3–13, 1987.

Nunn JF, Chanarin I: Editorial—nitrous oxide and vitamin B_{12}. *Br J Anaesth* 50:1089–1090, 1978.

Nunn JF, Sharer NM, Gorchein A, Jones JA, Wickramasinghe SN: Megaloblastic haemopoiesis after multiple short-term exposure to nitrous oxide. *Lancet* 1:1379—1381, 1982.

O'Sullivan H, Jennings F, Ward K, McCann S, Scott JM, Weir DG: Human bone marrow biochemical function and megaloblastic hematopoiesis after nitrous oxide anesthesia. *Anesthesiology* 55:645–649, 1981.

Phirman JR, Shapiro HM: Modification of nitrous oxide-induced intracranial hypertension by prior induction of anesthesia. *Anesthesiology* 46:150–151, 1977.

Price HL: Myocardial depression by nitrous oxide and its reversal by Ca^{++}. *Anesthesiology* 44:211–215, 1976.

Prys-Roberts C: Principles of treatment of poisoning by higher oxides of nitrogen. *Br J Anaesth* 39:432–437, 1967.

Rosen MA, Roizen MF, Eger EI, Glass RH, Martin M, Dandekar PV, Dailey PA, Litt L: The effect of nitrous oxide on in vitro fertilization success rate. *Anesthesiology* 67:42–44, 1987.

Saidman LJ, Eger EI: Effect of nitrous oxide and of narcotic premedication on the alveolar concentration of halothane required for anesthesia. *Anesthesiology* 25:302–306, 1964.

Severinghaus JW: The rate of uptake of nitrous oxide in man. *J Clin Invest* 33:1183–1189, 1954.

Smith NT, Calverley RK, Prys-Roberts C, Eger EI, Jones CW: Impact of nitrous oxide on the circulation during enflurane anesthesia in man. *Anesthesiology* 48:345–349, 1978.

Smith NT, Corbascio AN: The cardiovascular effects of nitrous oxide during halothane anesthesia in the dog. *Anesthesiology* 27:560–566, 1966.

Smith NT, Eger EI, Stoelting RK, Whayne TF,

Cullen D, Kadis LB: The cardiovascular and sympathomimetic responses to the addition of nitrous oxide to halothane in man. *Anesthesiology* 32:410–421, 1970.

Stanley TH, Kawamura R, Graves C: Effects of nitrous oxide on volume and pressure of endotracheal cuffs. *Anesthesiology* 41:256–262, 1974.

Stoelting RK, Gibbs PS: Hemodynamic effects of morphine and morphine-nitrous oxide in valvular heart disease and coronary artery disease. *Anesthesiology* 38:45–52, 1973.

Sweeney B, Bingham RM, Amos RJ, Petty AC, Cole PV: Toxicity of bone marrow in dentists exposed to nitrous oxide. *Br Med J* 291:567–569, 1985.

Vieira E, Cleaton-Jones P, Moyes D: Effects of low intermittent concentrations of nitrous oxide on the developing rat fetus. *Br J Anaesth* 55:67–69, 1983.

Wong KC, Martin WE, Hornbein TF, Freund FG, Everett J: The cardiovascular effects of morphine sulfate with oxygen and with nitrous oxide in man. *Anesthesiology* 38:542–549, 1973.

Neuromuscular Blocking Agents

MARGARET WOOD

Although curare was brought to Europe from South America by Charles Waterton in 1825, muscle relaxants were not used in routine clinical practice until over 100 years later when safe techniques of artificial respiration and a standardized preparation of curare became available. Today, a large number of muscle relaxants are in clinical use whose pharmacologic effects vary according to the specificity of their receptor blocking properties and the mechanism by which they produce neuromuscular block.

In addition to the established nondepolarizing muscle relaxants of long duration of action (pancuronium and tubocurarine) and the depolarizing muscle relaxant succinylcholine of short duration of action, new muscle relaxants have been and are being introduced into anesthetic practice in an attempt to provide improvement in the areas of duration of action, speed of onset, cumulation, and cardiovascular side effects. It is generally accepted that the undesirable side effects of succinylcholine due to its depolarizing mechanism of action mean that new compounds will be of the nondepolarizing class of agents. Two classes of compounds have produced new drugs with distinct advantages: the benzylisoquinolines, which include atracurium, mivacurium, and doxacurium, and the steroids, which include vecuronium and pipecuronium.

PHYSIOLOGY OF NEUROMUSCULAR TRANSMISSION

NEUROMUSCULAR JUNCTION

The neuromuscular junction is represented diagramatically in Figure 10.1 and can be seen to consist of a motor nerve terminal and skeletal muscle motor endplate, separated by the synaptic cleft that is filled with extracellular fluid. The motor nerve terminal is nonmyelinated and contains mitochondria, endoplasmic reticulum, and synaptic vesicles, all of which are concerned with the synthesis and storage of acetylcholine. The motor endplate is a highly folded membrane sit-

uated opposite the motor nerve terminal and separated by a gap of 200 to 300° A (the synaptic cleft) from the presynaptic membrane of the motor nerve terminal. Cholinergic receptors (acetylcholine binding sites) are located on both the presynaptic and postsynaptic membranes, and situated in close proximity to these receptors is the enzyme acetylcholinesterase. Plasma cholinesterase is present in the synaptic cleft.

SKELETAL MUSCLE CHOLINERGIC RECEPTOR

Cholinergic receptors are located on both the presynaptic (prejunctional) and postsynaptic (postjunctional) membranes. Although there is evidence that *presynaptic cholinergic receptors* are present at the motor nerve terminal and are different from postjunctional receptors, much less is known about them than the postjunctional nicotinic receptors of skeletal muscle.

The postjunctional nicotinic cholinergic receptors of the skeletal endplate are found on the shoulders of the postjunctional folds opposite the sites for acetylcholine release in the nerve terminal. Many receptors concentrate in this region (10,000 to 20,000/μm^2). The receptor is now known to be a protein with a molecular weight of 250,000 daltons. It consists of five glycoprotein subunits; alpha, beta, gamma, and delta (Figure 10.2). There are two alpha subunits and one each of the other three subunits. The subunits are arranged longitudinally to form a channel that allows the flow of ions down a concentration gradient. Sodium and calcium move into the muscle whereas potassium moves in the opposite direction. When acetylcholine (agonist) binds to the two alpha subunits of the acetylcholine receptor, the protein undergoes a conformational change that opens the channel so that cations pass through, the membrane becomes depolarized, and neuromuscular transmission occurs. Thus the cholinergic receptor has two main functions: (a) the recognition of the neurotransmitter, acetylcholine; and (b) the formation of an open ion channel

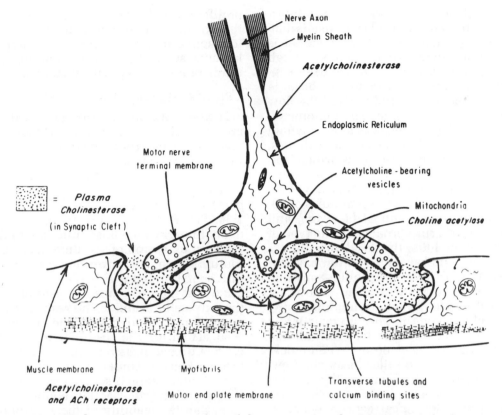

Figure 10.1.   Schematic representation of the neuromuscular junction.   The locations of important acetylcholine binding sites are shown in italics. With permission from Ali HH, Savarese JJ: Monitoring of Neuromuscular Function. *Anesthesiology* 45: 216–249, 1976.

that controls the flow of ions such as Na+, K+ and Ca^{2+} so that a change in membrane permeability results. Agonists and antagonists are able to bind to the alpha subunits. However, if only one alpha subunit is occupied by an agonist, the channel remains closed and depolarization cannot readily occur. Succinylcholine can bind to both alpha subunits so that the channel remains open. Competitive antagonists like d-tubocurarine bind to the alpha subunits, but the channel remains closed and the access of acetylcholine to the receptor is prevented. Blockade of neuromuscular transmission therefore occurs.

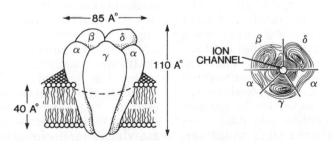

Figure 10.2.   Nicotinic acetylcholine receptor.   With permission from Taylor P: Are neuromuscular blocking agents more efficacious in pairs? *Anesthesiology* 63:1–3, 1985.

Many drugs have been shown to interfere with neuromuscular transmission; the extracellular end of the channel is wider than the part that extends through the cell membrane, and it has been suggested that large molecules can occlude or plug the channel and prevent the flow of ions through the channel, a phenomenon termed *channel blockade*. Channel blocking drugs include local anesthetics, some antibiotics, d-tubocurarine, and decamethonium. It is possible for some drugs to move into the channel and block ion movement when the channel is open, i.e., *simple open-channel blockade*, and examples of drugs producing this type of blockade include the local anesthetics (lidocaine, procaine) and the barbiturates. When the acetylcholine-activated channel closes with the molecule trapped inside the ion channel, *trapping channel blockade* is said to occur while another type of mechanism termed *closed-channel block* occurs when blockers bind to a site on the closed cholinergic receptor and effectively block flow once channel opening occurs. Thus two main pharmacological actions occur at the cholinergic receptor: (a) *competitive antagonism* and (b) *channel blockade*.

During prolonged exposure to acetylcholine, cholinergic receptors become refractory to additional agonist, i.e., *desensitization* occurs, from which recovery is slow. It is thought that when desensitization develops, receptors are able to bind agonists but the conformational state of the channel is such that it is not able to open.

Extrajunctional receptors are found on the membrane throughout the muscle but are normally not present in large numbers in active adult human muscle. When motor nerves are inactive, e.g., in patients with muscle denervation, traumatized skeletal muscle, spinal cord injury, stroke, or prolonged immobilization, these extrajunctional receptors proliferate. The extrajunctional receptors are markedly responsive to agonists such as succinylcholine and poorly responsive to antagonists such as d-tubocurarine. It has been suggested that the proliferation of extrajunctional receptors that results when nerve terminals are less active might account for the hyperkalemia seen after succinylcholine administration in this clinical setting.

RESTING MEMBRANE POTENTIAL

The resting membrane potential of muscle and nerve is maintained by the unequal distribution of potassium and sodium ions across the membrane. The more permeable ion is potassium and the ratio of potassium ions outside the cell to potassium ions inside the cell is about 1:30. The resting cell membrane is relatively impermeable to sodium due to the constant extrusion of sodium ions by the sodium pump. Potassium and protein are thus concentrated within the cell, and sodium and chloride ions are restricted to the extracellular fluid. The resting transmembrane potential is in the region of -90 mV, with the potential inside the muscle or nerve being negative relative to the exterior. Under these conditions, the cell membrane is said to be polarized. When a propagated action potential occurs, the permeability of the membrane to sodium and potassium ions increases and the transmembrane potential falls toward zero, with the interior of the fiber becoming positive with respect to the outside. Thus, the development of an action potential is associated with the inward movement of sodium ions followed by the outward movement of potassium ions.

ACETYLCHOLINE AND NEUROMUSCULAR TRANSMISSION

The transmitter substance at the neuromuscular junction is acetylcholine, a quaternary ammonium ester. Acetylcholine is synthesized in the motor nerve by the acetylation of choline under the control of the enzyme choline acetylase. The synthesized acetylcholine is then stored in synaptic vesicles at the motor nerve terminal and released into the synaptic cleft as "packets" or quanta, each of which contains at least 1000 molecules of acetylcholine. In the absence of stimulation, quanta are released randomly to produce miniature endplate potentials that can be recorded from the muscle endplate and are of the amplitude of 0.5 to 1.0 mV. These miniature endplate potentials represent the release of quanta of acetylcholine as each vesicle ruptures, but they produce insufficient voltage to reach the threshold required to initiate an action potential that triggers depolarization of the motor endplate.

However, the arrival of the nerve impulse produces the liberation of many hundred quanta of acetylcholine, which bind to the cholinergic receptors on the postsynaptic membrane causing an increase in the permeability of the membrane to sodium and potassium ions. This is followed by a fall in the transmembrane potential. Once the membrane potential is reduced from the resting value of -90 mV to the threshold potential of about -45 mV, an action potential develops and proceeds toward depolarization of the surrounding muscle membrane, and a propagated muscle action potential results. This action potential spreads over the surface of the muscle fiber initiating muscular contraction.

After binding to its receptors, acetylcholine is immediately hydrolyzed by acetylcholinesterase to acetic acid and choline. As the effect of the acetylcholine-receptor reaction diminishes, the membrane regains its initial permeability to sodium and potassium ions, and the membrane becomes repolarized. The hydrolysis of acetylcholine is said to be completed within 15 msec, leaving choline free to reenter the nerve for the resynthesis of acetylcholine.

Calcium ions must be present for the release of acetylcholine to occur. It is thought that depolarization opens calcium gates or channels in the motor nerve terminal membrane leading to an influx of calcium ions, which in turn are important in initiating the quantal release of acetylcholine from the synaptic vesicles into the synaptic cleft. It is possible that cyclic nucleotides are involved in the link between the nerve action potential and the entry of calcium ions into the nerve terminal. It is suggested that a nerve action potential activates adenylate cyclase in the nerve terminal membrane, which results in the conversion of ATP to cAMP (see Chapter 13). This acts on a protein kinase, which opens the calcium channel causing the synaptic vesicles to fuse with the nerve membrane and release acetylcholine. The cAMP is finally inactivated by phosphodiesterase. This theory would predict that adenylate cyclase activators such as prostaglandin E_1 and phosphodiesterase inhibitors such as theophylline derivatives would increase neuromuscular transmission, while calcium antagonists such as verapamil would be expected to decrease acetylcholine release. These effects have been confirmed in animal studies.

CLASSIFICATION OF NEUROMUSCULAR BLOCK

Muscle relaxants may be divided into two groups, nondepolarizing and depolarizing, according to the type of neuromuscular block that they produce: (*a*) nondepolarizing and (*b*) depolarizing.

(*a*) Nondepolarizing

This group of muscle relaxants includes d-Tubocurarine, pancuronium, gallamine, metocurine, alcuronium, fazadinium, atracurium and vecuronium. Nondepolarizing muscle relaxants can also be classified according to their duration of action:

Long-Acting

d-Tubocurarine	Gallamine
Metocurine	Pancuronium

Intermediate-Acting

Atracurium	Vecuronium

Doxacurium and pipecuronium are new long-acting nondepolarizing muscle relaxants, whereas mivacurium is a new short acting nondepolarizing muscle relaxant.

(*b*) Depolarizing

This group of muscle relaxants includes succinylcholine and decamethonium.

The extent of neuromuscular block produced by muscle relaxants can be affected by drugs and disease states, and the only clinically reliable method of assessing neuromuscular function is to stimulate a peripheral nerve using a peripheral nerve stimulator and observe or measure the response of the skeletal muscle. Other clinical tests such as the assessment of adequate ventilation and cough and airway maintenance by measurement of vital capacity and maximal inspiratory and expiratory force are also important at the termination of anesthesia and in the recovery room. The type of neuromuscular block present can be identified by the pattern of skeletal muscle responses evoked by single twitch, tetanus, continuous stimulaton, and train-of-four stimulation. For a description of the monitoring of neuromuscular function, the reader is referred to several reviews in the Bibliography at the end of the chapter. Three kinds of neuromuscular block can be differentiated clinically according to the pattern of the evoked muscle response to changes in frequency of nerve stimulation: nondepolarizing, depolarizing, and phase II or dual block.

Nondepolarizing Block (Competitive, Antagonist)

This type of block is caused by the nondepolarizing muscle relaxants. It is characterized by the absence of fasiculation, fade after slow (twitch) or fast (tetanic) rates of stimulation, fade with train-of-four stimulation at $2H_z$, posttetanic potentiation, antagonism by anticholinesterases, potentiation by nondepolarizing relaxants, and antagonism by depolarizing relaxants. Twitch depression results from the competitive blockade of postsynaptic cholinergic receptors whereas fade results from presynaptic effects. This type of block has also been termed competitive or antagonist neuromuscular block because nondepolarizing drugs bind to and occupy the cholinergic receptor on the postsynaptic membrane but do not themselves stimulate the receptor, hence, depolarization of the postsynaptic membrane by acetylcholine is prevented. This is an oversimplified concept, and, for example, d-tubocurarine also has presynaptic effects.

Depolarizing Block (Agonist) or Phase I Block.

This type of block follows the administration of succinylcholine and is characterized by muscle fasiculations preceding the onset of paralysis, absence of fade at slow and fast stimulation rates, a train-of-four ratio of greater than 0.7, no posttetanic potentiation, potentiation by anticholinesterases, antagonism by nondepolarizing relaxants, and potentiation by other depolarizing relaxants. In general depolarizing muscle relaxants imitate the action of acetylcholine and act as agonists at the cholinergic receptor; they bind to and stimulate the cholinergic receptor on the postsynaptic membrane, thus lowering the transmembrane potential and causing depolarization of the postsynaptic membrane. The reduction in membrane potential produced prevents the triggering of a propagated action potential by acetylcholine, and the muscle is unresponsive to further stimuli. The depolarization produced by succinylcholine lasts longer than that produced by acetylcholine, and a "depolarizing block" follows the initial depolarization whereby succinylcholine maintains the membrane in a depolarized state and prevents repolarization. It is important to note that the concentration of depolarizing relaxant required to maintain an 80 to 90% reduction in twitch height increases with continued exposure (tachyphylaxis).

Phase II, Dual Block, or Desensitization Block

A large dose or repeated administration of a depolarizing relaxant can cause the sensitivity of the cholinergic receptors on the motor endplate to change such that the typical depolarizing block changes to one that exhibits many of the classic characteristics of a nondepolarizing block. This alteration in characteristics is referred to as a phase II block (phase I is considered the original depolarizing block). Phase II block may reflect desensitization of postjunctional cholinergic receptors. Repetitive doses result in progressively less neuromuscular block (tachyphylaxis). It is characterized by poorly sustained tetanus, posttetanic facilitation, a train-of-four ratio of less than 0.3, and reversal of the block in some cases by anticholinesterase drugs. The use of train of four to diagnose the change of action of succinylcholine from a phase I to phase II block may be particularly useful. Succinylcholine is often administered as a single bolus dose when its rapid onset of action is required for a "rapid sequence" or "crash induction," and at this dose (1.0 to 1.5 mg/kg), phase II block is not likely to occur. Succinylcholine is still administered as a continuous infusion by some clinicians (2 to 15 mg/kg/hr is required for maintenance of 90% twitch depression) for periods of under 60 minutes, although phase II block is likely to result and recovery from phase II block is unpredictable. The use of succinylcholine by continuous infusion has markedly declined since the introduction of atracurium and vecuronium. Phase II block occurs more commonly in neonates and patients with myasthenia gravis. In addition, patients with atypical cholinesterase may develop a phase II block more readily after the administration of succinylcholine, possibly because the motor endplate is exposed to succinylcholine for a longer period of time due to reduced hydrolysis of the drug (see Chapter 5).

STRUCTURE-ACTIVITY RELATIONSHIP

The natural transmitter at the neuromuscular junction, acetylcholine, has a positively charged ammonium group that is attracted to the negatively charged cholinergic receptor site. This feature is common to the neuromuscular blocking drugs which also contain a quaternary monium group—four carbon radicals attached to one nitrogen atom.

$$CH_3 - N^+ - CH_2 \ldots\ldots R$$

with CH_3 groups and a 90 labeled above.

The majority of the nondepolarizing neuromuscular blocking drugs have two quaternary nitrogen groups, with the exception of d-tubocurarine and vecuronium, which are monoquaternary, and gallamine, which is triquaternary. The electrostatic attraction of the negatively charged cholinergic receptor for the positively charged quaternary ammonium group occurs not only at the neuromuscular junction but at cholinergic receptors throughout the body, e.g., at the vagus nerve endings (muscarinic receptors) and at autonomic ganglia (nicotinic receptors) (Table 10.1). The neuromuscular blocking agents show certain structural similarities to acetylcholine (Fig. 10.3). Succinylcholine is essentially two molecules of acetylcholine linked through the acetate and methyl groups whereas pancuronium possesses two acetylcholine like groups oriented on a steroid nucleus.

The specificity of a compound for either the cholinergic autonomic ganglionic receptor or the neuromuscular receptor is determined partly by the length of the carbon chain separating the two positively charged groups so that maximal ganglionic blockade occurs when five or six CH_2 groups intervene while intervention of ten CH_2 groups results in maximal neuromuscular blockade (Figure 10.4). This is seen clinically in that decamethonium (C10) is a depolarizing muscle relaxant whereas hexamethonium (C6) is a ganglionic blocking agent.

The shape and flexibility of the molecule is also important. Most receptor-stimulating molecules (agonists) such as succinylcholine are flexible, long, and slender and are able to bind to and activate the cholinergic receptor, producing depolarization like acetylcholine. Bulky and rigid molecules such as pancuro-

Table 10.1.
Cholinoceptive Sites

Site	Activators or Substrates	Inhibitors
Nicotinic Receptors		
(a)Neuromuscular junction	Nicotine, Tetraethylammonium Succinylcholine Decamethonium	d-Tubocurarine
(b)Autonomic ganglia	Dimethylphenylpiperazinium	Hexamethonium d-Tubocurarine
Muscarinic Receptors		
(Bowel, bladder, bronchi, sinus node of the heart, pupillary spinchter)	Muscarine	Atropine Gallamine* Pancuronium*
Esteratic Receptors		
(a)Active site of acetylcholinesterase	Acetylcholine Methacholine	Neostigmine Pyridostigmine Hexafluorenium
(b)Active site of plasma cholinesterase	Succinylcholine	Tetrahydroaminocrine Pancuronium

With permission from Savarese JJ, Philbin DM: Cardiovascular effects of neuromuscular blocking agents. *Int Anesth Clin* 17:1:13–54, 1979.
*The muscarinic inhibitory action of gallamine and pancuronium is limited to the SA node of the heart.

nium although similar in structure to acetylcholine cannot activate or stimulate the receptor themselves, but block the approach of acetylcholine and so they produce a nondepolarizing block by antagonism or receptor inhibition. Using this concept of a muscle relaxant acting as either an agonist or antagonist at all cholinergic receptors, one more readily understands the clinical side effects of some of the muscle relaxants. Thus, tachycardia associated with pancuronium is due to inhibition (antagonism) of muscarinic receptors at the heart, the cardiac effects of succinylcholine (bradycardia) are due to activation or stimulation of cholinergic cardiac receptors. It is interesting that pancuronium has also been shown to be an inhibitor of plasma cholinesterase (Table 10.1). Hypotension after the administration of d-tubocurarine probably involves both autonomic ganglion blocking and histamine-releasing properties.

At one time, d-tubocurarine was thought to contain two quaternary nitro-

gen groups. Everett and coworkers have shown this structure to be incorrect, and d-tubocurarine is now believed to have one quaternary nitrogen group and a tertiary nitrogen group in equilibrium with a proton at physiological pH. As a bulky monoquaternary structure is more likely to produce autonomic ganglionic blockade than a bisquaternary compound, the new formula supports the autonomic ganglionic blocking properties of d-tubocurarine. The histamine-releasing properties of d-tubocurarine are probably due to the presence of the tertiary amine. In addition, the increased efficacy of d-tubocurarine in acidotic states may be explained on the basis that the basic tertiary amino group becomes more ionized as the hydrogen ion concentration increases.

Methylation of d-tubocurarine to produce metocurine or dimethyl tubocurarine (a bisquaternary compound) reduces the histamine-releasing and ganglion-blocking activities associated with d-tubocurarine and results in a muscle re-

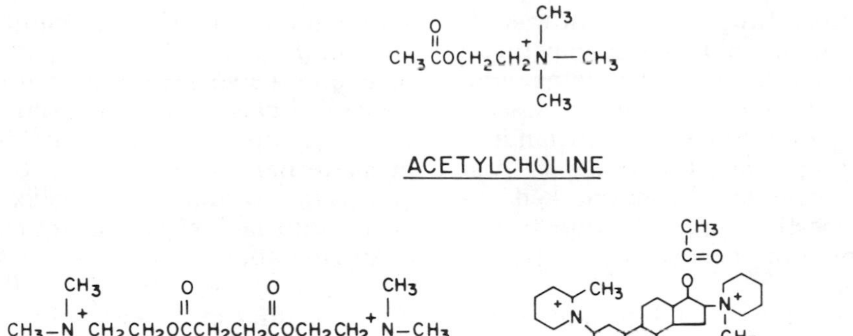

$$CH_3COCH_2CH_2\overset{+}{N}(CH_3)_3$$

ACETYLCHOLINE

SUCCINYLCHOLINE

PANCURONIUM

d - TUBOCURARINE

METOCURINE

GALLAMINE

Figure 10.3. Chemical structural similarity between acetylcholine and the neuromuscular blocking agents.

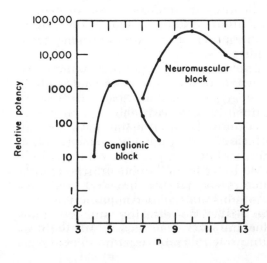

Figure 10.4. Structure-activity relationship data for ganglionic and neuromuscular block by polymethylene bismethonium compounds. The number of -Ch$_2$-groups between cationic groups is n; relative potency has logarithmic scale. Adapted with permission from Paton WDM, Zaimis EJ: The pharmacological actions of polymethylene bistrimethylamimonium salts. *Br J Pharmacol* 4:381–400, 1949.

laxant that is 3 times less potent than d-tubocurarine in blocking sympathetic and parasympathetic ganglia. In general, bisquaternary compounds do not possess strong ganglionic blocking or histamine-releasing properties. Gallamine (a tris-quaternary compound) has marked va-golytic properties, probably due to the presence of three positively charged ni-trogen atoms.

Many neuromuscular blocking agents possess two quaternary ammonium groups and at one time it was believed that the distance between the two qua-ternary centers was important in deter-mining the affinity of the muscle relaxant for the cholinergic receptor at the neu-romuscular junction, optimal competi-tive neuromuscular blocking action oc-curring when the two quaternary groups were 1.25 nm apart. However, d-tubocu-rarine has been shown to be a monoqua-ternary compound, gallamine is a triqua-ternary compound, and in the case of pancuronium the distance between the two quaternary groups is 1.108 nm. It is now believed that an interquaternary distance of 1.25 nm may confer optimal depolarizing activity but is not critical in competitive blockade.

Pancuronium is a steroid muscle relax-ant with two quaternary ammonium groups (Figure 10.3). Savage and cowork-ers recognized that the neuromuscular and vagolytic potencies of pancuronium were located separately on the A and D rings of the molecule, with the A ring being responsible for cardiac effects and the D ring for the neuromuscular effects. The intermediate-acting muscle relaxant vecuronium is structurally very similar to pancuronium but is a monoquaternary compound and does not possess the methyl group on the 2-piperidine nitro-gen of the A ring androstane nucleus (Figure 10.5). This difference in chemical structure is thought to be responsible for the lack of important autonomic side ef-fects associated with vecuronium. Al-though vecuronium is very hydrophilic, the monoquaternary ammonium group makes vecuronium more lipophilic than pancuronium, resulting in a more rapid onset of action and shorter duration of

action than that of pancuronium. Atra-curium (Figure 10.5) developed by Sten-lake and coworkers represents a new structural class of neuromuscular block-ing drugs, the benzylisoquinolines. It is a bisquaternary compound with methyl groups that confer muscle relaxant prop-erties with lack of significant cardiovas-cular side effects at therapeutic doses.

Figures 10.3 and 10.5 show the struc-tural formulae of the clinically important neuromuscular blocking agents.

PHARMACOKINETICS

Most of the muscle relaxants have one to three quaternary ammonium groups and are therefore almost completely ion-ized at physiological pH, highly water soluble, and only very slightly lipid sol-uble. They thus have a limited volume of distribution and do not readily cross the placenta or blood-brain barrier.

Peak concentrations are achieved rap-idly following intravenous administra-tion, after which the concentration falls rapidly due to extravascular distribution $(t_{1/2_\alpha})$. When equilibrium has been achieved between drug in blood and drug in tissues, the concentration falls more slowly due to elimination by excretion and/or metabolism (elimination phase) (Figure 10.6). Table 10.2 lists the phar-macokinetic parameters of the nondepo-larizing muscle relaxants, and Table 10.3 summarizes the routes of elimination for the nondepolarizing muscle relaxants, indicating the relative extent of urinary and biliary excretion and, in the case of vecuronium and pancuronium, meta-bolism.

Knowledge of the pharmacokinetic pa-rameters of the muscle relaxants in both healthy patients and those with disease states allows the calculation of the appro-priate dose for administration by bolus or infusion. The volume of distribtution at steady state (Vd_{ss}) is that volume calcu-lated to contain all of the drug at equilib-rium once mixing has occurred (see Chapter 1), or the total amount of drug in the body at the same time divided by the concentration in plasma. Thus, the dose of muscle relaxant required to achieve a

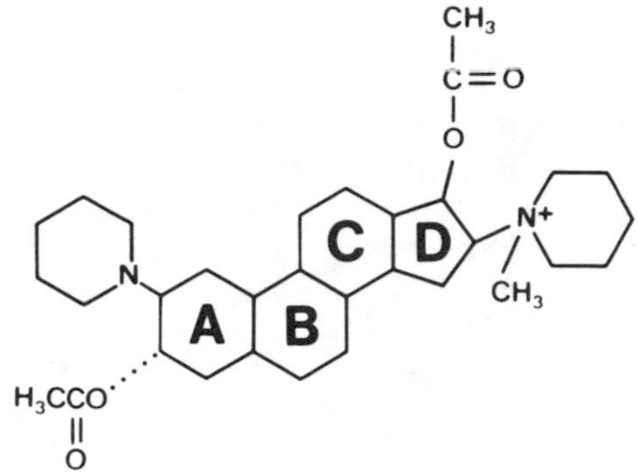

Vecuronium

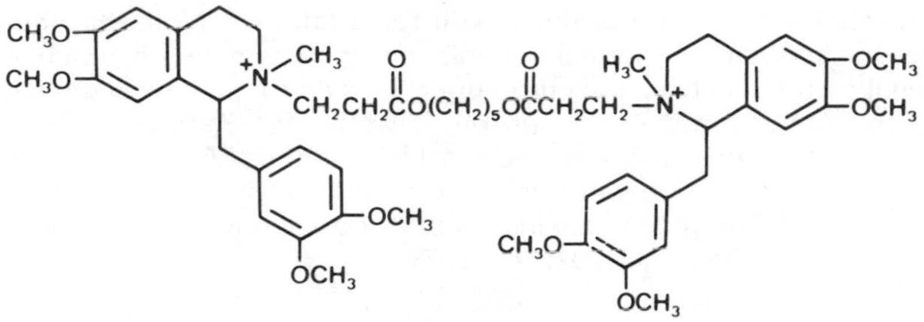

Atracurium

Figure 10.5. Chemical structure of the intermediate-acting neuromuscular blocking drugs, atracurium and vecuronium. Vecuronium, a monoquaternary steroid, is structurally similar to pancuronium and atracurium is a bisquaternary isoquinolinium compound.

therapeutic concentration (Cp) is equal to the product of the volume of distribution and the desired plasma concentration ($Vd_{ss} \times Cp$) (see page 11). Similarly, the infusion rate is calculated (see page 10) from the equation

Steady State Plasma Concentration (C_{ss})

$$= \frac{\text{Infusion rate}}{\text{Clearance}}$$

An increase in volume of distribution, perhaps as a consequence of altered protein binding in liver disease, would therefore lead to an increased initial bolus dose requirement to achieve neuromuscular blockade whereas decreased clearance would require a reduced infu-

sion rate or intermittent doses to be given at less frequent intervals. Table 10.4 gives required infusion rates and therapeutic plasma concentrations for the neuromuscular blocking agents in order to achieve 95% paralysis.

Although volatile anesthetics have been reported to inhibit drug metabolism and to reduce hepatic blood flow, there is no evidence that volatile anesthetics affect the pharmacokinetics of the muscle relaxants.

Pharmacokinetic factors responsible for interindividual variation in response to the muscle relaxants are discussed in a later section, "Factors Affecting Neuromuscular Blockade." Table 10.5 summarizes the pharmacokinetics of the non-

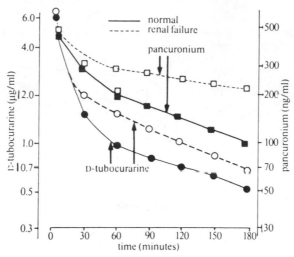

Figure 10.6.   Rates at which the plasma concentrations of d-tubocurarine and pancuronium fall in normal patients and in those with renal failure.   Note that the decay rates for both drugs are the same in normal patients, but the decay rate is much slower in patients with renal failure receiving pancuronium. The data for pancuronium were obtained with permission from McLeod K, Watson MJ, Rawlins MD: Pharmacokinetics of pancuronim in patients with normal and impaired renal function. *Br J Anaesth* 48:341–345, 1976; and the data for d-tubocurarine were obtained with permission from Miller RD, Matteo RS, Benet LZ, Sohn YJ: The pharmacokinetics of d-tubocurarine in man with and without renal failure. *J Pharmacol Exp Ther* 202:1–7, 1977.

depolarizing muscle relaxants in liver and renal disease.

TUBOCURARINE

The pharmacokinetic characteristics of d-tubocurarine in humans are given in Table 10.2. Due to its high degree of ionization and water solubility, d-tubocurarine is excreted mainly by the kidneys (Table 10.3). It is also excreted in the bile, and ligation of the renal pedicles in dogs increases the proportion excreted in the bile in 24 hours from 11 to 39% Metabolism does not play an important

Table 10.2.
Pharmacokinetic Parameters of the Nondepolarizing Muscle Relaxants

Parameter	d-Tubocurarine	Pancuronium	Metocurine	Gallamine	Atracurium	Vecuronium
Vd(ml/kg)	290–300	240–260	422–460	290	150–180	199–280
Distribution $t_{1/2}$ (min)	4.8–6.4	10–13	1.9*	16.1	2.0	7.5
Terminal $t_{1/2}$ (min)	84–119	114–146	217*	150	17–22	24–92
Cl (ml/kg/min)	2.2–2.6	1.9–2.1	1.05–1.4	1.6	5.0–6.0	3.6–6.7

Most of the data is taken with permission from Ramzan MI, Somogyi AA, Walker JA, Shanks CA, Triggs EJ: Clinical pharmacokinetics of the non-depolarizing muscle relaxants. *Clin Pharmacokinet* 6:25–60, 1981; Ward S, Neill AM, Weatherley BC, Corall IM: Pharmacokinetics of atracurium besylate in healthy patients after a single IV bolus dose. *Br J Anaesth* 55:113–118, 1983; and Lynam DP, Cronnelly R, Castagnoli, Canfell C, Caldwell J, Arden J, Miller RD: The pharmacodynamics and pharmacokinetics of vecuronium in patients anesthetized with isoflurane with normal renal function or with renal failure. *Anesthesiology* 69:227–231, 1988.
*Elimination t½ using three-compartment model.

Table 10.3.
Elimination of Nondepolarizing Muscle Relaxants in Healthy Patients

Drug	Unchanged Drug in Urine %	Metabolites in Urine %	Unchanged Drug in Bile %
d-Tubocurarine	38–44		11.8
Pancuronium	46	5–10	5–10
Metocurine	52		2.1
Gallamine	89–100		
Vecuronium	10–25	5	30–50

Data with permission from Meijer DKF, Weitering JG, Vermeer GA, Scaf AHJ: Comparative pharmacokinetics of d-tubocurarine and metocurine. *Anesthesiology* 51:402–407, 1979; Miller RD, Matteo RS, Benet L, Sohn YJ. The pharmacokinetics of d-tubocurarine in man with and without renal failure. *J Pharmacol Exp Ther* 202:1–7, 1977; Agoston S, Vermeer GA, Kerston VW, Scaf AHJ: A preliminary investigation of the renal and hepatic excretion of gallamine triethiodide in man. *Br J Anaesth* 50:345–349, 1978; Duvaldestin P, Agoston S, Henzel D, Kerston VW, Desmonts JM: Pancuronium pharmacokinetics in patients with liver cirrhosis. *Br J Anaesth* 50:1131–1136, 1978; Bencini AF, Scaf AHJ, Sohn YJ, Meistelman C, Lienhart A, Kersten UW, Schwarz S, Agoston S: Disposition and urinary excretion of vecuronium bromide in anesthetized patients with normal renal function or renal failure. *Anesth Analg* 65:245–251, 1986.

role in the elimination of d-tubocurarine.

A dose of 0.3 mg/kg in an adult produces nondepolarizing neuromuscular block that lasts about 51 minutes from the time of injection to 50% recovery of neuromuscular transmission and 74 minutes to 90% recovery. Serum d-tubocurarine concentrations have been found to correlate with twitch tension of the adductor muscle of the thumb during both inhalational and narcotic-nitrous oxide anesthesia, and it has been shown that twitch tension starts to recover at serum d-tubocurarine concentrations of about 0.70 mcg/ml. At 50% recovery of the twitch response, the concentration of d-tubocurarine is 0.45 mcg/ml, whereas complete recovery occurs at a serum d-tubocurarine concentration of 0.20 mcg/ml.

During continuous intravenous infusion of d-tubocurarine (rapid infusion of 16.8 mcg/kg/min over 10 minutes followed by 1.2 mcg/kg/min to the end of surgery) to achieve steady state plasma

Table 10.4.
Therapeutic Concentrations and Infusion Rates of Muscle Relaxants Required to Maintain 95% Paralysis

Relaxant	Plasma Concentration(μg/ml)	Calculated Infusion Rate* (μg/kg/min)
Alcuronium	0.8	1.0
Atracurium	1.3	7.2
Gallamine	10.0	13.0
Metocurine	0.6	0.78
Pancuronium	0.3	0.48
Tubocurarine	1.1	2.1
Vecuronium	0.2	0.92

With permission from Shanks CA: Pharmacokinetics of the nondepolarizing neuromuscular relaxants applied to calculation of bolus and infusion dosage regimens. *Anesthesiology* 64:72–86, 1986.
*The infusion rate is calculated from a knowledge of plasma clearance and therapeutic concentration for each relaxant. Infusion rate = therapeutic concentration × clearance.

Table 10.5.
Pharmacokinetics of the Nondepolarizing Muscle Relaxants in Renal and Liver Disease States

Muscle Relaxant	Volume of Distribution (L/kg)	Terminal Elimination Half-Life (min)	Clearance (ml/kg/min)
Renal Disease			
Pancuronium	0.24–0.30	257–489	0.3–0.9
Gallamine	0.29	752	0.24
Metocurine	0.30	684	0.38
Tubocurarine		330	
Vecuronium	0.24–0.35	68–97	2.5–4.5
Atracurium	0.17–0.22	18–24	6.3–6.7
Liver Disease—Biliary Obstruction			
Gallamine	0.25	160	1.2
Pancuronium	0.31–0.43	24–270	1.1–1.5
Liver Disease—Cirrhosis			
Pancuronium	0.35	208	1.5
Vecuronium	0.23	84	2.7

Most of the data is from Shanks CA: Pharmacokinetics of the nondepolarizing neuromuscular relaxants applied to calculation of bolus and infusion dosage regimens. *Anesthesiology* 64:72–86, 1986.

concentrations (Cp_{ss}), the distribution half-life is 6.2 minutes during nitrous oxide-narcotic anesthesia and 6.4 minutes during halothane anesthesia (0.5 to 0.7%), and the elimination half-life is 119 minutes during nitrous oxide-narcotic anesthesia and 104 minutes during halothane anesthesia. Thus, halothane anesthesia does not appreciably after the pharmacokinetics of d-tubocurarine in comparison with nitrous oxide-narcotic anesthiesia. However, halothane anesthesia decreases the plasma concentration of d-tubocurarine required to produce 50% neuromuscular blockage, i.e., 50% pharmacologic effect. The plasma concentration of d-tubocurarine required to produce 50% paralysis has been termed $Cp_{ss}(50)$; $Cp_{ss}(50)$ is 0.6 mcg/ml during nitrous oxide anesthesia, 0.36 mcg/ml during halothane (0.5 to 0.7%) anesthesia, and is further reduced to 0.22 mcg/ml during 1.0 to 1.2% halothane administration.

The plasma protein binding of d-tubocurarine is approximately 45% in normal adults (Table 10.6). A correlation between gamma globulin concentrations and d-tubocurarine requirements has been noted, and increased d-tubocurarine requirements have been reported in patients who are liable to have elevated gamma globulin levels, such as those with hepatic disease and bilharzial cirrhosis. The importance to the anesthetist of protein binding is that decreased binding increases the amount of free drug available to exert pharmacologic effect, thereby theoretically increasing neuromuscular blockade. Tubocurarine exhibits the highest percentage of protein binding, and this is not altered by liver, cardiac, or renal disease. The binding of d-tubocurarine is less in the neonate than in the adult (Table 10.6). Alterations in plasma protein binding are unlikely to be important in explaining individual variation in response to muscle relaxants inasmuch as none are highly protein bound.

Renal failure can profoundly affect the pharmacokinetics of the muscle relaxants. Determination of plasma concentrations of d-tubocurarine after the administration of 0.5 mg/kg to patients with and without renal function indicates that the plasma concentration remains elevated longer in patients without renal function (Figure 10.6). In renal failure the terminal elimination half-life is prolonged to 330 minutes, and only 13 to 15% of the injected dose is excreted unchanged in the urine as opposed to 38 to 44% in normal subjects (Table 10.3). For both d-tubocurarine and pancuronium, there is no change in the plasma concentration of drug required to produce neuromuscular blockade, indicating no pharmacodynamic change at the neuromuscular junction.

PANCURONIUM

The pharmacokinetic parameters of pancuronium are given in Table 10.2 Pancuronium elimination incorporates renal, biliary, and biotransformation routes of clearance (Table 10.3.). After 0.95 mg/kg of pancuronium intravenously, 37 to 44% of the administered dose is eliminated in the urine and 11% is excreted in the bile over the 30-hour postinjection period. Thus, renal elimination is the major excretory pathway in man, but some biliary elimination does occur. The clearance of pancuronium is reduced in patients with renal failure (Figure 10.6 and Table 10.5) resulting in increased duration of neuromuscular blockade. Pancuronium disposition is also altered in patients with hepatic dysfunction. Patients with total biliary obstruction and hepatic cirrhosis have an increased volume of distribution, prolonged elimination half-life, and reduced plasma clearance (Table 10.5). These alterations in pharmacokinetics are associated with a prolongation of neuromuscular blockade.

Pancuronium does not bind extensively to plasma proteins; the free fraction (unbound) is about 90% in normal adults (Table 10.6).

Although d-tubocurarine is excreted in the unchanged form, metabolism of pancuronium does occur. About 10 to 40% of an intravenous dose of pancuronium is metabolized by deacetylation to 3-hydroxy, 17-hydroxy, and 3,17-dihydroxy derivatives. Of the metabolites, the 3-hydroxy derivative possesses the most muscle-relaxant activity, being half as potent as pancuronium, whereas the other metabolites have only minimal relaxant activity. As much as 25% of the 3-hydroxy but less than 5% of the 17 and 3,17 dihydroxy derivatives are found in urine and bile. Pancuronium is 2 times more potent than the 3-hydroxy derivative, 50 times more potent than the 17-hydroxy analog, and 54 times more potent than the 3,17 dihydroxy compound as a neuromuscular blocking agent. The pharmacokinetic values of the metabolites of pancuronium are similar to those of the parent compound, and 3-hydroxy and 3,17 dihydroxy pancuronium have a sim-

Table 10.6.
Plasma Protein Binding of Nondepolarizing Muscle Relaxants

Subject	Percentage of Free d-Tubocurarine	Percentage of Free Metocurine	Percentage of Free Pancuronium	Percentage of Free Vecuronium
Neonate	68.7*	75.6*	91.0	
Mother	58.9	67.1	89.0	
Adult male	57.4	68.2	93.2	60
Adult nonpregnant female	54.6	64.9	88.9	
Renal failure			90.7	

From Wood M, Wood AJJ: Changes in plasma drug binding and alpha₁-acid glycoprotein in mother and newborn. *Clin Pharmacol Ther* 29:522–526, 1981; Wood M, Stone WJ, Wood AJJ: Plasma binding of pancuronium: Effect of age, sex and disease. *Anesth Analg* 62:29–32, 1983; and Duvaldestin P, Henzel D: Binding of tubocurarine, fazadinium, pancuronium and ORG NC45 to serum proteins in normal man and in patients with cirrhosis. *Br J Anaesth* 54:513–516, 1982.
*Significantly different from mother.

ilar duration of action; 17-hydroxy pancuronium has a shorter duration of
action.

Like d-tubocurarine, the serum concentration of pancuronium correlates
with the intensity of neuromuscular
blockade. Neuromuscular transmission
at the adductor muscle of the thumb
starts to recover at a serum pancuronium
concentration of about 0.2 mcg/ml and
recovery of twitch tension to 24, 50, and
75% of control values occurs at serum
concentrations of 0.13, 0.11, and 0.10
mcg/ml, respectively.

METOCURINE

The pharmacokinetic parameters of
metocurine are given in Table 10.2. After
administration of ^{14}C-metocurine (0.05
mg/kg) to patients anesthetized with
thiopental and nitrous oxide, the plasma
disappearance is triexponential, with a
terminal half-life of 217 minutes.

Animal studies indicate that the kidney is the primary excretory organ for
metocurine, but studies in humans have
shown that urinary excretion accounts
for less than 50% or the administered
dose. However, metocurine undergoes no
appreciable biliary excretion; after 48
hours only 2% of the injected dose is excreted in the bile (Table 10.3). Glucuronidation does not appear to be an alternative pathway for the elimination of
metocurine, and to date no metabolites
have been detected. In clinical concentrations about 24% of metocurine is
bound to plasma proteins (Table 10.6).
The effect of renal and hepatic disease on
the elimination of metocurine is given in
Table 10.5.

GALLAMINE

The disposition of gallamine in humans is summarized in Tables 10.2 and
10.3. Renal elimination is extremely
important, and animal experiments
have demonstrated that only minimal
amounts of gallamine are excreted in the
bile, even after bilateral renal pedicle ligation. Therefore, gallamine should not
be administered to patients with impaired renal function.

ATRACURIUM

The chemical degradation of quaternary ammonium salts by Hofmann elimination was first described in 1851,
around the same time that Claud Bernard
described the neuromuscular blocking effect of curare. This elimination pathway
normally requires treatment with a
strong alkali such as sodium hydroxide
at 100°C. By altering the chemical structure of various ammonium compounds
Stenlake and coworkers were eventually
able to synthesize a series of compounds
in which degradation was favored at
lower pH and temperature, i.e., physiological conditions (pH 7.4, 37°C). As a result, atracurium was introduced into
clinical practice as a bisquaternary muscle relaxant, with highly selective neuromuscular blocking properties and
rapidly metabolized *in vivo* to nonqua-
ternary components at physiological pH
and temperature. Atracurium is degraded by Hofmann elimination and
ester hydrolysis to components that are
clinically inactive.

Chemical inactivation is extremely
rapid; Hofmann elimination at the quaternary nitrogen yields laudanosine and
the monoquaternary acrylate whereas
ester hydrolysis gives monoquaternary
acid alcohol (Figure 10.7). Thus, the degradation of atracurium is relatively short
with an elimination half-life of about 20
min. The pharmacokinetic profile of atracurium makes it a muscle relaxant of intermediate duration and suitable for use
by continuous infusion.

The pharmacokinetic parameters for
the disposition of atracurium are given in
Table 10.2, and Figure 10.8 shows the decline in plasma concentration of atracurium and the rapid appearance of its derivatives, laudanosine and the monoquaternary alcohol. Further analysis of
kinetic data has suggested that Hofmann
degradation is not the principal elimination pathway and that ester hydrolysis
may be more important than was originally thought. In addition, it has been
calculated that more than one-half (61%)
of the clearance of atracurium results
from possible "organ" (renal and he-

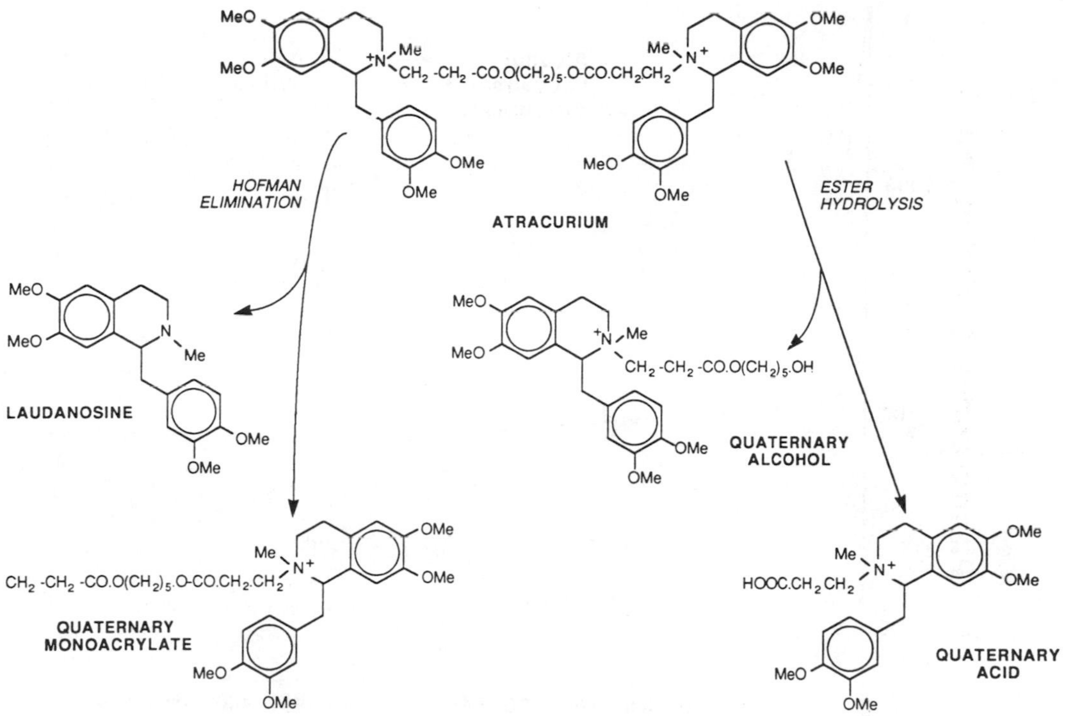

Figure 10.7. Metabolism of atracurium. With permission from Stenlake JB, Waigh RD, Urwin J, Dewar GH, Coker GG: Atracurium: conception and inception. *Br J Anaesth* 55:3S–10S, 1983.

patic)-based elimination in the central compartment. Other laboratory work has indicated that atracurium may be inactivated by a nucleophile substitution reaction to form laudanosine and an acrylate.

Atracurium is metabolized by ester hydrolysis independent of plasma cholinesterase responsible for succinylcholine inactivation. The rates of atracurium degradation are not different when the drug is incubated in plasma from normal patients or genetically deficient homozygotes for succinylcholine with almost no cholinesterase activity, and it is safe to administer atracurium to patients with low or abnormal cholinesterase. The duration of action is independent of renal and hepatic function.

Although laudanosine, one of the principal metabolites of atracurium, has no neuromuscular blocking effects, it can enter the central nervous system and at high concentrations produce central stimulation and seizure-like activity in

animals. This is not likely after usual therapeutic doses in humans. Halothane anesthetic requirments are, however, increased and the minimum alveolar concentration (MAC) for halothane has been shown to be increased when atracurium is given.

VECURONIUM

Vecuronium is metabolized by deacetylation (like pancuronium) in the liver to its metabolites, 3-hydroxyvecuronium, 17-hydroxyvecuronium, and 3,17-dihydroxyvecuronium. The 3-hydroxyvecuronium metabolite is almost as potent as the parent compound in the dog and cat. The other two derivatives have less than $\frac{1}{10}$ the neuromuscular blocking properties of vecuronium. Only small amounts of these metabolites (5% as the 3-hydroxy metabolite) have, however, been detected in humans, with 10 to 25% of the injected dose of vecuronium being excreted unchanged in the urine and 30 to 50% excreted unchanged in the bile

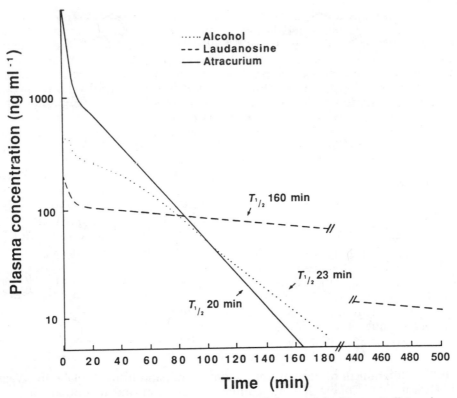

Figure 10.8.   Pharmacokinetics of atracurium and its metabolites.   Fall in plasma concentration of atracurium and its derivatives laudanosine and the monoquaternary alcohol after a bolus dose of atracurium of 0.3 mg/kg to a healthy patient. With permission from Ward S, Weatherley BC: Pharmacokinetics of atracurium and its metabolites. *Br J Anaesth* 58:6S–10S, 1986.

(Table 10.3). The pharmacokinetic parameters of vecuronium are given in Table 10.2. The relatively short elimination half-life and rapid clearance are reflected in the fact that vecuronium (like atracurium) is a muscle relaxant of intermediate duration of action.

SUCCINYLCHOLINE

The short duration of action of succinylcholine is due to its rapid metabolism. It is hydrolyzed by the enzyme plasma cholinesterase in two stages; in the first stage, succinyldicholine is broken down to choline and succinylmonocholine, and in the second, succinylmonocholine is hydrolyzed to choline and succinic acid (Figure 10.9). Succinylmonocholine has only about ½₀ to ⅛₀ the neuromuscular blocking activity of succinylcholine.

After an intravenous injection of 1.0

mg/kg to an adult, nearly all of the succinylcholine is metabolized within 1 minute, if one assumes the zero order (see Chapter 1) rate of hydrolysis determined in vitro of 27 mg succinylcholine/liter of adult plasma/minute. However, the rapid metabolism of succinylcholine has made it difficult to obtain accurate pharmacokinetic information in man, and most studies have been in animals or in vitro. Recently, in vivo studies in man have demonstrated that the in vivo rate of hydrolysis may be much lower than expected when compared with in vitro estimations, and it is likely that succinylcholine exists in the active form in the blood for at least 3 minutes. With the circulation of the left arm occluded by a tourniquet, succinylcholine was administered intravenously (1.0 mg/kg) into the right hand, and the twitch response of both arms, was monitored for neuro-muscular blockade. When the circulation was restored to the occluded arm 3 min-utes after injection, neuromuscular blockade was produced in the arm whose circulation had been obstructed. Thus, considerable recirculation of the drug oc-curs even 3 minutes after injection. Therefore, the in vivo rate of disappear-ance of succinylcholine from the plasma may be as low as 3 to 7 mg/L.

FACTORS AFFECTING NEUROMUSCULAR BLOCKADE

Drug Interactions

There are many drugs apart from those used during anesthesia that are known to interfere with neuromuscular transmis-sion, and these may interact with the muscle relaxants. Although these drugs in themselves do not usually cause clin-ically evident neuromuscular blockade, they may be responsible for prolongation of neuromuscular paralysis at the end of surgery, postoperative respiratory de-pression, drug-induced myasthenic dis-orders, and the unmasking or aggravation of myasthenia gravis. Mechanisms re-sponsible for such drug interactions in-clude presynaptic inhibition of the prop-agation of the nerve action potential, impaired release of acetylcholine due to deficient storage, synthesis or release of the neurotransmitter from the motor nerve terminal, postsynaptic receptor block, and combined presynaptic and postsynaptic block.

ANTIOBIOTICS

Neomycin, streptomycin, dihydro-streptomycin, kanamycin, gentamycin, polymyxin A, polymyxin B, colistin, lin-comycin, and tetracycline have all been implicated as interacting with and in-creasing the action of the nondepolariz-ing agents. The mechanism of action is not the same for all antibiotics, and it is possible for an antibiotic to have a pre-synaptic effect, postsynaptic effect, or both. It is thought that streptomycin and other aminoglycoside antibiotics produce neuromuscular blockade in a manner similar to that of magnesium by inhibi-tion of acetylcholine release from the presynaptic nerve terminal and to a smaller extent by stabilzation of the post-junctional membrane. Antibiotics that are known to increase the action of suc-cinylcholine include neomycin, strepto-mycin, kanamycin, polymyxin B, and co-listin, and antibiotics that are thought to be devoid of neuromuscular effects are penicillin, chloramphenicol, and the cephalosporins.

Aminoglycoside-induced neuromus-cular blockade is sometimes partially an-tagonized by calcium and neostigmine, but neuromuscular block produced by polymyxin B is augmented by neostig-mine and is not reversed by calcium. 4-Aminopyridine has been shown to antag-onize the neuromuscular block induced by neomycin and polymyxin B. Table 10.7 summarizes the effects of antibiotics on neuromuscular transmission and the interactions between antibiotics and muscle relaxants.

ANTICHOLINESTERASES

The interaction between the anticho-linesterases and the neuromuscular blocking agents is discussed in Chapter 5. Echothiopate, tetrahydroaminoacrine, hexafluornium, procaine, trimetaphan, phenelzine, chlorpromazine, and some

STEP I SUCCINYLCHOLINE $\xrightarrow{\text{Pseudocholinesterase}}$ SUCCINYLMONOCHOLINE + CHOLINE

STEP II SUCCINYLMONOCHOLINE $\xrightarrow[\text{Specific Liver Esterase}]{\text{Pseudocholinesterase}}$ SUCCINIC ACID + CHOLINE

Figure 10.9. Hydrolysis of succinylcholine.

Table 10.7.
Interaction of Antibiotics, Muscle Relaxants, Neostigmine, and Calcium§

Antibiotic	Neuromuscular Block from Antibiotic Alone Antagonized by		Increase in Neuromuscular Block of		Neuromuscular Block from Antibiotic-dTc Antagonzed by	
	Neostigmine	Calcium	dTc†	SCh‡	Neostigmine	Calcium
Neomycin	Sometimes	Sometimes	Yes	Yes	Usually	Usually
Streptomycin	Sometimes	Sometimes	Yes	Yes	Yes	Usually
Gentamycin	Sometimes	Yes	yes	§	Sometimes	Yes
Kanamycin	Sometimes	Sometimes	Yes	Yes	Sometimes	Sometimes
Paromomycin	Yes	Yes	Yes	§	Yes	Yes
Viomycin	Yes	Yes	Yes	§	Yes	Yes
Polymyxin A	No	No	Yes	§	No	No
Polymyxin B	No‖	No	Yes	Yes	No‖	No
Colistin	No	Sometimes	Yes	Yes	No	Sometimes
Tetracycline	No	§	Yes	No	Partially	Partially
Lincomycin	Partially	Partially	Yes	§	Partially	Partially
Cindamycin	Partially	Partially	Yes	§	Partially	Partially

With permission from Miller RD: Antagonism of neuromuscular blockade. *Anesthesiology* 44:318–329, 1976.
†d-Tubocurarine.
‡Succinylcholine.
§Not studied.
‖Block augmented by neostigmine.

insecticides all inhibit plasma cholinesterase, leading to a possibly prolonged response to succinylcholine.

CARDIOVASCULAR DRUGS

Antiarrhythmic agents may modify the action of muscle relaxants, and quinidine, procainamide, and propranolol have all been shown to augment d-tubocurarine-induced blockade in cats. Quinidine has been reported to unmask or worsen the symptoms of myasthenia gravis and to cause postoperative respiratory depression after the use of muscle relaxants. Furosemide and other diuretics, such as thiazides and ethacrynic acid, intensify the effects of nondepolarizing muscle relaxants, possibly because of diuresis-induced reduction in the volume of distribution and associated electrolyte imbalance, such as hypokalemia. Laboratory experiments show that low doses of diuretics augment and high doses antagonize the block produced by d-tubocurarine, suggesting that diuretics such as furosemide and the thiazides may

have a biomodal effect at the neuromuscular junction. One possible explanation for this effect is that low doses of furosemide appear to inhibit protein kinases, whereas large doses inhibit phosphodiesterase. Large doses of furosemide have been shown to antagonize pancuronium-induced neuromuscular blockade in neurosurgical patients. It is interesting that aminophylline, a phosphodiesterase inhibitor, can antagonize tubocurarine- and pancuronium-induced blockade and improve the strength of patients with myasthenia gravis. Continuous intravenous infusion of nitroglycerin in the cat has been shown to potentiate the neuromuscular block produced by pancuronium (but not by d-tubocurarine and succinylcholine); the significance of this is not yet clear.

LOCAL ANESTHETICS

The local anesthetics, procaine and lidocaine, enhance the neuromuscular block produced by nondepolarizing and depolarizing muscle relaxants.

OTHER DRUGS

Phenytoin has been shown to interfere with neuromuscular transmission, and exacerbation of myasthenia gravis by this drug has been reported. Lithium augments the effects of both depolarizing and nondepolarizing muscle relaxants and reportedly unmasks myasthenia gravis. Laboratory experiments have demonstrated that lithium potentiates the actions of pancuronium, succinylcholine, and decamethonium, but not those of d-tubocurarine and gallamine. It is not clear exactly how lithium produces neuromuscular block, but mechanisms that have been postulated include a depressant action on electrophysiological phenomena (lithium ions being substituted for sodium ions at a presynaptic level), interference with acetylcholine synthesis and/or release, and, in addition, a postsynaptic effect. Chlorpromazine has been shown to potentiate nondepolarizing relaxants. The administration of steroids may lead to a transient worsening of symptoms in patients with myasthenia gravis, but the mechanism of interference with neuromuscular transmission is unknown. Antagonism of pancuronium-induced blockade by hydrocortisone has also been reported. D-penicillamine, which is used in the treatment of Wilson's disease, may cause a myasthenia gravis-like syndrome. These patients have elevated serum levels of antibody to acetylcholine receptors, suggesting that an immunological mechanism is involved in this drug-induced syndrome. Azathioprine antagonizes nondepolarizing neuromuscular blockade, possibly by inhibiting phosphodiesterase.

Calcium ions play an important role in the presynaptic release of acetylcholine, and prolonged neuromuscular blockade has been reported after calcium antagonist administration during anesthesia with concurrent nondepolarizing neuromuscular blockade. Ketamine potentiates neuromuscular blockade produced by tubocurarine and atracurium, but not that produced by pancuronium or succinylcholine. Although the mechanism is not clear, in vitro studies have demonstrated that ketamine decreases the presynaptic release of acetylcholine and reduces the sensitivty of the motor endplate to acetylcholine.

Inhalation Anesthetic Agents

All of the inhalation agents augment both the degree and duration of the neuromuscular block induced by the nondepolarizing muscle relaxants. Possible mechanisms by which they may exert their effect include depression of the central nervous system, presynaptic inhibition of acetylcholine mobilization and release, postsynaptic receptor desensitization, or an action upon the muscle at some point distal to the cholinergic receptor. Waud has demonstrated that the inhalational anesthetic agents depress carbachol-induced depolarization of the motor endplate in a dose-related fashion, 1.0 minimum alveolar concentration (MAC) of halothane and enflurane producing about 19 and 40% depression, respectively. Only when the anesthetic concentration is sufficient to depress depolarization by 50% will an anesthetic itself depress the twitch response. Therefore, although at MAC, halothane and enflurane do not produce clinically measurable neuromuscular blockade, endplate sensitivity is decreased. Thus with an increasing dose of anesthetic, d-tubocurarine requirements are decreased. Figure 10.10 compares fractional twitch height *versus* d-tubocurarine concentration dose-response curves in the presence of halothane, diethyl ether, and enflurane at concentrations equal to MAC during studies on isolated guinea pig nerve-muscle preparations. The anesthetics shift the dose-response curves to the left indicating that lower d-tubocurarine concentrations are required to reduce twitch height.

The administration of 1.25 MAC halothane as compared with a nitrous oxide-narcotic regimen decreases d-tubocurarine dose requirements by about 50% in humans, whereas the administration of 1.25 MAC enflurane results in the patient requiring only 30% as much d-tubocura-

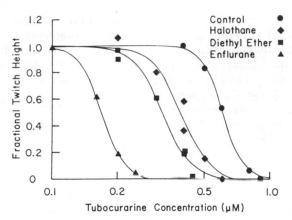

Figure 10.10. Effects of anesthetics on tubocurarine dose-response curve. *Ordinate:* twitch heights expressed as fraction of control values. *Abscissa:* d-tubocurarine concentrations (μM). Anesthetic concentrations were equal to MAC. Note that all the anesthetics shifted the dose-response curve to the left of the control curve, i.e., a lower d-tubocurarine concentration is required to block the twitch response and in addition that each anesthetic causes a different degree of shift. With permission from Waud BE: Decrease in dose requirements of d-tubocurarine by volatile anesthestics. *Anesthesiology* 51:298–302, 1979.

rine as would have been necessary with the nitrous oxide-narcotic technique. Similar results have also been obtained for pancuronium. Enflurane and isoflurane augment d-tubocurarine and pancuronium-induced block about twice as much as does an equipotent concentration of halothane. Clinical studies thus suggest that inhalational anesthetics augment nondepolarizing relaxants in a dose-dependent manner in the following decreasing order: isoflurane and enflurane > halothane > nitrous oxide-narcotic anesthesia. Thus, increasing depth of inhalational anesthesia decreases the serum concentration of msucle relaxant required to produce paralysis.

Volatile anesthetics also potentiate the intermediate-acting neuromuscular blocking agents, atracurium and vecuronium, but the effect is less than that produced with the long-acting relaxant drugs, d-tubocurarine and pancuronium. Enflurane is the most potent volatile agent (followed by isoflurane and then halothane) in augmenting a vecuronium-induced neuromuscular block. The augmentation of vecuronium- or atracurium-induced neuromuscular blockade by enflurane and isoflurane is only 20 to

30% greater than the augmentation produced by halothane or a nitrous oxide-narcotic technique, and increasing the anesthetic concentration from 1.2 MAC to 2.2 MAC decreases the ED_{50} (dose-depressing twitch tension by 50%) of vecuronium 51, 33, and 18% during enflurane, isoflurane, and halothane, respectively. The ED_{50} for d-tubocurarine and pancuronium is decreased about 62 and 57%, respectively, for similar increases in halothane end-tidal concentration and 30 and 70% respectively, for similar increases in anesthetic end-tidal concentration for isoflurane. Thus, increasing the concentration of volatile anesthetic has less effect on the neuromuscular blockade produced by vecuronium than on that produced by the long-acting muscle relaxants.

Vecuronium infusion rates to produce 90% depression of control muscle twitch tension are similar for patients given enflurane (0.28 μg/kg/min) and isoflurane (0.30 μg/kg/min), but lower than required for patients receiving fentanyl (0.92 μg/kg/min). The plasma concentration producing 90% twitch depression ($Cpss_{90}$) was 70 ng/ml in patients receiving enflurane, 72 ng/ml in patients receiving isoflurane, but much higher in those receiving fentanyl anesthesia (165 ng/ml). Thus, patients receiving isoflurane and enflurane require lower infusion rates (and plasma concentrations) to achieve 90% neuromuscular blockade than those receiving fentanyl. Because vecuronium clearance is the same during the three anesthetic regimens, the enhancement of vecuronium-induced neuromuscular blockade by isoflurane and enflurane is due to a pharmacodynamic rather than a pharmacokinetic change.

Atracurium-induced neuromuscular blockade is augmented by the volatile anesthetics, halothane and enflurane, but the magnitude is less than that associated with the long-acting neuromuscular relaxants. The dose-depressing twitch tension 50% (ED_{50}) is 77, 70, 68, and 83 μg/kg during halothane, enflurane, isoflurane, and fentanyl-nitrous oxide, respectively. Thus the potency of atracurium does not differ by more than 20% for all four anesthetic regimens. The mechanism by which atracurium and vecuronium are less affected by choice of anesthetic than are the long-acting relaxants tubocurarine and pancuronium is not known.

Electrolytes

Generation of action potentials by muscle and nerve follow changes in the conductance of their membranes to sodium and potassium, and normal neuromuscular function depends on the maintenance of the correct ratio between intracellular and extracellular ionic concentrations. Therefore, one can predict that abnormalities of electrolyte balance would affect neuromuscular transmission. An acute decrease in the extracellular potassium concentration will tend to increase the endplate transmembrane potential, causing hyperpolarization and increased resistance to depolarization, and greater sensitivity to the nondepolarizing muscle relaxants. Conversely, an increased extracellular potassium concentration lowers the resting endplate transmembrane potential and thereby partially depolarizes the mem-

brane, which should increase the effects of the depolarizing agents and oppose the action of the nondepolarizing drugs. Studies in cats have demonstrated that diuretic-induced chronic hypokalemia reduces the pancuronium requirements for neuromuscular blockade and that more neostigmine is required for antagonism.

The release of acetylcholine from the motor nerve terminal is also affected by calcium and magnesium ion concentrations, which have opposing effects. Calcium increases the quantal release of acetylcholine from the nerve terminal, decreases the sensitivity of the postjunctional membrane to transmitter, and enhances the excitation-contraction coupling mechanism of muscle. In contrast, magnesium decreases acetylcholine release and reduces the sensitivity of the postjunctional membrane to acetylcholine. Consequently, the action of the nondepolarizing muscle relaxants can be accentuated by low calcium and high magnesium levels. In addition, magnesium augments the block produced by depolarizing relaxants. Therefore, the dose of muscle relaxant should be reduced in patients with toxemia of pregnancy receiving magnesium therapy.

Acid-Base Balance

Respiratory acidosis enhances d-tubocurarine- and pancuronium-induced neuromuscular block and opposes reversal by neostigmine. The changes observed in metabolic acidosis and respiratory and metabolic alkalosis have yielded conflicting reports, but laboratory studies appear to indicate that in the presence of respiratory acidosis and metabolic alkalosis the antagonism by neostigmine of d-tubocurarine- and pancuronium-induced neuromuscular blockade is opposed.

In cats, acidosis augments and alkalosis lessens a vecuronium-induced neuromuscular blockade. In humans, a respiratory acidosis will increase and prolong neuromuscular blockade produced by vecuronium. In animals, both respiratory and metabolic acidosis increases and respiratory and metabolic alkalosis decreases an atracurium-induced neuromuscular blockade.

Hypothermia

Early studies suggested that hypothermia increased the magnitude and duration of depolarization block but diminished the response to nondepolarizing muscle relaxants. More recent work has not confirmed these results although it is now recognized that hypothermia produces profound pharmacokinetic and pharmacodynamic changes. In cats, hypothermia to 34° and 28°C prolongs the neuromuscular blockade produced by both d-tubocurarine and pancuronium. Hepatic and renal elimination of both pancuronium and d-tubocurarine is delayed, and, in addition, the metabolism of pancuronium is reduced. Hypothermia also appears to increase the sensitivity of the neuromuscular junction to pancuronium; the plasma concentration of pancuronium required for twitch tension depression of a similar order was less at 29°C than at 38°C. However, in contrast, a higher plasma concentration of d-tubocurarine was necessary to produce neuromuscular blockade at 28°C than at 39°C. The reason for this difference is as yet unknown.

Hypothermia prolongs the duration of action of atracurium and vecuronium and decreases the infusion rate required to maintain a constant degree of neuromuscular blockade. The augmentation of neuromuscular blockade may be due to decreased metabolism of vecuronium and atracurium during hypothermia.

Disease States

The effect of *renal* disease on the pharmacokinetics of the nondepolarizing muscle relaxants is summarized in Table 10.5. Gallamine and metocurine are almost entirely dependent on renal excretion, and Figure 10.6 shows the increased plasma concentrations of d-tubocurarine and pancuronium found in patients with impaired renal function. All of the long-acting muscle relaxants are largely dependent on the kidney for elimination,

and the introduction of the nondepolarizing muscle relaxants of intermediate duration, atracurium and vecuronium, has been a major advance in the management of patients with renal dysfunction.

No differences have been found in atracurium pharmacokinetics and pharmacodynamics in patients with normal renal function and those with renal failure, probably due to the unique mode of elimination of atracurium. Atracurium kinetic values for elimination half-life of 20 minutes, clearance 5.8 ml/min/kg, and volume of distribution (Vd_β) 141 ml/kg have been reported for patients with chronic renal failure. These are similar to values seen in normal individuals, (Table 10.2). Measurable amounts of the two metabolites, laudanosine and the monoquaternary alcohol, are produced when atracurium is given to patients with renal failure; laudanosine (peak concentration 0.27 μg/ml; elimination half-life 234 minutes) and the monoquaternary alcohol (peak concentration 0.43 μg/ml; elimination half-life 39 minutes) result. The elimination half-life of laudanosine is 197 minutes in normal patients and 234 minutes in patients with renal failure and is therefore not substantially affected by renal failure. Laboratory experiments in dogs have indicated that convulsions do not occur at plasma laudanosine concentrations of less than 17 μg/ml so that atracurium appears safe for use in patients with severe renal disease. Anephric patients also exhibit the ability to distribute and eliminate atracurium normally. When atracurium was given to patients with acute renal failure in the intensive care unit by intravenous infusion, no differences were found between the pharmacokinetic parameters derived for atracurium in patients with abnormal or normal renal function, but laudanosine elimination half-life was prolonged in patients with renal failure. In patients with renal failure there also appears to be greater variation in plasma laudanosine concentrations, but the highest value (758 ng/ml) was considerably less than the purported toxic level (17 μg/ml) for the dog. Thus, in the inensive care unit setting, atracurium has been administered for long periods of time to patients with renal dysfunction without producing laudanosine concentrations high enough to cause convulsions. Laudanosine does not have neuromuscular blocking effects. In the operating room, during a continuous intravenous infusion of atracurium to maintain a therapeutic plasma concentration of 2 μg/ml, laudanosine concentrations of 1 μg/ml would be predicted to be attained in patients with normal renal function and 1.6 μg/ml in patients with renal impairment. In summary, the pharmacokinetics and pharmacodynamics of atracurium are not affected by renal dysfunction, and atracurium is a drug of choice for these patients.

The disposition of vecuronium is marginally affected by renal failure. Bencini has demonstrated that the pharmacokinetic parameters of vecuronium are similar in patients with or without renal failure and no vecuronium metabolites were measured in the plasma, while Lynam and coworkers have shown that clearance is reduced (5.29 ml/kg/min in normal patients; 3.08 ml/kg/min in patients with absent renal function) and elimination half-life is prolonged (52 minutes in normal patients and 83 minutes in patients with absent renal function) leading to prolonged neuromuscular blockade in the renal failure group. No changes were found in drug distribution. No change in sensitivity to vecuronium has been demonstrated in pateints with renal failure. A modest cumulative effect has been demonstrated when vecuronium is given to patients in renal failure, and careful monitoring of neuromuscular blockade is required.

The effect of *hepatic* disease on the disposition of the nondepolarizing muscle relaxants is summarized in Table 10.5. Most of the long-acting nondepolarizing muscle relaxants are excreted unchanged in the urine, with biliary excretion presenting an alternative route of elimination. However, pancuronium is metabolized by the liver, 15 to 40% of the administered dose undergoing deacetylation and biliary excretion by the liver in humans. Liver disease has been shown

to affect the disposition of pancuronium; the distribution and elimination half-lives are increased in patients with cirrhosis. These changes are accompanied by an increased volume of distribution and reduced plasma clearance. The high volume of distribution in these patients means that there is an increased volume of body fluid in which pancuronium is distributed so that a larger initial dose may be required to achieve a given degree of neuromuscular blockade. However, once the neuromuscular block has been achieved, it will last longer due to delayed elimination.

Hofmann elimination and hydrolysis make the clearance of atracurium unaffected by hepatic disease. Patients with fulminant hepatic failure exhibit the same pharmacokinetic values as normal patients and no differences in sensitivity have been reported. In cirrhotic patients, although the elimination half-life and clearance of atracurium is unaltered, the volume of distribution (V_1 and Vd_β) is increased. However, although the clearance of the metabolite laudanosine is unaffected by cirrhosis (8.3 m/kg/min in controls and 6.9 ml/kg/min in cirrhotics), the elimination half-life is prolonged (168 minutes in controls, 277 minutes in cirrhotics), accompanied by an increase in volume of distribution. Other workers have also shown that in patients with severe hepatic disease, the elimination of the atracurium metabolite is prolonged (terminal elimination half-life of 560 minutes), but peak concentrations are similar to those seen in healthy patients and those with renal disease. Thus, an intravenous infusion of atracurium should be administered with care in patients with hepatic dysfunction, inasmuch as the elimination half-life of laudanosine is much longer than that of atracurium and might be expected to increase over time with the administration of multiple doses or an intravenous infusion. Atracurium has been given by intravenous infusion to effectively and safely provide neuromuscular blockade for patients undergoing liver transplantation.

Thirty to 50% of an injected dose of vecuronium is eliminated in the bile (Table

10.3) so one might predict that the duration of vecuronium would be prolonged in patients with liver disease, and indeed, vecuronium plasma clearance is reduced in patients with cirrhosis and the elimination half-life is prolonged, resulting in a prolongation of neuromuscular blockade. Vecuronium plasma clearance was 4.26 ml/min/kg in healthy patients and 2.73 ml/kg/min in cirrhotics, whereas the elimination half-life was 58 minutes in controls and 84 minutes in the patients with cirrhosis. The distribution volumes of vecuronium in cirrhotic patients are unchanged. Vecuronium has a longer duration of action in cirrhotic patients and should be used with caution in patients with hepatic dysfunction with careful monitoring of neuromuscular function. Thus atracurium is the only nondepolarizing muscle relaxant whose pharmacokinetics are not affected by renal and hepatic disease.

Plasma cholinesterase is synthesized in the liver so that levels may be diminished in advanced liver disease. The short duration of action of succinylcholine is due to hydrolysis of the drug by this enzyme, and a prolonged response may occur in patients with advanced hepatic failure.

The response of patients with **neuromuscular** disease to the muscle relaxants is often unpredictable so that neuromuscular function should be monitored intraoperatively. Patients suffering from myasthenia gravis are very sensitive to nondepolarizing muscle relaxants but resistant to depolarizing drugs, and they may readily develop a phase II block. Small doses of atracurium and vecuronium have been used safely in myasthenic patients and may be used cautiously if deep inhalational anesthesia is to be avoided. Patients with the myasthenic Eaton-Lambert syndrome (an association of advanced carcinomatous conditions, such as oat cell carcinoma of the bronchus and motor neuropathy) are very sensitive to both depolarizing and nondepolarizing muscle relaxant drugs. Patients with amyotrophic lateral sclerosis, syringomyelia, and other lower motor neuron lesions have defective neuromuscular transmission and nerve conduction and may exhibit an exaggerated response to nodepolarizing muscle relaxants. In familial periodic paralysis, the response to muscle relaxants is unpredictable and their use should probably be avoided. Patients with myotonia dystrophica and myotonia congenita exhibit a generalized muscle spasm after the administration of depolarizing drugs, which is not relieved by d-tubocurarine.

The **burned** patient sometimes exhibits an increased requirement for nondepolarizing muscle relaxants, but the mechanism remains unclear. Pharmacokinetic changes, such as alterations in protein binding or volume of distribution, are not important. It has been suggested that extrajunctional cholinergic receptors increase in number after thermal injury. Succinylcholine should be avoided in the burned patient because succinylcholine causes hyperkalemia in these patients, which may lead to arrhythmias or even cardiac arrest.

Age

It has been recognized for many years that neonates are more sensitive to nondepolarizing muscle relaxants and that the response of the small infant to some extent resembles that of the adult myasthenia patient. Electromyographic studies of myoneural function have shown that the responses of children older than 12 weeks are similar to those of adults, whereas infants less than 12 weeks of age have less mature responses, suggesting that the infant myoneural junction continues to develop after birth. Changes in body composition and renal and hepatic function continue to occur with development and produce age-related variations in the disposition of relaxants, e.g., extracellular fluid volume decreases with age and might be expected to lead to age-related changes in distributional volume.

Bennett and his coworkers have shown that the neonate at birth is more sensitive to pancuronium and d-tubocurarine, and that the potency ratio of pancuronium as compared with d-tubocurarine ranges from 1:1 at birth to 6:1 at 28 days. The dose of pancuronium required for the production of apnea and muscle relaxation at 1 day of age was 49 μg/kg during nitrous oxide anesthesia and by 4 weeks the dose requirement had increased to 90 μg/kg. The increased sensitivity of the neonate to the nondepolarizing muscle relaxants and the wide interindividual variability in dose requirements have led to the use of titration regimens to prevent overdosage. The dose should be reduced if prematurity, acidosis, or hypothermia is present or if an inhalational anesthetic agent is coadministered.

The pharmacodynamics and kinetics of d-tubocurarine have been investigated in neonates, infants, and children when it was shown that the neonate was indeed more sensitive to d-tubocurarine than were adults. The plasma level of d-tubocurarine at which 50% depression of twitch height occurred ($Cpss_{50}$) was lower in neonates and infants under 1 year of age than were values obtained for children and adults, indicating that neonates and infants have an increased sensitivity to d-tubocurarine. The steady state distributional volume (Vd_{ss}) was greater in neonates than infants, children, and adults, so that despite the increased sensitivity, initial relaxant dose size should not differ with age. The elimination half-life was longer in neonates than other groups and plasma clearance did not differ with age. The longer elimination half-life resulted from the larger distribution volume, and thus second and subsequent doses should be required at less frequent intervals.

During anesthesia for infants and children, similar age-related changes as those found for d-tubocurarine have been shown for vecuronium. Volume of distribution at steady state (Vd_{ss}) was larger in infants and children and was accompanied by prolonged elimination. Sensitivity was reduced in the infants; $Cpss_{50}$ was lower in infants (57 ng/ml) than in children (110 ng/ml). Clearance was unchanged and was similar in infants, children, and adults. Thus, as for tubocurarine, the age-related changes in volume of distribution and sensitivity

cancel each other out so that initial dose requirements are the same. Thus, the ED_{50} (dose producing 50% depression of twitch tension) is similar for all age groups (16.5, 19.0, and 15.0 μg/kg for infants, children, and adults, respectively) but the duration of neuromuscular blockade and recovery time is much longer in infants than in children.

The novel routes of elimination of atracurium result in atracurium pharmacokinetics in infants differing from those described for other muscle relaxants. Atracurium pharmacokinetic studies in infants and children are conflicting, but one study has demonstrated a decrease in volume of distribution with increasing age accompanied by a greater clearance for infants than children; distribution and elimination half-lives tended to be shorter. However, pharmacodynamic studies suggest that dose requirements (ED_{95}—dose required to produce 95% neuromuscular blockade) are reduced in neonates and infants, so that sensitivity is increased in this group of patients. There is greater variability in response to atracurium in the newborn than in older infants, so that the initial dose should be reduced and titrated to clinical effect.

In contrast to the increased sensitivity demonstrated for the nondepolarizing relaxants, clinical anesthesiologists have recognized for many years that neonates are resistant to the depolarizing muscle relaxant succinylcholine and that increased doses are required to produce adequate relaxation for endotracheal intubation. The dose producing 90% depression of twitch height (ED_{90}) is larger in neonates and infants compared with children, being 0.5, 0.6, 0.35, and 0.29 mg/kg, respectively, for neonates, infants, children, and adults. Thus neonates and infants require about twice as much succinylcholine as adults, and children require 20% more.

At the other extreme of life, muscle relaxant pharmacology is altered in the elderly, and dosage adjustments are required in some instances. With both d-tubocurarine and metocurine, the elderly exhibit a decreased clearance, decreased volume of distribtuion, and prolonged elimination half-life, but no change in sensitivity. Thus, the intitial dose and subsequent doses should be reduced in elderly patients.

McLeod and colleagues demonstrated a number of years ago that pancuronium clearance is progressively reduced with increasing patient age, probably related to decreased renal function in the elderly. However, in contrast more recently Rupp et al. have shown no statistically significant effect of increasing age on pancuronium's volume of distribution, elimination half-life, or clearance.

It is interesting that atracurium with alternative routes of degradation does not appear to require any age-related dosage reduction. However, the dose required of vecuronium to maintain a constant level of neuromuscular blockade when given by infusion is reduced, and once the infusion is stopped, the rate of recovery is prolonged in elderly patients. Volume of distribution (Vd_{ss}) and clearance of vecuronium are less in older patients than young adults, with no difference in elimination half-life. However, the steady state plasma concentration of pancuronium and vecuronium producing 50% depression of twitch tension ($Cpss_{50}$) is the same in young and elderly patients, indicating that elderly patients do not differ from young patients in their pharmacodynamic response to either vecuronium or pancuronium. Thus, pharmacokinetic rather than pharmcodynamic differences must account for any reduction in dosage requirments of vecuronium and pancuronium in the elderly population.

CARDIOVASCULAR EFFECTS

Although the main site of action of the neuromuscular blocking agents is the nicotinic receptor of striated muscle, they may act at other cholinergic receptor sites throughout the body, such as nicotinic receptors in autonomic ganglia and the muscarinic receptors in the heart. The nondepolarizing muscle relaxants vary with respect to their relative potency in producing blockade of sympathetic autonomic ganglia and cardiac

muscarinic (vagal) receptors. Figure 10.11 depicts dose response curves for the long-acting nondepolarizing muscle relaxants d-tubocurarine, metocurine, gallamine, and pancuronium in cats for neuromuscular, vagal, and sympathetic blockade. Undesirable cardiovascular effects of the long-acting muscle relaxants are thus due to histamine release, ganglionic blockade, cardiac antimuscarinic effect, and/or sympathetic nervous stimulation. At clinical doses of d-tubocurarine, some degree of blockade of sympathetic ganglia and the adrenal medulla nearly always occurs, resulting in a fall in blood pressure. The hypotension associated with d-tubocurarine administration, however, is due mainly to histamine release and is accompanied by a fall in systemic vascular resistance. Metocurine may also decrease blood pressure by histamine release, although hypotension is less frequently associated with metocurine than d-tubocurarine, because metocurine does not produce sympathetic blockade or vagal inhibition at doses required to produce neuromuscular blockade, and its highly specific and potent effect at the neuromuscular junction results in metocurine producing the least circulatory side effects of the long-acting muscle relaxants (Figure 10.11). Thus, metocurine does not usually cause a decrease in arterial pressure in humans.

Pancuronium and gallamine are frequently associated with a modest (10 to 15% increase) tachycardia and hypertension. When a nondepolarizing muscle relaxant antagonizes the effects of acetylcholine released by vagal postganglionic nerves in the heart, arterial hypertension and tachycardia result. Figure 10.11 shows that tachycardia is almost invariably associated with gallamine-induced neuromuscular blockade, whereas the vagolytic effect of pancuronium does not usually become evident until a high degree of neuromuscular block is achieved.

The effects of pancuronium on the sympathetic nervous system are more complex than simply inhibition of cardiac muscarinic receptors (vagolytic effect). Pancuronium is able to block muscarinic receptors on sympathetic

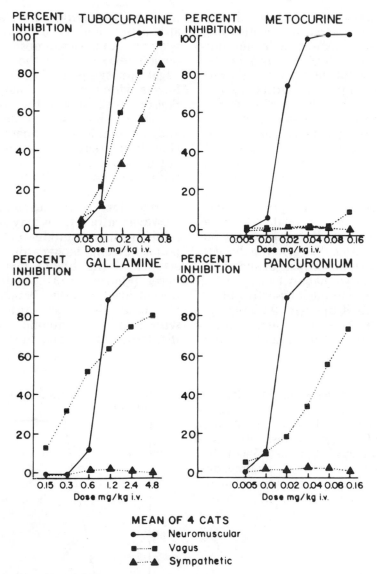

Figure 10.11. **Cardiovascular effects of the nondepolarizing muscle relaxants in cats.** Dose-response curves of d-tubocurarine, metocurine, gallamine and pancuronium for neuromuscular, vagal and sympathetic blockade in cats. From Hughes R, Chapple DJ: Effects of nondepolarizing neuromuscular blocking agents on peripheral autonomic mechanisms in cats. *Br J Anaesth* 48:59–67, 1976.

postganglionic nerve terminals. These receptors function as part of a negative feedback mechanism to modulate or prevent excess catecholamine release, in a manner analogous to the presynaptic adrenergic receptors. Thus, blockade by pancuronium results in increased norepinephrine release. Pancuronium can

also block M_i inhibitory muscarinic receptors found in interneurons of sympathetic ganglia, leading to enhanced sympathetic activity. Finally, pancuronium may also stimulate norepinephrine release from adrenergic nerve terminals and inhibit catecholamine reuptake from sympathetic nerve endings. Thus, in addition to an increase in heart rate due to vagal inhibition, pancuronium also exhibits stimulatory sympathetic nervous system effects that together may be responsible in part for the myocardial ischemia produced in patients with coronary artery disease, when heart rate is elevated after pancuronium administration.

The depolarizing (agonist) muscle relaxant succinylcholine is said to mimic the action of acetylcholine at nicotinic and muscarinic receptors. Therefore, one might predict that succinylcholine would increase "vagal tone" and produce bradycardia. This effect is related to dose and rate of administration, and it may be blocked by atropine. (See also the discussion of cardiovascular effects of succinylcholine later in the chapter.)

It is thus clear that the long-acting muscle relaxants elicit undesirable hemodynamic side effects with a narrow autonomic margin of safety. In contrast, the intermediate-acting muscle relaxants, atracurium and vecuronium, possess a *wide* margin between doses that produce muscle relaxation and those that produce vagal and sympathetic effects, i.e., they have a wide autonomic margin of safety. Figure 10.12 shows the dose-response curves for blockade of neuromuscular and autonomic mechanisms for atracurium in monkeys. Vecuronium and atracurium do not produce vagal or sympathetic nervous inhibition in humans when given in therapeutic doses required for neuromuscular blockade. However, atracurium may release histamine in humans producing transient hypotension and tachycardia in some instances at the higher level of clinical doses (Figure 10.13). Vecuronium does not release histamine. Pancuronium may attenuate the bradycardia associated with high-dose narcotic regimens, and the failure of atracurium and vecuro-

Figure 10.12. Cardiovascular effects of atracurium in monkeys. Dose-response curves showing blockade of neuromuscular and autonomic mechanisms by atracurium in monkeys. With permission from Hughes R, Chapple DJ: The pharmacology of atracurium: a new competitive neuromuscular blocking agent. *Br J Anaesth* 53:31–44, 1981.

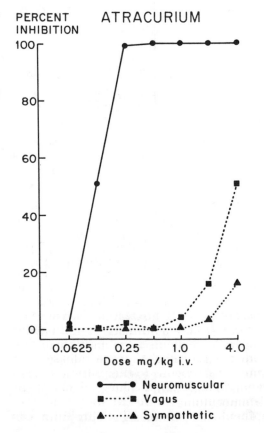

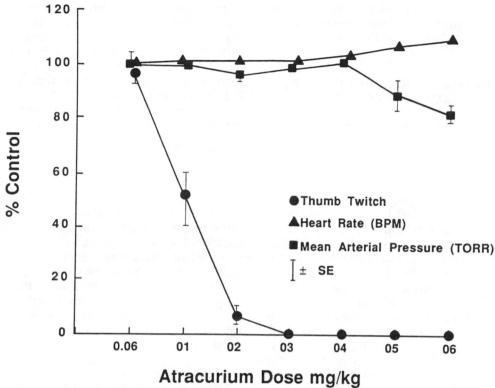

Figure 10.13.   Cardiovascular effects of atracurium in humans.   Means neuromuscular, heart rate, and blood pressure responses to atracurium at various doses. With permission from Basta S, Ali HH, Savarese JS, Sunder N, Gionfriddo M, Cloutier G, Lineberry C, Cato AE: Clinical pharmacology of atracurium besylate (BW 33A): a new nondepolarizing muscle relaxant. *Anaesth Analg* 61:723–729, 1982.

nium to increase heart rate may be associated with bradycardia when patients concomitantly receive high doses of opioids, such as sufentanil.

HISTAMINE RELEASE

Tubocurarine, metocurine, and succinylcholine have all been shown to cause histamine release in humans. Histamine release is less common with pancuronium and alcuronium, although isolated cases of possible histamine release associated with the administration of pancuronium and alcuronium have been reported. It is wise to avoid the use of dtubocurarine in patients with a history of asthma, skin allergy, or pheochromocytoma.

The most common sign of histamine re-

lease seen after the use of d-tubocurarine is erythema of the upper chest and face, whereas bronchospasm only occasionally occurs. Histamine release may contribute to the hypotensive effect of d-tubocurarine.

Vecuronium does not cause histamine release; however, large doses of atracurium (3 times the ED_{95}, i.e., 3 times the dose required to depress baseline twitch by 95%) given rapidly may elicit histamine release and produce hypotension. Thus, the ability of atracurium to release histamine is approximately one-half that of metocurine and less than one-third that of tubocurarine. Slowing the rate of administration of atracurium prevents histamine release and associated hemodynamic effects. The use of H_1 and H_2 receptor blocking agents can attenuate histamine-induced circulatory effects after d-tubocurarine and atracurium administration, in a similar fashion to that elicited for morphine.

INDIVIDUAL NEUROMUSCULAR BLOCKING AGENTS

Long-Acting Nondepolarizing Muscle Relaxants

d-TUBOCURARINE

d-Tubocurarine was one of the first muscle relaxants to be introduced into clinical practice but is rarely used today. Its structural formula is given in Figure 10.3. The main disadvantage of d-tubocurarine is its hypotensive action, caused principally by a fall in peripheral resistance due to autonomic ganglionic blockade and histamine release.

Suggested Dosage and Administration. An intravenous dose of 0.6 mg/kg may be administered to adults to facilitate endotracheal intubation whereas 0.3 to 0.5 mg/kg intravenously is a satisfactory dose for the maintenance of relaxation during nitrous oxide-narcotic anesthesia. The dose should be reduced further to 0.2 to 0.3 mg/kg if halothane and to 0.1 to 0.15 mg/kg if enflurane is administered in conjunction with the muscle relaxant.

PANCURONIUM

Pancuronium is a synthetic bisquaternary aminosteroid with no hormonal activity. Its structural formula is given in Figure 10.3. It is about 5 to 7 times as potent as d-tubocurarine. Pancuronium increases heart rate and arterial blood pressure without causing a fall in stroke volume. Total peripheral resistance is unchanged. Its cardiovascular stability may be due to a positive inotropic effect on the heart, stimulation of cardiac sympathetic ganglia, inhibition of catecholamine reuptake, or direct stimulation of sympathetic activity. There is minimal histamine release. It appears to be a safe neuromuscular blocking agent for use in patients susceptible to malignant hyperpyrexia.

Suggested Dosage and Administration. The dose of pancuronium required to pro-

duce satisfactory conditions for endotracheal intubation in adults is 0.06 to 0.1 mg/kg. For the production of muscular relaxation during surgery, 0.04 to 0.08 mg may be administered intravenously. The intravenous dose should be reduced to 0.03 to 0.06 mg/kg or 0.02 to 0.04 mg/kg during halothane or enflurane anesthesia, respectively.

GALLAMINE

The structural formula of gallamine is given in Figure 10.3. The main disadvantage of gallamine is that it nearly always produces a marked tachycardia, which lasts longer than the duration of the neuromuscular block. It is excreted unchanged by the kidney, and is therefore best avoided in patients with renal failure. Gallamine is also unsuitable for prolonged surgery because repeated doses result in a cumulation effect. Histamine release is minimal. Gallamine is rarely used today.

METOCURINE

Metocurine (formerly dimethyltubocurarine) is a nondepolarizing muscle relaxant that was reintroduced into clinical practice in 1977. Its structural formula is given in Figure 10.3. It is about 1 to 2 times more potent than d-tubocurarine as a neuromuscular blocking agent, but at neuromuscular blocking doses, metocurine does not cause inhibition of vagal transmission or sympathetic ganglionic blockade (Figure 10.11) and, therefore, produces minimal hemodynamic changes in humans. The relatively stable heart rate and blood pressure make metocurine a useful agent for patients with coronary artery disease and hypertension.

Suggested Dosage and Administration. The recommended dose for relaxation during nitrous oxide-narcotic anesthesia is 0.2 to 0.3 mg/kg whereas 0.25 to 0.4 mg/kg may be required to facilitate endotracheal intubation.

ALCURONIUM

Alcuronium is a nondepolarizing relaxant that is prepared from toxiferine, an alkaloid of calabash curare, by the substitution of an allyl group in each of the two quaternary ammonium groups. Alcuronium is about twice as potent as d-tubocurarine, but its duration of action is shorter. Muscular relaxation occurs 2 to 4 minutes after the injection of 0.2 mg/kg and lasts about 15 to 20 minutes. Like d-tubocurarine it may cause a fall in blood pressure but does not cause histamine release. There is no evidence of any significant metabolism of alcuronium and most of the drug is excreted unchanged in the urine, so it should be used cautiously in the presence of impaired renal function.

FAZADINIUM

Fazadinium is a rapidly acting nondepolarizing neuromuscular relaxant that has a shorter duration of action than both d-tubocurarine and pancuronium. Fazadinium, 1 mg/kg, provides better intubating conditions than 0.1 mg/kg of pancuronium during the first minute after administration but does not act as rapidly as succinylcholine. Therefore, in obstetric and emergency anesthetic practice, succinylcholine still remains the drug of choice. Animal studies have shown that fazadinium is extensively metabolized to inactive metabolites.

Intermediate-Acting Nondepolarizing Muscle Relaxants

The intermediate-acting nondepolarizing muscle relaxants, atracurium and vecuronium, were introduced into anesthetic practice in 1984. These drugs have about one-third the duration of action of the long-acting nondepolarizing muscle relaxants and exhibit minimal to absent cardiovascular effects. Atracurium and vecuronium have a similar rate of onset of neuromuscular blockade when compared with the long-acting nondepolarizing muscle relaxants, so they have not replaced succinylcholine when rapid intubation is required within 60 seconds, e.g., in emergency and obstetric anesthesia. Neuromuscular blockade produced by atracurium and vecuronium is readily antagonized by the anticholinesterases within 20 minutes of administration of a paralyzing dose. The intermediate duration of action associated with atracurium and vecuronium is reflected by their relatively high plasma clearance.

ATRACURIUM

Atracurium is an intermediate-acting nondepolarizing muscle relaxant; the chemical structure is shown in Figure 10.5. When given in doses producing 95% twitch height depression (ED_{95} = 0.2 mg/kg), the total duration of block is about 30 to 45 minutes from injection to 95% recovery of twitch height. Larger doses to produce good conditions for tracheal intubation (twice ED_{95}) are required, when the duration of action is increased to about 64 minutes. The onset of action is not as short as that of succinylcholine. The unique pharmacokinetic properties of atracurium make it an ideal agent to be used in patients with renal and hepatic disease. Cardiovascular stability is good, but atracurium does cause histamine release when given in larger doses. Atracurium rarely causes cardiovascular effects if a dose less than 0.5 mg/kg is given. Atracurium lacks cumulative effects.

Suggested Dosage and Administration. The recommended initial intravenous dose of atracurium is 0.4 to 0.5 mg/kg; the dose should be reduced by approximately one-third if administered during steady state isoflurane or enflurane anesthesia. Incremental doses of 0.08 to 0.10 mg/kg may be given to provide maintenance of neuromuscular blockade. Atracurium may be given by continuous infusion at a rate of 6 to 8 μg/kg/min to provide stable neuromuscular blockade during surgery. The infusion rate should be reduced by 20 to 30% during inhalational anesthesia.

VECURONIUM

Vecuronium, a monoquaternary analog of the steroid relaxant pancuronium, is an intermediate-acting nondepolarizing muscle relaxant; the structural formula is given in Figure 10.5. The ED_{95} (dose required to produce 95% suppression of twitch height) is 0.05 mg/kg and the duration of action is 30 minutes. Thus, the potency is equal to or slightly greater than that of pancuronium. If twice the ED_{95} is given, the duration of action increases to 45 minutes. Vecuronium has a wide autonomic margin of safety and does not produce undesirable hemodynamic effects. The onset of action is similar to atracurium and not as short as succinylcholine.

Suggested Dosage and Administration. An initial dose of 0.08 to 0.10 mg/kg produces good intubation conditions within 2.5 to 3 minutes and maximal neuromuscular blockade within 3 to 5 minutes of administration. If succinylcholine is given for intubation, an initial dose of 0.04 to 0.06 mg/kg of vecuronium is recommended. Suggested incremental doses are 0.010 to 0.015 mg/kg. The dose should be reduced during volatile anesthesia by about 20 to 30%. Vecuronium can be administered by continuous intravenous infusion when the recommended infusion dosage is 1 to 2 µg/kg/min during balanced anesthesia.

Depolarizing Muscle Relaxants

SUCCINYLCHOLINE

This depolarizing muscle relaxant has a short duration of action due to its rapid enzymatic hydrolysis by plasma cholinesterase (Figure 10.9). When given intravenously (0.5 to 1.0 mg/kg), it has an onset of action in about 30 seconds and a duration of action of 3 to 5 minutes. The short duration of action makes succinylcholine a particularly useful agent for endotracheal intubation. Thus succinylcholine has retained widespread use over the last 30 years because of its short onset and brief duration of action despite its many side effects. The structural formula of succinylcholine is given in Figure 10.3. Unfortunately, succinylcholine has some potentially harmful side effects that may contraindicate its use in certain clinical situations.

SIDE EFFECTS

Potassium Release. In normal healthy individuals, succinylcholine causes the serum potassium to rise by a small amount (0.5 mEq/L) due to the rapid mobilization of potassium from the intracellular to the extracellular fluid compartment. However, in certain circumstances, large potassium shifts occur that may cause ventricular arrhythmias, ventricular fibrillation, and possible cardiac arrest in susceptible individuals (Figure 10.14). Succinylcholine should be avoided in patients suffering from burns, uremia, massive muscle trauma, denervation injuries, lower motor neuron lesions, spinal cord injury, upper motor neuron lesions, and tetanus. A hyperkalemic response is likely in individuals whose muscles have been denervated by either nerve damage or burns. Denervated muscle exhibits a hypersensitivity to depolarizing agents so that depolarization produces a large potassium efflux that raises serum potassium levels. The potentially dangerous flux of potassium after succinylcholine administration is not seen immediately after injury but may occur 5 to 15 days after injury and persist for 2 to 3 months after burns or trauma and 3 to 6 months after neurological lesions.

Serum potassium concentrations after succinylcholine administration in patients with renal failure increase to a similar extent as in normal subjects. Thus the use of succinylcholine in patients with severe renal disease but normal serum potassium is appropriate when emergency "rapid" intubation is essential; in other situations the nondepolarizing muscle relaxants, atracurium or vecuronium, are preferable.

The beta$_2$-adrenergic receptor is important in the regulation of serum potassium levels (see page 412), and beta-adrenergic blockade has been shown to lead to an increase in potassium levels. The normal increase in potassium induced by succinylcholine is exaggerated in the presence of propranolol in dogs. However, the importance of this laboratory finding in humans perioperatively is unknown.

Muscle Pains. Postsuccinylcholine muscle pains can be an uncomfortable side effect as they are often worst in patients undergoing short surgical procedures who are allowed to be ambulatory on the

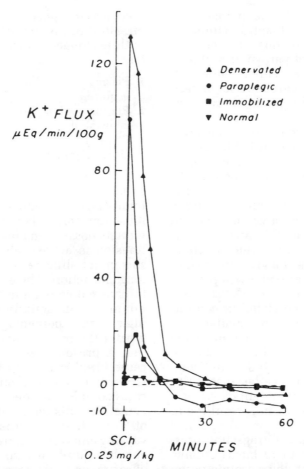

K⁺ FLUX
μEq/min/100g

▲ Denervated
● Paraplegic
■ Immobilized
▼ Normal

SCh
0.25 mg/kg

MINUTES

Figure 10.14. Potassium flux after succinylcholine administration associated with denervation, paraplegia, and immobilization in dogs. With permission from Gronert GA, Theye RA: Pathophysiology of hyperkalemia induced by succinylcholine. *Anesthesiology* 43:89–99, 1975.

day of surgery. The pains chiefly occur in the shoulder girdle, rib cage, and neck. A small preceding dose of a nondepolarizing muscle relaxant reduces the incidence of muscle fasiculations and muscle pains, but if a large dose is administered it may be difficult to obtain excellent muscle relaxation and the time to onset of paralysis is prolonged.

Cardiac Effects. Bradycardia, junctional arrhythmias, and even cardiac arrest have been reported after succinylcholine administration. Succinylcholine may thus mimic the effects of acetylcholine at cardiac receptors to produce a bradycardia. A slight increase in arterial blood pressure and bradycardia are more likely to occur after repetitive administration. In some adult patients, a tachycardia has been reported after the first dose, whereas in children, a bradycardia may occur after the first dose of succinylcholine. The fact that bradycardia is more common after repeated doses suggests that a metabolite of succinylcholine (e.g., succinylmonocholine) may be responsible for the negative chronotropic effects. It is possible that succinylcholine produces its cardiovascular effects via the cholinergic nicotinic receptors in the parasympathetic ganglia of the heart and also the postganglionic cholinergic muscarinic receptors of the heart inasmuch as atropine and trimethaphan attenuate the response. Experimental studies have suggested that direct perfusion of the sinoatrial node with succinylcholine produces a positive chronotropic effect, which is blocked by pindolol, whereas succinylmonocholine (a metabolite of succinylcholine) produces a negative chronotropic effect, which is blocked by atropine. Succinylcholine also exhibited a biphasic action; small doses produced a bradycardia and large doses an increase in heart rate. The cardiac effects are more likely to occur after large or repeated doses in children and if atropine has been omitted from the premedication. Although as discussed above, the mechanism is unknown, atropine will prevent or ameliorate these effects.

Ocular Effects. Succinylcholine administration causes a rise in intraocular pressure, possibly due to contraction of the extraocular muscles. Succinylcholine should, therefore, be avoided in penetrating injuries of the eye because a rise in intraocular pressure might cause prolapse of the vitreous humor, resulting in loss of vision.

Intragastric Pressure. Intragastric pressure increases of 7 to 12 cm H_2O have been recorded after the administration of succinylcholine, which theoretically might be sufficient to cause gastric regurgitation. However, most anesthetists consider the technique of "crash intubation" using succinylcholine to facilitate intubation justified in certain emergency situations when rapid intubation is required to prevent aspiration.

Malignant Hyperpyrexia or Hyperthermia. Succinylcholine can trigger the development of the malignant hyperpyrexia syndrome. This disease is characterized by a rapid rise in heat production, muscular rigidity, marked lactic acid and carbon dioxide production, and increased oxygen consumption resulting in hyperthermia, hyperkalemia, respiratory and metabolic acidosis, and myoglobinuria. **Dantrolene** has become the drug of choice in the treatment of malignant hyperthermia and is discussed at the end of this chapter.

Prolonged Apnea. Succinylcholine administration is occasionally associated with prolonged apnea. This may be due to:

1. Plasma cholinesterase deficiency—acquired
2. Plasma cholinesterase abnormality—congenital
3. Phase II block
4. Drug interactions

If plasma cholinesterase activity is deficient or abnormal, succinylcholine hydrolysis is reduced and prolonged muscular paralysis results. Certain individuals possess an abnormal type of cholinesterase whose ability to hydrolyze succinylcholine is reduced and so prolongs its action. The enzyme differs from the normal enzyme in the percentage inhibition of its activity by dibucaine: the higher the percentage inhibition the greater the proportion of normal enzyme that is present (see Chapter 5). A dibucaine number above 80 (80% inhibition) is normal, whereas one below 20 indicates complete absence of the normal enzyme. Patients with a dibucaine number of 30 to 70 are heterozygotes possessing varying amounts of normal and abnormal enzyme. Routine laboratory estimations of serum cholinesterase levels do not differentiate between the normal and atypical enzyme. Plasma cholinesterase is discussed further in Chapter 5.

If serious respiratory depression occurs after the use of succinylcholine, the patient's respiration should be controlled, and peripheral nerve stimulation should be performed to establish whether the depression is of central or peripheral origin and, if the depression is peripheral, the nature of the block. Later, a plasma cholinesterase estimation and dibucaine number estimation should be performed and, if an abnormality is detected, the patient's family should be investigated.

The action of succinylcholine is prolonged by interaction with other drugs, many of which have anticholinesterase activity; procaine, lidocaine, procainamide, propanidid, quinidine, cytotoxic agents, neostigmine, hexafluorenium, and tetrahydroaminoacrine have all been reported as prolonging the action of succinylcholine.

Suggested Dosage and Administration. For a brief period of paralysis, e.g., to facilitate intubation, the usual intravenous dose is 0.5 to 1.0 mg/kg. Succinylcholine may also be administered as a continuous intravenous infusion prepared by diluting 500 mg succinylcholine in 500 ml of solution (0.1% solution). The dose requirement varies from patient to patient and the progress of the neuromuscular block must be monitored using a peripheral nerve stimulator to avoid the development of a phase II block.

DECAMETHONIUM

Decamethonium is a depolarizing muscle relaxant that is little used today because tachyphylaxis and a phase II block readily occur. The duration of action of decamethonium is longer than that of succinylcholine, being about 30 to 40 minutes.

NEW MUSCLE RELAXANTS

Two new long-acting muscle relaxants, doxacurium and pipecuronium, and a short-acting muscle relaxant, mivacurium, are currently undergoing clinical trials. Pancuronium, a muscle relaxant of long duration, exhibits cardiovascular side effects so that the introduction of long-acting muscle relaxants such as doxacurium and pipecuronium that have minimal or absent cardiovascular effects will be an important advance. Mivacurium is a short-acting muscle relaxant of under 30 minutes duration, but, in contrast to succinylcholine, is a nondepolarizing relaxant.

PIPECURONIUM

Pipecuronium bromide is a long-acting nondepolarizing neuromuscular relaxant that does not exhibit cardiovascular effects. It is an analog of pancuronium, but the two charged quaternary nitrogens are arranged more peripherally on the pipecuronium molecule than on the pancuronium molecule. It does not release histamine.

Its neuromuscular potency is similar to or slightly greater (1 to 1.5) than that of pancuronium. The ED_{95} (dose required to produce 95% depression of twitch height) is 0.05 mg/kg and the intubating dose (twice the ED_{95}) is 0.08 to 0.1 mg/kg. Pipecuronium and pancuronium have a similar onset and duration of action. Volatile anesthetics potentiate the effects of pipecuronium. Pharmacokinetic studies after the administration of pipecuronium (0.07 mg/kg) yield values of 309 ml/kg, 137 minutes, and 2.4 ml/kg/min for volume of distribution (Vd_{ss}), elimination half-life, and clearance, respectively. These findings suggest that pipecuronium has a faster clearance and larger volume of distribution than pancuronium. It is 32% bound to plasma proteins in the rat. Plasma concentrations of pipecuronium are higher in patients with renal failure, with a 33% reduction in clearance and a prolonged elimination half-life. Vd_{ss} was larger in patients with renal failure. Thus, pipecuronium may be less suitable for use in patients with renal failure than vecuronium or atracurium. The kidney appears to be an important route of elimination for pipecuronium in the dog.

DOXACURIUM

Doxacurium is a long-acting nondepolarizing new neuromuscular relaxant with a duration of action similar to that of pancuronium. It is a bisquaternary benzylisoquinolinium diester, with a chemical structure similar to that of atracurium. It is not susceptible to Hofmann degradation. Doxacurium is approximately twice as potent as pancuronium at the neuromuscular junction and the ED_{95} is 0.02 to 0.03 mg/kg. It is devoid of cardiovascular effects and does not appear to cause histamine release when administered in clinical doses. Doxacurium has been administered to patients undergoing coronary artery bypass grafting and valvular replacement. When given in doses 3 times the ED_{95}, it did not elicit clinically important hemodynamic effects. It therefore has a wide autonomic margin of safety. Volatile anesthetics enhance the degree of neuromuscular blockade produced by doxacurium, with isoflurane augmenting blockade more than halothane.

MIVACURIUM

Mivacurium is a nondepolarizing neuromuscular blocking agent with a short duration of action. It is rapidly hydrolyzed by plasma cholinesterase; the rate of hydrolysis *in vitro* using plasma cholinesterase is 1.76 μmol/hr, i.e., approximatoly 88% of the rate of succinylcholine. Mivacurium is a bisbenzylisoquinolinium diester compound. The response of patients with abnormal genotypes for cholinesterase appears to show no clear pattern, but abnormal responses have been reported in some patients.

The ED_{95} for neuromuscular blockade is 0.08 mg/kg. The rapid rate of hydrolysis suggests that mivacurium undergoes rapid clearance with a short elimination half-life and so would be an ideal agent for short surgical procedures. When given in a dose suitable for tracheal intubation (i.e., twice the ED_{95}), the duration of action of mivacurium is twice that of succinylcholine and 33 to 50% that of equipotent doses of atracurium and vecuronium. Neuromuscular blockade is readily antagonized by the anticholinesterase group of drugs.

Preliminary data suggest that mivacurium produces minimal cardiovascular effects up to a dose of twice the ED_{95}. Doses greater than this when administered rapidly may produce adverse cardiovascular effects. A transient decrease in blood pressure has been described, probably due to histamine release. Mivacurium administered in doses of 0.15 to 0.25 mg/kg over 60 seconds to cardiac patients produces few significant hemodynamic effects, but a small number of patients exhibit transient hypotension when given doses greater than 0.15 mg/kg, i.e., twice the ED_{95}.

When mivacurium is given by continuous intravenous infusion, the steady state infusion rate necessary to maintain 95% twitch suppression is 8.3 μg/kg/min for mivacurium as compared with 7.9 μg/kg/min for atracurium and 1.2 μg/kg/min for vecuronium. Recovery times

after stopping the mivacurium infusion is about 50% of the recovery time for equivalent infusions of atracurium and 40 to 50% of those for vecuronium. It is interesting that there is a significant correlation between mivacurium infusion rate and plasma cholinesterase activity. Mivacurium exhibits ideal pharmacologic characteristics for administration by continuous infusion and does not appear to show cumulation. However, some workers have suggested that slight cumulation may occur at higher doses. Volatile anesthetics augment mivacurium-induced neuromuscular blockade. Mivacurium does not appear to have a faster onset of action than the intermediate-acting nondepolarizing neuromuscular blocking agents; the onset time is longer than that of succinylcholine so it is unlikely to replace succinylcholine when rapid and effective intubation is required in emergency situations. However, its short duration of action may be of advantage in the outpatient anesthesia setting.

DANTROLENE

Dantrolene is a lipid-soluble hydantoin (Figure 10.15) that was introduced as a skeletal muscle relaxant for use in chronic disorders of muscle spasticity such as spinal cord injury, stroke, and cerebral palsy. However, dantrolene is used by anesthesiologists for the management of malignant hyperthermia. Dantrolene is poorly soluble in water and once its efficacy in the treatment of malignant hyperthermia was recognized an intravenous preparation was developed. Dantrolene is supplied in ampules containing 20 mg of lyophilized dantrolene sodium (powder) together with mannitol (3G, to improve solubility) and sodium hydroxide to yield a solution of pH 9.5, when the contents are dissolved in 60 ml of water. The final concentration of the parenteral preparation is 0.33 mg/ml. *Azumolene*, a new investigational dantrolene analog that antagonizes halothane and caffeine contracture, has greater water solubility.

The introduction of dantrolene for the treatment of malignant hyperthermia has been instrumental in reducing mortality

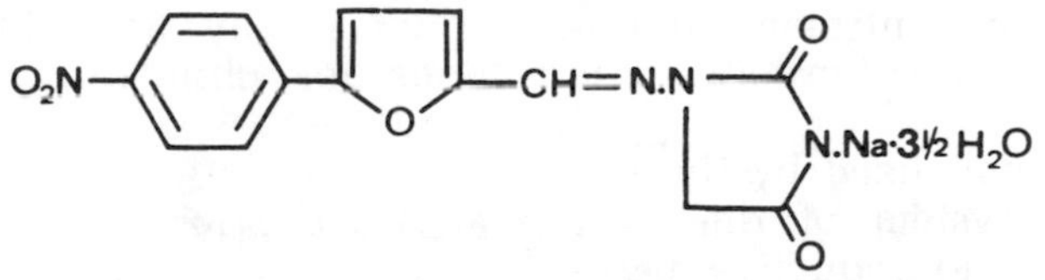

Dantrolene

Figure 10.15.   Chemical structure of dantrolene.

from around 80% in the 1960s to about 7% at the present time. Harrison (1975) first gave dantrolene 1.0 mg/kg intravenously to malignant hyperthermia susceptible (MHS) swine after the halothane-induced syndrome was well established with muscle rigor, acidosis, and hyperthermia. This reduced mortality to give a survival rate of 88%. Further studies have confirmed these findings, and dantrolene is today the therapeutic agent of choice in malignant hyperthermia in humans.

Pharmacology. Dantrolene relaxes skeletal muscle. In malignant hyperthermia-susceptible (MHS) individuals there is a failure of excitation-contraction coupling due to a defect of calcium-storing membranes, possibly the sarcoplasmic reticulum or sarcolemma or both, resulting in a rise in myoplasmic calcium leading to sustained contracture and rigidity. Dantrolene inhibits the calcium influx induced by electrical stimulation or potassium-induced depolarization and inhibits the augmented caffeine-induced contracture in MHS muscle. The mechanism and site of action of dantrolene is not completely understood, but it is postulated that dantrolene depresses the rate and amount of calcium release from the sarcoplasmic reticulum or increases calcium uptake into the sarcoplasmic reticulum. Laboratory studies in MHS swine have shown that halothane-induced depolarization of skeletal muscle sarcolemma is reduced by dantrolene. Dantrolene also has effects on vascular and heart muscle, as well as skeletal muscle. Although the mode of action of dantrolene is not clear, dantrolene provides life-saving treatment for MHS individuals.

Pharmacokinetics. After oral administration of dantrolene, about 20% of the dose is absorbed and peak concentrations are achieved in about 6 hours. Intravenous administration of dantrolene (2.4 mg/kg) to adults yields a blood concentration 5 minutes after the infusion is given of 5.36 μg/ml and an elimination half-life ($t_{1/2\beta}$) of 12.0 hours. Blood concentrations exceed 2.0 μg/ml for approximately 6 hours. Therapeutic blood concentrations are generally accepted to be above 3.0 μg/ml, inasmuch as the twitch response is maximally depressed when dantrolene blood concentrations are above 2.5 to 3.0 μg/ml. Dantrolene concentrations 24 hours after administration are 1.7 μg/ml, when patients report a subjective sensation of weakness. At 48 hours, the residual blood dantrolene concentration is only 0.3 μg/ml. In children, when the same intravenous dose of dantrolene is given, maximal dantrolene concentrations are 6.0 μg/ml, and 5 minutes after the infusion the concentration is 5.37 μg/ml. The elimination half-life is 10.0 hours, clearance is 0.64 ml/min/kg, and volume of distribution (Vd_{SS}) is reported to be 0.54 L/kg. Effective blood concentrations were achieved for over 4 hours after dantrolene administration. Thus, a single intravenous dose of dantrolene of 2.4 mg/kg produces blood concentrations that exceed 3.0 μg/ml for about 6 hours, and if continued prophylaxis is required a second dose (1.2 mg/kg) should be given 6 hours after the first dose.

Dantrolene is metabolized to a metabolite, 5-OH dantrolene (see below), which is 50% as effective as dantrolene in depressing twitch response. The peak blood concentration of this metabolite is achieved 7 hours after dantrolene administration, and the elimination half-life is 9.0 hours.

Dantrolene is metabolized by the microsomal oxidase system of the liver through oxidative and reductive pathways. Hydroxylation of the hydantoin rings forms 5-hydroxydantrolene (5-OH dantrolene) whereas reduction of the nitro-moiety of the benzene ring yields aminodantrolene, which is then acetylated.

Suggested Dosage and Administration. Effective therapeutic concentrations of dantrolene are achieved for the treatment of malignant hyperthermia after the administration of 2.4 mg/kg. During a crisis, this dose may be repeated at 15-minute intervals until clinical improvement is achieved or a total dose of 10 mg/kg has been given. Some anesthesiologists recommend a second dose of 2.4 mg/kg dantrolene 12 hours after the first dose because malignant hyperthermia may recur in the postoperative period.

Preanesthetic medication with dantrolene to MHS patients is controversial, and many advocate no prophylactic administration of dantrolene to avoid the side effects. Preoperative oral administration 2 to 4 days before surgery is no longer advocated, and if dantrolene is to be given to prevent the occurrence of malignant hyperthermia in MHS individuals, it should be administered in a dose of 2.4 mg/kg. intravenously during induction of anesthesia.

Toxicity, Precautions, and Contraindications. Dantrolene may cause dizziness, dysarthria, lightheadedness, and drowsiness. Hepatic dysfunction has been reported after chronic oral therapy. Oral dantrolene sodium prophylaxis for malignant hyperthermia may cause clinically significant muscle weakness.

Dantrolene elevates serum potassium. Dantrolene and verapamil when given together have been shown to cause severe myocardial depression in dogs and hyperkalemia with cardiovascular collapse in swine. Because verapamil, a calcium antagonist, has been advocated for the treatment of malignant hyperpyrexia, this drug interaction demonstrated in animals may have important implications for clinical management of the syndrome.

BIBLIOGRAPHY

Physiology of Neuromuscular Transmission

Dreyer F: Acetylcholine receptor. Br J Anesth 54:115–130, 1982.

Engbaek J, Ostergaard D, Viby-Mogensen J: Double burst stimulation (DBS): a new pattern of nerve stimulation to identify residual neuromuscular block. Br J Anaesth 62:274–270, 1989.

Miller RD: Editorial: How should residual neuromuscular blockade be detected? Anesthesiology 70:379–380, 1989.

Standaert FG: Release of transmitter at the neuromuscular junction. Br J Anaesth 54:131–145, 1982.

Standaert FG, Dretchen KL: Cyclic nucleotides in neuromuscular transmission. Anesth Analg 60:91–99, 1981.

Standaert FG: Dretchen KL, Skirboll LR, Morgenroth VH: A role of cyclic nucleotides in neuromuscular transmission. J Pharmacol Exp Ther 199:553–544, 1976.

Taylor P: Are neuromuscular blocking agents more efficacious in pairs? Anesthesiology 63:1–3, 1985

Waud BE, Waud DR: Interaction among agents that block end-plate depolarization competitively. Anesthesiology 63:4–15, 1985.

Drug Interactions

Anderson KA, Marshall RJ: Interactions between calcium entry blockers and vecuronium bromide in anaesthetized cats. Br J Anaesth 57:775–781, 1985.

Argov Z, Mastaglia FL: Disorders of neuromuscular transmission caused by drugs. N Engl J Med 301:409–413, 1979.

Azar I, Cottrell J, Gupta B, Turndorf H: Furosemide facilitates recovery of evoked twitch response after pancuronium. Anesth Analg 59:55–57, 1980.

Bordon H, Clarke MT, Katz H: The use of pancuronium bromide in patients receiving lithium carbonate. Can Anaesth Soc J 21:79–82, 1974.

Ghoneim MM, Long JP: The interaction between magnesium and other neuromuscular blocking agents. Anesthesiology 32:23–27, 1970.

Glisson SN, El-Etr AA, Lim R: Prolongation of pancuronium induced neuromuscular blockade by intravenous infusion of nitroglycerin. Anesthesiology 51:47–49, 1979.

Harrah MD, Way WL, Katzung B: The interaction of d-tubocurarine with antiarrhythmic drugs. Anesthesiology 33:406–410, 1970.

Havdala HS, Borison FL, Diamond BI: Potential hazards and applications of lithium in anesthesiology. Anesthesiology 50:534–537, 1979.

Hill GE, Wong KC, Hodges MR: Lithium carbonate and neuromuscular blocking agents. Anesthesiology 46:122–126, 1977.

Krieg N, Rutten JMJ, Drul JF, Booij LHDJ: Preliminary review of the interactions of ORG NC45 with anaesthetics and antibiotics in animals. Br J Anaesth 52:33S–36S, 1980.

McIndewar IC, Marshall RJ: Interactions between the neuromuscular blocking drug ORG NC45 and some anaesthetic, analgesic and antimicrobial agents. Br J Anaesth 53:785–791, 1981.

Miller RD, Sohn YJ, Matteo RS: Enhancement of d-tubocurarine neuromuscular blockade by diuretics in man. Anesthesiology 45:442–445, 1976.

Miller RD, Way WL, Katzung G: The potentiation of neuromuscular blocking agents by quinidine. Anesthesiology 28:1036–1041, 1967.

Pittinger C, Adamson R: Antibiotic blockade of neuromuscular function. Ann Rev Pharmacol 12:169–184, 1972.

Pittinger CB, Eryasa Y, Adamson R: Antibiotic-induced paralysis. Anesth Analg (Cleve) 49:487–501, 1970.

Toft P, Helbo-Hansen S: Interaction of ketamine with atracurium. Br J Anaesth 62:319–320, 1989.

Pharmacokinetics

Agoston S, Crul JF, Kersten UW, Scaf AHJ: Relationship of the serum concentration of pancuronium to its neuromuscular activity in man. Anesthesiology 47:509–512, 1977.

Bencini AF, Scaf AHJ, Sohn YJ, Meistelman C, Lienhart A, Kersten UW, Schwarz S, Agoston S: Disposition and urinary excretion of vecuronium bromide in anesthetized patients with normal renal function or renal failure. Anesth Analg 65:245–251, 1986.

Brandon BW, Stiller RL, Cook DR, Woelfel SK, Chadravorti S, Lai A: Pharmacokinetics of atracurium in anaesthetized infants and children. Br J Anaesth 58:1210–1213, 1986.

Chapple DJ, Miller AA, Ward JB, Wheatley PL: Cardiovascular and neurological effects of laudanosine. Br J Anaesth 59:218–225, 1987.

Cook DR, Wingard LB, Taylor FH: Pharmacokinetics of succinylcholine in infants, children and adults. Clin Pharmacol Ther 20:493–498, 1976.

Cronnelly R, Fisher DM, Miller RD, Gencarelli P, Nguyen-Gruenke L, Castagnoli N: Pharmacokinetics and pharmacodynamics of vecuronium (ORG NC45) and pancuronium in anaesthetized humans. Anesthesiology 58:405–408, 1983.

DeBros FM, Lai A, Scott R, deBros J, Batson AG, Goudsouzien N, Ali HH, Cosimi AB, Savarese JJ: Pharmacokinetics and pharmacodynamics of atracurium during isoflurane anesthesia in normal and anephric patients. Anesth Analg 65:743–746, 1986.

Donati F: Atracurium, pharmacokinetics and metabolites. Can J Anaesth 36:257–261, 1989.

Duvaldestin P: Pharmacokinetics in intravenous anaesthetic practice. Clin Pharmacokinet 6:61–82, 1981.

Duvaldestin P, Agoston S, Henzel D, Kerseten UW, Desmonts JM: Pancuronium pharmacokinetics in patients with liver cirrhosis. Br J Anaesth 50:1131–1136, 1978.

Fahey MR, Morris RB, Miller RD, Nguyen TL, Upton RA: Pharmacokinetics of ORG NC45 (Norcuron) in patients with and without renal failure. Br J Anaesth 53:1049–1052, 1981.

Fahey MR, Rupp SM, Canfell C, Fisher DM, Miller RD, Sharma M, Castagnoli K, Hennis PJ: Effect of renal failure on laudanosine excretion in man. Br J Anaesth 57:1049–1051, 1985.

Fahey MR, Rupp SM, Fisher DM, Miller RD, Sharma M, Canfell C, Castagnoli K, Hennis PJ: The pharmacokinetics and pharmacodynamics of atracurium in patients with and without renal failure. Anesthesiology 61:699–702, 1984.

Farman JV, Turner JM, Blanloeil Y: Atracurium infusion in liver transplantation. Br J Anaesth 58:96S–102S, 1986.

Feldman SA, Cohen EN, Golling RC: The excretion of gallamine in the dog. Anesthesiology 30:593–598, 1969.

Fisher DM, Canfell PC, Fahey MR, Rosen JI, Rupp SM, Sheiner LB, Miller RD: Elimination of atracurium in humans: contribution of Hofmann elimination and ester hydrolysis versus organ-based elimination. Anesthesiology 65:6–12, 1986.

Fisher DM, Castagnoli K, Miller RD: Vecuronium kinetics and dynamics in anesthetized infants and children. Clin Pharmacol Ther 37:402–406, 1985.

Fisher DM, Miller RD: Neuromuscular effects of vecuronium (ORG NC45) in infants and children during N_2O, halothane anesthesia. Anesthesiology 58:519–523, 1983.

Fisher DM, O'Keeffe C, Stanski DR, Cronnelly R, Miller RD, Gregory GA: Pharmacokinetics and pharmacodynamics of d-tubocurarine in infants, children, and adults. Anesthesiology 57:203–208, 1982.

Fleischli G, Cohen EN: An analog computer simulation for the distribution of d-tubocurarine. Anesthesiology 27:64–69, 1966.

Gibaldi M, Levy G, Hayton W: Kinetics of the elimination and neuromuscular blocking effect of d-tubocurarine in man. Anesthesiology 36:213–219, 1972.

Hobbiger F, Peck AW: Hydrolysis of suxamethonium by different types of plasma. Br J Pharmacol 37:258–271, 1969.

Holst-Larsen H: The hydrolysis of suxamethonium in human blood. Br J Anaesth 48:887–891, 1976.

Hunter JM, Jones RS, Utting JE: Comparison of vecuronium, atracurium and tubocurarine in normal patients and in patients with no renal function. Br J Anaesth 56:941–950, 1984.

Hunter JM, Parker CJR, Bell CF, Jones RS, Utting JE: The use of different doses of vecuronium in patients with liver dysfunction. Br J Anaesth 57:758–764, 1985.

Ingram MD, Sclabassi RJ, Cook DR, Stiller RL, Bennett MH: Cardiovascular and electroencephalographic effects of laudanosine in "nephrectomized" cats. Br J Anesth 58:14S–18S, 1986.

Lebrault C, Berger JL, D'Hollander AA, Gomeni R, Henzel D, Duvaldestin P: Pharmacokinetics and pharmacodynamics of vecuronium (ORG NC45) in patients with cirrhosis. Anesthesiology 62:601–605, 1985.

Lebrault C, Duvaldestin P, Henzel D, Chauvin M, Guesnon P: Pharmacokinetics and pharmacodynamics of vecuronium in patients with cholestasis. Br J Anaesth 58:983–987, 1986.

Lepage JY, Malinge M, Cozian A, Pinaud M, Blanloeil Y, Souron R: Vecuronium and atracurium in patients with end-stage renal failure. Br J Anaesth 59:1004–1010, 1987.

Lynam DP, Cronnelly R, Castagnoli KP, Canfell PC, Caldwell J, Arden J, Miller RD: The pharmacodynamics and pharmacokinetics of vecuronium in patients anesthetized with isoflurane with normal renal function or with renal failure. Anesthesiology 69:227–231, 1988.

Martyn JAJ, Matteo RS, Greenblatt DJ, Lebowitz PW, Savarese JJ: Pharmacokinetics of d-tubocurarine in patients with thermal injury. Anesth Analg 61:241–246, 1982.

Matteo RS, Backus WW, McDaniel DD, Brotherton WP, Abraham R, Diaz J: Pharmacokinetics and pharmacodynamics of d-tubocurarine and metocurine in the elderly. Anesth Analg 64:23–29, 1985.

Matteo RS, Spector S, Horowitz PE: Relationship of serum d-tubocurarine concentration to neuromuscular blockade in man. Anesthesiology 41:440–443, 1974.

McLeod K, Watson MJ, Rawlins SMD: Pharmacokinetics of pancuronium in patients with normal and impaired renal function. Br J Anaesth 48:341–345, 1976.

Meakin G, McKiernan EP, Morris P, Baker RD: Dose response curves for suxamethonium in neonates, infants and children. Br J Anaesth 62:655–658, 1989.

Meijer DKF, Weitering JG, Vermeer GA, Scaf AHJ: Comparative pharmacokinetics of d-tubocurarine and metocurine in man. Anesthesiology 51:402–407, 1979.

Meijer DKF, Weitering JG, Vonk RJ: Hepatic uptake and biliary excretion of d-tubocurarine and trimethyltubocurarine in the rat in vivo and in isolated perfused rat livers. J Pharmacol Exp Ther 198:229–239, 1976.

Meistelman C, Lienhart A, Leveque C, Bitker MO, Pigot B, Viars P: Pharmacology of vecuronium in patients with end-stage renal failure. Eur J Anaesth 3:153–158, 1986.

Merrett RA, Thompson CW, Webb FW: In vitro degradation of atracurium in human plasma. Br J Anaesth 55:61–66, 1983.

Miller RD, Agoston S, Booij LHD, Kerston U, Crul JF, Ham J: Comparative potency and pharmacokinetics of pancuronium and its metabolites in anesthetized man. J Pharmacol Exp Ther 207:539–543, 1978.

Miller RD, Agoston S, VanderPol F, Booij LHD, Crul JH, Ham J: Hypothermia and the pharmacokinetics and pharmacodynamics of pancuronium in the cat. J Pharmacol Exp Ther 207:532–538, 1978.

Miller RD, Matteo RS, Benet LZ, Sohn YJ: The pharmacokinetics of d-tubocurarine in man and without renal failure. J Pharmacol Exp Ther 202:1–7, 1977.

Miller RD: Pharmacokinetics of competitive muscle relaxants. Br J Anaesth 54:161–167, 1982.

Miller RD: Pharmacokinetics of atracurium and other nondepolarizing neuromuscular blocking agents in normal patients and those with renal or hepatic dysfunction. Br J Anaesth 58:11S–13S, 1986.

Miller RD, Roderick LL: Pancuronium-induced neuromuscular blockade, and its antagonism by

neostigmine, at 29, 37, and 41°C. Anesthesiology 46:333–335, 1977.

Nigrovic V, Auen M. Wajskol A: Enzymatic hydrolysis of atracurium in vivo. Anesthesiology 62:606–609, 1985.

Nigrovic V, Klaunig JE, Smith SL, Schultz NE: Potentiation of atracurium toxicity in isolated rat hepatocytes by inhibition of its hydrolytic degradation pathway. Anesth Analg 66:512–516, 1987.

Nigrovic V, Pandya JB, Auen M, Wajskol A: Inactivation of atracurium in humans and rat plasma. Anesth Analg 64:1047–1052, 1985.

Parker CJR, Hunter JM: Pharmacokinetics of atracurium and laudanosine in patients with hepatic cirrhosis. Br J Anaesth 62:177–183, 1989.

Parker CJR, Jones JE, Hunter JM: Disposition of infusions of atracurium and its metabolite, laudanosine, in patients in renal and respiratory failure in an ITU. Br J Anaesth 61:531–540, 1988.

Ramzan IM, Shanks CA, Triggs EJ: Pharmacokinetics and pharmacodynamics of gallamine triethiodide in patients with total biliary obstruction. Anesth Analg 60:289–296, 1981.

Ramzan MI, Somogyi AA, Walker JS, Shanks CA, Triggs EJ: Clinical pharmacokinetics of the non-depolarizing muscle relaxants. Clin Pharmacokinet 6:25–60, 1981.

Rupp SM, Castagnoli KP, Fisher DM, Miller RD: Pancuronium and vecuronium pharmacokinetics and pharmacodynamics in younger and elderly adults. Anesthesiology 67:45–49, 1987.

Scheepstra GL, Vree TB, Crul JF, VandePol F, Reekers-Ketting J: Convulsive effects and pharmacokinetics of laudanosine in the rat. Eur J Anaesth 3:371–383, 1986.

Shanks CA: Pharmacokinetics of the nondepolarizing neuromuscular relaxants applied to calculation of bolus and infusion dosage regiments. Anesthesiology 64:72–86, 1986.

Shanks CA, Avram MJ, Fragen RJ, O'Hara DA: Pharmacokinetics and pharmacodynamics of vecuronium administered by bolus and infusion during halothane or balanced anesthesia. Clin Pharmacol Ther 42:459–464, 1987.

Shanks CA, Avram MJ, Ronai AK, Bowsher DJ: The pharmacokinetics of d-tubocurarine with surgery involving salvaged autologous blood. Anesthesiology 62:161–165, 1985.

Shanks CA, Somogyi AA, Triggs EJ: Dose-response and plasma concentration-response relationship of pancuronium in man. Anesthesiology 51:111–118, 1979.

Sheiner LB, Stanski DR, Vozeh S, Miller RD, Ham J: Simultaneous modeling of pharmacokinetics and pharmacodynamics: application to d-tubocurarine. Clin Pharmacol Ther 25:358–371, 1979.

Somogyi AA, Shanks CA, Triggs EJ: Clinical pharmacokinetics of pancuronium bromide. Eur J Clin Pharmacol 10:367–372, 1976.

Somogyi AA, Shanks CA, Triggs EJ: Disposition kinetics of Pancuronium bromide in patients with total biliary obstruction. Br J Anaesth 49:1103–1107, 1977.

Somogyi AA, Shanks CA, Triggs EJ: The effect of renal failure on the disposition and neuromuscular blocking action of pancuronium bromide. Eur J Clin Pharmacol 12:23–29, 1977.

Stanski DR, Ham J, Miller RD, Sheiner LB: Pharmacokinetics and pharmacodynamics of d-tubocurarine during nitrous oxide-narcotic and halothane anesthesia in man. Anesthesiology 51:235–241, 1979.

Stanski DR, Ham J, Miller RD, Sheiner LB: Time-dependent increase in sensitivity to d-tubocurarine during enflurane anesthesia in man. Anesthesiology 52:483–487, 1980.

Stiller RL, Cook DR, Chakravorti S: In vitro degradation of atracurium in human plasma. Br J Anaesth 57:1085–1088, 1985.

Thompson JM: Pancuronium binding by serum proteins. Anaesthesia 31:219–227, 1976.

Tsui D, Graham GG, Torda TA: The pharmacokinetics of atracurium isomers in vitro and in humans. Anesthesiology 67:722–728, 1987.

Upton RA, Nguyen TL, Miller RD, Castagnoli N: Renal and biliary elimination of vecuronium (ORG NC45) and pancuronium in rats. Anesth Analg 61:313–316, 1982.

Ward S, Boheimer N, Weatherley BC, Simmonds RJ, Dopson TA: Pharmacokinetics of atracurium and its metabolites in patients with normal renal function and in patients in renal failure. Br J Anaesth 59:697–706, 1987.

Ward S, Neill EAM: Pharmacokinetics of atracurium in acute hepatic failure (with acute renal failure). Br J Anaesth 55:1169–1172, 1983.

Ward S, Neill EAM, Weatherley BC, Corall IM: Pharmacokinetics of atracurium besylate in healthy patients (after a single IV bolus dose). Br J Anesth 55:113–118, 1983.

Ward S, Weatherley BC: Pharmacokinetics of atracurium and its metabolites. Br J Anaesth 58:6S–10S, 1986.

Waser PG, Wiederkehr H, Sin-Ren AC, Kaiser-Schoenenberger E: Distribution and kinetics of ^{14}C-vecuronium in rats and mice. Br J Anaesth 59:1044–1051, 1987.

Weinstein JA, Matteo RS, Ornstein E, Schwartz AE, Goldstoff M, Thal G: Pharmacodynamics of vecuronium and atracurium in the obese surgical patient. Anesth Analg 67:1149–1153, 1988.

Wood M, Wood AJJ: Changes in plasma drug binding and alpha$_1$-acid glycoprotein in mother and newborn. Clin Pharmacol Ther 29:522–526, 1981.

Wood M, Stone WJ, Wood AJJ: Plasma binding of pancuronium—effect of age, sex and disease. Anesthesiology 62:29–32, 1983.

Factors Affecting Neuromuscular Blockade

Bennett EJ, Ignacio A, Patel K. Grundy EM, Salem MR: Tubocurarine and the neonate. Br J Anaesth 48:687-688, 1976.

Bennett RJ, Ramamurthy S, Dalal FY, Salem MR. Pancuronium and the neonate. Br J Anaesth 47:75-78, 1975.

Brandom BW, Cook DR, Woelfel SK, Rudd GD, Fehr B, Lineberry CG: Atracurium infusion requirements in children during halothane, isoflurane, and narcotic anesthesia. Anesth Analg 64:471-476, 1985.

Brandom BW, Woelfel SK, Cook DR, Fehr BL,

Rudd GD: Clinical pharmacology of atracurium in infants. Anesth Analg 63:309-312, 1984.

Cannon JE, Fahey MR, Castagnoli KP, Furuta T, Canfell PC, Sharma M, Miller RD: Continuous infusion of vecuronium: the effects of anesthetic agents. Anesthesiology 57:503-506, 1987.

Cook DR: Muscle relaxants in infants and children. Anesth Analg 60:335-343, 1981.

D'Hollander AA, Luyckx C, Barvais L, deVille A: Clinical evaluation of atracurium besylate requirements for stable muscle relaxation during surgery: lack of age related effects. Anesthesiology 59:237-240, 1983.

D'Hollander A. Massaux F, Nevelsteen M, Agoston S: Age-dependent dose-response relationship of ORG NC 45 in anesthetized patients. Br J Anaesth 54:653-626, 1982.

Ellis FR: Neuromuscular disease and anesthesia. Br J Anaesth 46:603-612, 1974.

Fisher DM, O'Keeffe C, Stanski DR, Cronnelly R, Miller RD, Gregory GA: Pharmacokinetics and pharmacodynamics of d-tubocurarine in infants, children, and adults. Anesthesiology 57:203-208, 1982.

Fogdall RP, Miller RD: Neuromuscular effects of enflurane, alone and in combination with d-tubocurarine, pancuronium and succinylcholine in man. Anesthesiology 42:173-178, 1975.

Goudsouzian NG: Atracurium in infants and children. Br J Anaesth 58:23S–28S, 1986.

Goudsouzian NG, Liu LMP: The neuromuscular response of infants to a continuous infusion of succinylcholine. Anesthesiology 60:97–101, 1984.

Goudsouzian N. Liu LMP, Gionfriddo M, Rudd GD: Neuromuscular effects of atracurium in infants and children. Anesthesiology 62:75–79, 1985.

Ham J, Miller RD, Benet LZ, Matteo RS, Roderick LL: Pharmacokinetics and pharmacodynamics of d-tubocurarine during hypothermia in the cat. Anesthesiology 49:324–329, 1978.

Ham J, Miller RD, Sheiner LB, Matteo RS: Dosage schedule independence of d-tubocurarine pharmacokinetics, pharmacodynamics and recovery of neuromuscular function. Anesthesiology 50:528–533, 1979.

Hughes R: The influence of changes in acid-base balance on neuromuscular blockade in cats. Br J Anesth 42:658–668, 1970.

Hughes R, Payne JP: Interaction of halothane with nondepolarizing neuromuscular blocking drugs in man. Br J Clin Pharmacol 7:485–490, 1979

Matteo RS, Lieberman IG, Salanitre E, McDaniel DD, Diaz J: Distribution, elimination, and action of d-tubocurarine in neonates, infants, children and adults. Anesth Analg 63:799–804, 1984.

McLeod K, Hull CJ, Watson MJ: Effects of ageing on the pharmacokinetics of pancuronium. Br J Anaesth 47:435–438, 1979.

Meretoja OA, Wirtavouri K: Influence of age on the dose-response relationship of atracurium in pediatric patients. Acta Anaesthesiol Scand 32:614–618, 1988.

Miller RD, Crique M, Eger EI: Duration of halothane anesthesia and neuromuscular blockade with d-tubocurarine. Anesthesiology 44:206–210, 1976.

Miller RD, Eger EI, Way WL, Stevens WC, Dolan WM: Comparative neuromuscular effects of forane and halothane alone and in combination with d-tubocurarine in man. *Anesthesiology* 35:38–42, 1971.

Miller RD, Roderick LL: Acid-base balance and neostigmine antagonism of pancuronium neuromuscular blockade. *Br J Anaesth* 50:317–324, 1978.

Miller RD, Van Nyhuis LS, Eger EI, Way WL: The effect of acid-base balance on neostigmine antagonism of d-tubocurarine-induced neurosmuscular blockade. *Anesthesiology* 42:377–383, 1975.

Miller RD, Way WL, Dolan WM, Stevens WC, Eger EI: The dependence of pancuronium and d-tubocurarine induced neuromuscular blockade on alveolar concentration of halothane and forane. *Anesthesiology* 37:573–581, 1972.

Nightingale DA: Use of atracurium in neonatal anesthesia. *Br J Anaesth* 58:32S–36S, 1986.

Rupp SM, McChristian JW, Miller RD. Neuromuscular effects of atracurium during halothane-nitrous oxide and enflurane nitrous oxide anesthesia in humans *Anesthesiology* 63:16–19, 1985.

Rupp SM, Miller RD, Gencarelli PJ: Vecuronium-induced neuromuscular blockade during enflurane, isoflurane, and halothane anesthesia in humans. *Anesthesiology* 60:102–105, 1984.

Swen J, Gencarelli PJ, Koot HWJ: Vecuronium infusion dose requirements during fentanyl and halothane anesthesia in humans. *Anesth Analg* 64:411–414, 1985.

Waud BE: Decrease in dose requirements of d-tubocurarine by volatile anesthetics. *Anesthesiology* 51:298–302, 1979.

Waud BE: Serum d-tubocurarine concentration and twitch height. *Anesthesiology* 43:381–382, 1975.

Waud BE, Waud DR: The effects of diethyl ether, enflurane and isoflurane at the neuromuscular junction. *Anesthesiology* 42:275–280, 1975.

Cardiovascular Effects

Barnes PK, Brindle-Smith G, White WD, Tennant WR: Comparison of the effects of ORG NC45 and pancuronium bromide on the heart rate and arterial pressure in anesthetized rat. *Br J Anesth* 54:435–439, 1982.

Booij LHDJ, Edwards RP, Sohn YJ, Miller RD: Cardiovascular and neuromuscular effects of ORG NC 45, pancuronium, metocurine, and d-tubocurarine in dogs. *Anesth Analg* 59:26–30, 1980.

Bowman WC: Non-relaxant properties of neuromuscular blocking drugs. *Br J Anaesth* 54:147–160, 1982.

Fitzal S, Gilly H, Ilias W: Comparative investigations on the cardiovascular effects of ORG NC45 and pancuronium in dogs. *Br J Anaesth* 55:641–646, 1983.

Hilgenberg JC, Stoelting RK, Harris WA: Systemic vascular responses to atracurium during enflurane-nitrous oxide anesthesia in humans. *Anesthesiology* 58:242–244, 1983.

Hughes R, Chapple DJ: Cardiovascular and neuromuscular effects of dimethyltubocurarine in anesthetized cats and rhesus monkeys. *Br J Anaesth* 48:847–851, 1976.

Hughes R. Chapple DJ: Effects of nondepolarizing neuromuscular blocking agents on peripheral autonomic mechanisms in cats. *Br J Anaesth* 48:59–67, 1976.

Jacobs HK, Lim S, Salem MR, Rao TLK, Mathru M, Smith BD: Cardiac electrophysiologic effects of pancuronium. *Anaesth Analg* 64:693–699, 1985.

Kelman GR, Kennedy BR: Cardiovascular effects of pancuronium in man. *Br J Anaesth* 43:335–338, 1971.

Lee C, Yang E, Lippmann, M: Constrictive effect of pancuronium on capacitance vessels. *Br J Anaesth* 52:261–263, 1980.

Marshall IG, Gibb AJ, Durant NN: Neuromuscular and vagal blocking actions of pancuronium bromide, its metabolites, and vecuronium bromide (ORG NC45) and its potential metabolites in the anesthetized cat. *Br J Anaesth* 55:703–714, 1983.

Morris RB, Cahalan MK, Miller RD, Wilkinson PL, Quasha AL, Robinson SL: The cardiovascular effects of vecuronium (ORG NC45) and pancuronium in patients undergoing coronary artery bypass grafting. *Anaesthesiology* 58:438–440, 1983.

Moyers JR, Carter JG, Fehr BL, Lineberry CC, Sokoll MD, Shimosato S: Circulatory effects of atracurium in patients with cardiovascular disease. *Br J Anaesth* 58:83S–88S, 1986.

Pedersen T, Engbaek J, Ording H, Viby-Mogensen J: Effect of vecuronium and pancuronium on cardiac performance and transmural myocardial perfusion during ketamine anesthesia. *Acta Anesthesiol Scand* 28:443–446, 1984.

Rupp SM, Fahey MR, Miller RD: Neuromuscular and cardiovascular effects of atracurium during nitrous oxide-fentanyl and nitrous oxide-isoflurane anesthesia. *Br J Anaesth* 55:67S–70S, 1983.

Salmenpera M. Peltola K. Takkunen O, Heinonen J: Cardiovascular effects of pancuronium and vecuronium during high-dose fentanyl anesthesia. *Anesth Analg* 62:1059–1064, 1983.

Saxena PR, Dhasmana KM, Prakash O: A comparison of systemic and regional hemodynamic effects of d-tubocurarine, pancuronium, and vecuronium. *Anesthesiology* 59:102–108, 1983.

Seed RF, Chamberlain JH: Myocardial stimulation by pancuronium bromide. *Br J Aanesth* 49:401–407, 1977.

Son LS, Waud BE, Waud DR: A comparison of the neuromuscular blocking and vagolytic effects of ORG NC45 and pancuronium. *Anesthesiology* 55:12–18, 1981.

Stoelting RK: The hemodynamic effects of pancuronium and d-tubocurarine in anesthetized patients. *Anesthesiology* 36:612–615, 1972.

Stoelting RK: Hemodynamic effects of gallamine during halothane-nitrous oxide anesthesia. *Anesthesiology* 39:645–647, 1973.

Stoelting RK: Hemodynamic effects of dimethyltubocurarine during nitrous oxide-halothane anesthesia. *Anaesth Analg (Cleve)* 53:513–515, 1974.

Histamine

Barnes PK, Renzy-Martin N. Thomas VJE, Watkins J: Plasma histamine levels following atracurium. *Anesthesia* 41:821–824, 1986.

Basta SJ, Savarese JJ, Ali HH, Moss J. Gionfriddo

M: Histamine-releasing potencies of atracurium, dimethyl tubocurarine and tubocurarine. *Br J Anaesth* 55:105S–106S, 1983.

Cannon JE, Fahey MR, Moss J, Miller RD: Large doses of vecuronium and plasma histamine concentrations. *Can J Anesth* 35:350–353, 1988.

Fisher MMcD, Munro I: Life-threatening anaphylactoid reactions to muscle relaxants. *Anesth Analg* 62:559–564, 1983.

Futo J, Kupferberg JP, Moss J, Fahey MR, Cannon JE, Miller RD: Vecuronium inhibits histamine N-methyltransferase. *Anesthesiology* 69:92–96, 1988.

Hosking MP, Lennon RL, Gronert GA: Combined H_1 and H_2 receptor blockade attenuates the cardiovascular effects of high-dose atracurium for rapid sequence endotracheal intubation. *Anesth Analg* 67:1089–1092, 1988.

Paton WDM: Histamine release by compounds of simple chemical structure. *Pharmacol Rev.* 9:269–328, 1957.

Robertson EN, Booij LHDJ, Fragen RJ, Crul JF: Intradermal histamine release by three muscle relaxants. *Acta Anesthesiol Scand* 27:203–205, 1983.

Watkins J: Histamine release and atracurium. *Br J Anaesth* 58:19S–22S, 1986.

Tubocurarine

Everett AJ, Lowe LA, Wilkinson S: Revision of the structure of (+) tubocurarine chloride and (+)-chondrocurine. *Chem Commun* 1020–1021, 1970.

King H: Curare Alkaloids. I. Tubocurarine. *J Chem Soc* 1381–1389, 1935.

Pancuronium

Katz RL: Clinical neuromuscular pharmacology of pancuronium. *Anesthesiology* 34:550–556, 1971.

Marshall IG, Gibb AJ, Durnt NN: Neuromuscular and vagal blocking actions of pancuronium bromide, its metabolites, and vecuronium bromide (ORG NC45) and its potential metabolities in the anesthestized cat. *Br J Anaesth* 55:703–714, 1983.

Gallamine

Agoston S, Vermeer GA, Kersten UW, Scaff AHJ: A preliminary investigation of the renal and hepatic excretion of gallamine triethiodide in man. *Br J Anesth* 50:345–349, 1978.

Metocurine

Savarese JJ, Ali HH, Antonio RP: The clinical pharmacology of metocurine. *Anesthesiology* 47:227–284, 1977.

Fazadinium

Simpson BR, Savage TM, Foley EI, Ross LA, Strunin L. Walton B, Maxwell MP, Harris DM: An azobis-arylimidazopyridinum derivative: a rapidly acting nondepolarizing muscle relaxant. *Lancet* 1:516–518, 1972.

Atracurium

Basta SJ, Ali HH, Savarese JJ, Sunder N, Gionfriddo M, Cloutier G, Lineberry C, Cato AE: Clinical pharmacology of atracurium besylate (BW 33A): a new non-depolarizing muscle relaxant. *Anesth Analg* 61:723–729, 1982.

Bell CF, Hunter JM, Jones RS, Utting JE: Use of atracurium and vecuronium in patients with oesophageal varices. *Br J Anaesth* 57:160–168, 1985.

Eager GM, Flynn PJ, Hughes R: Infusion of atracurium for long surgical procedures. *Br J Anaesth* 56:447–452, 1984.

Fisher DM, Sheiner LB: The value for organ-related clearance of atracurium: An over-calculation. *Anesthesiology* 66:102–103, 1987.

Griffiths RB, Hunter JM, Jones RS: Atracurium infusions in patients with renal failure in an ITU. *Anaesthesia* 41:375–381, 1986.

Hennis PJ, Fahey MR, Canfell PC, Shi WZ, Miller RD: Pharmacology of laudanosine in dogs. *Anesthesiology* 65:56–60, 1986.

Hilgenberg JC: Comparison of the pharmacology of vecuronium and atracurium with that of other currently available muscle relaxants. *Anesth Analg* 62:524–531, 1983.

Hilgenberg JC, Stoelting RK: Haemodynamic effects of atracurium in the presence of potent inhalation agents. *Br J Anaesth* 58:70S–74S, 1986.

Hughes R, Chapple DJ: The pharmacology of atracurium: A new competitive neuromuscular blocking agent. *Br J Anaesth* 53:31–44, 1981.

Katz RL, Stirt J, Murray AL, Lee C: Neuromuscular effects of atracurium in man. *Anesth Analg* 61:730–734, 1982.

Lanier WL, Milde JH, Michenfelder JD: The cerebral effects of pancuronium and atracurium in halothane-ancsthetized dogs. *Anaesthesiology* 63:589–597, 1985.

Maharaj RJ, Humphrey D, Kaplan N, Kadwa H, Plignaut P, Brock-Utne JG, Welsh N: Effects of atracurium on intraocular pressure. *Br J Anaesth* 56:459–462, 1984.

Miller RD, Rupp SM, Fisher DM, Cronnelly R, Fahey MR, Sohn YJ: Clinical pharmacology of vecuronium and atracurium. *Anesthesiology* 61:444–453, 1984.

Nigrovic V, Gallup W, Pandya J. Fry K: Generation of reactive metabolites during spontaneous degradation of atracurium in vivo. *Am J Med Sci* 297:12–17, 1989.

Nigrovic V, Smith S: Involvement of nucleophiles in the inactivation of atracurium. *Br J Anesth* 59:617–621, 1987.

Payne JP, Hughes R: Evaluation of atracurium in anesthetized man. *Br J Anaesth* 53:45–54, 1981.

Rupp SM, McChristian JW, Miller RD: Neuromuscular effects of atracurium during halothane-nitrous oxide and enflurane-nitrous oxide anesthesia in humans. *Anesthesiology* 63:16–19, 1985.

Savarese JJ: The new neuromuscular blocking drugs are here. *Anesthesiology* 55:1–3, 1981.

Schneider MJ, Stirt JA, Finholt DA: Atracurium, vecuronium, and intraocular pressure in humans. *Anesth Analg* 66:877–882, 1986.

Scott RPF, Goat VA: Atracurium: Its speed of onset, a comparison with suxamethonium. *Br J Anaesth* 54:909–911, 1982.

Scott RPF, Savarese JJ, Basta SJ, Embree P, Ali HH, Sunder H, Hoaglin DC: Clincial pharmacology of atracurium given in high dose. *Br J. Anaesth* 58:834–838, 1986.

Shi WZ, Fahey MR, Fisher DM, Miller RD, Canfell C, Eger EI: Laudanosine (A metabolite of atracurium) increases the minimum alveolar concentration of halothane in rabbits. *Anesthesiology* 63:584–588, 1985.

Sokoll MD, Gergis SD, Mehta M, Ali NM, Lineberry C: Safety and efficacy of atracurium (BW33A) in surgical patients receiving balanced or isoflurane anesthesia. *Anesthesiology* 58:450–455, 1985.

Sosis M, Larijani GE, Marr AT: Priming with atracurium. *Anesth Analg* 66:329–332, 1987.

Stenlake JB, Waigh RD, Urwin J, Dewar GH, Cokor GG: Atracurium; conception and inception. *Br J Anaesth* 55:3S–10S 1983.

Tateishi A, Zornow MH, Scheller MS, Canfell PC: Electroencephalographic effects of laudanosine in an animal model of epilepsy. *Br J Anaesth* 62:548–552, 1989.

Wadon AJ, Dogra S, Anand S: Atracurium infusion in the intensive care unit. *Br J Anaesth* 58:64S–67S, 1986.

Ward S, Wright DJ: Neuromuscular blockade in myasthenia gravis with atracurium besylate. *Anaesthesia* 39:51–53, 1984.

Vecuronium

Bencini AF, Houwertjes MC, Agoston S: Effects of hepatic uptake of vecuronium bromide and its putative metabolites on their neuromuscular blocking actions in the cat. *Br J Anaesth* 57:789–795, 1985.

Bencini A, Newton DEF: Rate of onset of good intubating conditions, respiratory depression and hand muscle paralysis after vecuronium. *Br J Anaesth* 56:959–965, 1984.

Bencini AF, Scaf AHJ, Agoston S, Houwertjes MC, Kersten UW: Disposition of vecuronium bromide in the cat. *Br J Anaesth* 57:782–788, 1985.

Bevan DR, Donati F, Gyasi H, Williams A: Vecuronium in renal failure. *Can Anaesth Soc J* 31:491–496, 1984.

Booij LHDJ, vanderPol F, Crul JF, Miller RD: Antagonism of ORG NC45 neuromuscular blockade by neostigmine, pyridostigmine, and 4-aminopyridine. *Anaesth Analg* 59:31–34, 1980.

Cody MW, Dormon FM: Recurarisation after vecuronium in a patient with renal failure. *Anaesthesia* 42:993–995, 1987.

Durant NN, Houwertjes MC, Crul JF: Comparison of the neuromuscular blocking properties of ORG NC45 and pancuronium in the rat, cat and rhesus monkey. *Br J Anaesth* 52:723–729, 1980.

Engbaek J. Ording H, Sorensen B, Viby-Mogensen J: Cardiac effects of vecuronium and pancuronium during halothane anaesthesia. *Br J Anaesth* 55:501–505, 1983.

Engbaek J, Ording H, Viby-Mogensen J: Neuromuscular blocking effects of vecuronium and pancuronium during halothane anesthesia. *Br J Anaesth* 55:497–500, 1983.

Fahey MR, Morris RB, Miller RD, Sohn YJ, Cronnelly R, Gencarelli P: Clinical pharmacology of ORG NC45 (Norcuron TM): a new nondepolarizing muscle relaxant. *Anesthesiology* 55:6–11, 1981.

Ferres CJ, Crean PM, Mirakhur RK: An evalua-

tion of ORG NC45 (vecuronium) in paediatric anaesthesia. *Anaesthesia* 38:943–947, 1983.

Fisher DM, Fahey MR, Cronnelly, Miller RD: Potency determiniation for vecuronium (ORG NC45): comparison of cumulative and single-dose techniques. *Anesthesiology* 57:309–310, 1982.

Gencarelli PJ, Miller RD: Antagonism of ORG NC45 (vecuronium) and pancuronium neuromuscular blockade by neostigmine. *Br J Anaesth* 54:53–55, 1982.

Gencarelli PJ, Swen J, Koot HWJ, Miller RD: Hypocarbia and spontaneous recovery from vecuronium neuromuscular blockade in anesthetized humans. *Anesth Analg* 63:608–610, 1984.

Gencarelli PJ, Swen J, Koot HWJ, Miller RD: The effects of hypercarbia and hypocarbia on pancuronium and vecuronium neuromuscular blockades in anesthetized humans. *Anesthesiology* 59:376–380, 1983.

Giffin JP, Hartung J, Cottrell JE, Capuano C, Shwiry B: Effect of vecuronium on intracranial pressure, mean arterial pressure and heart rate in cats. *Br J Anaesth* 58:441–443, 1986.

Hilgenberg JC: Comparison of the pharmacology of vecuronium and atracurium with that of other currently available muscle relaxants. *Anesth Analg* 62:524–531, 1983.

Jantzen JP, Hackett GH, Erdmann K, Ernshaw G: Effect of vecuronium on intraocular pressure. *Br J Anaesth* 58:433–436, 1986.

Kerr WJ, Baird WLM: Clinical studies on ORG NC45: comparison with pancuronium. *Br J Anaesth* 54:1159–1164, 1982.

Kunjappan VE, Brown EM, Alexander GD: Rapid sequence induction using vecuronium. *Anaesth Analg* 65:503–506, 1986.

Lennon RL, Olson RA, Gronert GA: Atracurium or vecuronium for rapid sequence endotracheal intubation. *Anesthesiology* 64:510–513, 1986.

Marshall IG, Agoston S, Booij LHDJ, Durant NN, Foldes FF: Pharmacology of ORG NC45 compared with other non-depolarizing neuromuscular blocking drugs. *Br J Anaesth* 52:11S–18S, 1980.

Meistelman C, Loose JP, Saint-Maurice C, Delleur MM, daSilva GL: Clinical pharmacology of vecuronium in children. *Br J Anaesth* 58:996–1000, 1986.

Miller RD, Rupp SM, Fisher DM, Cronnelly R, Fahey MR, Sohn YJ: Clinical pharmacology of vecuronium and atracurium. *Anesthesiology* 61:444–453, 1984.

Mirakhur RK, Ferres CJ, Clarke FSJ, Bali IM, Dundee JW: Clinical evaluation of ORG NC45. *Br J Anaesth* 55:119–124, 1983.

Musich J. Walts LF: Pulmonary aspiration after a priming dose of vecuronium. *Anesthesiology* 64:517–519, 1986.

Rosa G, Sanfilippo M, Vilardi V, Orfei P, Gasparetto A: Effects of vecuronium bromide on intracranial pressure and cerebral perfusion pressure. *Br J Anaesth* 58:437–440, 1986.

Rupp SM, Miller RD, Gencarelli PJ: Vecuronium-induced neuromuscular blockade during enflurane, isoflurane, and halothane anesthesia in humans. *Anaesthesiology* 60:102–105, 1984.

Savage DS, Sleigh T, Carlyle I: The emergence of ORG NC45, 1-[(2β,3α,5α,16β,17β)-3, 17-bis-(acetylosy)-2-(1-piperidinyl)-androstan-16-YL]-1-methylpiperidinium bromide, from the pancuronium series. *Br J Anaesth* 52:3S–9S, 1980.

Savarese JJ: The new neuromuscular blocking drugs are here. *Anaesthesiology* 55:1–3, 1981.

Smith CE, Donati F, Bevan DR: Cumulative dose-response with infusion: a technique to determine neuromuscular blocking potency of atracurium and vecuronium. *Clin Pharmacol Ther* 44:56–64, 1988.

Taboada JA, Rupp SM, Miller RD: Refining the priming principle for vecuronium during rapid-sequence induction of anesthesia. *Anesthesiology* 64:243–247, 1986.

Van der Veen F, Bencini A: Pharmacokinetics and pharmacodynamics of ORG NC45 in man. *Br J Anaesth* 52:37S–41S, 1980.

Succinylcholine

Anderson N: Changes in intragastric pressure following the administration of suxamethonium. *Br J Anaesth* 34:363–365, 1962.

Cook JH: The effect of suxamethonium on intraocular pressure. *Anaesthesia* 36:359–365, 1981.

Craythorne NWB, Rottenstein HS, Dripps RD: The effect of succinylcholine on intraocular pressure in adults, infants and children during general anesthesia. *Anesthesiology* 21:59–63, 1960.

d'Hollander AA, Agoston S, deVille A, Cuvelier F: Clinical and pharmacological actions of a bolus injection of suxamethonium: two phenomena of distinct duration. *Br J Anaesth* 55:131–134, 1983.

Durant NN, Katz RL: Suxamethonium. *Br J Anaesth* 54:195–209, 1982.

Gronert GA, Theye RA: Pathophysiology of hyperkalemia induced by succinylcholine. *Anesthesiology* 43:89–99, 1975.

Koide M, Waude BE: Serum potassium concentrations after succinylcholine in patients with renal failure. *Anesthesiology* 36:142–145, 1972.

Leighton BL, Cheek TG, Gross JB, Apfelbaum JL, Shantz BB, Gutsche BB, Rosenberg H: Succinylcholine pharmacodynamics in peripartum patients. *Anesthesiology* 64:202–205, 1986.

Lerman J, Chinyanga HM: The heart rate response to succinylcholine in children: a comparison of atropine and glycopyrrolate. *Can Anaesth Soc J* 30:377–381, 1983.

Masey SA, Glazebrook CW, Goat VA: Suxamethonium: a new look at pretreatment. *Br J Anaesth* 55:729–733, 1983.

McCammon RL, Stoelting RK: Exaggerated increase in serum potassium following succinylcholine in dogs with beta blockade. *Anesthesiology* 61:723–725, 1984.

Miller RD, Way WL, Hamilton WK, Layzer RB: Succinylcholine-induced hyperkalemia in patients with renal failure? *Anesthesiology* 36:138–141, 1972.

Silk E, King J, Whittaker M: Assay of cholinesterase in clinical chemistry. *Ann Clin Biochem* 16:57–75, 1979.

Yasuda I, Hirano T, Amaha K, Fudeta H, Obara S: Chronotropic effect of succinylcholine and succinylmonocholine on the sinoatrial node. *Anesthesiology* 57:289–292, 1982.

Dantrolene

Britt BA: Dantrolene. *Can Anaesth Soc J* 31:61–75, 1984.

Flewellen LEH, Nelson TE, Jones WP, Arens JF, Wagner DI: Dantrolene dose response in awake man: implications for management of malignant hyperthermia. *Anesthesiology* 59:275–280, 1983.

Harrison GG: Dantrolene—Dynamics and kinetics. *Br J Anaesth* 60:279–286, 1988.

Lerman J, McLeod ME, Strong HA: Pharmacokinetics of intravenous dantrolene in children. *Anesthesiology* 70:625–629, 1989.

SanJuan AC, Wong KC, Port JD: Hyperkalemia after dantrolene and verapamil-dantrolene administration in dogs. *Anesth Analg* 67:759–762, 1988.

Verburg MP, Oerlemans FTJJ, vanBennekom CA, Gielen MJM, deBruyn CHMM, Crul JF: In vivo induced malignant hyperthermia in pigs. I. Physiological and biochemical changes and the influence of dantrolene sodium. *Acta Anesthesiol Scand* 28:1–8, 1984.

Watson CB, Reierson N, Norfleet EA: Clinically significant muscle weakness induced by oral dantrolene sodium prophylaxis for malignant hyperthermia. *Anesthesiology* 65:312–314, 1986.

Doxacurium

Basta SJ, Savarese JJ, Ali HH, Embree PB, Schwartz AF, Rudd GD, Wasila WB: Clinical pharmacology of doxacurium chloride. *Anesthesiology* 69:478–486, 1988.

Coudsouzian NG, Alifimoff JK, Liu LMP, Foster V, McNulty B, Savarese JJ: Neuromuscular and cardiovascular effects of doxacurium in children anesthetized with halothane. *Br J Anaesth* 62:263–268, 1989.

Katz JA, Fragen RJ, Shanks CA, Dunn K, McNulty B, Rugg GD: Dose-repsonse relationships of doxacurium chloride in humans during anesthesia with nitrous oxide and fentanyl, enflurane, isoflurane, or halothane. *Anesthesiology* 70:432–436, 1989.

Lennon RL, Hosking MP, Houck PC, Rose SH, Wedel DJ, Gibson BE, Ascher JA, Rudd GD: Doxacurium chloride for neuromuscular blockade before tracheal intubation and surgery during nitrous oxide-oxygen-narcotic-enflurane anesthesia. *Anesth Analg* 68:253–260, 1989.

Murray DJ, Mehta MP, Choi WW, Forbes RB, Sokoll MD, Gergis SD, Rudd GD, Abou-Donia MM: The neuromuscular blocking and cardiovascular effects of doxacurium chloride in patients receiving nitrous oxide narcotic anesthesia. *Anesthesiology* 69:472–477, 1988.

Sarner JB, Brandom BW, Cook DR, Dong ML, Horn MC, Woelfel SK, Davis PJ, Rudd GD, Foster VJ, McNulty BF: Clinical pharmacology of doxacurium chloride (BW A938U) in children. *Anesth Analg* 67:303–306, 1988.

Scott RPF, Norman J: Doxacurium chloride: a preliminary clinical trial. *Br J Anaesth* 62:373–377, 1989.

Stoops CM, Curtis CA, Kovach DA, McGammon

RL, Stoelting RK, Warren TM, Miller D, Abou-Donia MM: Hemodynamic effects of doxacurium chloride in patients receiving oxygen sufentanil anesthesia for coronary artery bypass grafting or valve replacement. *Anesthesiology* 69:365–370, 1988.

Mivacurium

Ali HH, Savarese JJ, Embree PB, Basta SJ, Stout RG, Bottros LH, Weakly JN: Clinical pharmacology of mivacurium chloride (BW B1090U) infusion: comparison with vecuronium and atracurium. *Br J Anaesth* 61:541–546, 1988.

Brandom BW, Woelfel SK, Cook DR, Weber S, Powers DM, Weakly JN: Comparison of mivacurium and suxamethonium administered by bolus and infusion. *Br J Anaesth* 62:488–493, 1989.

Caldwell JE, Kitts JB, Heier T, Fahey MR, Lynam DP, Miller RD: The dose-response relationship of mivacurium chloride in humans during nitrous oxide-fentanyl or nitrous oxide-enflurane anesthesia. *Anesthesiology* 70:31–35, 1989.

Goudsouzian NG, Alifimoff JK, Eberly C, Smeets R, Griswold J, Miler V, NcNulty BF, Savarese JJ: Neuromuscular and cardiovascular effects of mivacurium in children. *Anesthesiology* 70:237–242, 1989.

Sarner JB, Brandom BW, Woelfel SK, Dong ML, Horn MC, Cook DR, McNulty BF, Foster VJ: Clinical pharmacology of mivacurium chloride (BW B1090U) in children during nitrous oxide-halothane and nitrous oxide-narcotic anesthesia. *Anesth Analg* 68:116–121, 1989.

Savarese JJ, Ali HH, Basta SJ, Embree PB, Scott RPF, Sunder N, Weakly JN, Wastila WB, El-Sayad HA: The clinical neuromuscular pharmacology of mivacurium chloride (BW B1090U). *Anesthesiology* 69:723–732, 1988.

Savarese JJ, Ali HH, Basta SJ, Scott RPF, Embree PB, Wastila WB, Abou-Donia MM, Gelb C: The cardiovascular effects of mivacurium chloride (BW B1090U) in patients receiving nitrous oxide-opiate-barbiturate anesthesia. *Anesthesiology* 70:386–394, 1989.

Stoops CM, Curtis CA, Kovach DA, McCammon FL, Stoelting RK, Warren TM, Miller D, Bopp SK, Jugovic DJ, Abou-Donia MM: Hemodynamic effects of mivacurium chloride administered to patients during oxygen-sufentanil anesthesia for coronary artery bypass grafting or valve replacement. *Anesth Analg* 68:333–339, 1989.

Weber S, Brandom BW, Powers DM, Sarner JB, Woelfel SK, Cook DR, Foster VJ, McNulty BF, Weakly JN: Mivacurium chloride (BW B1090U)-induced neuromuscular blockade during nitrous oxide-isoflurane and nitrous oxide-narcotic anesthesia in adult surgical patients. *Anesth Analg* 67:495–499, 1988.

Pipecuronium

Caldwell JE, Canfell PC, Castagnoli KP, Lynam DP, Fahey MR, Fisher DM, Miller RD: The influence of renal failure on the pharmacokinetics and duration of action of pipecuronium bromide in patients anesthetized with halothane and nitrous oxide. *Anesthesiology* 70:7–12, 1989.

Caldwell JE, Castagnoli KP, Canfell PC Fahey MR, Lynam DP, Fisher DM, Miller RD: Pipecuronium and pancuronium: comparison of pharmacokinetics and duration of action. *Br J Anaesth* 61:693–697, 1988.

Deam RD, Soni N: Effects of pipecuronium and pancuronium on the isolated rabbit heart. *Br J Anaesth* 62:287–289, 1989.

Tassonyi E. Neidhart P, Pittet JF, Morel DR, Gemperle M: Cardiovascular effects of pipecuronium and pancuronium in patients undergoing coronary artery bypass grafting. *Anesthesiology* 69:793–796, 1988.

Wierda JMKH, Richardson FJ, Agoston S: Dose-response relation and time course of action of pipecuronium bromide in humans anesthetized with nitrous oxide and isoflurane, halothane, or droperidol and fentanyl. *Anesth Analg* 68:208–213, 1989.

General

Ali HH, Savarese JJ: Monitoring of neuromuscular function. *Anesthesiology* 45:216–249, 1976.

Deacock AR, Hargrove RL: The influence of certain ganglionic blocking agents on neuromuscular transmission. *Br J Anaesth* 34:357–362, 1962.

Hunter JM: Adverse effects of neuromuscular blocking drugs. *Br J Anaesth* 59:46–60, 1987.

11

Local Anesthetic Agents

MARGARET WOOD

Local anesthetics are drugs that produce reversible depression of nerve conduction when applied to the nerve fiber. Cocaine was the first local anesthetic discovered; the topical local anesthetic properties of cocaine were described by Freud and Koller in 1884, and in 1885, Halsted demonstrated that cocaine could prevent conduction in nerve trunks.

During the first half of the twentieth century, a search for synthetic substitutes for cocaine was carried out, and most of the compounds synthesized were ester derivatives of benzoic acid. Procaine was synthesized in 1905. In 1943, Löfgren synthesized lidocaine, which is an amide derivative of diethylamino acetic acid. Since that time, all of the new local anesthetic agents that have been introduced into clinical practice have been amino-amides with the exception of chloroprocaine.

PHYSIOLOGY OF NERVE CONDUCTION

The ionic mechanism of nerve conduction provides a basis for the understanding of the mechanism of action of the local anesthetics, since local anesthetics block the transmission or conduction of nerve impulses (action potentials) along peripheral nerves that signal pain to the central nervous system. Cytoplasm inside the nerve cell and axon contains positively charged potassium ions and negatively charged protein ions. Although the potassium ions are able to diffuse through the surrounding membranes, the protein ions cannot. Outside in the extracellular fluid, positively charged sodium ions and negatively charged chloride ions are present, both of which are able to diffuse through the membrane into the cell, but the sodium is immediately extruded via the sodium pump. Thus, the only freely diffusible ions are potassium from inside and chloride from outside the membrane. Inside the membrane, the potassium concentration is high and the chloride concentration is low, while outside, the chloride concentration is high and the potassium concentration is low. The high concentration of potassium ions inside the membrane will tend to diffuse outwards along a concentration gradient and is held inside the membrane by an excess of negatively charged ions; an electrical potential therefore exists whereby the inside is negative with respect to the outside. The magnitude of this potential is in the region of -60 to -90 mV.

When a nerve impulse passes along a nerve, the membrane suddenly becomes permeable to sodium ions which move into the inside, making the inside positive ($+40$ mV) with respect to the outside, so that the total action or spike potential is about 110 mV. Thus, the generation of the action potential is associated with increased sodium conductance. The membrane then ceases to be permeable to sodium and becomes permeable to potassium, so that potassium ions flow from the inside to the outside and the membrane potential returns to its resting level of -60 to -90 mV. Thus, the nerve has gained sodium ions and lost potassium ions; these are reexchanged during a slow recovery period.

MECHANISM OF ACTION OF LOCAL ANESTHETICS

As discussed in the previous section, the transmission of nerve impulses is dependent upon a wave of depolarization passing down the axonal membrane, followed by repolarization. The axonal membrane consists of a phospholipid bilayer which has pores or ion-specific channels through which ions pass. Most channels have a "gate" which regulates the passage of ions through them. It is thought that the increase in sodium permeability associated with depolarization results from the opening of sodium channels in the cell membrane, so that an action potential propagation involves an initial opening of sodium channels ("activation") followed by spontaneous closing ("inactivation") of sodium channels and concurrent opening of potassium channels. The initial opening of a few sodium channels brings about the opening of more channels, producing further membrane depolarization—a cascade effect. Ion channels are selective for a particular ion that is preferentially carried through the channel; for example, sodium channels transport Na^+ 12 times better than potassium ions, while lithium ions pass through the Na^+ channel as well as Na^+ ions (see page 588).

A wide range of drugs and substances has been shown to block sodium channels, such as biotoxins (tetrodotoxin), phenothiazines, anticonvulsants, antiarrhythmics, and local anesthetic agents. Local anesthetics cause sodium channel blockade by reducing the permeability of the cell membrane to sodium ions so that, although the resting and threshold potential is unaffected, there is marked depression of the rate of depolarization such that it fails to reach the threshold potential. A propagated action potential, therefore, does not occur and neural blockade results.

It is postulated that local anesthetic diffuses through the lipid cell membrane into the axoplasm, where it ionizes again. Sodium channel blockade is probably a result of binding to a specific "receptor" site in or near the sodium channel. Drugs may access this binding site either through the hydrophilic pore or via the lipid bilayer. The action of some racemic local anesthetics is stereospecific.

Blockade of the sodium channel is thought to result from interaction of drug (in this case local anesthetic) with a specific receptor-like site associated with the sodium channel. One widely accepted model for drug blockade of ion channels is the *modulated receptor hypothesis*, which suggests that affinity of the receptor is modulated by the channel state, i.e., open, inactivated, or resting (Fig. 11.1). Normally during the generation of each action potential, the sodium channel changes from rested-closed to open-activated to inactivated-closed. Generally, local anesthetics have low affinity for the resting sodium channel and high affinity for the open or inactivated channel.

Sodium channels recover much more slowly after an action potential when the nerve is exposed to local anesthetic than would occur in the drug-free state. Because of this slow recovery, there may not be enough time between repeated nerve action potentials for full recovery to occur. During the action potential when the channel is open, the local anesthetic exhibits high affinity for the receptor but, after the action potential is over, the sodium channel develops a lower-affinity state and some drug then unbinds from the receptor. If another action potential arrives before all the drug has unbound from the receptor, an additional increment of blocking will occur. An increase in the stimulus frequency increases the degree of block ("use" or frequency-dependent block). Most local anesthetics therefore produce a much greater degree of nerve blockade at higher degrees of firing. This phenomenon is called *frequency-dependent local anesthetic blockade*. The extent and time course of frequency-dependent blockade are related not only to the relative affinity (binding) of the various channel receptors for local anesthetic, but also to ease of access by the drug to the channel receptor.

The *guarded receptor* hypothesis has been advanced as an alternative to the modulated receptor hypothesis to explain local anesthetic action. In the modulated receptor theory, receptor affinity for local anesthetic changes from low to high depending on the conformation state of the sodium channel, but in the guarded receptor hypothesis, the affinity is constantly high, but access of local anesthetic to the receptor is limited by channel "gates."

Thus, in summary, local anesthetics block nerve action potentials by binding to sodium channels and preventing their opening. It is important to remember that local anesthetics exert effects not only on nerves, but should they gain inadvertent access to the circulation, on cardiac sodium channels as well. Subtle differences in the receptor kinetics of various local anesthetics at the sodium channel in cardiac tissues may have serious con-

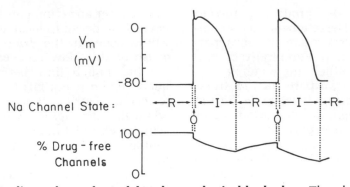

Figure 11.1.   Sodium channels and local anesthetic blockade.   The degree of sodium channel blockade is dependent on the state of the sodium channel. Schematic diagram illustrating time-dependent changes in sodium channel states *(middle)* and block of sodium channels *(bottom)* associated with the cardiac action potential *(top)* in the presence of a local anesthetic drug. The *top trace* shows two simulated ventricular muscular action potentials. V_m, transmembrane voltage. The drug (local anesthetic) binds to sodium channels in open *(O)* and inactivated *(I)* states but has a very low affinity for channels in the rested *(R)* state. As indicated *(middle)*, sodium channels are in the rested state during diastole, open transiently during the action potential upstroke, and in an inactivated (closed) state during the action potential plateau. As indicated at the *bottom,* all channels are in a drug-free state after a long rest, i.e., no binding, but drug binding to open and inactivated channels develops during the action potential. Drug dissociation during diastole is time dependent and incomplete, resulting in an accumulation of drug-associated (blocked) channels with successive beats. "Use" or frequency-dependent blockade (reduction in V_{max}, i.e., the maximum upstroke velocity of the action potential) results whenever the block that develops during an action potential has not enough time to fully dissipate during diastole. The block development can result from local anesthetic binding to open *(O)* sodium channels (during the upstroke of the action potential), from drug binding to inactivated *(I)* sodium channels (during the plateau of the action potential), or from drug binding to channels in both states. (With permission from Clarkson CW, Hondeghem LM: Mechanism for bupivacaine depression of cardiac conduction: fast block of sodium channels during the action potential with slow recovery from block during diastole. *Anesthesiology* 62:396–405, 1985.)

sequences for toxicity (see later in the chapter).

NERVE FIBER SIZE AND EFFECT OF LOCAL ANESTHETIC

There are two types of nerve fiber, myelinated and nonmyelinated. In the myelinated nerve fiber, the central axon is surrounded by a myelin sheath and an outer neurilemmal sheath. In the non-myelinated nerve, the myelin sheath is absent and the neurilemmal sheath is the only covering of the axon. The myelin sheath is interrupted at about 1-mm intervals at the nodes of Ranvier. In the myelinated nerve fibers, the depolarization process leaps from one node of Ranvier to the next. This is known as saltatory conduction and gives an increase in conduction velocity.

Nerve fibers vary in both size and conduction velocity and have been divided into A, B, and C groups (Table 11.1). The group A fibers are myelinated fibers found in sensory and motor nerves and have been further subdivided into α, β, γ, and δ on the basis of nerve fiber diameter. The group B fibers are myelinated preganglionic autonomic nerve fibers. Type C nerve fibers are nonmyelinated fibers, responsible for pain and temperature

Table 11.1.
Classification of Nerve Fibers

Nerve fiber	Myelination	Diameter (μm)	Conduction velocity (m/sec)	Function
A-α	Heavily	15–20	70–120	Motor
A-β	Moderately	5–12	30–70	Touch and pressure
A-γ	Moderately	5–10	30–70	Proprioception
A-σ	Lightly	2–5	12–30	Pain and temperature
B	Lightly	1–4	3–15	Preganglionic autonomic
C	No	0.5–1.0	0.5–2.0	Pain and temperature

functions. The velocity of conduction is proportional to fiber diameter. The largest myelinated fibers with a diameter of 20 μm conduct at 120 m per second, while C fibers have a slower conduction velocity of about 1 to 2 m per second.

As a general rule, the greater the diameter of the nerve fiber, the higher the concentration of local anesthetic required to produce conduction blockade, and thus, smaller nerve fibers are more sensitive to the action of local anesthetic than are large fibers. There is, therefore, a definite order of onset of blockade for the different nerve fiber types within a nerve trunk. Following epidural and major peripheral nerve or plexus blockade, increased skin temperature is the first sign of blockade (B fibers). This is followed by loss of pain and temperature due to A-δ and C fiber blockade. Proprioception (A-γ) and touch (A-β) fibers are then blocked by higher concentrations of local anesthetic, while the highest concentrations are required for motor blockade (A-α).

STRUCTURE-ACTIVITY RELATIONSHIP

Chemical compounds that possess local anesthetic activity have certain structural features in common. Löfgren first noted that almost all the local anesthetics are composed of hydrophilic and hydrophobic (lipophilic) components, separated by an intermediate chain (Fig. 11.2). The hydrophilic group is generally a secondary or tertiary amine, while the hydrophobic group is usually an aromatic

residue. Therefore, a local anesthetic can be depicted as:

Aromatic group—Intermediate Amine group
(lipophilic)   chain— (hydrophilic)

Linkage to the aromatic group has provided a means for classification of the local anesthetics. Local anesthetics with an ester linkage between the aromatic residue and the intermediate chain are known as **amino-esters;** examples of local anesthetics in this group include procaine, chloroprocaine, and tetracaine. Local anesthetics with an amide linkage between the aromatic group and the intermediate chain are known as **amino-amides** and include lidocaine, mepiva-

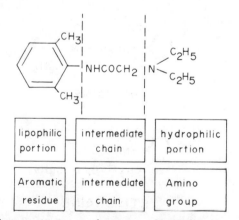

lipophilic portion	intermediate chain	hydrophilic portion
Aromatic residue	intermediate chain	Amino group

Figure 11.2. Lofgren's scheme for true local anesthetic agents, illustrated by lidocaine. (With permission from Takman BH: The chemistry of local anaesthetic agents: classification of blocking agents. *Br J Anaesth* 47:183–190, 1975.)

caine, bupivacaine, and etidocaine. The structural formulae of some of the commonly administered local anesthetics are given in Fig. 11.3. The type of linkage to the aromatic group is an important determinant of biodegradation; the ester compounds are readily hydrolyzed in plasma by pseudocholinesterase, while the amide local anesthetics are more slowly metabolized in the liver.

Structural alterations in the molecule produce physicochemical changes that can alter anesthetic potency and toxicity. Lipid solubility is an important determi-

nant of anesthetic potency; changes in either the aromatic or amine portion of a local anesthetic can alter lipid solubility and thereby affect anesthetic potency. In addition, lengthening the intermediate chain tends to increase anesthetic potency, until a critical length is reached after which potency usually declines. Increase in degree of protein binding is thought to increase the duration of local anesthetic activity. Thus, the addition of a butyl group to the aromatic residue of the ester local anesthetic procaine increases lipid solubility and protein bind-

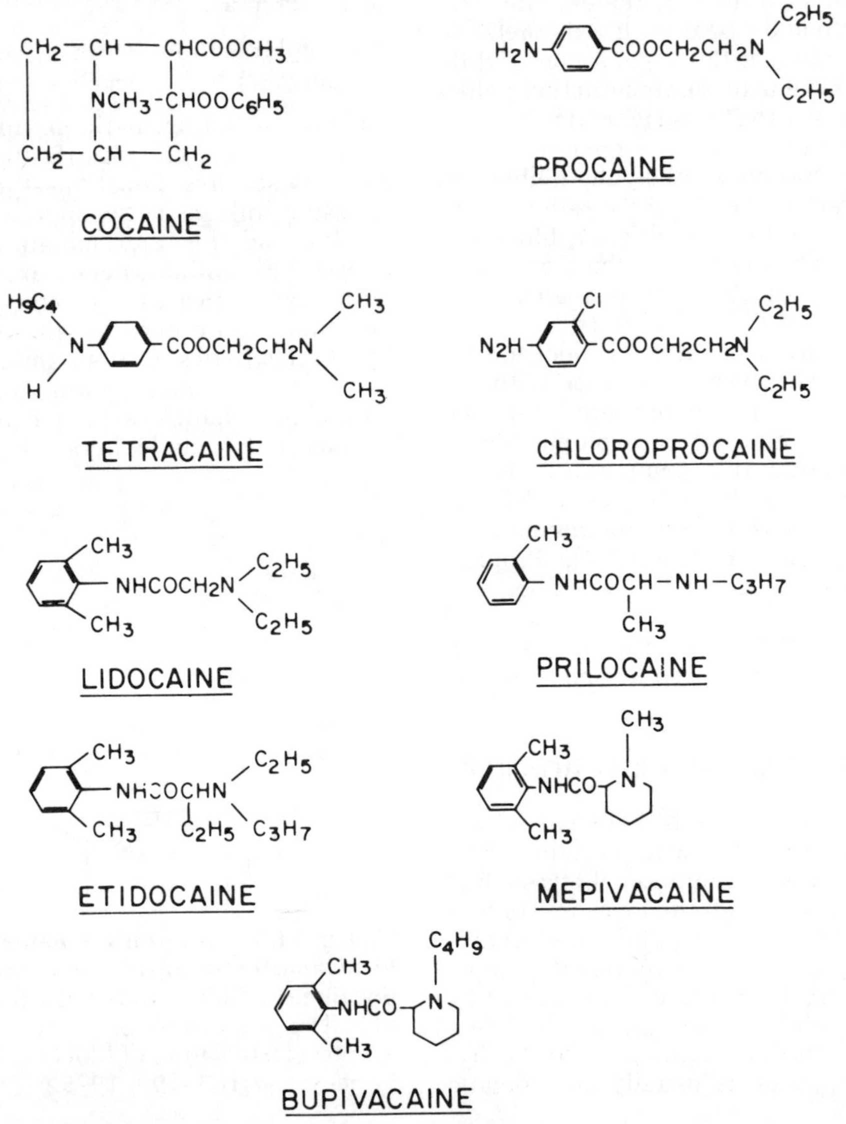

Figure 11.3.   Structural formulae of some local anesthetics.

ing, resulting in the compound tetra-caine, which has greater anesthetic potency and longer duration of action. Similarly, the addition of a butyl group to the amine portion of mepivacaine results in the compound bupivacaine (more lipid soluble and highly protein bound), which has greater anesthetic potency and longer duration of action than mepivacaine.

Mepivacaine, prilocaine, bupivacaine, and etidocaine have an asymmetric carbon atom and therefore can exist in two stereoisomeric forms, having different pharmacodynamic and pharmacokinetic properties. These local anesthetics are administered clinically as racemates. Lidocaine does not exist as a stereoisomer.

PHYSICOCHEMICAL PROPERTIES AND LOCAL ANESTHETIC ACTION

The pharmacological action of the local anesthetics is influenced by lipid solubility, plasma binding, and the dissociation constant.

Lipid Solubility

Highly lipid-soluble drugs readily penetrate cell membranes. In general, the highly lipid-soluble local anesthetic agents are the most potent and have a longer duration of action.

Protein Binding

Increased duration of anesthetic action correlates with high plasma binding. Al-though protein binding reduces the amount of free drug that is available for diffusion, it is thought to provide a depot for maintenance of neural blockade. It has always been assumed that a relationship exists between plasma protein binding of local anesthetics and degree of binding to neuronal membrane proteins. Laboratory studies have indeed shown that poorly protein-bound local anesthetics are washed out rapidly from isolated nerve preparations, whereas highly protein-bound local anesthetics such as bupivacaine are removed at a slower rate.

Dissociation Constant (pKa)

The degree of ionization has an important influence on drug distribution and action because it is only the nonionized form that readily crosses cell membranes. The degree of ionization of a substance depends on the nature of the substance (acid or base), its dissociation constant (pKa), and the pH of the medium in which it is present. The pKa of a drug is the pH at which it is 50% ionized and 50% unionized (see Chapter 1). A weak base is more ionized in an acidic solution and, thus, decreasing the pH will increase the ionization of the base. Local anesthetics are weak bases with pKa values that range from 7.6 to 8.9 (Table 11.2). Local anesthetics with a pKa near physiological pH (7.4) have a greater amount of drug in the nonionized form (which more readily diffuses across the nerve sheath

Table 11.2.
Physiocochemical Properties of Some Local Anesthetics

Agent	Molecular weight	pKa* (25°C)	Partition coefficient† (lipid solubility)	Plasma protein binding (%)	Relative potency
Procaine	236	8.9	0.02		1
Chloroprocaine	271	8.7	0.14		1
Tetracaine	264	8.5	4.1		8
Prilocaine	220	7.9	0.9		2
Mepivacaine	246	7.6	0.8	75	2
Lidocaine	234	7.9	2.9	60–75	2
Bupivacaine	288	8.1	28	90–97	8
Etidocaine	276	7.7	141	94–97	6

*pKa, dissociation constant.
†Heptane/buffer (pH = 7.4).

and membrane to its site of action) than local anesthetics with a higher pKa. Local anesthetics with a higher pKa will be more ionized at physiological pH and thus will have less nonionized drug available to penetrate the nerve sheath and membrane. Therefore, local anesthetics with pKa values close to physiological pH tend to have a more rapid onset of action.

Factors that promote local extracellular acidosis, for example, infection, increase drug ionization and therefore reduce local anesthetic diffusion toward and penetration of the nerve membrane.

Table 11.2 lists the physicochemical properties of some of the local anesthetic agents.

POTENCY AND DURATION OF ACTION

Local anesthetics have also been classified on the basis of anesthetic potency and duration of action.

1. **Short duration of action and low anesthetic potency.**
   Procaine
   Chloroprocaine
2. **Intermediate duration of action and anesthetic potency.**
   Lidocaine
   Mepivacaine
   Prilocaine
   Cocaine
3. **Long duration of action and high anesthetic potency.**
   Bupivacaine
   Tetracaine
   Etidocaine

PHARMACOKINETICS

The uptake and distribution of the local anesthetics are of vital importance to the anesthesiologist because systemic toxicity following regional anesthesia depends on the balance between the rate processes involved in drug absorption and systemic disposition (Fig. 11.4). The pharmacokinetics of local anesthetics can be divided into two processes: absorption kinetics and systemic disposition kinetics.

Absorption Kinetics

Most pharmacokinetic studies of local anesthetics in humans have involved the measurement of blood concentrations over a period of time following drug administration as a part of a regional procedure. However, it is important to realize that these drug concentration-time profiles are a function of both absorption and disposition, the two processes occurring simultaneously. Thus, plasma concentrations of local anesthetics depend on absorption from the injection site, tissue distribution, metabolism, and excretion. Knowledge of the pharmacokinetic parameters following intravenous infusion alone allows the separation of absorption and disposition kinetics, and the absolute rate of drug absorption can then be calculated. Determinants of systemic absorption include physicochemical properties of the local anesthetic agent itself, dosage, route of injection, addition of vasoconstrictor to the injected solution, vasoactive properties of the

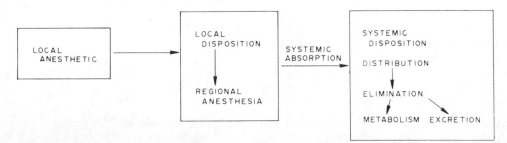

Figure 11.4. Fate of local anesthetics.

local anesthetic, and pathophysiological factors such as disease processes.

Systemic absorption following epidural injection has been shown to be a biphasic process. Figure 11.5 depicts the absorption of lidocaine and etidocaine following epidural injection, where it can be seen that net absorption from the epidural space of the long-acting, more lipid-soluble, highly protein-bound anesthetic (etidocaine) is slower probably due to a greater retention in fat and tissues of the epidural space. It is also apparent that epinephrine has less influence on the uptake and anesthetic duration of the longer-acting agents. The slower overall absorption of the longer-acting drugs has obvious important implications for systemic toxicity. Studies measuring the net absorption of local anesthetic from the epidural space have been extended to

allow the calculation of local and systemic accumulation of anesthetic during intermittent injection and continuous epidural administration, and they indicate that systemic accumulation will tend to be faster with the shorter-acting anesthetics, while local accumulation will tend to be faster and greater with the longer-acting anesthetics (Figs. 11.6 and 11.7).

The systemic absorption of lidocaine and bupivacaine from both the epidural and subarachnoid space has been determined in surgical patients. The rate of absorption was shown to be a biphasic process (fast and slow), with the contribution of the later slow phase being greater for bupivacaine than for lidocaine after epidural injection (Table 11.3). It is thought that the more lipid-soluble bupivacaine is taken up by extradural fat

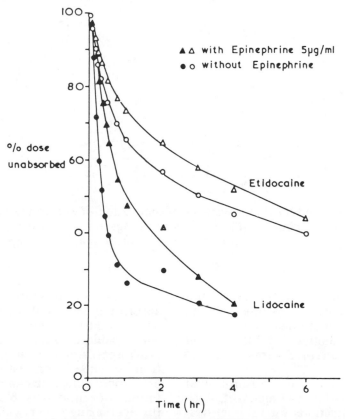

Figure 11.5. Systemic absorption of etidocaine and lidocaine after extradural injection in volunteers. (With permission from Tucker GT, Mather LE: Pharmacokinetics of local anaesthetic agents. *Br J Anaesth* 47:213–224, 1975.)

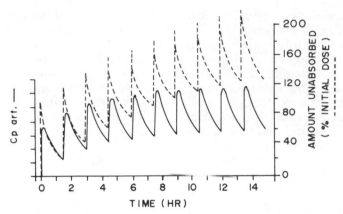

Figure 11.6.   Predicted local and systemic accumulation of lidocaine during a multiple extradural injection regimen.   (Plain solution; dosage interval, 1.5 hr.) (With permission from Tucker GT, Mather LE: Pharmacokinetics of local anaesthetic agents. *Br J Anaesth* 47:213–224, 1975.)

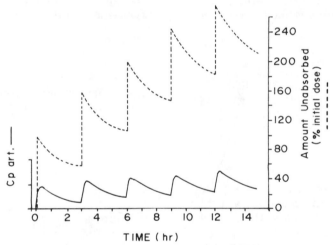

Figure 11.7.   Predicted local and systemic accumulation of etidocaine during a multiple extradural injection regimen.   (Plain solution; dosage interval, 3 hr). (With permission from Tucker GT, Mather LE: Pharmacokinetics of local anaesthetic agents. *Br J Anaesth* 47:213–224, 1975.)

and neural tissue, resulting in a relatively slower release into the systemic circulation. These studies thus seem to confirm the predictions of Mather and Tucker illustrated in Figures 11.6 and 11.7.

Differences in the rate of absorption of different anesthetics are important, since they have implications for rational dosage during continuous epidural infusions or multiple dosing over a prolonged period of time.

The site of injection affects systemic absorption of local anesthetic agents, since blood flow and the presence of tissue capable of binding local anesthetics are imporrtant determinants of uptake from the site of administration. The highest blood concentrations are generally found after intercostal block, followed by (in decreasing order) caudal block, epidural block, brachial plexus block, sciatic-femoral block, and subcutaneous infiltration. Figure 11.8 shows the mean

Table 11.3.
Absorption of Lidocaine and Bupivacaine from the Subarachnoid and Epidural Space in Surgical Patients

	Lidocaine		Bupivacaine	
	Subarachnoid	Epidural	Subarachnoid	Epidural
Fast				
F_1*		0.38	0.35	0.29
$t_{1/2\alpha1}$ (min)‡		9.3	50	8
Slow				
F_2*		0.58	0.61	0.64
$t_{1/2\alpha2}$ (min)‡	71	82	408	371
F†	1.03	0.96	0.96	0.91

Simultaneous investigation of absorption and disposition using the technique of combining regional injection of unlabeled drug with simultaneous intravenous injection of the deuterated stable isotope allows calculation of rate of absorption. The absorption of bupivacaine from the subarachnoid space was characterized as two first-order absorption processes, yielding a fast and slow half-life,‡ while the absorption of lidocaine was monoexponential. The time course for absorption of both bupivacaine and lidocaine from the epidural space was biexponential, yielding two half-lives.* The fractions of the dose absorbed in the fast and slow processes are F_1 and F_2, respectively, while F† represents total systemic availability. Note the more rapid absorption of bupivacaine when given by epidural injection than subarachnoid injection. This is related to the increased vascularity of the epidural space. (With permission from Burm AGL, VanKleef JW, Vermeulen NPE, Olthof G, Briemer DD, Spierdijk J: Pharmacokinetics of lidocaine and bupivacaine following subarachnoid administration in surgical patients: simultaneous investigation of absorption and disposition kinetics using stable isotopes. *Anesthesiology* 69:584–592, 1988; and Burm AGL, Vermeulen NPE, De Boer AG, Van Kleef JW, Spierdijk J, Breimer DD: Pharmacokinetics of lidocaine and bupivacaine in surgical patients following epidural administration: simultaneous investigation of absorption and disposition kinetics using stable isotopes. *Clin Pharmacokinet* 13:191–203, 1987.)

maximum plasma mepivacaine concentrations attained for various types of regional block, where the highest value was obtained for intercostal nerve block with 2% plain solution and the lowest for caudal block with 1% solution plus epinephrine. Higher concentrations of local anesthetic solutions are associated with higher maximum plasma concentrations.

The addition of a vasoconstrictor agent to local anesthetic solution reduces the rate of systemic absorption and thereby reduces peak plasma local anesthetic concentrations (Fig. 11.8). Epinephrine concentrations greater than 1:200,000 (5 μg/ml) produce little advantage in further reducing peak plasma local anesthetic concentrations and may, in addition, cause adverse sympathomimetic side effects.

Peak blood or plasma concentrations of lidocaine and bupivacaine after administration for various regional procedures are given in Tables 11.4 and 11.5. The re-

lationship between cardiovascular and central nervous system toxicity and blood concentrations of lidocaine is depicted in Figure 11.9. When bupivacaine was administered intravenously to five subjects (10 mg/min for 8 to 12.5 minutes), all the subjects exhibited lightheadedness, circumoral numbness, and disorientation, while four showed signs of central nervous system toxicity such as muscular twitching, nystagmus, and slurred speech. None of the subjects had convulsions. During the period of the infusion, the mean plasma bupivacaine concentration for the five subjects was 2.24 μg/ml. Other studies have confirmed that symptoms of central nervous system toxicity occur at plasma bupivacaine concentrations of about 2.0 to 2.6 μg/ml. However, plasma bupivacaine concentrations as high as 4 μg/ml have been observed during prolonged epidural infusions without signs of serious toxicity. It has been suggested that the post-

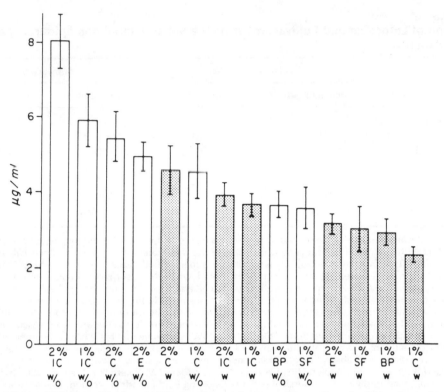

Figure 11.8.   Relationship between mean maximum plasma level of mepivacaine (Cp. $\pm$ SEM) and route of injection.   *IC,* intercostal; *C,* caudal; *E,* epidural; *BP,* brachial plexus; *SF,* sciatic/femoral; *w/o,* plain solution; *w,* plus epinephrine (1:200,000; *stippled blocks*). (With permission from Tucker GT, Moore DC, Bridenbaugh PO, Bridenbaugh LD, Thompson GE: Systemic absorption of mepivacaine in commonly used regional block procedures. *Anesthesiology* 37:277–287, 1972.)

operative increase in α_1-acid glycoprotein observed after trauma and surgery increases bupivacaine binding, thereby reducing free (active) concentrations.

Systemic Disposition Kinetics

Following absorption from the site of injection into the systemic circulation, local anesthetics first undergo distribution from the blood into interstitial and cellular fluids, followed by elimination which is mainly by metabolism and to a small extent by renal excretion (Fig. 11.4).

Drug distribution is influenced by physicochemical properties such as lipid solubility, plasma protein binding, and degree of ionization as well as physiological factors such as regional blood flow.

Important determinants of local anesthetic distribution include plasma drug binding and acid-base balance. The longer-acting amide anesthetic agents exhibit higher plasma protein binding than the shorter-acting agents (Table 11.2). In addition, these drugs also bind to red blood cells, and blood/plasma drug concentration ratios are inversely related to plasma binding (see Chapter 1 for discussion of significance of whole blood to plasma concentration ratios). The principal binding protein for many of the basic amide local anesthetics is α_1-acid glycoprotein, and the reduced binding of lidocaine in the neonate is due in part to their lower levels of α_1-acid glycoprotein (see Chapter 12). Bupivacaine also binds avidly to α_1-acid glycoprotein. The effects of protein binding and acid-base balance

Table 11.4.
Maximum Blood or Plasma Concentrations of Lidocaine after Administration for Regional Anesthesia

Route	Dose (mg)	Concentration (%)	Venous blood (B) or plasma (P) concentration (μg/ml)
Endotracheal	400	4	1.07 (B)
	400	4	0.77 (P)
	2 mg/kg	4	1.7–2.4 (B)
Brachial plexus	400*	2	~3.4 (P)
	400*	2 with epinephrine	~2.4 (P)
	6.2 mg/kg	1.5 with epinephrine	2.5 (P)
Intercostal block	400	1	6.0 (P)
	400	1 with epinephrine	4.9)P)
	400	4	8.42 (P)
Peridural	300–550	2	1.7–9.4 (B)
	300–680	2 with epinephrine	1.0–4.4 (B)
	200	2	3.3 (P)
	400	2	4.27 (P)
	400	2 with epinephrine	3.0 (P)
Caudal	6.6 mg/kg	1.5	1.8 (P)

Data with permission from Tucker GT, Mather LE: Clinical pharmacokinetics of local anesthetics. *Clin Pharma cokinet* 4:241–278, 1979.
*With bupivacaine.

Table 11.5.
Maximum Blood or Plasma Concentrations of Bupivacaine after Administration for Regional Anesthesia

Route	Dose (mg)	Concentration (%)	Venous blood (B) or plasma (P) concentration (μg/ml)
Pudendal	25	0.25 with epinephrine	0.31 (P)
Brachial plexus	300	0.5 with epinephrine	1.55 (P)
	150*	0.75	~1.0 (P)
	150*	0.75 with epinephrine	~0.5 (P)
Intercostal block	400	0.5 with epinephrine	2.5 (P)
	70	0.5 with epinephrine	0.26 (B)
Peridural	150	0.5 with epinephrine	1.14 (P)
	150	0.5	1.26 (P)
	225	0.75 with epinephrine	2.33 (P)
	70–100	0.5 with epinephrine	0.33 (B)
	25	0.25 with epinephrine	0.16 (P)
	150	0.75 with epinephrine	1.19 (P)
	225	0.75 with epinephrine	1.25 (P)

Data with permission from Tucker GT, Mather LE: Clinical pharmacokinetics of local anesthetics. *Clin Pharma-cokinet* 4:241–278, 1979.
*With chloroprocaine.

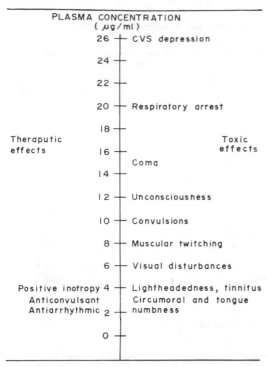

PLASMA CONCENTRATION
(μg/ml)

26 — CVS depression

24 —

22 —

20 — Respiratory arrest

18 —

Theraputic   Toxic
effects   16 —   effects

           Coma
14 —

12 — Unconsciousness

10 — Convulsions

8 — Muscular twitching

6 — Visual disturbances

Positive inotropy 4 — Lightheadedness, tinnitus
Anticonvulsant   Circumoral and tongue
Antiarrhythmic 2 — numbness

0 —

Figure 11.9.   The relationship between lidocaine plasma concentration and pharmacological effect. (With permission from Mather LE, Cousins MJ: Local anaesthetics and their current clinical use. *Drugs* 18:185–205, 1979.)

on local anesthetic distribution and membrane transfer are discussed in Chapters 1 and 12.

The pharmacokinetic parameters describing the disposition of the important amide local anesthetics are given in Table 11.6. Clearance of the amide agents depends on metabolism to a large extent, since renal excretion of unchanged drug

accounts for less than 1 to 5% of the administered dose.

Lidocaine has the characteristics of a high extraction drug, having a high hepatic "first pass" extraction which results in very poor bioavailability (35%) (see Chapter 1). Thus, because it is so avidly removed as it passes through the liver, its hepatic clearance is dependent on liver blood flow. The clearance of lidocaine is, therefore, reduced in disease states such as cardiac failure, which reduce liver blood flow. This will result in higher plasma concentrations following lidocaine use in such patients. A further pharmacokinetic change in cardiac failure is the reduction in the volume of distribution (see Chapters 1 and 16). Age is also a determinant of lidocaine disposition; clearance does not appear to differ in elderly and young patients, but the elderly have a longer terminal half-life and an increased volume of distribution. The effects of cardiac, renal, and hepatic disease on the disposition of lidocaine and the calculation of dosing regimens in these situations are discussed in Chapter 16, when this drug is used as an antiarrhythmic agent.

The amide-type anesthetics are metabolized chiefly in the liver, and renal clearance of unchanged local amide anesthetic is low. Lidocaine undergoes N-dealkylation to yield monoethylglycinexylidide (MEGX) which, in turn, is followed by secondary N-dealkylation to give glycinexylidide (GX) or hydrolysis to yield 2,6-xylidine. 2,6-Xylidine is further metabolized to 4-hydroxy-2,6-xylidine, which then appears in the urine. Direct amide hydrolysis of lidocaine also

Table 11.6.
Pharmacokinetic Parameters of Some Amide Local Anesthetics

Parameter	Lidocaine	Mepivacaine	Bupivacaine	Etidocaine
Vd_{ss}* (L)	91	84	73	134
Terminal $t_{1/2}$ (hr)	1.6	1.9	2.7	2.7
Clearance, CL (L/min)	0.95	0.78	0.58	1.11

With permission from Tucker GT: Pharmacokinetics of local anaesthetics. *Br J Anaesth* 58:717–731, 1986.
*Vd_{ss}, volume of distribution at steady state.

occurs. MEGX and GX are found in significant concentrations in the blood of patients receiving lidocaine. These metabolites have pharmacological activity. MEGX is metabolized in the liver and has a terminal elimination half-life of about 120 minutes, while GX has an elimination half-life of 10 hours. Mepivacaine is metabolized to the N-demethylated derivative 2,6-pipecoloxylidide (PPX), and conjugates of the 3-hydroxy and 4-hydroxy compounds are also found in the urine. Prilocaine undergoes metabolism to yield o-toluidine which, in turn, is metabolized to 4- and 6-hydroxytoluidine. 6-Hydroxytoluidine is believed to be responsible for the methemoglobinemia which occurs following high doses of prilocaine in humans. Data on the metabolism of bupivacaine are limited, but bupivacaine is known to be metabolized to PPX.

The ester-type local anesthetics are cleared in both plasma and liver, undergoing rapid hydrolysis by plasma cholinesterase. The rates of metabolism vary markedly for the different agents. Chloroprocaine exhibits the most rapid rate of hydrolysis (4.7 μmol/ml/hour) as compared to 1.1 μmol/ml/hour for procaine and 0.3 μmol/ml/hour for tetracaine. This has obvious implications for toxicity; chloroprocaine is the least toxic of the ester-type local anesthetics, while tetracaine is the most toxic agent.

Procaine is hydrolyzed by plasma cholinesterase to paraaminobenzoic acid and diethylaminoethanol. The in vitro half-life of procaine is reported as varying between 39 and 43 seconds and is prolonged in renal and hepatic disease. Chloroprocaine is hydrolyzed by plasma cholinesterase to give 2-chloroparaaminobenzoic acid (CABA) and diethylaminoethanol. The in vitro half-life of chloroprocaine after it has been added to plasma obtained from men, nonpregnant and pregnant women, and umbilical cords at the time of delivery is given in Table 11.7, showing altered rates of in vitro metabolism in individual subjects. Plasma cholinesterase activity in newborn infants is about 50% that of adults and does not reach adult levels until

Table 11.7.
In Vitro Half-Life in Plasma of Chloroprocaine

Subject	$t_{1/2}$ (sec)
Pregnant females (7)*	20.9 ± 5.8†
Umbilical cord (7)	42.6 ± 11.2
Males (6)	20.6 ± 4.1
Nonpregnant females (5)	25.2 ± 3.7
Homozygous atypical cholinesterase carriers (10)	106.0 ± 45.0

With permission from O'Brien JE, Abbey V, Hinsvark ON, Perel J, Finster M: Metabolism and measurement of chloroprocaine, an ester type local anesthetic. *J Pharm Sci* 66:75–78, 1979.
*Numbers in parentheses, number of subjects.
†Mean ± SD.

about 1 year of age. (Chloroprocaine is also hydrolyzed at a slower rate in blood from homozygous atypical cholinesterase carriers; Table 11.7.) Because of its rapid hydrolysis, it is difficult to measure plasma concentrations of chloroprocaine directly. However, when chloroprocaine is added directly to plasma, it disappears rapidly, with an in vitro half-life measured in seconds. In vivo, however, following epidural administration, absorption continues for a prolonged period after administration, resulting in a more prolonged apparent half-life; the mean maternal in vivo half-life of chloroprocaine after epidural anesthesia has been shown to be 3.1 minutes and to range from 1.5 to 64 minutes.

Bupivacaine and neostigmine inhibit chloroprocaine hydrolysis in vitro, while there is both clinical and laboratory evidence that chloroprocaine or its metabolite decreases the efficacy of bupivacaine.

The pharmacokinetics and placental transfer of local anesthetics in obstetric anesthetic practice are discussed in Chapter 12.

PHARMACOLOGICAL EFFECTS

Local anesthetics have clinically important effects on the central nervous system, cardiovascular system, and neuromuscular junction.

Central Nervous System

Local anesthetics readily cross the blood-brain barrier causing central nervous system stimulation, followed at higher doses by depression. The severity of the central nervous system effects correlates with plasma concentration for the local anesthetic lidocaine (Fig. 11.9). At nontoxic plasma concentrations, minimal central nervous system effects are evident. The earliest signs of toxicity are circumoral and tongue numbness, which may proceed to tinnitus, nystagmus, and dizziness. Further elevations in plasma concentration cause central nervous system excitation, such as restlessness and tremor. These signs are a warning that blood concentrations are close to toxic levels. Further increases in plasma concentration lead to convulsions, coma, and cardiorespiratory arrest.

Cardiovascular System

Local anesthetics exert effects on cardiac muscle and on the peripheral vascular smooth muscle causing peripheral arteriolar dilation and myocardial depression. At toxic concentrations, the combined effects of peripheral vasodilation, decreased myocardial contractility, and depressant effects on cardiac rate and conduction lead to circulatory collapse and cardiac arrest. The electrophysiological effects of bupivacaine and lidocaine and their relative cardiotoxicity are discussed later in the chapter.

Lidocaine plasma concentrations of 2 to 5 μg/ml cause mild peripheral vasodilation, with slight or no changes in myocardial contractility, diastolic volume, and cardiac output. Lidocaine concentrations of 5 to 10 μg/ml cause a progressive decrease in myocardial contractility, increase in diastolic volume, and decrease in cardiac output, while levels above 10 μg/ml cause depression of peripheral vascular resistance and a marked decrease in myocardial contractility resulting in profound hypotension. The cardiovascular effects of the local anesthetics

are not usually evident after most regional anesthetic procedures, unless inadvertent systemic injection and the attainment of high blood concentrations occur.

Some local anesthetics have a quinidine-like action on the heart. Procaine resembles quinidine in that it increases the refractory period, raises the threshold for stimulation, and prolongs conduction time. Although procaine is unsuitable for use as an antiarrhythmic agent, procainamide is of therapeutic importance in the management of abnormalities of cardiac rhythm (see Chapter 16).

Neuromuscular Junction

Local anesthetics can affect transmission at the neuromuscular junction and, in certain situations, potentiate the effects of the depolarizing and nondepolarizing muscle relaxants (see Chapter 10).

TOXICITY OF LOCAL ANESTHETICS

Once local anesthetics are absorbed into the circulation, they can cause systemic toxicity. The most common causes of adverse reactions to local anesthetics are accidental intravascular injection and overdosage. Local anesthetics exert toxic effects on the cardiovascular and central nervous systems in particular, and the correlation of adverse effects and blood concentrations for lidocaine are given in Figure 11.9. Toxic blood concentrations may result in convulsions, followed by respiratory depression, coma, and cardiovascular collapse. Treatment of toxic reactions includes management of the airway and administration of oxygen, while convulsions may be treated by diazepam or thiopental. Rarely, convulsions may persist, and a neuromuscular relaxant may be required. Cardiovascular depression should be treated by elevation of the legs and administration of a vasopressor agent such as ephedrine (15 to 30 mg) in the first instance. Hypoxia and acidosis should be immediately corrected, and prolonged inotropic support may be required. Atropine may be needed to reverse bradycardia.

Cardiotoxicity

During the late 1970s and early 1980s in the United States, cases were described in which the use of bupivacaine (especially high concentrations of 0.75%) was associated with profound cardiovascular depression and even death in some instances. Many of these patients were pregnant. A special feature of these cases was that cardiovascular depression and arrhythmias, such as ventricular fibrillation, occurred early and were resistant to therapy. During the same period, several cases of death due to intravenous regional anesthesia (Bier's block) using bupivacaine were reported in the United Kingdom. These case reports alerted anesthesiologists to the possibility that the more potent local anesthetics, such as bupivacaine and etidocaine, might be more cardiotoxic than other local anes-

thetics, such as lidocaine. Local anesthetic-induced myocardial toxicity is rare in clinical practice, because of the large dose of drug necessary to produce this effect and because usually the signs and symptoms of central nervous system toxicity precede the cardiovascular effects, thus alerting the physician to the possibility of toxicity.

CC/CNS RATIO

The ratio of dosage or blood levels required to produce irreversible cardiovascular collapse to the dosage or blood levels required to elicit convulsions, i.e., central nervous system toxicity, has been termed the CC/CNS ratio and has been shown to be lower for bupivacaine and etidocaine than for lidocaine in adult sheep (Fig. 11.10). The CC/CNS dose ratio for lidocaine is about 7.0, indicating

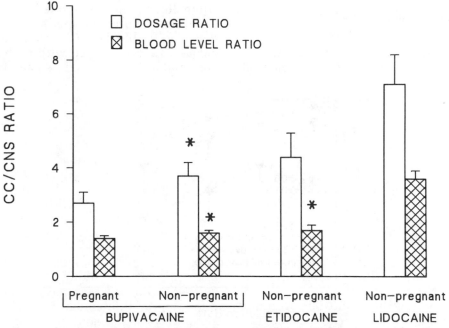

Figure 11.10. Bupivacaine and lidocaine toxicity in pregnant and nonpregnant sheep. Comparison of bupivacaine doses and blood concentrations associated with the onset of circulatory collapse and convulsions (*CC/CNS* ratio) with those of lidocaine, indicating that a narrower margin of safety exists for bupivacaine than lidocaine in nonpregnant sheep. *, significantly different from lidocaine. (Data from Morishima HO, Pedersen H, Finster M, Hiraoka H, Tsuiji A, Feldman HS, Arthur GR, Covino BG: Bupivacaine toxicity in pregnant and nonpregnant ewes. *Anesthesiology* 63:134–139, 1985; and Morishima HO, Pedersen H, Finster M, Sakuma K, Bruce SL, Gutsche BB, Stark RI, Covino BG: Toxicity of lidocaine in adult, newborn, and fetal sheep. *Anesthesiology* 55:57–61, 1981.)

that 7 times as much drug is needed to induce irreversible cardiovascular collapse as is required to produce convulsions, thus providing the warning of convulsions well before cardiovascular collapse occurs. In contrast, the CC/CNS dose ratio in pregnant sheep for bupivacaine is even lower, i.e., 2.7. Similar results exist for CC/CNS blood level ratios, when narrower CC/CNS ratios have been shown for bupivacaine and etidocaine than lidocaine. In addition, myocardial tissue levels of various local anesthetics determined at the time of irreversible cardiovascular collapse have shown that bupivacaine and etidocaine myocardial tissue/blood concentration ratios are higher than those obtained for lidocaine. Other studies have shown that the myocardial uptake of bupivacaine and lidocaine is similar but that bupivacaine is removed from the myocardium much more slowly than lidocaine.

ELECTROPHYSIOLOGICAL EFFECTS— VENTRICULAR ARRHYTHMIAS

Local anesthetics have been known for many years to exert electrophysiological effects on the heart, and lidocaine has been widely used as an antiarrhythmic agent. Local anesthetics depress the maximal rate of increase of the cardiac action potential (V_{max}, maximum upstroke velocity of the action potential) in a dose-dependent manner. V_{max} is a direct measure of the fast inward sodium current. Clarkson and Hondeghem have shown that in vitro both lidocaine and bupivacaine, like other anesthetics, depress V_{max}. However, the state and rate-dependent block for the two agents are dissimilar. Lidocaine binds to both open and inactivated channels and dissociates from the channel rapidly after an action potential. On the other hand, bupivacaine binds only to inactivated channels and dissociates more slowly (Fig. 11.11). Such differences are likely to be due to differences in the physicochemical properties of the two drugs, i.e., lipid solubility and protein binding. It is interesting that, when lidocaine was applied to bupivacaine-treated preparations, sodium channels were unblocked. Clarkson and Hondeghem suggested that, with each action potential, lidocaine occupied any free re-

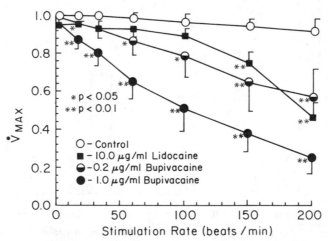

Figure 11.11. Mechanism for bupivacaine depression of cardiac conduction. The effect of bupivacaine and lidocaine on V_{max} (the maximum upstroke velocity of the cardiac action potential) at different stimulation rates. Bupivacaine markedly depresses the rapid phase of depolarization (V_{max}) in isolated guinea pig ventricular muscle preparations. In addition, the rate of recovery from a steady-state block was slower for bupivacaine than lidocaine. (With permission from Clarkson SW, Hondeghem LM: Mechanism for bupivacaine depression of cardiac conduction: fast block of sodium channels during the action potential with slow recovery from block during diastole. *Anesthesiology* 62:396–405, 1985.)

ceptors when channels were open and thereby prevented bupivacaine block of inactivated channels. Since recovery from lidocaine block was fast, repeated stimulations resulted in fewer bupivacaine-blocked channels. This finding may be important for the treatment of bupivacaine-induced cardiac toxicity. Thus, the differences in the manner in which lidocaine and bupivacaine block cardiac sodium channels (i.e., differences in their affinity for and duration of binding to sodium channels) may be fundamental to the relative cardiotoxicity of lidocaine and bupivacaine.

In the in vivo situation, a reduction in V_{max} will result in prolongation of the PR and QRS interval on the electrocardiogram, and it is interesting that differences between lidocaine and bupivacaine have also been demonstrated in their effects on conducting tissue. Bupivacaine and etidocaine cause nodal and ventricular arrhythmias and wide QRS complexes at plasma concentrations associated with central nervous system toxicity, while lidocaine does not. Reiz and Nath injected lidocaine and bupivacaine directly into the coronary arteries of pigs and showed that bupivacaine caused QRS prolongation at much lower doses than lidocaine; comparable prolongations of the QRS interval with bupivacaine and lidocaine were obtained at a 1:16 dose ratio. However, depression of left ventricular contractility occurred in a dose-dependent fashion that reflected the drugs' anesthetic potency (bupivacaine/lidocaine = 4:1). Sudden ventricular fibrillation was caused by both lidocaine and bupivacaine again at a ratio of about 1:16. Thus, many of these animal studies appear to show that bupivacaine is more likely to have deleterious effects on conducting tissue and myocardial ventricular muscle than lidocaine. Although all local anesthetics exert a dose-dependent negative inotropic action, the more potent local anesthetics, such as bupivacaine, appear to depress myocardial contractility at lower doses and concentrations than less potent local anesthetics, such as lidocaine.

CARDIOTOXICITY AND PREGNANCY

The majority of clinical reports of bupivacaine cardiotoxicity have been in pregnant patients. It is possible that the pregnant patient may be more susceptible to the toxic effects of local anesthetics; the CC/CNS dosage ratio for bupivacaine is lower in pregnant than in nonpregnant sheep (Fig. 11.10).

RESUSCITATION

Many of the reported cases of cardiotoxicity have described difficulty in cardiac resuscitation. Rapid correction of acidosis and hypoxia is important, and treatment of central nervous system (CNS) toxicity, such as convulsions, is imperative. The drug treatment of ventricular fibrillation occurring as a result of bupivacaine is difficult; lidocaine and bupivacaine may have additive CNS effects, but there is evidence that lidocaine may be effective in this situation (see Chapter 16). Bretylium has been advocated as it has been shown to be effective in laboratory studies, and the cardiac arrhythmias may be of the reentrant type.

ACIDOSIS AND HYPOXIA

Acidosis and hypoxia markedly potentiate the cardiovascular toxicity of bupivacaine, perhaps more than lidocaine.

Neurotoxicity

Although the potential neurotoxicity of local anesthetics has been of concern to anesthesiologists for many years, the agents used clinically rarely result in localized nerve damage. Large epidemiological studies of spinal anesthesia attest to the safety of this technique. However, animal studies in the laboratory show that local anesthetics can cause neurotoxicity at concentrations much higher than those employed clinically.

The potential neurotoxicity of chloroprocaine became the subject of considerable debate, when cases of prolonged sensory and motor deficits following inadvertent subarachnoid injection of chloroprocaine intended for epidural anesthesia appeared in the literature in 1980 and after. Animal studies that followed in an attempt to clarify the issue yielded contradictory results, some studies demonstrating neurologic deficits while others failed to confirm these observations. The local neural toxicity of chloroprocaine is now believed to be due to the antioxidant sodium bisulfite present as a preservative, and perhaps the low pH of the anesthetic solution. Commercial preparations of chloroprocaine containing sodium bisulfite result in paralysis in rabbits when injected intrathecally, while pure chloroprocaine does not. Sodium bisulfite alone administered into the subarachnoid space is associated with paralysis. Isolated nerve studies have also shown that the combination of a low pH and bisulfite may be responsible for irreversible conduction blockade. Chloroprocaine itself, therefore, does not appear to be neurotoxic. **Pure chloroprocaine** (sodium bisulfite and methylparaben free) is now available for epidural use, while chloroprocaine with methylparaben is available in multiple-dose vials for infiltration block only.

Hypersensitivity

Hypersensitivity is extremely rare and may be manifest as localized edema, urticaria, bronchospasm, and anaphylaxis. Dermatitis may occur following skin application or as contact dermatitis in dentists. Ester derivatives of paraaminobenzoic acid cause most of the hypersensitivity reactions, and hypersensitivity to the amide local anesthetics is unusual, although hypersensitivity to lidocaine has been reported.

USE OF VASOCONSTRICTORS

All local anesthetics except cocaine cause peripheral vasodilation by direct relaxation of blood vessel smooth muscle. Cocaine inhibits the uptake of norepinephrine by the adrenergic nerve terminal, thus potentiating the action of catecholamines, and unlike other local anesthetics, causes vasoconstriction and mydriasis. The vasodilator property of the local anesthetics enhances their vascular absorption; addition of a vasoconstrictor to the local anesthetic solution decreases vascular absorption, resulting in the drug being in contact with nerve tissue for a longer period of time, thus prolonging the period of conduction blockade. In clinical practice, local anesthetic solutions usually contain epinephrine, at a concentration of 5 μg/ml (1:200,000 dilution). Epinephrine decreases the rate of absorption of local anesthetic into the systemic circulation, not only prolonging the duration of blockade but also reducing systemic toxicity.

Some of the vasoconstrictor agent may itself be absorbed into the systemic circulation, and about 10 minutes after the use of local anesthetic solution containing epinephrine, sympathomimetic effects may be evident. The use of vasoconstrictors is contraindicated in nerve blocks to areas supplied by end arteries which have limited collateral circulation (such as digits, hand, feet, and penis) and in certain disease states such as hypertension and thyrotoxicosis.

INDIVIDUAL LOCAL ANESTHETICS: ESTERS

Cocaine, procaine, tetracaine, and chloroprocaine have ester linkages in their intermediate chain and are hydrolyzed at varying rates by plasma pseudocholinesterase. Cocaine is an ester of benzoic acid, while the remainder of the esters are derivatives of paraaminobenzoic acid.

Cocaine

Cocaine is an alkaloid obtained from the leaves of *Erythroxylon coca* (coca tree) which is indigenous to Peru and Bolivia. The leaves have been chewed by natives of these South American countries for centuries because of the ability of cocaine to produce euphoria and to increase capacity for muscular work due to sympathetic and central nervous system stimulation. It is an ester of benzoic acid, and its structural formula is given in Figure 11.3.

CENTRAL NERVOUS SYSTEM

Cocaine stimulates the central nervous system; in low doses it produces a feeling of well-being and euphoria accompanied in some cases by excitement and restlessness. Higher doses cause convulsions, coma, medullary depression, and death due to respiratory failure. Cocaine stimulates the vomiting center.

CARDIOVASCULAR SYSTEM

Cocaine blocks the uptake of catecholamines at adrenergic nerve endings and, thus, enhances the effects of both sympathetic nervous system stimulation and endogenously and exogenously administered catecholamines. Cocaine causes vasoconstriction and mydriasis, probably due to sympathetic stimulation. Bradycardia due to central vagal stimulation may occur after small doses, while moderate doses cause central and peripheral sympathetic stimulation resulting in tachycardia, peripheral vasoconstriction, and hypertension. Larger doses may cause direct myocardial depression, ventricular fibrillation, and death.

LOCAL ANESTHETIC EFFECTS

Cocaine blocks nerve conduction when applied directly to nerve tissue and, thus, can be used for surface anesthesia. Although cocaine was once widely used for ophthalmological procedures, it is not used for this purpose today, because it causes sloughing of the corneal epithelium and raises intraocular pressure. The toxic and addictive properties of cocaine make cocaine unsuitable for parenteral use, and today it is only used for topical anesthesia.

SUGGESTED DOSAGE AND ADMINISTRATION

Cocaine USP and cocaine hydrochloride USP are preparations of the alkaloid available *only* for surface anesthesia. Solutions employed for surface anesthesia vary from 1.0 to 10.0%; 4 to 5% concentration is recommended for mucous membranes of the mouth, nose, and throat. Cocaine causes vasoconstriction, and the use of epinephrine with cocaine is not only unnecessary but potentially dangerous in that cocaine "sensitizes" the heart to catecholamines.

TOXICITY, PRECAUTIONS, AND CONTRAINDICATIONS

Cocaine is a drug of addiction. Overdosage may cause sympathetic nervous system stimulation, excitement, restlessness, headache, and vomiting.

Procaine

Procaine is a derivative of paraaminobenzoic acid and was synthesized by Einhorn in 1905. Its structural formula is given in Figure 11.3. It has a short duration of action. Its high pKa (Table 11.2) makes it highly ionized at plasma pH and, thus, it has poor spreading or penetrating properties. Procaine has vasodilator activity, is rapidly absorbed following parenteral administration, and does not remain long at the site of injection. It is, therefore, ineffective as a surface anesthetic. In order to delay systemic absorption, vasoconstrictor drugs are often added to procaine solutions. The pharmacological actions of procaine are similar to those of local anesthetics in general. Procaine has antiarrhythmic, quinidine-like effects, but is unsuitable for clinical use because of its central nervous system toxicity and rapid biotransformation. Procainamide, a congener of procaine, has been developed as an effective oral antiarrhythmic agent (see Chapter 16).

DRUG INTERACTIONS

Procaine is hydrolyzed to produce paraaminobenzoic acid, which antagonizes the pharmacological action of the sulfonamides. Procaine may prolong the effect of succinylcholine, since both drugs are metabolized by the same enzyme (see Chapters 5 and 10). Anticholinesterase drugs increase the toxicity of normally safe doses of procaine by inhibiting its degradation: the metabolism of procaine is also reduced in patients with genetic abnormalities of plasma cholinesterase.

SUGGESTED DOSAGE AND ADMINISTRATION

Procaine is little used today as a local anesthetic. However, it may be used as a 1 or 2% solution with epinephrine for infiltration and nerve block and as a 5% solution mixed with an equal volume of 5% dextrose for spinal anesthesia. Procaine has also been used to treat patients developing malignant hyperpyrexia and to prolong the action of other drugs, by forming poorly soluble salts or conjugates, for example, procaine penicillin G.

Chloroprocaine

Chloroprocaine is a halogenated derivative of procaine, and its structural formula is given in Figure 11.3. Chloroprocaine has pharmacological properties similar to procaine. The rapid plasma hydrolysis of chloroprocaine results in low toxicity and a short duration of action. Its onset of action is about 6 to 12 minutes, and the duration of anesthesia is about 30 to 60 minutes, depending on the amount of local anesthetic used.

SUGGESTED DOSAGE AND ADMINISTRATION

The maximum single recommended doses* of chloroprocaine with and without epinephrine (1:200,000) are 1000 and 800 mg, respectively. Chloroprocaine is available as 1.0, 2.0, and 3.0% solutions. It is ineffective for topical anesthesia. A 1.0% solution is suitable for infiltration anesthesia, when it has a duration of anesthesia of about 45 to 60 minutes (70 to 80 minutes with epinephrine). For peripheral nerve block, a 1.0% solution may be employed; the duration of anesthesia is only 45 minutes (70 minutes

---

*Maximum suggested safe doses of local anesthetics stated here are a guide to clinical use, and no single maximum safe dose exists for an individual local anesthetic. The upper limit of safe dosage is quoted for regional procedures (not subarachnoid block), and if that dose were to be administered intravenously, serious toxicity would ensue. In addition, these dosages should not be injected into highly vascular areas.

with epinephrine). A 2.0 or 3.0% solution may be used for epidural and caudal blockade, when the duration of action is 30 to 45 minutes (70 minutes with the addition of epinephrine, 1:200,000). Low toxicity, short duration of action, rapid metabolism, and low fetal/neonatal blood levels make chloroprocaine a suitable anesthetic for obstetric practice (see Chapter 12).

The use of chloroprocaine for epidural anesthesia has declined because of reports of neurotoxicity following accidental subarachnoid injection. The local neurotoxicity of chloroprocaine may be due to the preservative, sodium bisulfite, and pure chloroprocaine (sodium bisulfite and methyl paraben free) is now available for epidural use.

Tetracaine

Tetracaine is an ester of paraaminobenzoic acid, and its structural formula is given in Figure 11.3. It is a potent, long-acting local anesthetic, which is hydrolyzed by plasma pseudocholinesterase at a much slower rate than the shorter-acting local anesthetics, procaine and chloroprocaine. Paraaminobenzoic acid is a metabolite. Its pharmacological effects are similar to those of local anesthetics in general, which have been described earlier in this chapter.

SUGGESTED DOSAGE AND ADMINISTRATION

Solutions of 1.0% tetracaine are available for spinal anesthesia, when the dose varies from 5.0 to 20.0 mg; tetracaine is mixed with distilled water (hypobaric spinal anesthesia), 10% dextrose (hyperbaric spinal anesthesia), or cerebrospinal fluid (isobaric spinal anesthesia). The onset of blockade occurs within about 10 minutes, and the duration of anesthesia is 60 to 90 minutes. It is a useful local anesthetic agent when the amide group of local anesthetics are contraindicated, for example, in malignant hyperpyrexia. The maximum suggested therapeutic dose is 1.0 to 1.5 mg/kg or 100 mg for an average (70 kg) healthy adult patient.

INDIVIDUAL LOCAL ANESTHETICS: AMIDES

Lidocaine

The structural formula and physicochemical properties are given in Figure 11.3 and Table 11.2, respectively. Lidocaine has a rapid onset of action and intermediate potency and duration of action. It is one of the most widely used local anesthetics.

SUGGESTED DOSAGE AND ADMINISTRATION

Lidocaine is effective for the production of analgesia by infiltration, nerve, epidural, caudal, and spinal block, and topical application. It is often used with epinephrine to prolong the action and reduce the rate of systemic absorption. A 4% solution is recommended for topical application to the oropharynx and tracheobronchial tree in adults, while a 2% solution is also available for infants. A 2% viscous solution is sometimes used for topical application to the mouth. The onset of action following topical application is 5 minutes, with a duration of action of 15 to 30 minutes. Lidocaine can be used for infiltration anesthesia with a solution of 0.5 to 1.0%, with or without epinephrine. Onset of anesthesia is rapid, and duration of anesthesia is 75 minutes without epinephrine and 400 minutes with epinephrine using the 1.0% local anesthetic solution. Lidocaine is also employed for peripheral nerve blockade, as a 0.5 to 1.0% solution with or without epinephrine. Onset of anesthesia for a major nerve block, such as brachial plexus block, occurs within 5 to 15 minutes of administration and lasts for about 60 minutes without epinephrine and 120 minutes with epinephrine. Lidocaine for epidural and caudal block is administered as a 1.0 to 2.0% solution with or without epinephrine, depending on the degree of sensory and motor block required. Onset of blockade results in 5 to 20 minutes, with a duration of action of about 60 minutes without epinephrine and 100 minutes with epinephrine. Lidocaine has also been employed for spinal anesthesia, where it has a rapid onset and the duration of anesthesia is about 60 minutes without epinephrine and about 90 minutes with epinephrine. It is administered as a 5% solution in 7.5% dextrose.

The upper limit for safe dosage in the adult is 200 to 400 mg without epinephrine and 500 mg with epinephrine or 7.0 mg/kg. Lidocaine, 400 mg, injected into the epidural space results in blood concentrations in the range of 2.0 to 4 μg/ml. Toxic symptoms occur at blood concentrations above 5 μg/ml (Fig. 11.9), and convulsions are associated with blood concentrations of 10 μg/ml. The intravenous use of lidocaine in the treatment of cardiac dysrhythmias is discussed in Chapter 16.

Mepivacaine

The structural formula and physicochemical properties of mepivacaine are given in Figure 11.3 and Table 11.2, respectively. It is a local anesthetic of the amide type and is used for infiltration, nerve, epidural, and caudal block but is ineffective topically. It has a similar potency and speed of onset as lidocaine, but slightly longer duration of action, and is administered in doses and concentrations similar to those of lidocaine. The upper limit of safe dosage in the adult for mepivacaine is 400 mg (500 mg with epinephrine) or 7.0 mg/kg. For reasons outlined in Chapter 12, mepivacaine is not a satisfactory agent in obstetric anesthetic practice.

Prilocaine

The structural formula and physicochemical properties appear in Figure 11.3 and Table 11.2, respectively. Prilocaine is equipotent to lidocaine, but its duration of action is longer, and it is less toxic. It can be used for all types of blockade in concentrations similar to those of lidocaine. The upper limit of safe dosage is 400 to 500 mg (600 mg with epinephrine) or 8.0 mg/kg. Prilocaine undergoes rapid hepatic metabolism to *o*-toluidine, which is thought to cause methemoglobinemia when high doses of prilocaine (above 600 mg) are administered. The metabolite *o*-toluidine is thought to be responsible for the oxidation of hemoglobin to methemoglobin. Methemoglobinemia can be successfully treated by the intravenous administration of methylene blue, 1.0 mg/kg.

Bupivacaine

The structural formula and physicochemical properties of bupivacaine are given in Figure 11.3 and Table 11.2. Its structure is the same as that of mepivacaine, with the exception that a butyl group replaces the methyl group on the amino nitrogen. It is about 4 times more potent than lidocaine and has a prolonged duration of action. Its speed of onset is slower than that of mepivacaine and lidocaine.

SUGGESTED DOSAGE AND ADMINISTRATION

Bupivacaine is administered for the production of infiltration anesthesia in concentrations of 0.125 to 0.25% with or without epinephrine. Onset of anesthesia is reasonably rapid, and duration of anesthesia is 200 minutes (400 minutes with epinephrine). For peripheral nerve block, 0.25 to 0.5% solutions with and without epinephrine are employed. The onset of action is slow (10 to 20 minutes). Duration of anesthesia is about 400 minutes, and the addition of epinephrine only marginally increases duration of effect. Bupivacaine is very popular for production of epidural blockade when solutions of 0.25 to 0.5% are employed with or without epinephrine.

The obstetric use of bupivacaine has been rarely associated with sudden cardiovascular collapse following accidental systemic administration and is discussed earlier in the chapter. Bupivacaine solutions, 0.75%, are no longer recommended for obstetric use in the United States. Bupivacaine has recently been advocated for spinal anesthesia, when doses of 5 to 20 mg produce anesthesia of similar duration to tetracaine, i.e., 2 to 4 hours. Isobaric and hyperbaric solutions of 0.5% and 0.75% bupivacaine have been extensively investigated for surgical procedures performed under subarachnoid blockade. Each 1.0 ml of bupivacaine for spinal use (Marcaine spinal) contains 7.5 mg of bupivacaine chloride and 82.5 mg of dextrose and can be used with or without epinephrine. The upper limit of safe bupivacaine dosage in the adult is 150 mg without epinephrine and 200 mg with epinephrine or 2.0 mg/kg.

Etidocaine

Etidocaine (Figure 11.3) is a long-acting derivative of lidocaine, and its physicochemical properties are described in Table 11.2. It can be seen that, although etidocaine is structurally similar to lidocaine, it differs in certain physicochemical properties and possesses a greater degree of lipid solubility and plasma protein binding capacity. It is about 2 to 3 times more potent than lidocaine but less toxic than bupivacaine. Etidocaine has a similar onset of action to that of lidocaine, but a more prolonged duration of action. Etidocaine is effective for infiltration anesthesia, peripheral nerve block, and epidural and caudal blockade. Etidocaine produces a high degree of motor blockade when administered into the epidural space. The upper limit of safe dosage in the adult is 300 mg (400 mg with epinephrine) or 4.0 mg/kg. Etidocaine is available as a 0.5 and 1.0% solution with and without epinephrine and a 1.5% solution with epinephrine.

EMLA

A new topical local anesthetic ointment or cream (EMLA) containing a eutectic mixture of lidocaine and prilocaine has been developed to produce dermal analgesia. A *eutectic* mixture is one which has a melting point lower than each individual constituent, so that a mixture of lidocaine and prilocaine is an oil at temperatures above 16°C. Consequently, 80% of the emulsion droplets in EMLA cream is local anesthetic base, and it is no longer necessary to dissolve or dilute the drug. Normally, local anesthetics have little effect on intact skin, since the ability to penetrate the skin requires high concentrations of local anesthetic, and previous topical emulsions have at the most 20% of the drug in the base form. EMLA (eutectic mixture of local anesthetics) is a formulation in which the active agents are present in greater concentrations than would be possible with either base alone. EMLA may be particularly useful to anesthesiologists to reduce the pain of venipuncture, especially in children.

BIBLIOGRAPHY

General

Bengtsson M, Edstrom HH, Lofstrom JB: Spinal analgesia with bupivacaine, mepivacaine, and tetracaine. *Acta Anaesthesiol Scand* 17:278–283, 1983.

Blair MR: Cardiovascular pharmacology of local anesthetics. *Br J Anaesth* 47:247–252, 1975.

Bromage PR: Physiology and pharmacology of epidural analgesia. *Anesthesiology* 28:592–622, 1967.

Bromage PR, Burfoot MF, Crowell DE, Truant AP: Quality of epidural blockade. III. Carbonated local anaesthetic solutions. *Br J Anaesth* 39:197–208, 1967.

Concepcion M, Covino BG: Rational use of local anaesthetics. *Drugs* 27:256–270, 1984.

Covino BG: New developments in the field of local anesthetics and the scientific basis for their clinical use. *Acta Anaesthesiol Scand* 26:242–249, 1982.

Covino BG: Pharmacology of local anaesthetic agents. *Br J Anaesth* 58:701–716, 1986.

DeJong RH: Differential nerve block by local anesthetics. *Anesthesiology* 53:443–444, 1980.

Evers H, VonDarde O, Juhlin L, Ohlsen L, Vinnars E: Dermal effects of compositions based on the eutectic mixture of lignocaine and prilocaine (EMLA): studies in volunteers. *Br J Anaesth* 57:997–1005, 1985.

Gissen AJ, Covino BG, Gregus J: Differential sensitivity of fast and slow fibers in mammalian nerve. II. Margin of safety for nerve transmission. *Anesth Analg* 61:561–569, 1982.

Greene NM: Uptake and elimination of local anesthetics during spinal anesthesia. *Anesth Analg* 62:1013–1024, 1983.

Jack JJB: Physiology of peripheral nerve fibres in relation to their size. *Br J Anaesth* 47:173–182, 1975.

Jorfeldt L, Lofstrom B, Pernow B, Persson B, Wahren J, Widman B: The effect of local anaesthetics on the central circulation and respiration in man and dog. *Acta Anaesthesiol Scand* 12:153–169, 1968.

Lund PC, Cwik JC, Gannon FT: Extradural anaesthesia: choice of local anaesthetic agents. *Br J Anaesth* 47:313–321, 1975.

Maunuksela EL, Korpela R: Double-blind evaluation of a lignocaine-prilocaine cream (EMLA) in children. *Br J Anaesth* 58:1242–1245, 1986.

Moore DC: Spinal anesthesia: bupivacaine compared with tetracaine. *Anesth Analg* 59:743–750, 1980.

Moore DC, Bridenbaugh LD, Thompson GE, Balfour RI, Horton WG: Factors determining dosages of amide-type local anesthetic drugs. *Anesthesiology* 47:263–268, 1977.

Stanton-Hicks M, Murphy TM, Bonica JJ, Berges PU, Mather LE, Tucker GT: Effects of peridural block. V. Properties, circulatory effects, and blood levels of etidocaine and lidocaine. *Anesthesiology* 42:398–407, 1975.

Swerdlow M, Jones R: The duration of action of bupivacaine, prilocaine, and lignocaine. *Br J Anaesth* 42:335–339, 1970.

Takman BH: The chemistry of local anaesthetic agents: classification of blocking agents. *Br J Anaesth* 47:183–190, 1975.

Wildsmith JAW: Peripheral nerve and local anaesthetic drugs. *Br J Anaesth* 58:692–700, 1986.

Wildsmith JAW, Strichartz GR: Local anaesthetic drugs—an historical perspective. *Br J Anaesth* 56:937–939, 1984.

Willatts DG, Reynolds F: Comparison of the vasoactivity of amide and ester local anaesthetics. An intradermal study. *Br J Anaesth* 57:1006–1011, 1985.

Mechanism of Action

Catterall WA: Common modes of drug action on Na$^+$ channels: local anesthetics, antiarrhythmics, and anticonvulsants. *Trends Pharmacol Sci* 8:57–65, 1987.

Clarkson CW, Hondeghem LM: Mechanism for bupivacaine depression of cardiac conduction: fast block of sodium channels during the action potential with slow recovery from block during diastole. *Anesthesiology* 62:396–405, 1985.

Courtney KR: Local anesthetics. Molecular basis of drug action in anesthesia. *Int Anesthesiol Clin* 26:239–247, 1983.

Kendig JJ: Clinical implications of the modulated receptor hypothesis: local anesthetics and the heart. *Anesthesiology* 62:382–384, 1985.

Lee AG: A consumers' guide to models of local anesthetic action. *Anesthesiology* 51:64–71, 1979.

Pharmacokinetics

Arthur GR, Scott DHT, Boyes RN, Scott DB: Pharmacokinetic and clinical pharmacological studies with mepivacaine and prilocaine. *Br J Anaesth* 51:481–485, 1979.

Benowitz ML, Meister W: Clinical pharmacokinetics of lignocaine. *Clin Pharmacokinet* 3:177–201, 1978.

Benowitz N, Forsyth RP, Melmon KL, Rowland M: Lidocaine disposition kinetics in monkey and man. I. Prediction by a perfusion model. *Clin Pharmacol Ther* 16:87–98, 1974.

Boyes RN: A review of the metabolism of amide local anaesthetic agents. *Br J Anaesth* 47:225–230, 1975.

Boyes RN, Scott DB, Jebson PJ, Godman MJ, Julian DG: Pharmacokinetics of lidocaine in man. *Clin Pharmacol Ther* 12:105–116, 1971.

Braid DP, Scott DB: The systemic absorption of local analgesic drugs. *Br J Anaesth* 37:394–404, 1965.

Burm AGL, VanKleef JW, Gladines MP, Spierdijk J, Breimer DD: Plasma concentrations of lidocaine and bupivacaine after subarachnoid administration. *Anesthesiology* 59:191–195, 1983.

Burm AGL, VanKleef JW, Gladines MPRR, Olthof G, Spierdijk J: Epidural anesthesia with lidocaine and bupivacaine: effects of epinephrine on the plasma concentration profiles. *Anesth Analg* 65:1281–1284, 1986.

Burm AGL, VanKleef JW, Vermeulen NPE, Olthof G, Briemer DD, Spierdijk J: Pharmacokinetics of lidocaine and bupivacaine following subarachnoid administration in surgical patients: simultaneous investigation of absorption and disposition kinetics using stable isotopes. *Anesthesiology* 69:584–592, 1988.

Corke BC, Carlson CG, Dettbarn WD: The influence of 2-chloroprocaine on the subsequent analgesic potency of bupivacaine. *Anesthesiology* 60:25–27, 1984.

DeJong RH, Heavner JE, Oliveira L: Intravascular lidocaine compartment: kinetics of bolus injection. *Anesthesiology* 37:495–497, 1972.

Finholt DA, Stirt JA, DiFazio CA, Moscicki JC: Lidocaine pharmacokinetics in children during general anesthesia. *Anesth Analg* 65:279–282, 1986.

Greene NM: Blood levels of local anesthetics during spinal and epidural anesthesia. *Anesth Analg* 58:357–359, 1979.

Inoue R, Suganuma T, Echizen H, Ishizake T, Kushida K, Tomono Y: Plasma concentrations of lidocaine and its principal metabolites during intermittent epidural anesthesia. *Anesthesiology* 63:304–310, 1985.

Kuhnert BR, Kuhnert PM, Philipson EH, Syracuse CD, Kaine CJ, Yun C-h: The half-life of 2-chloroprocaine. *Anesth Analg* 65:273–278, 1986.

Kuhnert BR, Kuhnert PM, Prochaska AL, Gross TL: Plasma levels of 2-chloroprocaine in obstetric patients and their neonates after epidural anesthesia. *Anesthesiology* 53:21–25, 1980.

Loo JCK, Riegelman S: A new method for calculating the intrinsic absorption rate of drugs. *J Pharm Sci* 57:918–928, 1968.

Lund PC, Bush DF, Covino BG: Determinants of etidocaine concentration in the blood. *Anesthesiology* 42:497–503, 1975.

Mather LE, Long GJ, Thomas J: The intravenous toxicity and clearance of bupivacaine in man. *Clin Pharmacol Ther* 12:935–943, 1971.

Mather LE, Tucker GT, Murphy TM, Stanton-Hicks Md'A, Bonica JJ: The effects of adding adrenaline to etidocaine and lignocaine in extradural anaesthesia. II. Pharmacokinetics. *Br J Anaesth* 48:989–994, 1976.

Moore DC, Balfour RI, Fitzgibbons D: Convulsive arterial plasma levels of bupivacaine and the response to diazepam therapy. *Anesthesiology* 50:454–456, 1979.

Moore DC, Mather LE, Bridenbaugh PO, Bridenbaugh LD, Balfour RI, Lysons DF, Horton WG: Arterial and venous plasma levels of bupivacaine following epidural and intercostal nerve blocks. *Anesthesiology* 45:39–45, 1976.

Murphy TM, Mather LE, Stanton-Hicks Md'A, Bonica JJ, Tucker GT: The effects of adding adrenaline to etidocaine and lignocaine in extradural anaesthesia. I. Block characteristics and cardiovascular effects. *Br J Anaesth* 48:893–898, 1976.

O'Brien JE, Abbey V, Hinsvark O, Perel J, Finster F: Metabolism and measurement of chloroprocaine, an ester-type local anesthetic. *J Pharm Sci* 68:75–78, 1979.

Raj PP, Ohlweiler D, Hitt BA, Denson DD: Kinetics of local anesthetic esters and the effects of adjuvant drugs on 2-chloroprocaine hydrolysis. *Anesthesiology* 53:307–314, 1980.

Thomson PD, Melmon KL, Richardson JA, Cohn K, Steinbrunn W, Cudihee R, Rowland M: Lidocaine pharmacokinetics in advanced heart failure, liver disease, and renal failure in humans. *Ann Intern Med* 78:499–508, 1973.

Tucker GR, Boyes RN, Bridenbaugh PO, Moore DC: Binding of anilide-type local anesthetics in human plasma. I. Relationships between binding, physicochemical properties, and anesthetic activity. *Anesthesiology* 33:287–303, 1970.

Tucker GT: Pharmacokinetics of local anaesthetics. *Br J Anaesth* 58:717–731, 1986.

Tucker GT, Boas RA: Pharmacokinetic aspects of intravenous regional anesthesia. *Anesthesiology* 34:538–459, 1971.

Tucker GT, Mather LE: Pharmacology of local anesthetic agents. Pharmacokinetics of local anaesthetic agents. *Br J Anaesth* 47:213–224, 1975.

Tucker GT, Mather LE: Clinical pharmacokinetics of local anaesthetics. *Clin Pharmacokinet* 4:241–278, 1979.

Tucker GT, Moore DC, Bridenbaugh PO, Bridenbaugh LD, Thompson GE: Systemic absorption of mepivacaine in commonly used regional block procedures. *Anesthesiology* 37:277–287, 1972.

Usubiaga JE, Moya F, Wikinski JA, Wikinski R, Usubiaga LE: Relationship between the passage of local anaesthetics across the blood-brain barrier and their effects on the central nervous system. *Br J Anaesth* 39:943–947, 1967.

Widman B: Plasma concentration of local anaesthetic agents in regard to absorption, distribution, and elimination with special reference to bupivacaine. *Br J Anaesth* 47:231–236, 1975.

Wiklund L, Berlin-Wahlen A: Splanchnic elimination and systemic toxicity of bupivacaine and etidocaine in man. *Acta Anaesthesiol Scand* 21:521–528, 1977.

Wilkinson GR, Lund PC: Bupivacaine levels in plasma and cerebrospinal fluid following epidural administration. *Anesthesiology* 33:482–486, 1970.

Toxicity

Braid DP, Scott DB: Dosage of lignocaine in epidural block in relation to toxicity. *Br J Anaesth* 38:596–602, 1966.

Brown DT, Beamish D, Wildsmith JA: Allergic reaction to an amide local anaesthetic. *Br J Anaesth* 53:435–437, 1981.

Chadwick HS: Toxicity and resuscitation in lidocaine- or bupivacaine-infused cats. *Anesthesiology* 63:385–390, 1985.

Covino BG: Editorial—potential neurotoxicity of local anaesthetic agents. *Can Anaesth Soc J* 30:111–116, 1983.

Editorial: Cardiotoxicity of local anaesthetic drugs. *Lancet* 2:1192–1193, 1986.

Edouard A, Berdeaux A, Langloys J, Samii K, Giudicelli JF, Noviant Y: Effects of lidocaine on myocardial contractility and baroreflex control of heart rate in conscious dogs. *Anesthesiology* 64:316–321, 1986.

Gregg RV, Turner PA, Denson DD, Stuebing RC, Sehlhorst CS, Forsberg T: Does diazepam really induce the cardiotoxic effects of intravenous bupivacaine? *Anesth Analg* 67:9–14, 1988.

Hotvedt R, Refsum H, Helgesen KG: Cardiac electrophysiologic and hemodynamic effects related to plasma levels of bupivacaine in the dog. *Anesth Analg* 64:388–394, 1985.

Kasten GW, Martin ST: Bupivacaine cardiovascular toxicity: comparison of treatment with bretylium and lidocaine. *Anesth Analg* 64:911–916, 1985.

Kotelko DM, Shnider SM, Dailey PA, Brizgys RV, Levinson G, Shapiro WA, Kolke M, Rosen MA: Bupivacaine-induced cardiac arrhythmias in sheep. *Anesthesiology* 60:10–18, 1984.

Li DF, Bahar M, Cole G, Rosen M: Neurological toxicity of the subarachnoid infusion of bupivacaine, lignocaine, or 2-chloroprocaine in the rat. *Br J Anaesth* 57:424–429, 1985.

Liu P, Feldman HS, Covino BM, Giasi R, Covino GB: Acute cardiovascular toxicity of intravenous amide local anesthetics in anesthetized ventilated dogs. *Anesth Analg* 61:317–322, 1982.

Lynch C III: Depression of myocardial contractility in vitro by bupivacaine, etidocaine, and lidocaine. *Anesth Analg* 65:551–559, 1986.

Marx GF: Cardiotoxicity of local anesthetics—the plot thickens. *Anesthesiology* 60:3–5, 1984.

Moller RA, Covino BG: Cardiac electrophysiologic effects of lidocaine and bupivacaine. *Anesth Analg* 67:107–114, 1988.

Morishima HO, Pedersen H, Finster M, Feldman HS, Covino BG: Etidocaine toxicity in the adult, newborn, and fetal sheep. *Anesthesiology* 58:342–346, 1983.

Morishima HO, Pedersen H, Finster M, Hiraoka H, Tsuiji A, Feldman HS, Arthur GR, Covino BG: Bupivacaine toxicity in pregnant and nonpregnant ewes. *Anesthesiology* 63:134–139, 1985.

Morishima HO, Pedersen H, Finster M, Sakuma K, Bruce SL, Gutsche BB, Start RI, Covino BG: Toxicity of lidocaine in adult, newborn, and fetal sheep. *Anesthesiology* 55:57–61, 1981.

Myers RR, Kalichman MW, Reisner LS, Powell HC: Neurotoxicity of local anesthetics: altered perineurial permeability, edema, and nerve fiber injury. *Anesthesiology* 64:29–35, 1986.

Nancarrow C, Runciman WB, Mather LE, Upton RN, Plummer JL: The influence of acidosis on the distribution of lidocaine and bupivacaine into the myocardium and brain of the sheep. *Anesth Analg* 66:925–935, 1987.

Nath S, Haggmark S, Johansson G, Reiz S: Differential depressant and electrophysiologic cardiotoxicity of local anesthetics: an experimental study with special reference to lidocaine and bupivacaine. *Anesth Analg* 65:1263–1270, 1986.

Ready LB, Plumer MH, Haschke RH, Austin E, Sumi SM: Neurotoxicity of intrathecal local anesthetics in rabbits. *Anesthesiology* 63:364–370, 1985.

Reiz S, Nath S: Cardiotoxicity of local anaesthetic agents. *Br J Anaesth* 58:736–746, 1986.

Sage DJ, Feldman HS, Arthur GR, Datta S, Ferretti AM, Norway SB, Covino BG: Influence of lidocaine and bupivacaine on isolated guinea pig atria in the presence of acidosis and hypoxia. *Anesth Analg* 63:1–7, 1984.

Scott DB: Evaluation of the toxicity of local anaesthetic agents in man. *Br J Anaesth* 47:56–61, 1975.

Scott DB: Evaluation of clinical tolerance of local anaesthetic agents. *Br J Anaesth* 47:328–331, 1975.

Scott DB: Toxic effects of local anaesthetic agents on the central nervous system. *Br J Anaesth* 58:732–735, 1986.

Scott DB: Toxicity caused by local anaesthetic drugs. *Br J Anaesth* 53:553–554, 1981.

Tanz RD, Heskett T, Loehning RW, Fairfax CA: Comparative cardiotoxicity of bupivacaine and lidocaine in the isolated perfused mammalian heart. *Anesth Analg* 63:549–556, 1984.

Wang BC, Hillman DE, Spielholz NI, Turndorf H: Chronic neurological deficits and Nesacaine-CE—an effect of the anesthetic, 2-chloroprocaine, or the antioxidant, sodium bisulfite? *Anesth Analg* 63:445–447, 1984.

Wheeler DM, Bradley WL, Woods WT Jr: The electrophysiologic actions of lidocaine and bupivacaine in the isolated, perfused canine heart. *Anesthesiology* 68:201–212, 1988.

12

Drugs and Obstetric Anesthesia

BARRY C. CORKE

With the widespread application of techniques for measuring drug concentrations in plasma, it quickly became apparent that the placenta provides only a partial barrier to substances administered to the mother. The fact that clinically significant effects are not detected in the fetus does not imply that no placental transfer has occurred. It is, therefore, important that anesthesiologists who administer drugs to the mother during the perinatal period be aware of the principles involved in the placental transfer of drugs and the likely effects upon the neonate should significant transfer occur.

The problems occurring in the perinatal period with relation to the administration of drugs to the mother are by no means solely related to placental transfer. Alteration in the mother's normal physiology by the drug may be of significance to the fetus. For example, local anesthetics administered to the mother for regional anesthesia during parturition may cause maternal hypotension, which reduces placental blood flow causing fetal distress. It is important, therefore, not only to consider placental transfer when drugs are given during pregnancy and childbirth, but also any direct physiological effects they have on the mother which may indirectly affect the fetus. In addition, the disposition of many drugs is altered in the pregnant patient, due to changes in both drug distribution and elimination.

PASSAGE OF DRUGS ACROSS THE PLACENTA

Drugs reach the fetus by passage across the placenta, which is supplied with maternal blood from the uterine arteries, while two umbilical arteries (arising from the fetal internal iliac arteries) carry fetal blood to the placenta, and a single umbilical vein returns blood to the fetus (Fig. 12.1). The exchange of oxygen, carbon dioxide, and drugs between the maternal arterial and umbilical venous blood occurs across the intervillous spaces of the placenta to the fetal capillaries. The transfer of drugs across the placenta occurs by one of the following general processes:

SIMPLE DIFFUSION

Diffusion of drugs occurs through the placental membrane down a concentration gradient or, in the case of gases, a pressure gradient. It is the principal method by which most drugs cross the placenta.

PINOCYTOSIS

Microscopic invaginations of the cell wall engulf drops of extracellular fluid and solutes which are carried through in the resulting vacuoles.

ACTIVE TRANSPORT

Active transport involving carrier processes requires the expenditure of energy and may occur against a concentration gradient.

Changes in the placenta that occur as pregnancy advances, such as the increase in placental blood flow to 10 to 20% of maternal cardiac output, result in a larger proportion of drug transfer in late pregnancy than during early pregnancy.

Factors Affecting the Passage of Drugs across the Placenta

The transplacental passage of drugs is dependent on several important factors: lipid solubility; degree of drug ionization; molecular weight; protein binding; drug concentration gradients; maternal and fetal blood pH; and placental and fetal drug metabolism. Drug transfer across the placenta occurs mostly by diffusion, which is governed by the Fick diffusion equation:

$$\frac{\dot{Q}}{t} = ka\,\frac{(Cm - Cf)}{D}$$

where

$\frac{Q}{t}$ = quantity of drug diffusion in unit time;

a = the surface area over which diffusion is occurring

$(Cm - Cf$ = concentration gradient between the maternal (Cm) and fetal circulation (Cf);

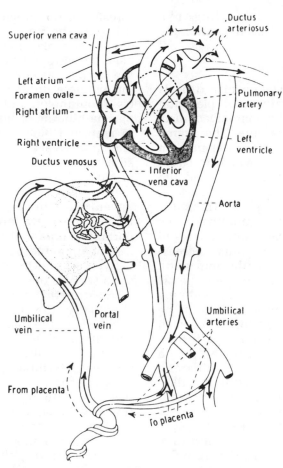

Figure 12.1.   The fetal circulation. (With permission from Ganong WF: *Review of Medical Physiology,* Lange Medical Publications, Los Altos, California, 1973, p 459, ed 7.)

D = thickness of the membrane;
k = diffusion coefficient or constant.

The diffusion constant of a compound is a function of its solubility in the membrane, its molecular weight and, in the case of a weak electrolyte, its degree of ionization. D, a, and k are constants, and it is useful to combine those constants to form k_{diff}, the rate constant of diffusion, in the simplified equation:

$$\frac{\dot{Q}}{t} = K_{diff}(Cm - Cf)$$

MOLECULAR WEIGHT

As a general principle, the larger the molecule the less likely placental trans-

fer is to occur. Compounds with a molecular weight below 600 readily cross the placenta, whereas the placenta is relatively impermeable to those above 1000. The majority of drugs given to the mother during labor have molecular weights in the region of 250 to 450, and so other factors are of more importance in determining placental transfer.

LIPID SOLUBILITY

Compounds possessing a high degree of lipid solubility diffuse readily across the placenta, while water-soluble, highly ionized compounds pass more slowly. Thus, poorly lipid-soluble quaternary bases such as *d*-tubocurarine cross the placenta in only limited amounts, whereas highly lipid-soluble drugs like thiopental cross the placenta extremely rapidly.

DEGREE OF IONIZATION

The degree of ionization of a drug is an important determinant of placental transfer because only nonionized drug readily crosses the placenta. The degree of ionization of a substance depends on the nature of the substance (acid or base), its dissociation constant (pKa), and the pH of the medium in which it is present. The pKa of a drug is the pH at which it is 50% ionized and 50% unionized (see Chapter 1). A weak base is more ionized in an acidic solution and, thus, decreasing the pH will increase the ionization of the base (see Chapter 1). When the pH values on two sides of a lipid membrane are the same, the concentrations of the ionized and nonionized forms on each side will be the same when equilibrium is achieved. However, when the pH on either side of the membrane is different, weak acids will accumulate on the alkaline side, while weak bases will accumulate on the acidic side because only the nonionized form crosses the lipid membrane and achieves equilibrium. Maternal and fetal blood pH may influence the degree of ionization and hence placental transfer of a drug. The pH of umbilical vessel blood is normally 0.10 to 0.15 units lower than that of maternal blood, and consequently there is a small pH gradient across the placenta. Basic drugs are, thus, more ionized in the fetus, while acidic drugs tend to be more ionized in maternal blood. The concentration of unionized basic drug is higher in maternal blood as compared with fetal blood, and as it is nonionized drug that diffuses across the placenta most readily, there will be a net transfer of basic drug from mother to fetus. If the fetus becomes increasingly acidotic during labor and delivery, then some of the basic local anesthetics may accumulate in the more acid fetal blood.

PROTEIN BINDING

The degree of plasma binding of a drug has an important effect on placental transfer in the pregnant patient because it is only the free or unbound drug that crosses the placenta. Many drugs have been found to have decreased binding in the neonate as compared to the mother, for example, local anesthetics, antibiotics, propranolol, and phenobarbital. The plasma binding of bupivacaine is higher in maternal blood than neonatal blood, and at delivery following the epidural administration of bupivacaine to the mother, the total umbilical venous plasma concentration of bupivacaine is lower than the total maternal venous plasma concentration. However, it is important to note that the concentration of free or unbound bupivacaine in umbilical venous and maternal venous plasma at delivery is the same. This is because it is free drug that crosses the placenta, and eventually the free concentration on each side of the placenta becomes equal. Therefore, differences in the protein binding of drugs in maternal and fetal plasma determine differences in *total* drug concentration on each side of the placenta, although the *free* concentrations are in fact equal (Fig. 12.2). As it is the free drug which is available for binding to receptor sites and exerting a drug's pharmacological effect, these effects should be similar in the mother and fetus in spite of the disparity in total drug levels.

Many drugs are bound to albumin in plasma. In addition, some basic drugs, for example, lidocaine, bupivacaine, and propranolol, have been shown to bind to α_1-acid glycoprotein, an acute phase reactant, which is known to increase nonspecifically in response to infection, inflammation, cancer, and trauma. The concentration of α_1-acid glycoprotein is lower in the fetus than the mother, thus accounting, at least in part, for the decreased binding of lidocaine and propranolol in the fetus (see Chapter 1).

PLACENTAL DRUG BIOTRANSFORMATION

The placenta contains a number of enzymes that are involved in drug biotransformation reactions, for example, monoamine oxidase and cholinesterase. The

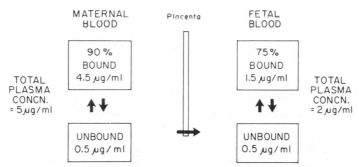

Figure 12.2.   The effect of protein binding on drug placental transfer.   Consider a theoretical drug which is 90% bound in the mother and 75% bound in the fetus. The free concentration in mother and fetus is equal at equilibrium (0.5 μg/ml), but the total concentration in the mother is higher than that in the fetus. (With permission from Scott DB: Analgesia in labour. *Br J Anaesth* 49:11–17, 1977.)

significance of these enzyme systems is unknown, but it has been postulated that they may play a role in protecting the fetus against compounds that the fetus cannot yet metabolize. It is also known that some drugs can be metabolized by the human placenta. The placental microsomal drug-metabolizing enzyme systems are similar to those in the liver, being capable of the basic processes of drug metabolism, such as, oxidation, reduction, hydrolysis, and conjugation.

Thus, high lipid solubility, low degree of ionization, low plasma binding, and low molecular weight are all important determinants of placental transfer of drugs.

DRUG UPTAKE AND DISTRIBUTION IN MOTHER AND FETUS

The disposition of drugs administered to the mother is influenced by many interrelated factors, and to facilitate pharmacokinetic modeling, the mother and fetus have been regarded as an integrated unit: the maternal-placental-fetal unit (Fig. 12.3).

Maternal Uptake and Distribution

During pregnancy, a number of striking biochemical and physiological changes take place which may influence drug disposition. Gastrointestinal motility is decreased, and the gastric emptying time may increase by 30 to 50%, both of which will alter the rate of drug absorption from the stomach and intestine. An indirect estimate of gastric emptying time can be obtained by studying the pharmacokinetics of acetaminophen absorption after an oral dose. Nimmo *et al.* have shown that absorption is normal in women early in labor (before they have received narcotic analgesics) and in postpartum patients. However, acetaminophen absorption is greatly delayed in women at a later stage in labor receiving narcotic analgesics, such as meperidine, heroin, and pentazocine, suggesting that the administration of narcotics during labor inhibits gastric emptying. Most of the delay in gastric emptying during labor can be attributed to the use of narcotic analgesics; advanced labor itself probably only produces a slight delay in gastric emptying. The absorption of acetaminophen in patients receiving no analgesics during labor and delivery is similar to that in patients undergoing epidural analgesia; thus, the slight delay in gastric emptying produced during advanced labor is unaffected by epidural analgesia. These observations have important implications for the obstetric anesthesiologist, one of whose main concerns is the prevention of maternal aspiration.

Drug distribution in the pregnant patient may differ from the nonpregnant patient due to a wide variety of factors, such as changes in maternal blood volume, cardiac output, tissue perfusion, hypoproteinemia, and the presence of

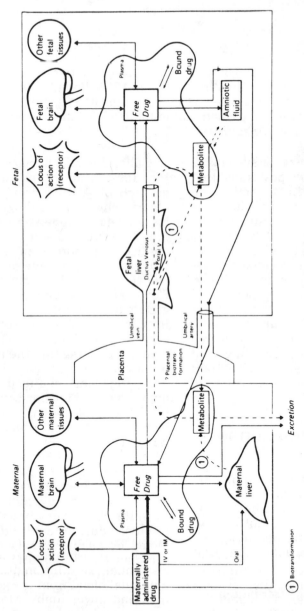

Figure 12.3. **Drug disposition in a model of the maternal-placental-fetal unit.** (With permission from Mirkin BL: In Boreus L (ed): *Fetal Pharmacology*. New York, Raven Press, 1973.)

the placental-fetal unit. Maternal blood volume increases during pregnancy, so that at term, it exceeds nonpregnant values by 30 to 40%. In addition, cardiac output increases by 30 to 40% during pregnancy and is greatly influenced by posture. Adoption of the supine posture during late pregnancy causes aortocaval obstruction by the gravid uterus, with a resultant decrease in venous return to the heart and fall in cardiac output. Plasma protein concentrations change during pregnancy; the plasma albumin concentration is lower in the pregnant woman at term than in the nonpregnant woman. These changes may modify drug binding in plasma, resulting in changes in drug distribution and possible increased placental transfer.

Drug elimination is also altered during pregnancy and childbirth. Liver biopsies taken during the first trimester of pregnancy in humans have shown a proliferation of smooth endoplasmic reticulum, indicating an increase in hepatic microsomal enzyme activity. Renal plasma flow and glomerular filtration rates increase during pregnancy, both of which might modify the renal clearance of drugs. Since creatinine clearance is increased about 50% during pregnancy, renal drug elimination might be expected to be increased, provided tubular reabsorption remains unchanged.

Relatively few pharmacokinetic studies have been conducted in obstetric patients because of practical difficulties. Table 12.1 lists the pharmacokinetic parameters that have been derived in pregnant women for some drugs of importance to the anesthesiologist.

The amount of drug transferred from the mother to the fetus depends, in part, on the free drug concentration in the maternal blood. This will be affected by dose, route, and duration of administration. In general, the larger the dose administered to the mother, the higher the maternal blood concentration. In late pregnancy, the reduced blood flow to the lower limbs due to venus pooling affects the absorption of drugs given intramuscularly into the thigh.

Uteroplacental blood flow at delivery is 500 to 700 ml/min, and about 80% of this perfuses the intervillous space. During uterine contractions, the intervillous blood supply is interrupted. The dynamics of blood flow to the uterus and placenta during labor and delivery influences the placental transfer of drugs that are administered as part of obstetric analgesia and anesthesia. If maternal placental blood flow is decreased, for example, during hypotension due to epidural blockade, drug transfer to the fetus may also decrease. A decrease in umbilical blood flow will similarly decrease the back transfer of drugs from the fetus to the mother.

The partial occlusion of the inferior vena cava by the enlarged uterus may result in the venous return being redirected via collateral channels, mainly the azygos and vertebral venous systems. The internal vertebral venous plexus becomes enlarged and engorged and so reduces the size of the epidural space, offering a possible explanation for the reduced dosage requirements of local anesthetic for epidural blockade during pregnancy.

Fetal Uptake and Distribution

A diagram of the fetal circulation is presented in Figure 12.1. Blood from the placental villi carrying nutrients, gases, and drugs from the mother enters the fetus via the umbilical vein and either perfuses the fetal liver or bypasses the liver and passes through the ductus venosus into the inferior vena cava. Thus, the fetal hepatic extraction of drugs protects the brain and myocardium of the fetus to some extent against high circulating drug concentrations. In addition, any drug transferred across the placenta also undergoes dilution due to admixture with fetal blood from the gastrointestinal tract and lower limbs. Most of the oxygenated umbilical venous blood from the placenta enters the heart where it is diverted to the left atrium via the foramen ovale. This better oxygenated blood then leaves the left ventricle to supply the

Table 12.1.
Pharmacokinetic Parameters in Pregnant Patients for Some Drugs of Importance to the Anesthesiologist

Drug	Half-life $(t_{1/2\beta})$ (hr)	Volume of distribution (Vd_β) (L)	Plasma clearance (CL) (ml/min)
Bupivacaine			
Pregnant	9.0–9.4*		
Nonpregnant	1.3		
Etidocalne			
Pregnant	5.10		861
Nonpregnant	5.46		588
Meperidine			
Pregnant	2.53–3.78	230–371	767–1190*
Nonpregnant	2.95–3.60	233	964–1060
Thiopental			
Pregnant	5.2–26*	196–564*	286–502*
Nonpregnant	7.1–11.5	57–233	127–150
Diazepam			
Pregnant	65*	149	28
Nonpregnant	35–46	78	20–30
Pancuronium			
Pregnant	1.9*	0.35†	78*
Nonpregnant	2.4	0.38†	62
Midazolam			
Pregnant	0.86	0.7†	9.0‡
Pregnant, labor	0.76	0.4*, †	6.5‡
Pregnant, cesarean section	0.78	0.9†	13.9*, ‡
Nonpregnant	0.98	0.8†	8.7‡
Theophylline			
Pregnant	6.5*	36.8*	57.7*, §
Nonpregnant	4.3	30.7	94.3§
Vecuronium			
Pregnant	0.6‖	0.25	6.4‡
Nonpregnant	1.18	0.27	5.2

Most of the data are taken from Cummings AJ: A survey of pharmacokinetic data from pregnant women. *Clin Pharmacokinet* 8:344–354, 1983.
*Significantly different from nonpregnant.
†V_d, L/kg.
‡ml/min/kg.
§Nonrenal clearance.
‖Nonpregnant and pregnant groups not compared.

head. Deoxygenated blood that returns to the right atrium via the superior vena cava is pumped through the pulmonary artery and ductus arteriosus to supply the lower trunk and umbilical arteries. These right to left shunts modify fetal drug uptake and distribution.

The concentration of drug returning to the placenta via the umbilical artery de-pends on many factors (maternal blood concentration, fetal uptake and distribution, plasma drug binding, and fetal metabolism and elimination), and it is important to differentiate between the drug concentration in umbilical venous and umbilical arterial blood. At the commencement of drug administration to the mother, only the umbilical vein carries any drug, and the umbilical artery is virtually free of drug. Later as equilibration is achieved, the umbilical venous blood will contain more drug than umbilical arterial blood, reflecting the dilution of drug in the fetal circulation and uptake by the fetal tissues. Figure 12.4 shows propranolol concentrations in maternal, umbilical venous, and umbilical arterial blood during continuous maternal intravenous infusion of propranolol to a pregnant sheep. There is a concentration gradient from maternal vein to umbilical vein, where the concentration is higher than the umbilical artery.

The human fetal liver has been shown from a very early stage to have an enzyme system capable of metabolizing drugs. At the third month of gestation, cytochrome P-450 is present in human fetal liver. Drug-metabolizing enzyme studies have shown that the fetal liver

can oxidize certain drugs, though in general fetal enzymatic activity is less than that of the adult. Conjugation reactions are also important for the metabolism and excretion of drugs. However, glucuronidation reactions appear to be limited in the human fetal liver and kidney. Glucuronyl transferase activity is extremely low in the human fetus, and attempts to induce glucuronyl transferase with phenobarbital or dexamethasone in laboratory animals have only been effective during late prenatal or postnatal life. After birth, reduced quantities of metabolizing enzymes, such as glucuronyl transferase, become significant. Thus, in the liver of the neonate, both phase I (hydroxylation, dealkylation) and phase II (conjugation) reactions are decreased in comparison with adults, so that drug metabolism is generally reduced in the newborn. Many drugs remain in the circula-

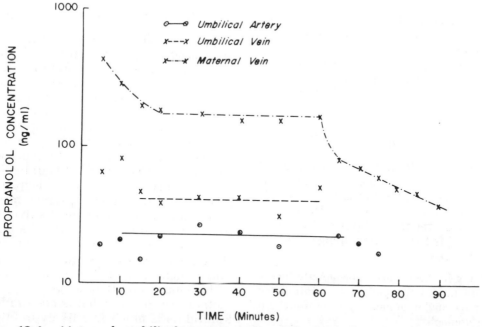

Figure 12.4. Maternal, umbilical, venous, and umbilical arterial propranolol concentrations during the continuous intravenous infusion of propranolol in the pregnant sheep. A loading dose of propranolol followed by a continuous intravenous infusion from 0 to 60 minutes was administered to the pregnant sheep. Note the rapid passage of drug across the placenta and the fall in maternal and fetal concentrations when the infusion was discontinued. (Data adapted from Wood M, Corke BR, Killam AP, Sundell H, Wood AJJ: A model for the simultaneous determination of the factors controlling fetal and maternal concentrations of either drugs or endogenous compounds. *Clin Res* 28:245A, 1980.)

tion for a prolonged time and can cause serious toxicity. Chloramphenicol and bilirubin, for example, both require conversion to glucuronides before excretion. Chloramphenicol can cause death due to circulatory collapse (gray baby syndrome) in premature babies who, as a result of failure of the liver to conjugate and of the kidney to excrete the drug, have high plasma chloramphenicol concentrations. The human fetal adrenal gland possesses the ability to catalyze certain important oxidation-reduction reactions. Renal glomerular filtration, tubular secretion, and reabsorption from the renal tubule are reduced at birth, so that for drugs whose main route of elimination is the kidney, excretion may be delayed in the neonate.

PROPHYLAXIS OF GASTRIC ACID ASPIRATION

Gastric acid aspiration remains a leading cause of maternal mortality, and pharmacologic regimens have been introduced in an attempt to reduce the likelihood of serious respiratory complications if aspiration occurs (Mendelson's syndrome).

Particulate Antacids

If an adequate dose of conventional antacid is administered at 2- to 3-hour intervals, it is possible to maintain the pH of gastric contents above the critical level of 2.5. More recently, the use of particulate antacids has been challenged for the following reasons:

1. Mixing in the stomach is generally inadequate unless the patient is manipulated through 360° to promote spread throughout the stomach.
2. Animal studies have shown that pulmonary damage, specifically a foreign body reaction, may be as severe following the aspiration of particulate antacids as it is from gastric acid.
3. Most importantly perhaps, deaths from aspiration have continued to occur in obstet-

ric patients despite what was thought to be adequate antacid prophylaxis.

Nonparticulate Antacids

Because the particulate nature of conventional antacids may be damaging, the use of nonparticulate compounds, such as sodium citrate, has become popular. The use of sodium citrate may be less effective in neutralizing the acidity of gastric contents and also increases gastric fluid volume. However, it has been shown that sodium citrate administration (30 ml) produces a gastric fluid pH of above 2.5 in the majority of patients (64 to 84%). This effect is very short lived and is adequate only for a period of 30 to 45 minutes. It must therefore be given just prior to the induction of anesthesia. Repeated administration should not be instituted as it is likely to produce gastrointestinal symptoms.

Histamine H_2-Receptor Antagonists

Both cimetidine and ranitidine have been used in obstetric patients in an attempt to maintain gastric fluid pH above 2.5. Cimetidine has been shown to be both safe and effective in raising gastric fluid pH above 2.5, and neurobehavioral studies have not revealed any effects upon the neonate. Ranitidine is also effective in raising gastric fluid pH and, since it is highly ionized, it is unlikely to cross the placenta to a large degree. Cimetidine inhibits the microsomal mixed-function oxidase system of the liver (see page 616), thereby prolonging the elimination of several drugs used in anesthesia; for example, it is possible that cimetidine might reduce the metabolism of amide local anesthetics given to the mother leading to higher concentrations. Ranitidine is much less likely to inhibit drug metabolism, and the use of ranitidine is preferable in the obstetric patient for prophylaxis of gastric acid aspiration.

The use of drugs, including prokinetic drugs, to reduce gastric volume and increase gastric fluid pH is further discussed in Chapters 5 and 23.

INDIVIDUAL DRUGS

Intravenus Anesthetic Agents

THIOPENTAL

As would be anticipated from the foregoing discussion, thiopental crosses the placenta rapidly and can be detected in the umbilical venous blood within 30 seconds of its administration to the mother. The level in the umbilical artery is always less than that found in the umbilical vein and reaches a maximum within 2 to 3 minutes. Figure 12.5 shows the concentrations of the thiobarbiturate, thiamylal, in mother and newborn following its administration during elective cesarean section. The placental transfer of thiopental has been studied during vaginal delivery and cesarean section and, although thiopental levels in the umbilical vessels were similar in both delivery groups, it was noted that the proportion of infants with an Apgar score at 1 minute of 7 or above was greater in the vaginal delivery group. It has been suggested that during vaginal delivery, uterine contractions and cord compression reduce the amount of thiopental reaching the fetus.

In the past, it has been suggested that the interval between the induction of anesthesia and delivery of the neonate (I-D interval) might affect neonatal outcome. It is unlikely that the baby can be delivered prior to the attainment of peak barbiturate levels in fetal blood (Fig. 12.5), and of greater importance during this period is the maintenance of a normal cardiac output in the mother, particularly avoiding aortacaval compression by the uterus. Oxygenation is also important, and the administration of 60% inspired concentration to the mother produces optimal neonatal outcome. If the above factors are taken into account, there is no evidence that extending the I-D interval to as long as 20 minutes produces any deleterious effects in the neonate.

KETAMINE

Other induction agents have been studied in an attempt to find an alternative to

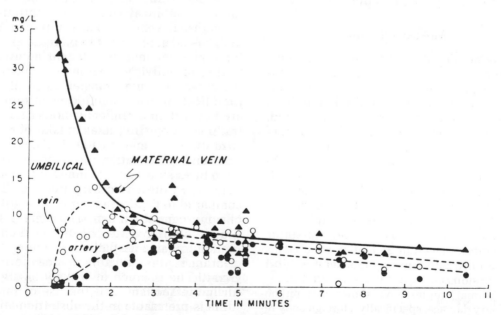

Figure 12.5. Thiamylal concentrations in maternal vein (▲), umbilical vein (○) and umbilical artery (●) following single injection (4 mg/kg) for cesarean section. (With permission from Kosaka Y, Takahashi T, Mark LC: Intravenous thiobarbiturate anesthesia for cesarean section. *Anesthesiology* 31:489–506, 1969.)

thiopental which might possess significant advantages. Ketamine has been advocated for use as an induction agent for general anesthesia and as an analgesic in the parturient patient. However, ketamine rapidly crosses the placenta and the plasma concentration in mixed cord blood is similar to the maternal venous level 1.5 to 6.5 minutes after administration to the mother. When used as an induction agent for cesarean section, it is generally administered intravenously in doses of 1 mg/kg, while to produce analgesia for a vaginal delivery, the dosage is reduced to 0.25 mg/kg to ensure that the mother remains awake. As in the nonpregnant patient, ketamine raises the arterial blood pressure by 15 to 25%, and it, therefore, should be avoided in the hypertensive patient. Despite this vasopressor effect, animal experiments have shown that the increase in maternal blood pressure is not associated with a reduction in uterine blood flow. In addition, ketamine is associated with an increase in uterine tone when administered to the pregnant patient at term.

Muscle Relaxants

The nondepolarizing muscle relaxants, which are quaternary ammonium compounds, are highly ionized at physiological pH and possess low lipid solubility; therefore placental transfer is limited. However, they all cross the placenta when used during the administration of anesthesia for cesarean section, but without demonstrable effect on the neonate. If very large doses of muscle relaxants are administered to the mother during a short period of time, for example d-tubocurarine in the management of status epilepticus, placental transfer becomes important, and the neonate may exhibit depression of neuromuscular function.

SUCCINYLCHOLINE

Succinylcholine may be administered to the pregnant woman in normal clinical doses without producing pharmacological effects in the neonate. Problems have arisen, however, when the mother has a congenital plasma cholinesterase abnor-

mality (see Chapter 5) which reduces succinylcholine hydrolysis. If the baby also inherits the abnormality, the increased amount of succinylcholine transferred across the placenta may produce significant neuromuscular block. The plasma cholinesterase activity in fetal or premature infant blood is only about half that of the adult. In addition, plasma cholinesterase levels fall about 20 to 30% in the mother during pregnancy. Little information is available on the placental transfer of succinylcholine in pregnant patients. After the injection of 2 mg/kg of radiolabeled succinylcholine into the maternal femoral vein of the monkey, maximum fetal concentrations of about 4% of the maximum maternal concentration are achieved in 5 to 10 minutes.

NONDEPOLARIZING RELAXANTS

Metocurine and pancuronium concentrations have been measured during anesthesia for cesarean section, and for both these drugs the umbilical vein concentration at delivery is lower than the maternal vein concentration; but the ratio of umbilical venous concentration to maternal venous concentration (UV/MV) has been observed to increase as the interval from muscle relaxant administration to delivery lengthens, indicating increased placental transfer. In addition, umbilical arterial blood concentrations are lower than umbilical venous concentrations, suggesting fetal uptake of pancuronium and metocurine. The distribution and elimination of pancuronium have been studied in women undergoing delivery by elective cesarean section and compared to findings obtained in a group of nonpregnant women. The mean half-life was shorter in the parturients than in the nonpregnant patients, while the clearance was greater in the former group. The volume of distribution was unchanged (Table 12.1).

The intermediate-duration nondepolarizing muscle relaxants, atracurium and vecuronium, have also been administered to pregnant patients, and the pharmacokinetic parameters are given in Table 12.1 The UV/M ratio is 0.11 for vecuronium, and similar values have been reported for atracurium; therefore, placental transfer is unlikely to lead to clinical effect in the neonate for either drug. The relatively short duration of action and freedom from cardiovascular side effects have made the intermediate-duration muscle relaxants useful agents in the parturient.

Local Anesthetics

Regional anesthesia involving the use of local anesthetics has achieved widespread popularity for the relief of maternal pain during labor and delivery. Factors affecting the placental transfer of the local anesthetics include protein binding, degree of ionization, and metabolism. Even though the incidence of serious adverse effects during spinal and epidural anesthesia is generally low, there is a risk of central nervous and cardiac toxicity in the newborn when local anesthetics are administered in the presence of fetal acidosis. Most local anesthetics are weak bases, and fetal acidosis may lead to "iontrapping" within the fetal circulation. Higher fetal blood concentrations of lidocaine have been observed during experimentally induced fetal acidosis in lambs, while high UV/MV concentration ratios of lidocaine and mepivacaine have been detected in neonates with umbilical artery pH values of 7.03 to 7.23. In addition, fetal plasma drug binding of local anesthetics may be decreased in the presence of fetal acidosis. Thus, even though UV/M total drug concentration ratios may be low, the fetus may have been exposed to clinically important free drug concentrations.

The local anesthetics have been divided into two groups:

1. Those possessing an **ester** linkage: procaine; chloroprocaine; tetracaine.
2. Those possessing an **amide** linkage: lidocaine, bupivacaine; mepivacaine.

ESTER LOCAL ANESTHETICS

The ester type of local anesthetics are metabolized by liver esterase and plasma cholinesterase at varying rates; the rate of hydrolysis proceeds extremely rapidly for chloroprocaine (4.7 μmol/ml/hour) and more slowly for tetracaine (0.3 μmol/ml/hour). The rate of hydrolysis will influence the duration of action as well as the degree of systemic toxicity. A drug such as chloroprocaine, which is hydrolyzed so rapidly that it has a maternal in vitro half-life of 21 seconds, inevitably has a limited degree of placental transfer, since drug which is present in the maternal circulation is metabolized before being able to cross the placenta. In addition, the products of hydrolysis [2-chloroaminobenzoic acid (CABA) and 2-diethylaminoethanol] are pharmacologically inactive. It is likely that metabolism of the ester group of local anesthetics occurs in the placenta, since the appropriate enzymes are known to be present in considerable quantities. Thus, the duration of action of chloroprocaine is short, and frequent injections are required during continuous epidural analgesia.

Plasma levels of chloroprocaine have been determined in obstetric patients and their newborns following epidural anesthesia for vaginal delivery and cesarean section. Low levels of chloroprocaine were detected in maternal plasma for at least 5 to 10 minutes after each epidural injection, and mean levels at delivery were between 23 and 51 ng/ml. CABA, the metabolic product of chloroprocaine, was present in the mother throughout labor. In addition, low concentrations of chloroprocaine (less than 17 ng/ml) were detectable in 50% of the umbilical venous and arterial blood samples, indicating that chloroprocaine does cross the placenta.

There is both clinical and experimental evidence that the prior administration of chloroprocaine interferes with the subsequent action of both bupivacaine and narcotics when they are administered epidurally. Clinically it has been demonstrated that even small doses of 2-chloroprocaine, such as would be administered as a test dose, reduce both the efficacy of bupivacaine and its length of action. Laboratory evidence suggests that one of the metabolites of 2-chloroprocaine interferes with the ability of bupivacaine to reach its site of activity on the nerve membrane.

There are as yet only clinical studies with respect to the effects of 2-chloroprocaine on the subsequent action of epidural narcotics. There does, however, appear to be a clinically important reduction in the efficacy of epidural narcotics, and it has been suggested that perhaps a metabolite of 2-chloroprocaine is a narcotic antagonist. Further clinical and laboratory studies are required to further define this potentially important drug interaction. The neurological toxicity of chloroprocaine is discussed in Chapter 11.

AMIDE LOCAL ANESTHETICS

The metabolism of the amide group of local anesthetics occurs mainly in the liver, and these drugs therefore tend to have longer half-lives. The placental transfer of the amide group of local anesthetics is influenced by two factors: (*a*) their degree of ionization at physiological pH and (*b*) their protein binding. There is an inverse correlation between the degree of plasma binding and the umbilical vein/maternal blood (UV/M) concentration ratio, suggesting that protein binding limits placental transfer (Table 12.2). However, although highly protein-bound drugs, such as bupivacaine (95%), tend to have low fetal/maternal total blood concentration ratios, free drug concentrations may be expected to be the same in the mother and baby once equilibrium is established (Fig. 12.2; see Chapter 1) and a low UV/M ratio does not always imply

low fetal drug exposure and low risk to the newborn. Animal studies have shown that the rate of transfer is lower for drugs that exhibit higher maternal plasma protein binding, but that if sufficient time is allowed for equilibrium to develop between mother and fetus, fetal accumulation of even highly bound drugs, such as bupivacaine and etidocaine, can occur.

The continuous administration of bupivacaine, lidocaine, or mepivacaine by the epidural route during labor and delivery always results in systemic accumulation and placental transfer. However, the extent of this accumulation appears to be much less for bupivacaine than for lidocaine or mepivacaine, so umbilical vein/maternal blood concentrations at delivery are higher following lidocaine and mepivacaine than bupivacaine. This is probably due to two factors, both of which limit the placental transfer of bupivacaine: *a* its protein binding and *b* its higher degree of ionization at physiological pH. (The pKa of bupivacaine is 8.05, as compared with 7.65 for mepivacaine and 7.85 for lidocaine.)

Peak concentrations of bupivacaine in maternal blood occur 10 to 60 minutes after epidural injection. The administration of bupivacaine without epinephrine in a dosage of 100 to 160 mg produces maternal blood concentrations in the region of 600 to 700 ng/ml and umbilical venous levels of about 200 ng/ml. The UV/MV ratio (the ratio at delivery of umbilical

Table 12.2.
Relationship between the Plasma Binding of Amide Local Anesthetics and UV/M Ratio

Local anesthetic	Percentage protein bound	Percent free fraction	UV/M ratio*
Prilocaine	55	45	1.00–1.18
Lidocaine	64	36	0.52–0.69
Mepivacaine	77	23	0.69–0.71
Etidocaine	94	6	0.14–0.35
Bupivacaine	95	5	0.31–0.44

Data from Poppers PJ: Evaluation of local anesthetic agents for regional anesthesia in obstetrics. *Br J Anaesth* 47(suppl):322–327, 1975.
*UV/M ratio, ratio at delivery of the concentration of local anesthetic in blood or plasma from the umbilical vein to the concentration of local anesthetic in blood from the mother. Those drugs which are least protein bound (highest percentage of free fraction) cross the placenta more readily resulting in a higher UV/M ratio.

venous to maternal venous blood concentrations) for bupivacaine is therefore between 0.2 and 0.4 and is not influenced by the dose-delivery interval (period of time between administration of the drug to the mother and delivery of the infant). However, the fetomaternal concentration ratios (the ratio of the concentration in fetal scalp blood to that in maternal venous blood) of bupivacaine rise to reach a constant value 30 minutes after epidural injection. The UA/MV drug concentration ratio (the ratio at delivery of umbilical arterial to maternal venous blood concentrations) rises with increasing time interval between epidural injection and delivery up to a time of 30 to 40 minutes, and thereafter is unrelated to the dose-delivery interval. In addition, the UA/UV blood concentration ratio (the ratio at delivery of umbilical arterial to umbilical venous blood concentrations) increases as the time between the last epidural injection of bupivacaine and delivery gets longer. It approaches a value of unity 60 minutes after administration, indicating fetal tissue uptake of bupivacaine during the preceding period.

Following the epidural administration of bupivacaine to the pregnant patient, the terminal half-life of bupivacaine in the mother is longer than in the nonpregnant adult, about 9 hours (Table 12.1). This may be due to reduced plasma binding leading to an increased volume of distribution or to continued absorption of bupivacaine in patients undergoing epidural anesthesia. The half-life of bupivacaine in the neonate is even more prolonged (Table 12.3). Maternal plasma bupivacaine levels are very low following subarachnoid injection, i.e., about 5% of those found during epidural bupivacaine anesthesia. Bupivacaine transplacental passage occurs in this situation, but only in very small amounts. Bupivacaine has the advantage of a long duration of action so that infrequent reinjections are required during continuous epidural anesthesia and, in addition, no detrimental effects have been observed on neurobehavioral assessment in the neonate.

The peridural administration of lidocaine or mepivacaine to women in labor results in umbilical concentrations at de-

Table 12.3.
Pharmacokinetic Parameters of Amide Local Anesthetics in the Neonate and Adult

Parameter	Lidocaine	Mepivacaine	Bupivacaine	Etidocaine
Percent bound				
Neonate	25	36	50–70	
Adult	55–65	75–80	85–95	90–95
Total concentration UV/MV ratio	0.5–0.7	0.5–0.7	0.1–0.4	0.2–0.5
V_d* (L/kg)				
Neonate	1.4–4.9	1.2–2.8		
Adult	0.2–1.0	0.6–1.5	0.8–1.6	1.5–1.8
$t_{1/2}$ (hr)				
Neonate	2.9–3.3	5.3–11.3	6.0–22.0	4.0–8.2
Adult	1.0–2.2	1.7–6.9	1.2–9.0	2.0–5.6
CL (L/hr/kg)				
Neonate	0.3–1.14	0.10–0.18		
Adult	0.3–1.09	0.17–1.10	0.3–0.5	0.75–1.15

With permission from Kanto J: Obstetric analgesia: clinical pharmacokinetic considerations. *Clin Pharmacokinet* 11:283–298, 1986.
*V_d, volume of distribution during the terminal elimination phase; $t_{1/2}$, terminal elimination half-life; CL total body clearance.

livery that are about 50 to 70% (lidocaine) and 70% (mepivacaine) of the maternal venous blood concentrations (i.e., UV/M ratios are 0.5 to 0.7 and 0.7, respectively; Table 12.2). The umbilical arterial blood concentration of lidocaine and mepivacaine is also lower than the umbilical venous concentration, indicating fetal uptake. Maternal plasma levels of lidocaine are lower after spinal anesthesia than epidural anesthesia, but lidocaine and its metabolites can be detected in neonatal urine, indicating neonatal exposure to lidocaine.

Thus, both lidocaine and mepivacaine are rapidly transferred to the fetus. There are reduced plasma protein binding and extensive fetal tissue distribution. The neonatal elimination half-life of mepivacaine and lidocaine is increased 2- to 3-fold compared to adults (Table 12.3). The decreased hepatic clearance of mepivacaine is partially compensated for by a higher renal clearance, secondary to decreased protein binding and tubular reabsorption. However, the hepatic clearance of lidocaine in the neonate is similar to that of the adult. The pharmacokinetic characteristics of mepivacaine make it less advantageous than lidocaine for obstetric analgesic practice. Lidocaine clearance is reduced in pregnant patients with preeclampsia compared with healthy pregnant patients.

The presence of epinephrine in local anesthetic solutions generally results in a decrease in blood concentration of local anesthetic, prolongation of regional blockade, and increased degree of motor blockade. The addition of epinephrine to lidocaine and mepivacaine as compared with plain local anesthetic solution lowers the total dose requirement, resulting in lower maternal and umbilical vessel blood concentrations and lower levels in the neonatal circulation during the first 4 hours after birth. There are, therefore, potential benefits to be obtained from the addition of epinephrine to lidocaine and mepivacaine, whereas there is little or no advantage to be gained from its addition to bupivacaine. However, it should also be noted that epinephrine in local anesthetic solution may prolong the length of the first stage due to its well-recognized tocolytic properties.

The half-life of lidocaine in the neonate following epidural injection to the mother is about 3 hours, while the half-life of mepivacaine in the neonate whose mother has received epidural mepivacaine is 9 hours.

The metabolism of bupivacaine occurs by N-dealkylation to the metabolite pipecolylxylidide (PPX), which is about one-eighth as potent and as toxic as the parent compound and is excreted in the urine. In the neonate, N-dealkylated PPX begins to appear at 12 hours and reaches peak concentration in the urine at 24 hours, indicating that the neonate is capable of metabolizing bupivacaine. PPX has been measured in maternal and umbilical venous blood samples at delivery when the UV/MV ratio was found to be in the range 0.7 to 0.95. The neonatal terminal elimination half-lives of bupivacaine and etidocaine are prolonged (Table 12.3), probably due to increased volume of distribution and reduced clearance.

The principal pathway of metabolism for lidocaine is by N-dealkylation to monoethylglycine xylidide (MEGX), with MEGX being only slightly less active than lidocaine. Amide hydrolysis of MEGX leads to the formation of the inactive compounds, xylidine and p-hydroxyxylidine. Amide hydrolysis of MEGX is extensive. Further dealkylation of MEGX to glycine xylidide (GX) also occurs. The newborn has the ability to metabolize lidocaine by similar pathways, and the metabolites of lidocaine are excreted in the urine of the newborn infant. However, the half-life of lidocaine in the newborn is longer (3 hours) than that of the nonpregnant adult (1.6 hours), indicating impaired elimination in the newborn infant (Table 12.3).

In the adult, mepivacaine undergoes both dealkylation and hydroxylation. Ring hydroxylation occurs as the primary reaction and results in the excretion of 15 to 20% of the drug as 3-hydroxymepivacaine and 10 to 14% as 4-hydroxymepivacaine. These metabolites are conjugated and then excreted in the urine. In the newborn, the metabolism of mepivacaine is markedly slower than that of the adult as it is unable to produce significant quantities of the ring-hydroxylated metabolites of mepivacaine. It, therefore, has to rely on renal excretion as the primary route of elimination. Therefore, the half-life of mepivacaine is about 9 hours in the newborn, about 5 times that of the adult. Thus, the neonate appears capable of carrying out the biotransformation of the local anesthetics, but the rate of metabolism and excretion is slower than that of the adult.

There have been reports of cardiac arrest or sudden cardiovascular collapse in parturients receiving bupivacaine to provide epidural analgesia and anesthesia. The cardiotoxicity of bupivacaine is fully discussed in Chapter 11. It now appears that the more potent local anesthetics, bupivacaine and etidocaine, are relatively more cardiotoxic than less potent agents such as lidocaine. The ratio of dose required for cardiovascular collapse and central nervous system toxicity (CC/CNS ratio) is lower for bupivacaine and etidocaine than for lidocaine. Pregnant animals are more sensitive to the cardiotoxic effects of bupivacaine, and ventricular arrhythmias are more likely to occur following toxic doses of bupivacaine than lidocaine. It is extremely important to stress that bupivacaine should be administered in fractionated incremental injections and not as a large dose via a bolus injection when epidural blockade is instituted. The 0.75% concentration of bupivacaine is no longer recommended for obstetric use.

Fetal bradycardia and acidosis are quite often associated with the administration of local anesthetics for paracervical block. Absorption of drugs from the vascular paracervical area is high, and peak maternal blood levels of lidocaine and mepivacaine (both without epinephrine) occur within 5 to 30 minutes after administration. Lidocaine concentrations in fetal scalp blood reach maximum values after 6 to 20 minutes. In some patients, it has been reported that the levels of mepivacaine and lidocaine were higher in fetal than maternal blood, and

studies have indicated that the UV/MV blood concentration for bupivacaine is higher after paracervical block than after epidural blockade. Adverse effects in the fetus following paracervical block are also related to the effect of high circulating local anesthetic concentrations on the myometrium; local anesthetics increase myometrial tonicity, thereby reducing placental blood flow with consequent fetal hypoxia, bradycardia, and acidosis.

Table 12.3 contrasts the pharmacokinetic parameters of amide local anesthetics in the neonate and adult.

Narcotic Analgesics

Although the narcotic analgesics are more than 95% ionized at physiological pH, the lipid-soluble nonionized fraction rapidly crosses the placenta to reach the fetus.

MEPERIDINE

Meperidine remains the most widely administered narcotic for the relief of maternal pain during labor and delivery. It may be administered by intramuscular injection (50 to 100 mg) or by intravenous injection (25 to 50 mg). The peak analgesic effect occurs within 40 to 60 minutes following intramuscular injection and 5 to 10 minutes following intravenous administration.

Narcotic analgesics have long been known to produce neonatal respiratory depression, but meperidine is thought to depress the infant's respiration less than morphine. It has been demonstrated, for example, that morphine shifts the carbon dioxide respiratory response curve of the newborn infant downwards and to the right to a greater extent than does meperidine (Fig. 12.6), and it has been suggested that the increased sensitivity of the newborn to morphine is due to an immature blood-brain barrier which permits a larger amount of morphine to gain access to receptor sites within the central nervous system.

The disposition of meperidine in pregnant patients during labor following intravenous injection has been studied and compared with healthy nonpregnant fe-

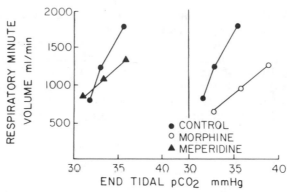

Figure 12.6. Effect of morphine and meperidine on the CO_2 response curve. (With permission from Way WL, Costley EC, Way EL: Respiratory sensitivity of the newborn infant to meperidine and morphine. *Clin Pharmacol Ther* 6:454–461, 1965.)

male subjects (Table 12.1). Clearance is reduced in labor, but similar to estimates reported for nonpregnant patients undergoing other surgical procedures. These effects were thought to be associated with the surgical stress of labor and delivery. However, other studies report no differences in pharmacokinetic parameters between pregnant and nonpregnant female subjects. Although pregnant and nonpregnant females metabolize meperidine similarly, it is evident that the neonate cannot n-demethylate meperidine to normeperidine as effectively as the adult. During the first 2 days of life, the neonate whose mother has received meperidine during labor excretes more parent compound than metabolite. During this 2-day period, the amount of meperidine excreted in the urine slowly decreases, but the urinary excretion of normeperidine falls more slowly, so that by the third day, more normeperidine than meperidine is excreted by the neonate. Thus, 3 days or longer are required for the infant to eliminate meperidine given to the mother during labor (Fig. 12.7). Umbilical cord/maternal venous blood concentration ratios of meperidine at delivery are in the region of 0.7 to 2.0; UV/MV and UA/MV blood concentration ratios increase with time following maternal meperidine administration and may reach values of greater than unity after 2 to 3 hours. In addition, it has been shown that the period of time between the intravenous injection of meperidine to the

mother and delivery (dose-delivery interval) has a critical effect on neonatal urine elimination of meperidine during the first 3 days of life. Neonatal excretion of meperidine appears to be greater when the dose-delivery interval is 2 to 3 hours, and much less if the dose-delivery interval is either longer or shorter.

Low fetal α_1-acid glycoprotein concentrations lead to low fetal plasma binding. The elimination half-life of meperidine is about 3 hours in the mother (Table 12.1) and 22 hours in the neonate.

Both spinal and epidurally administered narcotics have been used in the pregnant patient. In general, much lower dosages are required when narcotics are administered either spinally or epidurally than when given intravenously or intramuscularly. Therefore, placental transfer, although it will occur, is likely to be unimportant. Table 12.4 lists mean peak plasma concentrations of epidural and intrathecal narcotics when given to pregnant patients in labor.

Crawford has shown that, following an intravenous injection of meperidine to pregnant patients in labor, a greater proportion of the dose is transferred to the neonate than following intramuscular injection. Some animal studies have shown that epidural injection results in similar mean peak concentrations to those following intramuscular injection. Following meperidine (100 mg) given epidurally, maternal concentrations are higher than when given via the intramuscular

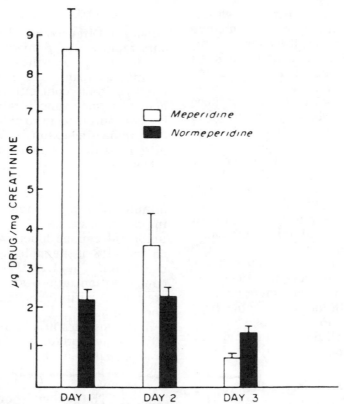

Figure 12.7.   Urinary excretion of meperidine and normeperidine by the neonate for 3 days postpartum.   (With permission from Kuhnert BR, Kuhnert PM, Prochaska AL, Sokol RJ: Meperidine disposition in mother, neonate, and nonpregnant females. *Clin Pharmacol Ther* 27:486–491, 1980.)

Table 12.4.
Plasma Concentrations of Narcotics after Epidural and Intrathecal Administration in Labor

Narcotic	Dose	Route of administration	C_{MAX}* (μg/L)	t_{MAX} (min)
Morphine	4 mg	Intramuscular	24.8	11.3
Morphine	4 mg	Epidural	12.5	20.8
Morphine + epinephrine	4 mg	Epidural	13.1	20.4
Morphine	0.02 mg/kg	Intrathecal	6	180
Meperidine	100 mg	Epidural	$\simeq$650	10
Meperidine	100 mg	Intramuscular	$\simeq$350	

With permission from Kanto J: Obstetric analgesia: clinical pharmacokinetic considerations. *Clin Pharmacokinet* 11:283–298, 1986.
*C_{MAX}, mean peak plasma concentration; t_{MAX}, time to peak plasma concentration.

route, probably due to increased vascularity of the epidural space in pregnancy (Table 12.4). However, it has been demonstrated that 25 mg of meperidine given as a single dose into the epidural space produced relief of labor pain with plasma concentrations of 45 to 188 μg/L; these are concentrations less than required to produce analgesia after intramuscular injection (about 350 μg/L; Table 12.4), suggesting that the primary site of action is in the spinal cord. When fentanyl was given via the epidural route as a single injection (150 to 250 μg), plasma drug concentrations 30 minutes later were low (0.01 to 1.1 ng/ml) and unlikely to cause respiratory depression.

Spinal and epidural narcotics given alone have not been adequate to control labor pain. However, techniques combining narcotics with local anesthetics have proved effective; for example, the combination of a small dose of fentanyl with a local anesthetic such as bupivacaine.

Inhalational Anesthetics

Pregnancy reduces anesthetic requirements. The minimum alveolar concentration (MAC) is reduced by up to 32% for methoxyflurane, 25% for halothane, and 40% for isoflurane during pregnancy; the mechanism is as yet undefined but is possibly related to increased levels of progesterone, which exerts a sedative effect.

The inhalational agents diffuse rapidly across the placenta because they are highly lipid soluble, unionized compounds. The degree of neonatal depression correlates with both maternal blood concentration and the time that the neonate has been exposed to the anesthetic agent. In addition, neonatal depression may also be due to physiological changes such as maternal hypotension or hypoxia produced by the inhalational anesthetic agent.

Halothane, enflurane, diethyl ether, and isoflurane have all been shown to cause uterine relaxation in a dose-related manner. Nitrous oxide and cyclopropane have little or no effect upon uterine activity.

NITROUS OXIDE

Placental transfer of nitrous oxide occurs rapidly, and Stenger found that as nitrous oxide anesthesia is continued during cesarean section after about 36 minutes, fetal concentrations approach maternal blood concentrations. The UA/UV concentration ratio at 36 minutes was 0.89, indicating extensive fetal uptake of nitrous oxide. The rapid transmission of nitrous oxide across the placenta has also been demonstrated by Marx and her coworkers, who found that, after 2 to 19 minutes of nitrous oxide anesthesia during cesarean section, the concentration in umbilical venous blood varied between 55 and 91% of the maternal arterial concentration. The UA/UV nitrous oxide concentration ratio again increased progressively with increasing duration of anesthesia.

A mixture of 50% nitrous oxide and 50% oxygen produces a significant degree of analgesia when administered during labor. It is more frequently inhaled by the patient intermittently with each contraction. The patient should be encouraged to breathe nitrous oxide before the onset of the painful contraction to allow the attainment of adequate nitrous oxide concentrations in the blood. Since nitrous oxide is relatively insoluble in blood (blood/gas partition coefficient is 0.47 at 37°C), blood levels rise rapidly, and a period of 45 to 50 seconds is sufficient time to produce an analgesic blood concentration (Fig. 12.8).

METHOXYFLURANE

Methoxyflurane at a concentration of 0.35% has been administered to provide analgesia during labor and delivery, although it is little used today. Methoxyflurane is highly soluble in blood (blood/gas partition coefficient is 13.0 at 37°C), and the time taken to achieve adequate maternal analgesic concentrations of methoxyflurane is longer than that associated with nitrous oxide (Fig. 12.8). The intermittent administration of methoxyflurane produces adequate analgesia without the same variation in blood concentrations of methoxyflurane that occur

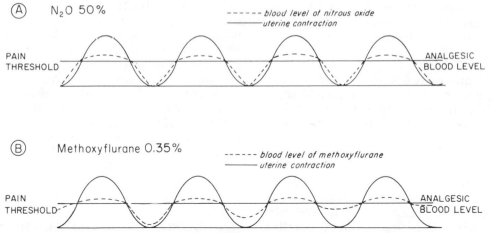

Figure 12.8.   Nitrous oxide and methoxyflurane as inhalation analgesic agents in obstetric patients.   Note that the level of nitrous oxide rises rapidly to reach analgesic blood levels and falls equally rapidly when inhalation ceases. Therefore, inhalation should be commenced prior to onset of contractions to achieve adequate analgesic levels. Methoxyflurane levels rise more slowly and consequently fall slowly allowing for some accumulation to occur leaving the baseline level close to the analgesic blood level.

with nitrous oxide administration (Fig. 12.8). Progressive accumulation results if administration is prolonged. Methoxyflurane (0.35%) does not appear to influence uterine contractility, but higher anesthetic concentrations (0.5 to 0.8%) cause uterine atony and postpartum bleeding.

Maternal and fetal plasma concentrations have been measured during the use of methoxyflurane for both analgesia and anesthesia, when UV/MA blood concentration ratios were reported as 0.5 to 0.7 at delivery. When methoxyflurane anesthesia followed the use of methoxyflurane analgesia, the incidence of neonatal depression was higher, and this was associated with higher umbilical venous blood levels of methoxyflurane at delivery.

It is well recognized that renal toxicity is associated with the metabolism of methoxyflurane to inorganic fluoride ion (see Chapter 9). Serum inorganic fluoride levels over 80 μmol/L are associated with high-output renal impairment, while levels over 50 μmol/L result in subclinical renal impairment with decreased concentrating ability of the renal

tubules. Maternal and neonatal inorganic fluoride levels are elevated following the use of methoxyflurane analgesia in pregnant patients, but not usually to nephrotoxic levels. Neonatal levels of serum inorganic fluoride at delivery following maternal methoxyflurane analgesia are in the range of 5 to 14 μmol/L and do not appear to produce any demonstrable renal impairment in the newborn.

HALOTHANE

Halothane is used to provide rapid profound uterine relaxation in certain emergency situations, such as during delivery of a second twin or during the attempted removal of a retained placenta.

Halothane at a concentration of 0.5 to 0.8% has been used as an adjunct to nitrous oxide-oxygen anesthesia during the course of cesarean section. It has been shown to reduce the incidence of maternal awareness which may occur during the administration of 60 to 70% nitrous oxide and has not been associated with uterine relaxation sufficient to increase postpartum blood loss. The administration of higher concentrations of halothane may cause maternal hypotension and postpartum bleeding.

ENFLURANE

Enflurane causes dose-related uterine relaxation such that administration of 3% enflurane is likely to produce a significant increase in postpartum bleeding.

ISOFLURANE

Isoflurane causes dose-dependent reduction in uterine contractility similar to that seen with halothane and enflurane at equipotent dosage. Since it possesses less myocardial depressant properties and a greater degree of analgesia, isoflurane is superior to halothane for administration during cesarean section. Its lack of seizure producing potential makes it superior to enflurane in obstetric practice. Current opinion regards a maternal inspired concentration of oxygen during general anesthesia of at least 50 percent to be optimal for the neonate. If this concentration of oxygen is administered with nitrous oxide alone the incidence of maternal awareness is unacceptably high. This problem can be eliminated by the use of low concentrations (i.e., 0.5 MAC) of one of the volatile anesthetic agents (viz isoflurane), without significantly interfering with myometrial contractility.

Other Drugs

MAGNESIUM

In the United States, magnesium sulfate is widely used in the management of preeclamptic toxemia and eclampsia. Magnesium has important effects on the central nervous system; hypermagnesemia causes depression of the central nervous system, while hypomagnesemia causes central nervous system irritability, disorientation, and convulsions. Excess magnesium in the extracellular fluid results in a decrease in acetylcholine release at the neuromuscular junction, reduces the sensitivity of the motor end plate to acetylcholine, and decreases the amplitude of the motor end plate poten-

tial. The administration of magnesium sulfate potentiates the neuromuscular blocking effect of both the depolarizing and nondepolarizing muscle relaxants, and their dosage should be reduced accordingly (see Chapter 10). The effects of excess magnesium ions at the neuromuscular junction are opposed by calcium.

Magnesium crosses the placenta, and the newborn may be drowsy and exhibit decreased muscle tone at delivery. The maternal administration of high doses of magnesium may result in neonatal hypoventilation requiring assisted ventilation.

A suggested regimen for the administration of magnesium sulfate during labor is to inject a bolus (4 g) intravenously, followed by the continuous intravenous infusion of a solution of magnesium sulfate (10 g/L) administered at a rate of 100 ml/hour (i.e., 1 g/hour).

The magnesium plasma level in normal subjects ranges from 1.5 to 2.2 mEq/L, while the therapeutic concentration range required to control the symptoms of preeclamptic toxemia is about 4.0 to 6.0 mEq/L. When treating patients with toxemia, it is important to monitor plasma magnesium concentrations and to ascertain the presence of deep tendon reflexes, since these are abolished when the plasma level reaches 10 mEq/L. Respiratory paralysis is possible when plasma levels reach 15 mEq/L.

OXYTOCICS

Oxytocic drugs possess the ability to stimulate the smooth muscle of the uterus and have been classified into three groups:

1. Oxytocin
2. Prostaglandins
3. Ergot derivatives

The oxytocic drugs are used by obstetricians to induce labor at term, correct postpartum uterine atony, treat postpartum bleeding, and induce therapeutic abortion.

The prostaglandin group of drugs is discussed in Chapter 24, and only oxytocin and the ergot derivatives will be discussed here.

Oxytocin is one of the polypeptide hormones of the posterior lobe of the pituitary gland. It stimulates uterine smooth muscle activity, increasing the frequency of existing contractions and raising the tone of the uterine musculature. In early pregnancy, the uterus is responsive to only high doses of oxytocin, whereas in the third trimester, there is a sharp rise in sensitivity culminating in the initiation of labor and delivery.

Oxytocin is prepared synthetically to limit antidiuretic and cardiovascular effects of contaminating vasopressin (ADH). However, synthetic oxytocin has also intrinsic antidiuretic properties, and cardiovascular effects may be manifest when high doses are administered. Synthetic oxytocin (Pitocin, Syntocinon) is usually administered intravenously, either as a bolus or continuous infusion, to stimulate and augment labor or to maintain uterine contraction and reduce bleeding from the uterus following delivery of the neonate and placenta. Oxytocin has marked but transient vasodilator effects when administered in large doses; a decrease in arterial blood pressure may occur, followed by a reflex-induced tachycardia and increase in cardiac output. The hypotensive effect is usually seen within 30 seconds of administration and seldom lasts beyond 10 minutes. Generally, there is no rebound hypertension. Transient electrocardiographic (ECG) changes such as T-wave flattening or inversion, prolongation of the QT interval, and tachycardia may be observed. Synthetic oxytocin also possesses antidiuretic activity and may cause water intoxication and dilutional hyponatremia when administered as a continuous intravenous infusion in an electrolyte-free solution over a prolonged period of time.

ERGOT DERIVATIVES

Ergot is the product of a fungus that grows on grasses, especially rye. The peripheral vascular effects of ergot led to epidemics of painful gangrene of the extremities during the Middle Ages due to the consumption of bread made from infected rye. A frequent complication of ergot poisoning (ergotism) was abortion.

Today, only a few purified ergot alkaloids are available for clinical use—ergonovine (Ergometrine), ergotamine, and methylergonovine. Ergonovine and oxytocin differ in their effect on the pregnant uterus. In moderate doses, oxytocin causes slow generalized contractions with a period of relaxation in between while moderate doses of ergonovine produce faster contractions superimposed on a tonic contraction. Higher doses of both drugs produce sustained tonic contraction. Thus, oxytocin is used for the induction of labor at term, while ergonovine is used only to prevent postpartum hemorrhage and is, therefore, administered after delivery. All the natural ergot alkaloids can cause a significant rise in blood pressure due to direct peripheral vasoconstriction; this is more marked with ergotamine than ergonovine or methylergonovine. Complications of ergonovine include nausea and vomiting and, rarely, hypertension. In addition, the ergot alkaloids also exhibit α-adrenergic blockade; ergotamine possesses significant α-adrenergic blocking effect, while ergonovine does not.

β_2-RECEPTOR AGONISTS

The knowledge that epinephrine inhibits uterine contractility led to the investigation of the use of β_2-receptor agonists to control premature labor (see Chapter 13). Administration of the β_2-agonists *terbutaline* and *ritodrine* to prevent preterm labor requires dosage to be titrated to clinical effect, i.e., until uterine contractions cease. At high doses, side effects include tachycardia, arrhythmias, and angina and may necessitate discontinuation of the drug. Pulmonary edema has also been reported in association with the use of β_2-receptor agonists in pregnancy, but the etiology remains controversial.

BIBLIOGRAPHY

Drug Uptake and Distribution in Mother and Fetus

Biehl D, Shnider SM, Levinson G, Callender K: Placental transfer of lidocaine: effects of fetal acidosis. *Anesthesiology* 48:409–412, 1978.

Finster M, Morishima HO, Boyes RN, Covino BG: The placental transfer of lidocaine and its uptake by fetal tissues. *Anesthesiology* 36:159–163, 1972.

Finster M, Pederson H: Placental transfer and fetal uptake of drugs. *Br J Anaesth* 51:25S–28S, 1979.

Green TP, O'Dea RF, Mirkin BL: Determinants of drug disposition and effect in the fetus. *Annu Rev Pharmacol Toxicol* 19:285–322, 1979.

Kennedy RL, Erenberg A, Robillard JE, Merkow A, Turner R: Effects of changes in maternal-fetal pH on the transplacental equilibrium of bupivacaine. *Anesthesiology* 51:50–54, 1979.

Kennedy RL, Miller RP, Bell JU, Doshi D, deSousa H, Kennedy MJ, Heald DL, David Y: Uptake and distribution of bupivacaine in fetal lambs. *Anesthesiology* 65:247–253, 1986.

Mill MD, Abramson FP: The significance of plasma protein binding on the fetal/maternal distribution of drugs at steady-state. *Clin Pharmacokinet* 14:156–170, 1988.

Mirkin BL: Perinatal pharmacology: placental transfer, fetal localization, and neonatal disposition of drugs. *Anesthesiology* 43:156–170, 1975.

Thomas J, Long G, Moore G, Morgan D: Plasma protein binding and placental transfer of bupivacaine. *Clin Pharmacol Ther* 19:426–434, 1976.

Tucker GT, Boyes RN, Bridenbaugh PO, Moore DC: Binding of anilide-type local anesthetic in human plasma. II. Implications in vivo, with special reference to transplacental distribution. *Anesthesiology* 33:304–314, 1970.

Vree TB, Reekers-Ketting JJ, Fragen RJ, Arts THM: Placental transfer of midazolam and its metabolite 1-hydroxymethylmidazolam in the pregnant ewe. *Anesth Analg* 63:31–34, 1984.

Wood M: Plasma drug binding: implications for anesthesiologists. *Anesth Analg* 65:786–804, 1986.

Wood M, Wood AJJ: Changes in plasma drug binding and α-acid glycoprotein in mother and newborn. *Clin Pharmacol Ther* 29:522-526, 1981.

Thiopental

Finster M, Mark LC, Morishima HD, Moya F, Perel JM, James LS, Dayton PG: Plasma thiopental concentrations in the newborn following delivery under thiopental-nitrous oxide anesthesia. *Am J Obstet Gynecol* 95:621–629, 1966.

Finster M, Morishima HO, Mark LC, Perel JM, Dayton PG, James LS: Tissue thiopental concentrations in the fetus and newborn. *Anesthesiology* 36:155–158, 1972.

Kosaka Y, Takahashi R, Mark LC: Intravenous thiobarbiturate anesthesia for cesarean section. *Anesthesiology* 31:489–506, 1969.

Muscle Relaxants

Cronnelly R, Fisher DM, Miller RD, Gencarelli P, Nguyen-Gruenke L, Castagnoli N: Pharmacokinetics and pharmacodynamics of vecuronium (ORG NC45) and pancuronium in anesthetized humans. *Anesthesiology* 58:405–508, 1983.

Dailey PA, Fisher DM, Shnider SM, Baysinger CL, Shinohara Y, Miller RD, Abboud TK, Kim KG: Pharmacokinetics, placental transfer, and neonatal effects of vecuronium and pancuronium administered during cesarean section. *Anesthesiology* 60:569–574, 1984.

Demetriou M, Depoix JP, Diakite B, Fromentin M, Duvaldestin P: Placental transfer of ORG NC 45 in women undergoing cesarean section. *Br J Anaesth* 54:643–645, 1982.

Flynn PJ, Frank M, Hughes R: Use of atracurium in caesarean section. *Br J Anaesth* 56:599–604, 1984.

Local Anesthetics

Chestnut DH, Geiger MW, Bates JN, et al.: The influence of pH-adjusted 2-chloroprocaine on the quality and duration of subsequent epidural bupivacaine during labor: a randomized, double-blind study. *Anesthesiology* A667, 1988.

Corke BC, Carlson CG, Dettborn WD: The influence of 2-chloroprocaine in the subsequent analgesic potency of bupivacaine. *Anesthesiology* 60:25–27, 1984.

Hodgkinson R, Husain FJ, Bluhm C: Reduced effectiveness of bupivacaine 0.5% to relieve labor pain after prior injection of chloroprocaine 2%. *Anesthesiology* 57:A201, 1982.

Ketalko DM, Thigpen JW, Shnider SM, et al.: Postoperative epidural morphine analgesia after various local anesthetics. *Anesthesiology* 59:A413, 1988.

Kuhnert BR, Kuhnert PM, Prochaska AL, Gross TL: Plasma levels of 2-chloroprocaine in obstetric patients and their neonates after epidural anesthesia. *Anesthesiology* 53:21–25, 1980.

Kuhnert BR, Zuspan KJ, Kuhnert PM, Syracuse CD, Brown DE: Bupivacaine disposition in mother, fetus, and neonate after spinal anesthesia for cesarean section. *Anesth Analg* 66:407–412, 1987.

Moore DC, Spierdijk J, VanKleef JD, Coleman RL, Love GF: Chloroprocaine neurotoxicity: four additional cases. *Anesth Analg* 61:155–159, 1982.

Morishima HO, Finster M, Pedersen H, Fukunaga A, Ronfeld RA, Vassallo HG, Covino BG: Pharmacokinetics of lidocaine in fetal and neonatal lambs and adult sheep. *Anesthesiology* 50:431–436, 1979.

Naulty JS, Hertwig L, Hunt CO: Durations of analgesia of epidural fentanyl following cesarean delivery—effects of local anesthetic drug selection. *Anesthesiology* 65:A180, 1986.

Pedersen H, Santos AC, Morishima HO, Finster M, Plosker H, Arthur GR, Covino BG: Does gestational age affect the pharmacokinetics and pharmacodynamics of lidocaine in mother and fetus? *Anesthesiology* 68:367–372, 1988.

Poppers PJ: Evaluation of local anesthetic agents for regional anaesthesia in obstetrics. *Br J Anaesth* 47:322–327, 1975.

Ralston HD, Shnider SM: The fetal and neonatal effects of regional anesthesia in obstetrics. *Anesthesiology* 48:34–64, 1978.

Ramanathan J, Bottorff M, Jeter J, Khalil M, Sibai GM: The pharmacokinetics and maternal and neonatal effects of epidural lidocaine in preeclampsia. *Anesth Analg* 65:120–126, 1986.

Ravindran RS, Bond VK, Tasch MD, Gupta CD, Luerssen TG: Prolonged neural blockade following regional analgesia with 2-chloroprocaine. *Anesth Analg* 59:447–451, 1980.

Reisner LS, Hochman BN, Plumer MH: Persistent neurologic deficit and adhesive arachnoiditis following intrathecal 2-chloroprocaine injection. *Anesth Analg* 59:452–454, 1980.

Reynolds F, Taylor G: Maternal and neonatal blood concentrations of bupivacaine. A comparison with lignocaine during continuous extradural analgesia. *Anaesthesia* 25:14–23, 1970.

Reynolds F, Taylor G: Plasma concentrations of bupivacaine during continuous epidural analgesia in labour: the effect of adrenaline. *Br J Anaesth* 43:436–440, 1971.

Santos C, Pedersen H, Morishima HO, Finster M, Arthur GR, Covino BG: Pharmacokinetics of lidocaine in nonpregnant and pregnant ewes. *Anesth Analg* 67:1154–1158, 1988.

Scanlon JW, Brown WU, Weiss JB, Alper MH: Neurobehavioural responses of newborn infants after maternal epidural anesthesia. *Anesthesiology* 40:121–128, 1974.

Scanlon JW, Ostheimer GW, Lurie AO, Brown WU, Weiss JB, Alper MH: Neurobehavioural responses and drug concentrations in newborns after maternal epidural anesthesia with bupivacaine. *Anesthesiology* 45:400–405, 1976.

Writer WDR, Davies JM, Strunin L: Editorial: Trial by media: the bupivacaine story. *Can Anaesth Soc J* 31:1–4, 1984.

Narcotic Analgesics

Beckett AH: Maternal and neonatal metabolism of analgesic drugs. *Br J Anaesth* 45(suppl):770–781, 1973.

Crawford JS, Rudofsky S: The placental transmission of pethidine. *Br J Anaesth* 37:929–933, 1965.

Nimmo WS, Wilson J, Prescott LF: Narcotic analgesics and delayed gastric emptying during labour. *Lancet* 1:890–893, 1975.

Szeto HH, Mann I, Bhakthavathsalan A, Liu M, Inturrisi CE: Meperidine pharmacokinetics in the maternal-fetal unit. *J Pharmacol Exp Ther* 206:448–459, 1978.

Tomson G, Garle RIM, Thalme B, Nisell H, Nylund L, Rane A: Maternal kinetics and transplacental passage of pethidine during labour. *Br J Clin Pharmacol* 13:653–659, 1982.

Way WL, Costley EC, Way EL: Respiratory sensitivity of the newborn infant to meperidine and morphine. *Clin Pharmacol Ther* 6:454–461, 1965.

Inhalational Anesthetics

Clark RB, Beard AG, Thompson DS, Barclay DL: Maternal and neonatal plasma inorganic fluoride levels after methoxyflurane analgesia for labor and delivery. *Anesthesiology* 45:88–91, 1976.

Clark RB, Cooper JO, Brown WE, Greifenstein FE: The effect of methoxyflurane on the foetus. *Br J Anaesth* 42:286–294, 1970.

Marx GF, Joshi CW, Orkin LR: Placental transmission of nitrous oxide. *Anesthesiology* 32:429–432, 1970.

Munson ES, Embro WJ: Enflurane, isoflurane, and halothane and isolated human uterine muscle. *Anesthesiology* 46:11–14, 1977.

Palahniuk RJ, Shnider SM, Eger EI: Pregnancy decreases the requirement for inhaled anesthetic agents. *Anesthesiology* 41:82–83, 1974.

Siker ES, Wolfson B, Dubnansky J, Fitting GM: Placental transfer of methoxyflurane. *Br J Anaesth* 40:588–592, 1968.

Magnesium

Gambling DR, Birmingham CL, Jenkins LC: Magnesium and the anaesthetist. *Can J Anaesth* 35:644–654, 1988.

β_2-Receptor Agonists

Caritis SN: Treatment of preterm labour. A review of the therapeutic options. *Drugs* 26:243–261, 1983.

Hutchings MJ, Paull JD, Wilson-Evered E, Morgan DJ: Pharmacokinetics and metabolism of salbutamol in premature labour. *Br J Clin Pharmacol* 24:69–75, 1987.

Pharmacokinetics

Belfrage P, Berlin A, Raabe N, Thalme B: Lumbar epidural analgesia with bupivacaine in labor. Drug concentration in maternal and neonatal blood at birth and during the first day of life. *Am J Obstet Gynecol* 123:839–844, 1975.

Belfrage P, Raabe N, Thalme B, Berlin A: Lumbar epidural analgesia with bupivacaine in labor. Determination of drug concentration and pH in fetal scalp blood, and continuous fetal heart rate monitoring. *Am J Obstet Gynecol* 121:360–365, 1975.

Blankenbaker WL, DiFazio CA, Berry FA: Lidocaine and its metabolites in the newborn. *Anesthesiology* 42:325–330, 1975.

Booth PN, Watson MJ, McLeod K: Pancuronium and the placental barrier. *Anaesthesia* 32:320–323, 1977.

Brown WU, Bell GC, Alper MH: Acidosis, local anesthetics, and newborns. *Obstet Gynecol* 48:27–30, 1976.

Brown WU, Bell GC, Lurie AO, Weiss JB, Scanlon JW, Alper MH: Newborn levels of lidocaine and mepivacaine in the first postnatal day following maternal epidural anesthesia. *Anesthesiology* 42:698–707, 1975.

Caldwell J, Moffatt JR, Smith RL, Lieberman BA, Cawston MO, Beard RW: Pharmacokinetics of bupivacaine administered epidurally during childbirth. *Br J Clin Pharmacol* 3:956P–957P, 1976.

Cummings AJ: A survey of pharmacokinetic data from pregnant women. *Clin Pharmacokinet* 8:344–354, 1983.

Cummings AJ, Whitelaw AGL: A study of conjugation and drug elimination in the human neonate. *Br J Clin Pharmacol* 12:511–515, 1981.

Datta S, Alper MH, Ostheimer GW, Brown WU, Weiss JB: Effects of maternal position on epidural anesthesia for cesarean section, acid-base status, and bupivacaine concentrations at delivery. *Anesthesiology* 50:205–209, 1979.

DiFazio CA: Metabolism of local anesthetics in the fetus, newborn, and adult. *Br J Anaesth* 51(suppl):29S–33S), 1979.

Duvaldestin P, Demetriou M, Henzel D, Desmonts JM: The placental transfer of pancuronium and its pharmacokinetics during caesarean section. *Acta Anaesthesiol Scand* 22:327–333, 1978.

Fox GS, Houle GL, Desjardins PD, Mercier G: Intrauterine fetal lidocaine concentrations during continuous epidural anesthesia. *Am J Obstet Gynecol* 110:896–899, 1971.

Frederiksen MC, Ruo TI, Chow MJ, Atkinson AJ: Theophylline pharmacokinetics in pregnancy. *Clin Pharmacol Ther* 40:321–328, 1986.

Hogg MIJ, Wiener PC, Rosen M, Mapleson WW: Urinary excretion and metabolism of pethidine and norpethidine in the newborn. *Br J Anaesth* 49:891–899, 1977.

Hyman MD, Shnider SM: Maternal and neonatal blood concentrations of bupivacaine associated with obstetrical conduction anesthesia. *Anesthesiology* 34:81–86, 1971.

Juchau MR, Chao ST, Omiecinski CJ: Drug metabolism by the human fetus. *Clin Pharmacokinet* 5:320–339, 1980.

Kanto J: Obstetric analgesia: clinical pharmacokinetic considerations. *Clin Pharmacokinet* 11:283–298, 1986.

Krauer B, Krauer F: Drug kinetics in pregnancy. *Clin Pharmacokinet* 2:167–181, 1977.

Kuhnert BR, Knapp DR, Kuhnert PM, Prochaska AL: Maternal and fetal and neonatal metabolism of lidocaine. *Clin Pharmacol Ther* 26:213–220, 1979.

Kuhnert BR, Kuhnert PM, Prochaska AL, Sokol RJ: Meperidine disposition in mother, neonate, and nonpregnant females. *Clin Pharmacol Ther* 27:486–491, 1980.

Kuhnert BR, Kuhnert PM, Tu AL, Lin DCK: Meperidine and normeperidine levels following meperidine administration during labor. II. Fetus and neonate. *Am J Obstet Gynecol* 133:909–914, 1979.

Kuhnert BR, Kuhnert PM, Tu AL, Lin DCK, Foltz RL: Meperidine and normeperidine levels following meperidine administration during labor. I. Mother. *Am J Obstet Gynecol* 133:904–908, 1979.

Kuhnert BR, Philipson EH, Pimental R, Kuhnert PM, Zuspan KJ, Syracuse CD: Lidocaine disposition in mother, fetus, and neonate after spinal anesthesia. *Anesth Analg* 65:139–144, 1986.

Magno R, Berlin A, Karlsson K, Kjellmer I: Anesthesia for cesarean section. IV. Placental transfer and neonatal elimination of bupivacaine following epidural anesthesia for elective cesarean section. *Acta Anaesthesiol Scand* 20:141–146, 1976.

Mitani GM, Steinberg I, Lien EJ, Harrison EC, Elkayam U: The pharmacokinetics of antiarrhythmic agents in pregnancy and lactation. *Clin Pharmacokinet* 12:253–291, 1987.

Morishima HO, Finster M, Pederson H, Fukunaga A, Ronfeld RA, Vassallo HG, Covino BG: Pharmacokinetics of lidocaine in fetal and neonatal lambs and adult sheep. *Anesthesiology* 50:431–436, 1979.

Morselli PL: Clinical pharmacokinetics in neonates. *Clin Pharmacokinet* 1:81–98, 1976.

Nation RL: Drug kinetics in childbirth. *Clin Pharmacokinet* 5:340–364, 1980.

Wilson CM, Dundee JW, Moore J, Howard PJ, Collier PS: A comparison of the early pharmacokinetics of midazolam in pregnant and nonpregnant women. *Anaesthesia* 42:1057–1062, 1987.

General

Aranda JV, Turmen T, Cote-Boileau T: Drug monitoring in the perinatal patient: uses and abuses. *Therapeutic Drug Monitoring* 2:39–49, 1980.

Besunder JB, Reed MD, Blumer JL: Principles of drug biodisposition in the neonate. A critical evaluation of the pharmacokinetic-pharmacodynamic interface (part I). *Clin Pharmacokinet* 14:189–216, 1988.

Besunder JB, Reed MD, Blumer JL: Principles of drug biodisposition in the neonate. A critical evaluation of the pharmacokinetic-pharmacodynamic interface (part II). *Clin Pharmacokinet* 14:261–286, 1988.

Morgan CA, Paull J: Drugs in obstetric anaesthesia, *Anaesth Intens Care* 8:278–288, 1980.

Rubin PC: Beta-blockers in pregnancy. *N Engl J Med* 305:1323–1326, 1981.

Whittaker M, Crawford JS, Lewis M: Some observations of levels of plasma cholinesterase activity within an obstetric population. *Anaesthesia* 43:42–45, 1988.

SECTION 3

CARDIOVASCULAR THERAPEUTICS

13

Drugs and the Sympathetic Nervous System

MARGARET WOOD

SELECTIVE β_2-RECEPTOR AGONISTS
   Metaproterenol
   Albuterol
   Terbutaline
   Fenoterol
   Ritodrine
   Isoetharine

THERAPEUTIC USES

NOREPINEPHRINE, EPINEPHRINE, AND THE SYMPATHOMIMETIC AMINES

The sympathomimetic drugs mimic the effects of stimulation of the sympathetic nervous system. They include:

1. **Norepinephrine** (levarterenol, noradrenaline). The transmitter at most sympathetic postganglionic adrenergic nerve terminals.
2. **Epinephrine** (adrenaline). The major hormone of the adrenal medulla.
3. **Dopamine.** The immediate precursor of norepinephrine found in high concentrations in sympathetic nerves and the adrenal medulla but also in the extrapyramidal nervous system.
4. **Isoproterenol** (isoprenaline). A synthetic catecholamine which does not occur in the body.

PHYSIOLOGY OF THE SYMPATHETIC NERVOUS SYSTEM

The autonomic nervous system is divided into two divisions, sympathetic and parasympathetic. The preganglionic fibers of the sympathetic nervous system arise from the thoracolumbar segments of the spinal cord, while the corresponding preganglionic fibers of the parasympathetic nervous system have a craniosacral origin. These preganglionic fibers synapse in autonomic ganglia from which arise postganglionic fibers that then innervate either adrenergic or cholinergic receptors situated throughout the body (Fig. 13.1). The neurotransmitter for the adrenergic receptor is norepinephrine, and the transmitter for the cholinergic receptors is acetylcholine. The adrenal medulla is embryologically and functionally homologous to the sympathetic autonomic ganglia, since the secretory chromaffin cells of the adrenal medulla originate from the same region of the neural crest as do the sympathetic ganglion cells, but differ in that the principal catecholamine released by the adrenal medulla is epinephrine and not norepinephrine.

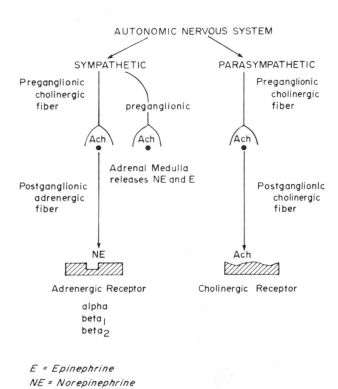

E = Epinephrine
NE = Norepinephrine
Ach = Acetyl choline

Figure 13.1.   Diagram of the autonomic nervous system.

Epinephrine, norepinephrine, and dopamine are all naturally occurring catecholamines while isoproterenol is a synthetic catecholamine. Norepinephrine is found mainly in the sympathetic nerves of the peripheral and central nervous system and acts locally on the effector cells in a wide variety of tissues—vascular smooth muscle, fat, liver, intestines, heart, spleen, adrenal medulla, and the brain and spinal cord. Dopamine, the immediate precursor of norepinephrine, is found in high concentrations in sympathetic nerves and also in the adrenal gland. In addition, dopamine is found in the eye and the brain. Investigations of the function of dopaminergic receptors in the basal ganglia of the brain have resulted in the use of levodopa in the treatment of Parkinson's disease. High concentrations of epinephrine are found in the adrenal medulla where the proportion of epinephrine to norepinephrine varies with age. In human adults, approximately 80% of adrenal medullary sympathomimetic amine is epinephrine, but in most fetal animals, norepinephrine is the predominant amine, with the proportion of epinephrine increasing with age.

STRUCTURE-ACTIVITY RELATIONSHIP

The chemical formulae of the important catecholamines are given in Figure 13.2. All have the common feature of the catechol nucleus, i.e., a benzene ring with adjacent hydroxyl (OH) substitutions and an ethylamine side chain. Phenylethylamine can be viewed as the parent compound consisting of a benzene ring and an aliphatic portion, ethylamine. Norepinephrine, epinephrine, and isoproterenol have hydroxyl groups substituted in positions 3 and 4 of the benzene ring. Since *O*-dihydroxybenzene is known as *catechol*, the term catecholamine has been applied to sympathomimetic amines that have hydroxyl substitutions in the benzene ring. The sympathomimetic drugs may be divided into catechol and noncatecholamines.

The structure-activity relationships of these compounds have been closely stud-

ied, and it is possible to predict their activity depending on the substitutions in the aromatic ring and the terminal amino group. The effects of substitution on the amino group are readily seen, for example, in the actions of catecholamines on the α- and β-receptors. Increase in the size of the substituent increases β-recep-

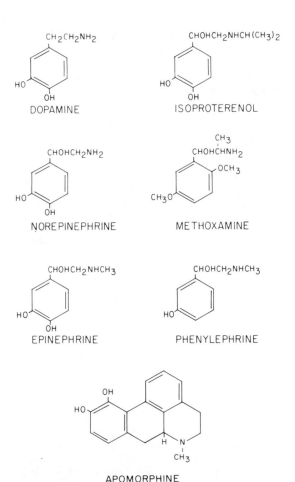

Figure 13.2. Chemical formulae of the important sympathomimetic amines.

tor activity. Norepinephrine has a free amino group and hence has weak β_2 activity. This is increased in epinephrine which has a methyl group addition, and maximum β_1 and β_2 activity is seen in isoproterenol with an isopropyl substituent. Conversely, α-receptor activity is greater the less the substitution on the terminal amino group and, thus, relative α activity is maximal in norepinephrine, less in epinephrine, and almost nonexistent in isoproterenol

Hydroxyl groups in positions 3 and 4 in the benzene ring favor α and β sympathetic activity. When both or one of these groups is missing, the overall potency is reduced.

The distance separating the aromatic ring from the terminal amino group is also important with the greatest sympathomimetic potency occurring when two carbon atoms separate the benzene ring from the amino group.

Drugs with hydroxyl groups in positions 3 and 4 on the benzene ring, i.e., *catechols*, can be metabolized by catechol-O-methyltransferase (COMT) as the name suggests, and drugs without substitution on the α-carbon atom can be metabolized by monoamine oxidase (MAO). Substitution on the α-carbon atom blocks oxidation by MAO, thus greatly prolonging the action of the non-catecholsympathomimetic amines (because they are also resistant to inactivation by COMT). Therefore, drugs without hydroxyl substitions on positions 3 and 4 of the benzene ring and with substitutions on the α-carbon atom, such as ephedrine and amphetamine, have a long duration of action, measured in hours rather than minutes.

Most potent sympathomimetic amines have a hydroxyl group on the β-carbon atom. The presence of this hydroxyl group creates a center of asymmetry around the β-carbon atom and allows two possible spatial arrangements around this carbon atom—stereoisomerism. Stereoisomers of epinephrine and norepinephrine with the levo($-$) configuration are much more potent than the dextro($+$) isomers. This striking stereospecificity for the adrenergic receptor

suggests that a specific three dimensional arrangement of the catecholamine is necessary for interaction with the receptor site.

SYNTHESIS, STORAGE, AND RELEASE OF THE CATECHOLAMINES

The **biosynthetic** pathways for the catecholamines are shown in Figure 13.3; norepinephrine is synthesized from the amino acid tyrosine by a series of enzyme-controlled steps, the rate-limiting step being that controlled by the enzyme tyrosine hydroxylase. At this point, norepinephrine synthesis can be controlled by either circulating norepinephrine concentrations acting as a feedback mechanism or drugs that are specific tyrosine hydroxylase inhibitors, such as α-methyltyrosine. Phenylethanolamine-N-methyltransferase (PNMT) is present expecially in the adrenal medulla and converts norepinephrine to epinephrine. None of the enzymes involved in the synthesis of the catecholamines is highly specific, and dopa decarboxylase, for example, can convert the drug α-methyldopa to α-methyldopamine which, in turn, is converted by dopamine β-hydroxylase to the "false transmitter," α-methylnorepinephrine.

The neurotransmitter norepinephrine is stored in dense core vesicles or granules at the sympathetic nerve terminal. These storage vesicles contain norepi-

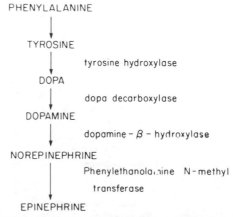

Figure 13.3.   Pathway for the biosynthesis of norepinephrine and epinephrine.

nephrine, dopamine β-hydroxylase, ATP, and a chromogranin, a protein necessary for catecholamine binding. The hydroxylation of tryrosine to dopa and the decarboxylation of dopa to dopamine take place in the cytoplasm, and dopamine then enters the storage granules where it is converted to norepinephrine.

The release of catecholamine from the granules at the nerve terminal occurs by the process of "exocytosis." The nerve action potential depolarizes the cell membrane and allows the passage of calcium ions into the nerve. This influx of calcium causes the vesicular membrane to fuse with the cell membrane, and the total contents of the vesicle, including norepinephrine, are released into the synaptic cleft.

Inactivation of the released catecholamine neurotransmitter is achieved by both reuptake and metabolism. A powerful pump mechanism is present at the adrenergic nerve terminal which allows norepinephrine to be taken up from the synaptic cleft back into the neuron. In most tissues, reuptake accounts for the removal of at least two-thirds of the released neurotransmitter and, therefore, is an important means of removal of nor-

epinephrine. In the neuron, most of the norepinephrine is then stored in the dense core vesicles, while a small amount is metabolized in the cytoplasm by monoamine oxidase (MAO).

METABOLISM AND DISPOSITION OF THE CATECHOLAMINES

The two enzymes that are important in the metabolism of the catecholamines are:

1. Monoamine oxidase (MAO)—oxidative deamination
2. Catechol-O-methyltransferase (COMT)— methylation

Monoamine oxidase is found in large amounts in the mitochondria of the sympathetic neurons as well as in the liver and the intestine. Catechol-O-methyltransferase appears to be localized exclusively outside the sympathetic neuron but in close proximity, and also in large amounts in the liver and kidneys. Once released from the postganglionic sympathetic neuron or adrenal medulla, the catecholamines bind to and activate the adrenergic receptor on the effector cell membrane. Norepinephrine that is not

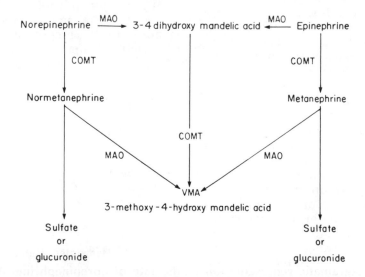

Figure 13.4.   The metabolic fate of norepinephrine and epinephrine.

taken back up into the adrenergic neuron enters the circulation where it is metabolized by COMT and MAO. The final major metabolic product of norepinephrine in man is 3-methoxy-4-hydroxymandelic acid (vanillyl mandelic acid, VMA) which is excreted in the urine, the quantitative excretion of which is used in the diagnosis of pheochromocytoma (Fig. 13.4). Figure 13.5 shows diagrammatically the fate of norepinephrine released at the sympathetic nerve ending. It is important to understand that the metabolic pathways are not the major processes involved in the fate of norepinephrine released at the sympathetic neuron or of exogenously administered catecholamines, but rather the reuptake

of catecholamines into the sympathetic nerve terminal.

THE ADRENERGIC RECEPTOR

Ahlquist in 1948 described two adrenergic receptors, α and β, and suggested that adrenergic receptors be classified according to the order of potency by which they are affected by sympathetic agonists and antagonists. Receptors which are stimulated by catecholamines with an order of potency of norepinephrine $\geq$ epinephrine $>$ isoproterenol are called α-receptors, and receptors that respond to catecholamines with an order of potency of isoproterenol $>$ epinephrine $\geq$ norepinephrine are called β-receptors.

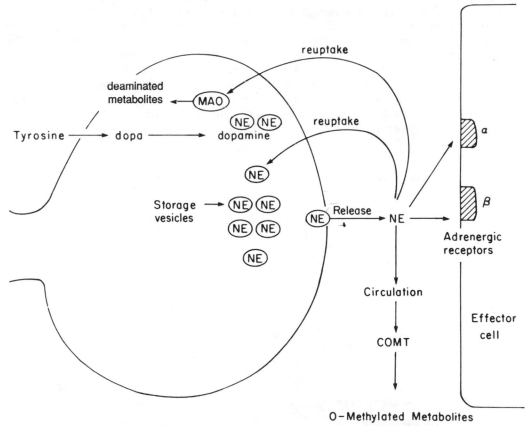

Figure 13.5.   Diagramatic representation of the fate of norepinephrine at the sympathetic nerve terminal. Norepinephrine (*NE*) is released from the nerve endings and acts on the adrenergic receptor. Some NE enters the circulation where it is *O*-methylated (COMT) and deaminated (MAO), but most NE is removed by reuptake into the neuron, where it is stored in the dense core vesicles or destroyed by MAO.

Table 13.1.
Classification of Adrenergic Receptors Based on Order of Potency of Agonists and Antagonists

	Receptor type			
	α	β_1	β_2	Dopamine
Agonists*	NE≥E>D>I	I>E>NE≥D	I>E>>NE>D	D≥EN>APO
Antagonists	Phenoxybenzamine	Propranolol†	Propranolol†	Haloperidol
	Phentolamine	Atenolol‡	Butoxamine	Phenothiazines
	Ergot alkaloids	Esmolol		
	Prazosin			

*NE, norepinephrine; E, epinephrine; D, dopamine; I, isoproterenol; EN, epinine; APO, apomorphine.
†and other nonselective β-blockers (see Table 14.1).
‡and other β-selective blockers (see Table 14.1).

Since then, the β-receptors have been divided into β_1 and β_2 depending on their relative response to epinephrine and norepinephrine (Table 13.1). The α-receptors have been subdivided into α_1 and α_2, and stimulation of postsynaptic α_1-receptors causes smooth muscle vasoconstriction and an increase in peripheral vascular resistance. The α_1-receptor is activated by the release of norepinephrine, and the norepinephrine released then stimulates the peripheral presynaptic α_2-receptor to inhibit further release of norepinephrine. So α_2 stimulation inhibits the release of norepinephrine itself and, thus, acts as a negative feedback mechanism (Fig. 13.6). Centrally, postsynaptic adrenergic receptors with α_2 characteristics have also been identified. Stimulation of these receptors appears to lower sympathetic outflow and results in a fall in blood pressure. This is the postulated mechanism for the hypotensive effect of clonidine. Hence, stimulation of α_2-receptors in the

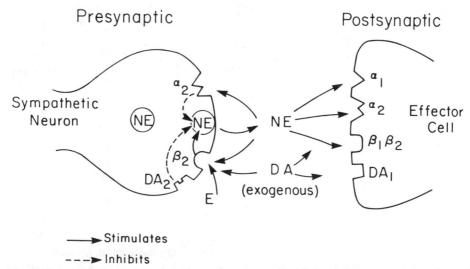

Figure 13.6. Location of adrenergic and dopaminergic receptors at the sympathetic nerve terminal. Norepinephrine stimulates α_1- and α_2-receptors at the postsynaptic site to produce vasoconstriction. Dopamine stimulates DA$_1$ receptors to result in vasodilation. Norepinephrine stimulates presynaptic α_2-receptors to inhibit the release of further norepinephrine. Dopamine activates presynaptic α_2- and presynaptic DA$_2$ receptors to inhibit norepinephrine release. *NE*, norepinephrine; *E*, epinephrine; *DA*, dopamine.

central nervous system reduces sympathetic outflow, while α_2 antagonism stimulates central nervous system sympathetic outflow.

Recently, great advances have been made in the elucidation of the nature of the β-receptor, even to the extent of amino acid sequencing of the receptor (see Fig. 3.3). Catecholamines or β agonists stimulate adenylate cyclase, which is located on the cytoplasmic face of the plasma membrane, and cyclic 3′,5′-adenosine monophosphate (cyclic AMP) is formed from ATP. The cyclic AMP which is formed is then released into the cytoplasm and acts to alter cellular function usually by phosphorylating an enzyme or protein. Thus, cyclic AMP is thought of as the "second messenger," while the circulating hormone (epinephrine, for example) is the first messenger traveling from the endocrine gland to its target cell. The receptor communicates with the adenylate cyclase component through an inhibitory or stimulatory guanine nucleotide regulatory protein (G protein, G_i and G_s, respectively). Receptor G protein adenylate cyclase communication and receptor function are discussed in detail in Chapter 3 and illustrated in Figures 3.2 and 3.4.

Subsequently, it has been realized that adenylate cyclase and cyclic AMP are not only involved in the mediation of the effects of the catecholamines, but also of a wide range of peptide hormones—insulin, glucagon, thyroid-stimulating hormone, adrenocorticotropic hormone, and parathyroid hormone. The concentration of cyclic AMP can also be increased by inhibition of the enzyme phosphodiesterase, the enzyme responsible for inactivating cyclic AMP to 5-AMP.

The methylxanthines, such as aminophylline and caffeine, are inhibitors of phosphodiesterase and, thus, allow the accumulation of cyclic AMP. It is interesting that aminophylline can produce effects, such as bronchodilation and increased myocardial contractility, that are also produced by catecholamines and are also mediated by a rise in cyclic AMP. However, this effect is produced only at high concentrations, and it is believed now that inhibition of phosphodiesterase may not be the major factor in producing the pharmacologic effects of aminophylline. The inotropic agents amrinone and milrinone are believed to exert a major part of their pharmacologic effect via inhibition of phosphodiesterase. The decrease in airway resistance caused by the β-agonists, isoproterenol and terbutaline, is accompanied by an increase in cyclic AMP.

The Dopamine Receptor

The dopaminergic receptor (DA) has been identified in the central nervous system and in renal and mesenteric blood vessels. There are, thus, multiple receptors that can recognize catecholamines: α-adrenergic; β-adrenergic; and dopaminergic. Dopamine receptors have been divided into two subtypes: DA_1 and DA_2 dopamine receptors. DA_1 receptors are found postsynaptically on the sympathetic nerve; stimulation of DA_1 receptors causes vasodilation of renal, mesenteric, coronary, and cerebral vessels. In addition, sodium excretion is increased. DA_2 receptors are located at the presynaptic level, and activation of these receptors inhibits norepinephrine release analogous to the inhibition of norepinephrine release produced by presynaptic α_2 stimulation. Stimulation of DA_2 receptors has also been shown to inhibit prolactin release and, to cause nausea

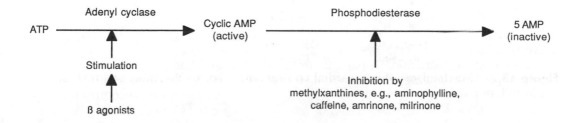

and vomiting, and explains the action of DA_2 antagonists such as metoclopramide (see page 89).

Figure 13.6 shows the location of adrenergic and dopamine receptors at the sympathetic nerve terminal. Dopamine increases myocardial contractility, heart rate, and atrioventricular conduction by stimulation of β_1-receptors but has no effect on β_2-receptors. Dopamine is an agonist at α_1- and α_2-adrenergic receptors to cause peripheral vasoconstriction. Dopamine also stimulates presynaptic DA_2 and α_2-adrenergic receptors to produce inhibition of norepinephrine release.

MECHANISMS OF ACTION OF INOTROPIC DRUGS

Myocardial muscle contains two contractile proteins, actin and myosin, which are under the control of two regulatory proteins, troponin and tropomyosin. The myocardium develops contractile force by forming cross-bridges between the actin and myosin myofilaments; these bridges generate a sliding motion, causing the actin and myosin filaments to interdigitate so that the cardiac muscle shortens or contracts. In the ab-

sence of calcium, the inhibitory protein tropomyosin prevents the interaction between actin and myosin. When increased intracellular levels of calcium are present (calcium binds to a specific site on the troponin complex), tropomyosin binds to troponin, and the conformational change in tropomyosin allows actin and myosin to interact, cross-bridges are formed, and contraction results. Thus, an increase in intracellular calcium initiates contraction.

The initial event in activating contraction of cardiac muscle is depolarization of the sarcolemma membrane. Fast sodium channels open, coinciding with the rapid upstroke of the cardiac action potential (Fig. 13.7). Depolarization of the cell membrane allows calcium to enter the cell via slow channels during the plateau phase of the action potential. This small amount of calcium then triggers a large calcium release from the sarcoplasmic reticulum to cause an abrupt rise in intracellular calcium concentration, which then reacts with the contractile proteins to initiate contraction. Relaxation occurs as calcium is taken up by the sarcoplasmic reticulum and finally transported out of the cell across the sarco-

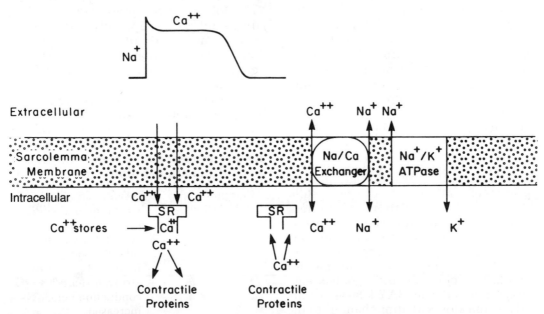

Figure 13.7.   Mechanisms of myocardial contraction.   For explanation, see text. *SR,* sarcoplasmic reticulum.

lemma to the extracellular space. Calcium enters the cell through slow calcium channels or through a sodium-calcium exchange mechanism (Fig. 13.7). The sodium pump (Na^+/K^+-ATPase) determines intracellular levels of calcium, sodium, and potassium. Inhibition of the sodium pump, for example, by digitalis glycosides raises the intracellular sodium concentration. The sodium-calcium exchanger then causes calcium to enter the cell in exchange for the increased intracellular sodium. The increased intracellular calcium is then stored in the sarcoplasmic reticulum for subsequent release.

Myocardial cyclic AMP is produced by the membrane-bound enzyme adenylate cyclase which is under the control of inhibitory and regulatory subunits (see Chapter 3). Cyclic AMP causes an increase in calcium influx through the slow channels via activation of protein kinases), thereby increasing myocardial contractility. As cyclic AMP is degraded by phosphodiesterases (cardiac phosphodiesterase III), inhibition of these enzymes results in elevated cyclic AMP concentrations, causing essentially the same physiological effects that occur with adenylate cyclase stimulation.

There is increasing evidence that α-adrenergic receptors in the myocardium may also be responsible for an increase in myocardial contractility. However, the side effects of α-agonists (vasoconstriction) preclude clinical use at the present time. Although the mechanism for α-agonist-induced increase in inotropy is not known, it is not due to an increase in cyclic AMP levels.

Intropic agents therefore increase myocardial contractility by either (a) increasing intracellular calcium during systole or (b) altering the sensitivity of contractile proteins to calcium. The administration of exogenous calcium increases calcium influx by increasing the ionic gradient across the slow calcium channel (Fig. 13.8). Calcium channel agonists, e.g., an experimental drug BAY k 8644, act directly at the slow calcium channel to increase intracellular calcium. Other inotropic drugs increase cyclic AMP by

stimulation of adenylate cyclase or by inhibition of phosphodiesterase. β-Adrenergic agonists (epinephrine, norepinephrine, isoproterenol, prenalterol, dopamine, and dobutamine) and partial agonists (such as xamoterol) stimulate adenylate cyclase, resulting in an increase in myocardial cyclic AMP, an increase in calcium influx via calcium channels, and an increase in myocardial contractility (Fig. 13.8). On the other hand, phosphodiesterase inhibitors, for example, the methylxanthines (theophylline) or the bipyridines (amrinone, milrinone), raise myocardial cyclic AMP by inhibiting the breakdown of cyclic AMP. Glucagon and histamine stimulate adenylate cyclase via cardiac membrane receptors linked to the adenylate cyclase system. Forskolin acts directly on adenylate cyclase to increase myocardial contractility. The mechanisms of action of theophylline and the methylxanthines are further discussed in Chapter 19. Inhibition of sodium-potassium ATPase by cardiac glycosides increases intracellular calcium (Fig. 13.8). Finally, the sensitivity of contractile proteins to calcium has been shown to be altered by some of the new positive intropic agents, e.g., *sulmazole*.

Figure 13.7 outlines the biochemical mechanisms of myocardial contraction, while Figure 13.8 illustrates the possible sites of action of the important inotropic agents.

PHYSIOLOGICAL EFFECTS OF THE SYMPATHOMIMETIC AMINES

The important effects of adrenergic receptor stimulation by the sympathomimetic drugs are as follows:

α-Receptor stimulation

β-Receptor stimulation, heart (predominantly β_1)
1. contractility increased
2. rate (SA node) increased
3. atrioventricular conduction velocity—increased
4. decreased refractory period

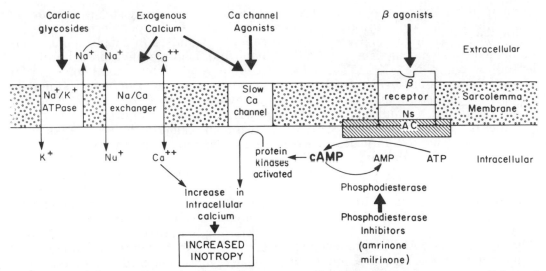

Figure 13.8. Site of action of inotropic agents. Inotropic agents raise intracellular calcium levels and thereby increase myocardial contractility. Circulating catecholamines (β-agonists) act on β-adrenergic receptors causing activation of adenylate cyclase (AC) resulting in increased cyclic AMP production. Myocardial cyclic AMP is produced by the membrane-bound enzyme adenylate cyclase, the activity of which is regulated by both inhibitory and stimulatory (N_s) subunits. Cyclic AMP increases intracellular calcium by activating protein kinases that are important for the phosphorylation of intracellular proteins. Calcium channel agonists (BAY k 8644) act at the calcium channel to increase calcium influx and consequently intracellular calcium concentrations. Intracellular cyclic AMP ($cAMP$) is broken down by phosphodiesterase so that the inhibition of phosphodiesterase leads to an increase in intracellular cAMP levels. Exogenous calcium leads to an increase in intracellular calcium by increasing the ionic gradient across the slow calcium channel. Digitalis glycosides inhibit sodium-potassium ATPase (the sodium pump) to increase intracellular calcium.

Vasoconstriction	Vasodilation (β_2)
Skin, abdominal viscera, gut	Skeletal muscle
Mydriasis	**Bronchial relaxation (β_2)**
	Uterine relaxation (β_2-receptor) if pregnant

Sympathetic effector cells may have α or β-receptors or both. For example, the smooth muscle of blood vessels that supply skeletal muscle has both α- and β-receptors. Low concentrations of epinephrine activate β-receptors and cause vasodilation, while higher concentrations activate α-receptors and cause vasoconstriction. The threshold concentration of epinephrine for stimulation of β-receptors is lower than that required for stimulation of α-receptors, but if sufficiently large doses are used, then stimulation of both α- and β-receptors

occurs, and then the α effect predominates.

β_1-Receptors are found in the heart, while β_2-receptors are found in the bronchi, vascular beds, and uterus. It has recently been shown that there are also β_2-adrenergic receptors in the heart, in both the atria and ventricles; stimulation of these receptors increases heart rate and myocardial contractility. Exogenously administered dopamine has α and β effects depending on dosage and acts also through stimulation of DA_1 receptors in renal and mesenteric beds producing vasodilation in these areas.

Norepinephrine is stored in the granules in adrenergic nerve endings in the myocardium. When sympathetic nerves to the heart are activated, norepinephrine as the neurotransmitter is released and stimulates β_1-adrenergic receptors on the myocardial cell surface. It is important to remember that norepinephrine is predominantly a β_1-agonist on the heart (it has predominantly α effects overall), so that the effect of sympathetic stimulation to the heart is mediated primarily via the β_1-receptor. If epinephrine were to be released, e.g., from the adrenal medulla, or administered exogenously, then β_2 cardiac stimulation would also occur. Drugs such as norepinephrine, epinephrine, and isoproterenol stimulate β_1-receptor sites in the myocardium directly, while some drugs such as dopamine stimulate the myocardium directly and, in addition, indirectly through the release of endogenous norepinephrine. Stimulation of the β_1-receptors in the heart produces an increase in heart rate (chronotropic effect), an increase in contractility (inotropic effect), and an increase in automaticity and conduction velocity. The metabolic effects (hyperglycemia, hyperlactidemia, hyperlipemia, and increased oxygen consumption) do not fall clearly into a simple α and β classification, but many of these effects appear to be mediated by β-receptors and are chiefly seen in response to epinephrine. In the intestine, sympathetic stimulation causes relaxation, decreased tone, and motility. These appear to be α and β effects as the presence of both an α and β blocking agent is required to antagonize the effects of epinephrine on the intestine. β_2-Receptors are also responsible for an important increase in potassium influx into cells, resulting in hypokalemia in response to epinephrine and selective β_2-agonists (see Fig. 14.5).

The adrenergic receptor activity of the most important sympathomimetic drugs is summarized below:

Epinephrine—has both α and β effects
Norepinephrine—has predominantly α effects
Isoproterenol—has both β_1 and β_2 effects.
Dopamine—has α and β effects depending on site and dose and dopaminergic effects on receptors in renal mesenteric beds.
Dobutamine—has predominantly β_1 effects

Knowledge of the repsonse to α and β stimulation makes it possible to predict the pharmacological effects of both the endogenous catecholamines and the synthetic sympathomimetic amines. Isoproterenol which acts mainly on β-receptors and has little α-effect causes an increase in heart rate and contraction, dilates skeletal muscle vascular beds (thus, causing a fall in mean blood pressure), and relaxes bronchial smooth muscle. One can also predict that phenylephrine which acts mainly on α-receptors and possesses little β-effect has almost no direct cardiac effect, does not relax bronchial muscle, but does cause a rise in mean blood pressure by contracting peripheral vascular beds and increasing peripheral resistance. A comparison of the effects of norepinephrine, epinephrine, isoproterenol, dopamine, and dobutamine is shown in Table 13.2, and the effects of the intravenous infusion of norepinephrine, epinephrine, isoproterenol, and dopamine in humans are shown in Figure 13.9.

Sympathomimetic agents may act *directly* on the adrenergic receptor (epinephrine, norepinephrine, isoproterenol, methoxamine) or *indirectly* by causing the release of norepinephrine (mephenteramine, methamphetamine, amphetamine, tyramine) or by both mechanisms (direct and indirect), i.e., *mixed* (ephedrine, metaraminol). Table 13.3 lists the commonly used sympathomimetic drugs, their mechanism of action, and their relative activity on α- and β-receptors.

DRUG INTERACTIONS AND THE SYMPATHETIC NERVOUS SYSTEM

Many drugs can modify the synthesis, uptake, release, and actions of the neurotransmitter norepinephrine at the adrenergic nerve terminal.

INTERFERENCE WITH NOREPINEPHRINE SYNTHESIS

α-Methyl-p-tyrosine (metyrosine) used in the management of pheochromocytoma prevents the conversion of tyrosine to dopa by inhibition of the rate-limiting

Table 13.2.
Comparison of the Effects of Norepinephrine, Epinephrine, Isoproterenol, Dopamine, and Dobutamine

Effect	Norepinephrine	Epinephrine	Isoproterenol	Dopamine	Dobutamine
Heart					
Rate	Slowed (reflex blood pressure rise)	Increased	Increased	Little change or increased	Little change
Myocardial contractility	Little effect	Increased	Increased	Increased	Increased
Cardiac output	Little effect or reduced	Increased	Increased	Increased	Increased
Automacity, conductivity	Increased	Much increased	Much increased	Increased	Increased slightly
Blood pressure					
Systolic	Rises	Rises	Little change or may fall	Increased at high doses, but little change or slightly decreased at lower doses	Slightly increased
Diastolic	Rises	Falls	Falls		Little change or increased
Mean	Rises	Rises	Falls		
Vascular beds					
Muscle	Constricted	Dilated	Dilated	Dilated or constricted	Dilated
Skin/viscera	Constricted	Constricted	Dilated	Dilated*	Dilated
Kidney	Constricted	Constricted	Constricted	Dilated*	Constricted
Coronary blood flow	Increased	Increased	Increased	Increased	Increased
Total peripheral resistance	Greatly increased	Increased	Decreased	Small increase	Small increase or no change
Bronchi	Little effect	Relaxed	Relaxed	No effect	Relaxed
Uterus (pregnant)	Increased tone	Relaxation	Relaxation	No effect	Relaxation

*Dopamine can cause both relaxation or contraction of vascular smooth muscle, depending on the degree of α- or β-adrenergic receptor stimulation which is dose related. In addition, dopamine stimulates specific dopaminergic receptors causing vasodilation of renal, mesenteric, and coronary vascular beds.

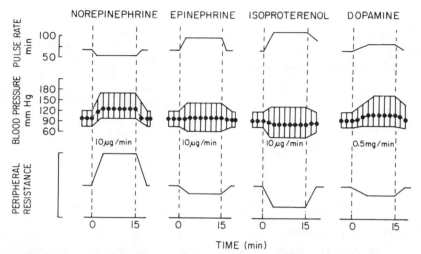

**Figure 13.9.   The effects of intravenous infusion of norepinephrine, epinephrine, isopro-
terenol, and dopamine in humans.**   Infusions were made intravenously during the time
indicated by the *broken lines*. (With permission from Allwood, MJ, Cobbold AF, Ginsburg
J: Peripheral vascular effects of noradrenaline, isoproprylnoradrenaline, and dopamine. *Br
Med Bull* 19:132–136, 1963.)

enzyme, tyrosine hydroxylase, and so results in reduction of catecholamine
synthesis.

α-Methyldopa is converted to α-meth-
ylnorepinephrine ("false transmitter") by
the enzyme system involved in the synthesis of norepinephrine.

BLOCKADE OF NOREPINEPHRINE
REUPTAKE

Imipramine and other tricyclic antidepressants, and cocaine inhibit norepinephrine reuptake, resulting in increased

amounts of norepinephrine being available at receptor sites.

Guanethidine enters the adrenergic
neuron by the reuptake mechanism causing the active release and then eventual
depletion of norepinephrine. This accounts for the hypertension and then hypotension, which occurs following the intravenous injection of guanethidine.

Reserpine prevents norepinephrine reuptake into the storage vesicle leading to
the destruction of norepinephrine by mitochondrial MAO and depletion from adrenergic terminals.

Table 13.3.
Commonly Used Sympathomimetic Drugs and Their Mechanism of Action

	Receptor type*		
Drug	α	β	Mechanism of action
Norepinephrine	++++	++	Direct
Epinephrine	+++	++++	Direct
Isoproterenol	0	++++	Direct
Phenylephrine	++++	+	Direct
Metaraminol	++++	+	Direct and indirect
Methoxamine	++++	0	Direct
Ephedrine	+	++	Direct and indirect
Dopamine	++	+++	Direct and indirect
Dobutamine	+	++++	

*α- and β-receptor activity: +, mild; ++, moderate; +++, great; ++++, greatest.

INTERFERENCE WITH THE RELEASE OF NOREPINEPHRINE

Bretylium prevents the release of norepinephrine from the sympathetic nerve terminal.

STIMULATION OF RECEPTORS BY α- OR β-RECEPTOR AGONISTS

BLOCKADE OF RECEPTORS BY α- OR β-RECEPTOR ANTAGONISTS

INHIBITION OF THE ENZYMATIC BREAKDOWN OF NOREPINEPHRINE BY MAO INHIBITORS, e.g., PARGYLINE, NIALAMIDE, TRANLCYPROMINE

Potentially dangerous hypertensive crises have been recorded when sympathomimetics have been given to patients receiving monoamine oxidase inhibitor antidepressants (MAO).

Monoamine Oxidase Inhibitor Antidepressants and Directly Acting Sympathomimetics. As monoamine oxidase only plays a minor role in terminating the action of norepinephrine released at sympathetic nerve endings and of injected norepinephrine and epinephrine (reuptake being the primary mechanism), one would theoretically expect that monoamine oxidase inhibitors would not potentiate the effects of exogenously administered directly acting catecholamines. Experiments have shown this to be true for norepinephrine but not for epinephrine. Results of experiments with isoproterenol have been variable.

Monoamine Oxidase Inhibitors and Indirectly Acting Sympathomimetics. In the presence of monoamine oxidase inhibitors, the concentration of norepinephrine free in the cytoplasm at the sympathetic nerve ending is much higher because of failure to break it down normally (see Fig. 13.5), and the administration of indirectly acting sympathomimetics, such as ephedrine and metaraminol, will lead to increased pharmacological effect. Hypertensive crises can, therefore, occur when an indirectly acting vasopressor is administered to a patient taking monoamine oxidase inhibitors. Hypertensive episodes have also been reported in patients under treatment with monoamine oxidase inhibiting antidepressants following the ingestion of food containing tyramine, such as cheese. Tyramine normally undergoes oxidative deamination in the liver, but because of MAO inhibition, these patients cannot break down tyramine and have elevated levels of this and other amines. As tyramine is an indirectly acting sympathomimetic agent, it produces severe hypertension by causing the release of norepinephrine that is present in excess at the sympathetic nerve endings. Therefore, the use of indirectly acting sympathomimetic amines should be avoided during general anesthesia in patients receiving monoamine oxidase inhibitor antidepressants.

MAOIs and their interactions with opioids, such as meperidine, are discussed on page 167, while the clinical pharmacology of MAOIs and anesthesia is discussed in detail in Chapter 21.

INDIVIDUAL SYMPATHOMIMETIC DRUGS

Epinephrine (Adrenaline)

In general, the pharmacological effects of epinephrine resemble the effects of stimulation of the sympathetic nervous system. Epinephrine is the key hormone involved in the body's "fight or flight" response to stress. The naturally occurring *l*-epinephrine is 10 times more potent that the *d*-isomer, levorotatory substitution on the β-carbon atom conferring the greater peripheral sympathetic activity as previously described.

CARDIOVASCULAR EFFECTS

The cardiovascular effects of epinephrine are due to the direct stimulation of both α- and β-adrenergic receptors. Stimulation of cardiac β-receptors causes an increase in heart rate and myocardial contractility. Cardial dysrhythmias including ventricular tachycardia and fibrillation may occur. Cardiac systole is shortened, cardiac output rises, and cardiac oxygen consumption is increased. Small doses of epinephrine stimulate β-adrenergic receptors in the peripheral vascular beds causing vasodilation, while moderate to large doses stimulate both α- and β-receptors. The α-receptors are less sensitive, but their effect predominates, so large doses of epinephrine cause vasoconstriction, an increase in peripheral resistance, and a rise in blood pressure. The blood vessels to skin, mucosa, and kidney are constricted due to the action of epinephrine on α-receptors, while if moderate doses of epinephrine are administered so that α and β stimulation occurs, the vasculature to skeletal muscle and splanchnic beds is dilated. When a bolus of epinephrine is given or an intravenous infusion is terminated, the β effect will persist after the α effect has ended, causing secondary hypotension. The hemodynamic effects of epinephrine are summarized in Table 13.2.

CENTRAL NERVOUS SYSTEM EFFECTS

Large doses may cause restlessness, anxiety, headache, and tremor.

RESPIRATORY EFFECTS

Epinephrine stimulates respiration due to an increase in central respiratory drive, but also due to its effects on the β_2-adrenergic receptors in the lung. It has a powerful bronchodilator action.

METABOLIC EFFECTS

Epinephrine raises blood glucose and free fatty acids. The lipolytic action is mediated by cyclic AMP via β-adrenergic receptors. Epinephrine also causes hypokalemia due to the β_2-mediated increase in potassium influx into cells.

SUGGESTED DOSAGE AND ADMINISTRATION

Epinephrine injection is available as a 1:1000 solution of epinephrine hydrochloride, i.e., 1-mg/ml adult dose—0.1 to 0.5 mg subcutaneously.

Epinephrine may be used during cardiac surgery to increase myocardial contractility when it is given as an intravenous infusion, titrated according to the patient's response, usually in the range of 0.01 to 0.1 μg/kg/min or 1 to 12 μg/min in the adult. A solution for intravenous infusion may be made by diluting 2 mg in 250 ml of fluid to yield a concentration of 8 μg/ml. Infusions of epinephrine have a dose-response relationship: 1 to 2 μg/min in the adult causes predominantly β effects, while 2 to 10 μg/min causes both α and β effects, and infusion of 10 to 16 μg/min causes predominantly α effects.

Cardiac emergencies: 2 to 5 ml of 1:10,000, i.e., 0.2 to 0.5 mg *intravenously* or 5 μg/kg *intravenously*.

Epinephrine for inhalational use: 1% solution of 1:100. i.e., 10 mg/ml. This should *not* be confused with the 1:1,000 solution.

Local anesthetics containing epinephrine 1:200,000 to 1:500,000 are often used to prolong the duration of action and intensity of effect of local anesthetics administered by local infiltration. Epinephrine administered by this route causes local vasoconstriction, thereby reducing the rate of absorption of the local anesthetic.

TOXICITY, PRECAUTIONS, AND CONTRAINDICATIONS

Epinephrine should be used cautiously in patients with hypertension and ischemic heart disease. Ventricular arrhythmias and ventricular fibrillation may follow the administration of epinephrine. Epinephrine should not be used in solutions of local anesthetics used for ring block of the finger as the consequent vasoconstriction may cause ischemia and gangrene.

Epinephrine and Anesthetic Agents. Volatile anesthetic agents sensitize the myocardium to circulating catecholamines, especially in the presence of hypoxia or hypercarbia, causing cardiac arrhythmias. Trichloroethylene, ethylchloride, cyclopropane, halothane, chloroform, and methoxyflurane have all been implicated. It has been suggested that there are two separate mechanisms by which catecholamines may cause ventricular arrhythmias during anesthesia: one is a reduction in supraventricular rate caused both directly by the general anesthetic agent and reflexly in response to the hypertensive effect of the catecholamine: the other mechanism is due to direct depression of the intraventricular conducting system by the inhalational anesthetic causing possible ventricular fibrillation. Of the anesthetics which are in use at the present time, halothane has the most pronounced cardiac sensitizing action. It is also thought that the mechanism is somehow related to the stimulation of β-adrenergic receptors in the heart, since β-receptor blockade consistently abolishes these arrhythmias. Therefore, adrenergic agents should be used extremely cautiously during inhalational anesthesia. When epinephrine has to be used for local hemostasis, the following schedule should be adhered to during halothane anesthesia:

1. Epinephrine concentrations no greater than 1:100,000 to 1:200,000 (1:200,000 is 5 μg/ml).
2. Total adult dose should not be greater than 10 ml of 1:100,000 solution in 10 minutes or
3. Total dose should not exceed 30 ml of 1:100,000 solution in 1 hour.

Although it is always difficult to suggest a safe dose of subcutaneous epinephrine, many anesthesiologists would consider 1 μg/kg of epinephrine to be reasonably safe during halothane anesthesia.

When enflurane was first introduced into anesthetic practice, it was suggested that a higher dose of epinephrine could be tolerated without causing ventricular arrhythmias than has since then been demonstrated. Therefore, although more epinephrine is required to produce ventricular irritability with enflurane than halothane, epinephrine should still be used cautiously during enflurane anesthesia (see Fig. 16.1). It has also been shown that lidocaine given with epinephrine affords extra protection. If an adrenergic agent is required to produce bronchodilation during general anesthesia, selective β_2 stimulators such as albuterol or terbutaline should be administered to minimize the cardiac stimulation.

Norepinephrine (Levarterenol, Noradrenaline)

Norepinephrine is the chemical neurotransmitter liberated by postganglionic adrenergic neurons and differs from epinephrine only by lacking the methyl substitution in the amino group (Table 13.1). As with epinephrine, the *l*-isomer is pharamacologically the most active.

CARDIOVASCULAR EFFECTS

The net effect of norepinephrine on the cardiovascular system depends not only on the adrenergic receptors stimulated, but also on the reflex responses elicited. Norepinephrine is a very powerful α-receptor stimulant and has weak β_1-receptor activity. The hemodynamic effects of norepinephrine are summarized in Table 13.2. Systolic and diastolic pressure increase, cardiac output is unchanged or decreased, and total peripheral resistance is greatly increased. The increased blood pressure stimulates baroreceptor activity and reflexly causes slowing of the heart. Marked vasoconstriction occurs. Renal, hepatic, and cerebral blood flow are all reduced. Muscle blood flow is reduced because, unlike epinephrine, small doses of norepinephrine do not cause vasodilation, and the blood vessels supplying skeletal muscle are constricted due to α-receptor stimulation.

RESPIRATORY EFFECTS

There is little bronchodilator effect.

SUGGESTED DOSAGE AND ADMINISTRATION

Levarterenol bitartrate injection is available as a 2% solution of the bitartrate equivalent to 0.1% of levarterenol base, i.e., 1 mg/ml.

Norepinephrine is usually given as an intravenous infusion obtained by diluting 2 ml (2 mg) of the 0.1% solution in 5000 ml of 5% dextrose solution giving a concentration of 4 μg/ml. The rate of infusion is adjusted to obtain the desired patient response; normally a rate of 2 to 4 μg of base per minute is required in the adult.

TOXICITY AND PRECAUTIONS

Norepinephrine must *not* be injected subcutaneously. Care is necessary to ensure that necrosis and sloughing do not occur at the site of intravenous injection due to extravasation. The infusion should preferably be administered through a central line.

Isoproterenol (Isoprenaline)

Isoproterenol is a synthetic catecholamine that acts almost exclusive on β-adrenergic receptors (both β_1 and β_2) and has no significant effect on α-receptors.

CARDIOVASCULAR EFFECTS

Isoproterenol stimulates the cardiac β_1-receptors, increasing heart rate, automacity, and contractility. It also lowers peripheral vascular resistance through β_2-receptor stimulation mainly in skeletal muscle but also in renal and mesenteric vascular beds, causing a fall in diastolic blood pressure. This results in an increased venous capacitance. Effects on blood pressure are variable depending on the dose administered. There is usually no change or a moderate fall in systolic blood pressure as well as a greater fall in diastolic blood pressure, leading to a fall in mean blood pressure. In the past, isoproterenol was used in the emergency management of patients with complete heart block, but the development of transvenous pacemakers has superseded its use in this situation. Isoproterenol is useful as an inotropic agent in patients with cardiac failure, especially those with valvular disease of the heart undergoing anesthesia who may functionally benefit from an increased heart rate and reduced venous capacitance filling. Newer inotropic agents such as dobutamine may prove preferable to isoproterenol in many situations where pharmacological support is required. However, if pulmonary bronchoconstriction is also present, e.g., pulmonary embolism, isoproterenol may still be a useful agent. Side effects that may occur are tachycardia, arrhythmias and hypotension. The hemodynamic effects of isoproterenol are summarized in Table 13.2.

RESPIRATORY EFFECTS

Marked bronchodilation occurs due to the stimulation of β_2-adrenergic receptors, and isoproterenol is a useful agent

in the treatment of bronchial asthma and drug-induced bronchoconstriction.

SUGGESTED DOSAGE AND ADMINISTRATION

Isoproterenol hydrochloride injection is available as a solution containing 10, 20, or 200 μg/ml.

An *intravenous* infusion can be made by diluting 1 mg of isoproterenol in 250 ml of fluid, giving a solution of 4 μg/ml. The rate of infusion should be titrated according to patient response, the usual rate being 0.01 to 0.1 μg/kg/min or 0.5 to 5.0 μg/min in the adult.

TOXICITY AND PRECAUTIONS

Side effects that may occur are tachycardia, ventricular arrhythmias, and hypotension. Aerosols containing isoproterenol are widely used at home by patients suffering from asthma. In many countries, including England and Australia, but not the United States, the mortality from asthma increased following the widespread introduction of these aerosols. The cause of death is not clear. Theories that have been suggested include: (a) excess stimulation of cardiac β_1-receptors giving rise to ventricular dysrhythmias; (b) hypoxemia despite improvement in bronchomotor tone due to ventilation/perfusion abnormalities; and (c) toxicity of the chlorofluorinated hydrocarbons used as propellants causing bronchoconstriction and cardiac arrhythmias. However, some of the cardiac side effects of isoproterenol may be reduced in these patients by the use of the newer selective β_2-receptor agonists, such as albuterol and terbutaline.

Dopamine

Dopamine differs from the other naturally occurring catecholamines in lacking a hydroxyl (OH) group on the side chain; i.e., it has no hydroxyl group on the β-carbon atom (Fig. 13.2). It is the immediate precursor of norepinephrine. Dopamine is used in the treatment of shock, hypotensive emergencies, and refractory congestive cardiac failure. In addition, dopamine is used at low infusion rates when only dopaminergic receptors are activated to improve renal perfusion and stimulate diuresis in oliguric patients.

CARDIOVASCULAR EFFECTS

Dopamine can cause both relaxation and contraction of vascular smooth muscle, depending on the dose administered. It differs from the other sympathomimetic agents in causing vasodilation in renal, mesenteric, coronary, and intracerebral vascular beds in dogs. This effect is not antagonized by β-adrenergic blocking agents, such as propranolol, but by butyrophenones (e.g., haloperidol), phenothiazines, and apomorphine. Demonstration of such selective antagonism supports the theory of a specific dopaminergic receptor in these vascular beds. When larger doses of dopamine are administered, the predominant effect is one of vasoconstriction which is antagonized by phentolamine and phenoxybenzamine. This suggests that the effect of dopamine at high doses appears to be mediated through stimulation of α-adrenergic receptors. Therefore, in healthy patients, the three infusion rates, low, medium, and high, elicit quite different cardiovascular responses and are used for different clinical therapeutic effects. The effect of *low* infusion rates of dopamine (0.1 to 2 μg/kg/min) is to stimulate dopaminergic receptors in the renal vessels causing increased renal blood flow, a rise in glomerular filtration rate, and sodium excretion. These effects are accompanied by little or no change in cardiac output or heart rate and are blocked by haloperidol. Reduction in blood pressure may occur due to inhibition of the sympathetic nervous system by stimulation of DA_2 receptors and by DA_1-induced vasodilation (Fig. 13.6). Dopamine, administered in low doses, is often used to improve renal blood flow and induce a diuresis in patients with oliguria and in surgical patients who have undergone procedures in which urine output may be decreased.

Infusion of dopamine at *medium* rates of 2 to 5 μg/kg/min stimulates β_1- and β_2-adrenoceptors causing an increase in myocardial contractility, stroke volume, and cardiac output. Heart rate is usually little changed. These effects are antagonized by propranolol. Medium infusion rates of dopamine are frequently used to provide inotropic support. If stimulation of α-adrenoceptors occurs, then vasoconstriction and an increase in afterload which would worsen heart failure may occur. A vasodilator, such as nitroglycerin or nitroprusside, is frequently administered with dopamine in this situation to provide vasodilation and a reduction in pulmonary wedge pressure.

High doses of dopamine (over 30 μg/kg/min) stimulate α-adrenoceptors, causing an increase in peripheral vascular resistance, decreased renal blood flow, and increase in peripheral vascular resistance, and an increased potential for arrhythmias. When higher doses of dopamine are administered that raise blood pressure, a reflex baroreceptor-mediated bradycardia may occur.

The intravenous administration of dopamine in doses that stimulate β-adrenoceptors (increasing cardiac output and contractility) causes an increase in coronary blood flow in dogs, without increasing myocardial oxygen utilization. However, dopamine will increase myocardial oxygen utilization if doses are administered that increase myocardial work by increased peripheral resistance and/or heart rate. Dopamine is a less powerful inotrope than epinephrine and isoproterenol, and in some patients in shock, dopamine may be ineffective. Norepinephrine is often used in combination with dopamine to produce an adequate perfusion pressure; nitroglycerin may then be added to this regimen.

SUGGESTED DOSAGE AND ADMINISTRATION

Dopamine is available for intravenous use as a solution of 40 mg/ml. An intravenous infusion can be made by diluting 200 mg of dopamine in 250 ml or 500 ml of solution to yield a final concentration of 800 μg/ml and 400 μg/ml, respectively. Dopamine should not be added to sodium bicarbonate or other alkaline intravenous solutions, since the drug is inactivated in alkaline solution. The rate of infusion should be titrated according to patient response, depending on the effect required. Starting at an initial rate of 0.1 μg/kg/min, the dose is gradually increased to 10 to 20 μg/kg/min or more if necessary.

TOXICITY, PRECAUTIONS, AND CONTRAINDICATIONS

Before dopamine is administered, it is important to ensure that the patient has an adequate circulating blood volume and that any hypovolemia has been corrected. Unwanted effects include nausea, vomiting, tachycardia, arrhythmias, angina, dyspnea, headache, and vasoconstriction resulting in hypertension. Dopamine should be administered via a central line where possible as extravasation may cause sloughing and necrosis in the surrounding tissues due to the α effects of high local concentrations. This can be treated with phentolamine. Contraindications to the use of dopamine include pheochromocytoma and cardiac dysrhythmias.

Dobutamine

Dobutamine is a synthetic derivative of isoproterenol that acts directly on β_1-receptors in the heart to increase myocardial contractility without greatly changing peripheral resistance or heart rate. Dobutamine appears to exert a more prominent inotropic than chronotropic action on the heart than isoproterenol, and it acts primarily on adrenergic β_1-receptors, whereas β_2- and α-receptors are only slightly stimulated. Its overall effect on total peripheral resistance is moderate, and one does not see large increases in blood pressure. Mild vasodilatory effects may be observed. Dobutamine does not stimulate renal dopaminergic receptors, so it does not possess the renal vasodilatory effects observed with dopamine.

Dobutamine exists as two stereoisomers; the (−)-isomer is more potent than the (+)-isomer at the α-adrenergic receptor, while the (+)-isomer is more potent than the (−)-isomer at the β-receptor. The commercially available preparation of dobutamine is a racemic mixture. Since stimulation of myocardial α-adrenergic receptors as well as β-adrenergic receptors leads to an increase in myocardial contractility, the effects of dobutamine are probably more complex than merely as a selective β_1-agonist. Dobutamine does not cause endogenous norepinephrine release, as has been shown for dopamine.

Dobutamine is a useful agent in low-output cardiac failure, hypotension secondary to decreased myocardial contractility, and during emergence from cardiopulmonary bypass. Dobutamine and dopamine have somewhat different cardiovascular effects and are often used together. Dobutamine is primarily an inotropic agent with modest peripheral vasodilating properties, whereas in contrast, dopamine is not only an inotrope but a vasopressor, increasing peripheral vascular resistance. Since dopamine administration usually increases not only cardiac output but also left ventricular filling pressures (when used in patients with congestive heart failure, cardiogenic shock, or after cardiac surgery) while, in contrast, systemic vascular resistance and filling pressures are little changed during dobutamine administration, the combination of dopamine and dobutamine has been advocated in order to limit the increase in left ventricular filling pressures induced by dopamine alone.

SUGGESTED DOSAGE AND ADMINISTRATION

Dobutamine should be given as a continuous intravenous infusion, the usual dose being 2.0 to 10 μg/kg/min, although doses above 30 μg/kg/min have been administered.

TOXICITY, PRECAUTIONS AND CONTRAINDICATIONS

Side effects include the development of arrhythmias, nausea, headache, angina, palpitations, and dyspnea. Tachycardia and ventricular dysrhythmias are less common with dobutamine than other β-adrenergic agonists.

Ephedrine

Ephedrine is a synthetic sympathomimetic amine that does not possess the catechol nucleus and, thus, is not metabolized by COMT (see p 379). It is the active principle of the plant Ma Huang and has been used for centuries in China. It is not prepared synthetically. Ephedrine stimulates α- and β-receptors and acts both directly and indirectly. Tachyphylaxis occurs.

CARDIOVASCULAR EFFECTS

Since ephedrine stimulates both α- and β-adrenergic receptors, its effects are similar to those of epinephrine, but they persist for much longer because of its resistance to the effects of COMT. Cardiac output and heart rate are increased. Systolic and diastolic blood pressure are increased, and pulse pressure is also increased. Renal and splanchnic blood flow are reduced, while coronary, cerebral, and skeletal muscle blood flows are increased.

RESPIRATORY EFFECTS

Respiration is stimulated and bronchodilation occurs due to stimulation of β_2-adrenergic receptors.

SUGGESTED DOSAGE AND ADMINISTRATION

Ephedrine is active when given by mouth, because it is resistant to MAO, the oral dose varying between 15 and 50 mg. Ephedrine can be given intramuscularly and intravenously, in doses of 10 to 15 mg in the adult.

TOXICITY, PRECAUTIONS, AND CONTRAINDICATIONS

The adverse effects associated with ephedrine are similar to those of epinephrine. Ephedrine should be used cautiously in patients with coronary artery disease.

Phenylephrine

Phenylephrine has strong α-receptor stimulating effects with weak β-receptor activity. It is a directly acting sympathomimetic.

CARDIOVASCULAR EFFECTS

The administration of phenylephrine causes a sharp rise in systolic and diastolic blood pressure. A reflex bradycardia that can be blocked by atropine occurs due to stimulation of the baroreceptors as occurs with all drugs that acutely raise blood pressure. The increase in blood pressure is largely due to the greatly increased peripheral resistance consequent on α-receptor stimulation. Cardiac output is either unchanged or slightly decreased. Renal, splanchnic, and cutaneous blood flows are all reduced.

SUGGESTED DOSAGE AND ADMINISTRATION

Phenylephrine hydrochloride is available for injection as a solution containing phenylephrine, 10 mg/ml. Phenylephrine may be administered intramuscularly or intravenously. For the treatment of hypotension during spinal anesthesia, 5 to 10 mg may be administered intramuscularly. If it is to be given intravenously, it should be administered as a continuous infusion. An infusion may be set up by diluting 10 mg of phenylephrine in 500 ml of 5% dextrose to yield a concentration of 20 μg/ml. Phenylephrine may be administered at an infusion rate of approximately 0.15 to 0.7 μg/kg/min, but the rate of infusion should be titrated according to the patient's response. Phenylephrine, 0.1 to 1.0 mg, may be given as a single intravenous injection, for example, during cardiopulmonary bypass to raise the mean perfusion pressure.

TOXICITY, PRECAUTIONS, AND CONTRAINDICATIONS

Care should be taken not to increase the rate of infusion too rapidly to produce hypertension. Arrhythmias are rare. Therapy should be discontinued slowly.

Methoxamine

Methoxamine is a potent vasopressor that exerts its effect almost entirely by α-receptor stimulation. Being already O-methylated, it cannot be inactivated by COMT and is not metabolized by MAO.

Therefore, methoxamine has a long duration of action.

CARDIOVASCULAR EFFECTS

Methoxamine causes a sharp and persistent rise in systolic and diastolic blood pressure due to increased peripheral vasoconstriction that may last from 1 to 2 hours. It has little effect on the heart, and cardiac output is usually unchanged or decreased. A reflex bradycardia commonly occurs. Renal blood flow is reduced. Methoxamine has been used in the treatment of hypotension during spinal anesthesia and to control paroxysmal atrial tachycardia probably through reflex vagal effects.

SUGGESTED DOSAGE AND ADMINISTRATION

Methoxamine hydrochloride injection: 10 to 20 mg/ml. Methoxamine may be given intramuscularly or intravenously, the dose varying between 10 to 20 mg intramuscularly, maximum effect being achieved within 20 minutes. Two to 10 mg may be administered slowly intravenously, in small increments.

TOXICITY, PRECAUTIONS, AND CONTRAINDICATIONS

Methoxamine should be given cautiously to patients with coronary artery disease or hypertension.

Other sympathomimetic amines include amphetamine, methamphetamine, mephentermine, and metaraminol.

Amrinone is a bipyridine derivative inotropic agent recently used in the treatment of congestive cardiac failure that improves hemodynamic indices without raising heart rate. Its mechanism of action is uncertain, but it does not seem to act through inhibition of sodium-potassium ATPase (like cardiac glycosides) or like catecholamines in stimulating adrenergic receptors and cyclic AMP generation. It is fully discussed later in this chapter.

Table 13.4 lists the concentrations and rates of administration of the clinically useful sympathomimetic amines.

Prenalterol

Prenalterol is a relatively selective β_1 agonist which has been used as an inotropic agent in the management of congestive heart failure. Heart rate is increased only slightly at inotropic doses. Other hemodynamic effects are predictable; myocardial contractility and cardiac output are increased, peripheral vascular resistance is increased, and tachyarrhythmias may occur. Prenalterol may be administered intravenously in bolus doses of 1.0 to 5.0 mg given slowly, or as an infusion of 0.5 mg/min per 70-kg body weight to a maximum of 20 mg. It has also been administered orally when bioavailability was found to be about 33% and the duration of action 4 to 6 hours.

Pirbuterol is a selective β_2-adrenoceptor agonist that, in addition to its use as a bronchodilator in obstructive airway disease (see Chapter 19), has also been used as an inotropic agent.

Xamoterol is a partial agonist at the β_1-adrenoceptor that also has been administered orally as a positive inotrope for the chronic treatment of cardiac failure.

OTHER POSITIVE INOTROPIC AGENTS

At the present time, considerable effort is being directed toward the development of positive inotropic agents that

Table 13.4.
Concentrations and Rates of Infusion of Sympathomimetic Amines

	Dose range $(mcg/kg^{-1}min^{-1})$	Aver. adult dose (mcg/min^{-1})	Dilution (mg/ml)
Epinephrine	0.01–0.1	2.0	2/250
Norepinephrine	0.05–0.25	4.0	2/500
Isoproterenol	0.01–0.1	2.0	1/250
Dopamine	0.5–>30	200	200/250
Dobutamine	0.5–20	200	250/500

possess both inotropic and vasodilatory effects. The toxicity of the most widely used orally administered inotrope, digitalis, is of course well recognized, and it is therefore important that any new drug developed should be available for oral as well as intravenous use. Positive inotropic agents with vasodilatory effects would be especially useful in the management of congestive cardiac failure and also following the termination of cardiopulmonary bypass during cardiac surgery when manipulation of cardiac preload and afterload in conjunction with increased contractility may markedly improve cardiac performance.

Amrinone

Amrinone is a bipyridine derivative which has been shown to possess both inotropic and vasodilatory effects. Its chemical structure is given in Figure 13.10. Amrinone is a nonglycoside, nonsympathomimetic positive inotropic agent that appears to exert the major part of its effect through inhibition of phosphodiesterase leading to increased concentrations of intracellular cyclic AMP (Fig. 13.8). Other mechanisms may also be important. Amrinone may also have synergistic inotropic effects with β-adrenergic agonists, since the latter stimulate cyclic AMP production while amrinone inhibits its degradation.

The drug has been shown to improve cardiac index, lower systemic vascular resistance, and reduce cardiac filling pressures, i.e., pulmonary artery occluded and right atrial pressures. Heart rate is unchanged generally or may increase slightly. In patients with congestive heart failure, amrinone does not increase myocardial oxygen consumption, which is either unchanged or decreased. Amrinone may thus be useful in the clinical setting of low cardiac output and high ventricular filling pressure.

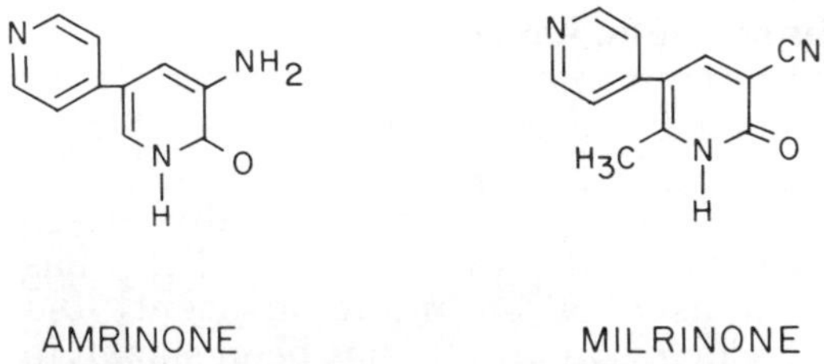

Amrinone is fairly rapidly and well absorbed after oral administration. Following the intravenous administration of amrinone, distribution is rapid with a distribution half-life of about 1.5 minutes, resulting in a rapid onset of action. Volume of distribution ($V_{d_{ss}}$) ranges from 1.3 to 1.5 L/kg. The terminal elimination half-life following intravenous bolus administration (0.8 to 2.2 mg/kg) is 2.6 hours. The clearance of amrinone ranges from 0.28 to 0.42 L/hour/kg in healthy individuals but, in chronic cardiac failure patients, it is decreased (0.12 to 0.18 L/hour/kg), resulting in a considerably prolonged elimination half-life (5.8 hours). A correlation has been demonstrated between the hemodynamic parameter of improvement in cardiac index and plasma amrinone concentrations in patients with cardiac failure. Although amrinone is conjugated in the liver, a large amount of the administered dose is excreted unchanged in the urine (26 to 30%).

Amrinone administration has produced marked hemodynamic improvements when given intravenously over a short period of time to patients with congestive cardiac failure. However, side effects of long-term oral administration include thrombocytopenia and gastrointestinal symptoms, such as nausea, vomiting, and abdominal pain, and amrinone is now recommended for intravenous use only and should only be given over a short period of time. The dose-dependent, cardiac-depressant effects of the volatile anesthetic agents, isoflurane and enflurane, are attenuated by amrinone in dogs, suggesting that amrinone might be a useful agent in the acute management of anesthetic-induced cardiovascular depression. Amrinone has also been shown in laboratory studies to reverse many of the cardiovascular effects of verapamil and propranolol, given either alone or in combination during isoflurane anesthesia.

The drug is given as a loading dose of 0.75 mg/kg intravenously over a period

AMRINONE   MILRINONE

Figure 13.10. Chemical formulae of amrinone and milrinone.

of 2 to 3 minutes, followed by an infusion of 5 to 10 µg/kg/min titrated to hemodynamic effect. The loading dose may be repeated 30 minutes after the first injection if required. Higher infusion rates have been administered, but the total daily dose of amrinone should not exceed 10 mg/kg. Since amrinone has vasodilatory effects, hypotension may occur, especially in patients with low cardiac filling pressures. When high infusion rates are administered, invasive cardiovascular monitoring is essential.

Milrinone

Milrinone is a bipyridine derivative with both inotropic and vasodilatory effects (Fig. 13.10). Like amrinone, the mechanism of action of milrinone is in part due to inhibition of phosphodiesterase with resultant increase in cyclic AMP (Fig. 13.8). Milrinone is 15 to 30 times more potent than its parent compound, amrinone, and has similar pharmacological properties. Milrinone improves cardiac performance by increasing myocardial contractility and by decreasing systemic vascular resistance. Left ventricular filling and pulmonary artery pressures are also decreased. Milrinone has been shown to be effective in the management of congestive cardiac failure after both intravenous and oral administration. The drug does not increase myocardial oxygen consumption.

Side effects observed with amrinone (thrombocytopenia and gastrointestinal complications) do not appear to be major adverse effects with milrinone and, therefore, milrinone may have a role in the chronic therapy of congestive heart failure.

Pharmacokinetic studies of milrinone have shown that the elimination half-life is about 0.8 hour and the volume of distribution about 0.3 L/kg. Clearance values are about 0.15 L/kg/hour. Bioavailability is about 85 to 92% after oral administration. The elimination half-life is prolonged in patients with severe renal failure and congestive heart failure. Milrinone may undergo active renal excretion.

Suggested dosage is a bolus intrave-

nous injection of 25 µg/kg or an infusion of up to 0.7 µg/kg/min. Maximal improvement has been observed with oral doses of 10 mg at 6-hour intervals.

Other New Inotropic Agents

Fenoxamine has pharmacological and hemodynamic effects that are similar to amrinone. It is a phosphodiesterase inhibitor. *Sulmazole* is another phosphodiesterase inhibitor with positive inotropic, chronotropic, and vasodilator effects. It has also been reported to increase the sensitivity of the myocardial contractile proteins to calcium. **Enoximone** and **piroximone** (phosphodiesterase inhibitors) are two other agents undergoing investigation for the treatment of chronic cardiac failure. Piroximone is the metabolite of enoximone.

Thus, it can be seen that many inotropic agents are currently being evaluated for the treatment of chronic cardiac failure.

Dopamine Analogs and Prodrugs

Dopamine, through activation of DA_1 receptors (vasodilation) and DA_2 receptors (inhibition of norepinephrine release from sympathetic neurons), lowers blood pressure when given in low doses (Fig. 13.6). Dopamine agonists are currently undergoing intensive investigation in the management of congestive heart failure and hypertension. Dopamine analogs and prodrugs may be effective in the management of congestive cardiac failure because, by decreasing sympathetic nervous system activity and causing vasodilation, cardiac output is increased without an increase in heart rate or decrease in renal blood flow. Their vasodilatory effects are also of benefit in the treatment of hypertension.

While it has been known for many years that the oral administration of **levodopa,** a drug used in Parkinson's syndrome (see page 122), has antihypertensive effects, it is only recently that it has been used as an inotropic agent, and levodopa given orally has been shown to cause significant improvement in patients with severe congestive cardiac failure. Levodopa is decarboxylated to dopamine, and it has been estimated that 1 to 1.5 g of levodopa orally is equivalent to an intravenous infusion of dopamine, 2 to 4 μg/kg/min. Blood pressure is decreased, and renal blood flow and sodium excretion are increased. **Ibopamine,** a derivative of deoxyepinephrine (epinine, N-methyldopamine), is an orally active positive inotropic drug with dopaminergic vasodilatory activity. It is converted to N-methyldopamine after oral ingestion.

The dopamine analog, **propylbutyl dopamine,** stimulates DA_2 and DA_1 receptors, but has weak α-receptor agonist activity and no β_1 or β_2 agonist effects. It has been used in the management of severe congestive cardiac failure (5 to 20 μg/kg/min) when, along with an increase in cardiac index, dose-related decreases in arterial blood pressure, cardiac filling pressures, and peripheral vascular resistance were observed. DA_1-mediated renal effects also occurred. Nausea and vomiting were important side effects. The drug has also been used to lower blood pressure in hypertensive patients. Another dopamine analog, **dopexamine,** is a DA_1 and DA_2 receptor agonist that also stimulates β_2- and, to a limited extent, β_1-receptors. It does not appear to stimulate α-receptors. Thus, in addition to its vasodilator and renal effects, dopexamine may also increase heart rate.

Fenoldopam is a selective agonist at the DA_1 receptor. This drug has also been used in the management of congestive heart failure and hypertension. Oral and intravenous forms are available.

Bromocriptine, in addition to its effects at serotonin receptors, exhibits marked DA_2 agonist effects and has been shown to lower blood pressure.

SELECTIVE β_2-RECEPTOR AGONISTS

By modifying the structure of isoproterenol (a β_1- and β_2-receptor stimulant), a series of compounds that can selectively activate either β_1-receptors in the heart or β_2-receptors in the lung can be produced. Increasingly bulky lipophilic groups added to the amino group of iso-

proterenol (Fig.13.11) increase the potency for β_2-receptor stimulation. Changing the hydroxyl substitution of isoproterenol from the 3, 4 to 3, 5 position in the benzene ring produces metaproterenol which retains its β_2-receptor stimulating properties, but loses β_1 agonist activity. Thus, a series of drugs have been developed that selectively stimulate β_2-receptors without activating β_1-receptors in the heart, thereby reducing the incidence of undesirable cardiac side effects. However, it should be remembered that these drugs do still have β_1 effects at high levels, so that increasing the dosage leads to tachycardia and ventricular dysrhythmias. Since it is now recognized that β_2-receptors are present in the heart, it is possible that these cardiac effects are in fact β_2 mediated. Drugs that are selective β_2-receptor agonists include *pirbuterol, metaproterenol* (orciprenaline), *(albuterol* (salbutamol), *terbutaline, fenoterol, ritodrine,* and *isoetharine.* They relax the smooth muscle of the bronchi, uterus, and vessels supplying skeletal muscle, but have less β_1-stimulating properties on the heart than isoproterenol. Doses of albuterol (salbutamol) that are equally effective as isoproterenol in producing bronchodilation are, therefore, less likely to produce tachycardia and dysrhythmias. Metaproterenol, ritodrine, terbutaline, and fenoterol have also been used to delay delivery in premature labor by producing uterine relaxation. However, larger doses are required than for bronchodilation, and side effects such as nervousness, hypotension, and tachycardia are more often seen.

THERAPEUTIC USES OF THE SYMPATHOMIMETIC AMINES

PHYSIOLOGICAL CONSIDERATIONS

Although the sympathomimetic amines are extremely useful therapeutic agents, they do have undesirable side effects. Those with predominantly β_1-receptor-stimulating properties are liable to increase heart rate and produce ventricular irritability, both of which are deleterious to myocardial function. α-Re-

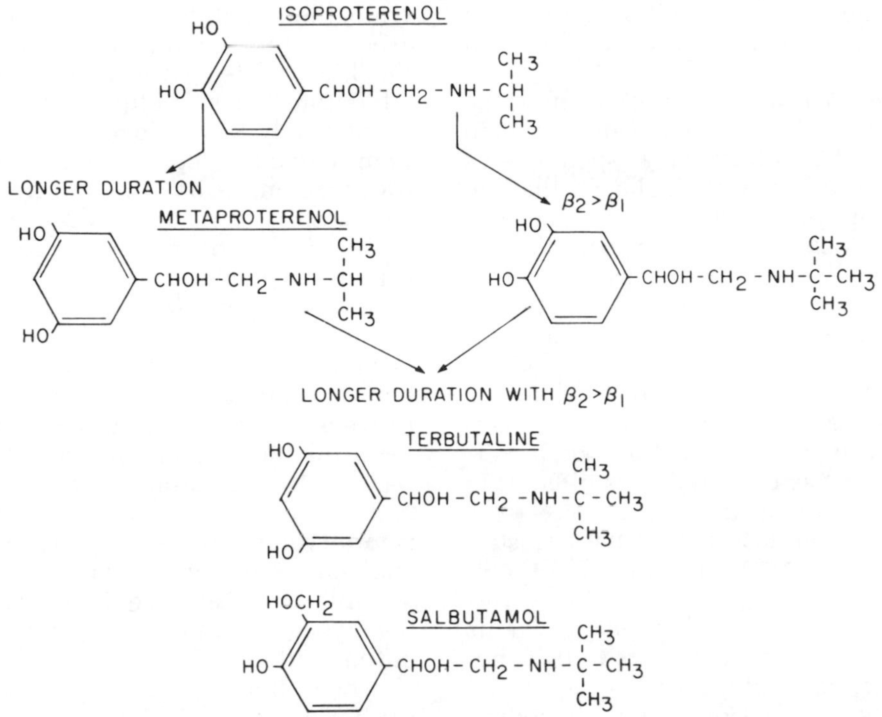

Figure 13.11 Molecular modifications of isoproterenol. (With permission from Mueller RA: Recent developments in the physiology of bronchomotor tone and the pharmacology of bronchodilators. Anesthesia and respiratory function. *Int Anesthesiol Clin* 15:140, 1977.)

ceptor agonists increase peripheral vascular resistance, leading to hypertension and reduced tissue perfusion, especially important to the kidneys.

Before a sympathomimetic agent is administered intravenously, hypo- and hypervolemia, hypoxemia, and abnormalities of acid-base and electrolyte balance should be corrected. The patient should also be monitored hemodynamically with measurement of central venous pressure and ideally with monitoring of pulmonary arterial and wedge pressure. In addition, measurement of cardiac output is also helpful.

Dopamine has become the inotrope of choice in the first instance in many clinical situations. It is a less powerful inotrope than epinephrine or norepinephrine but has vasodilating properties, and selectively increases renal blood flow, which can be extremely useful in the clinical setting of hypotension and reduced cardiac output.

Disadvantages of the more powerful

inotropic agents, such as epinephrine, are that in higher doses they act as α-receptor agonists and reduce both tissue perfusion and renal blood flow. Profound constriction of the renal vasculature bed over a long period may lead to renal failure. In addition, peripheral vasoconstriction limits peripheral tissue perfusion and results in tissue hypoxia and an increasing metabolic acidosis. Although the increase in peripheral resistance increases arterial blood pressure, it also increases myocardial work and oxygen utilization. Dysrhythmias including sinus tachycardia and ventricular dysrhythmias increase the work of the heart and may also reduce cardiac output. In patients with a low cardiac output, normal or low arterial pressure and high ventricular filling pressures with evidence of pulmonary venous engorgement, the combination of a vasodilator with an inotropic agent (e.g., sodium nitroprusside with low-dose dopamine), may be considered. Thus, it can be seen that hemodynamic monitoring makes a significant contribution to the choice of inotropic agent.

Cardiac Arrest. Epinephrine may be given for cardiac asystole in an attempt to promote the return of a spontaneous heart beat or, for ventricular fibrillation, to coarsen fibrillation prior to electrical countershock. Since the myocardium is "sensitized" to circulating catecholamines during inhalational anesthesia, the question of whether catecholamines such as epinephrine should be administered during cardiac arrest occurring under general anesthesia is controversial. However, in a situation where cardiac arrest has occurred, it is difficult to withhold epinephrine.

Epinephrine dose for cardiac arrest: 2 to 10 ml of 1:10,000 solution of epinephrine.

Hypotension. Sympathomimetic agents may be used as vasopressors to treat hypotension occurring during general and spinal anesthesia. However, with modern anesthetic practice, it is generally unnecessary and unwise (for reasons outlined above) to give a sympathomimetic agent during inhalational anesthesia. However, vasopressors such as methoxamine and ephedrine are frequently administered during spinal and epidural anesthesia to both prevent and treat the hypotension that can occur in this situation.

Anaphylactic Shock. Epinephrine is the drug of choice in the treatment of anaphylactic shock, which may be manifest by respiratory distress, vascular collapse, and shock. Pruritus, uticaria, and angioedema may also occur. Epinephrine should be administered subcutaneously, 0.2 to 0.5 ml of 1:1000 solution. Aminophylline may also be required to treat bronchospasm. Steroids and antihistamines may be required. Oxygen, either by mask or via an endotracheal tube, with controlled respiration may be necessary in severe cases. The anesthesiologist is most likely to be required to treat anaphylactic shock occurring during radiographic procedures when a reaction occurs to the diagnostic agent being used.

Acute Myocardial Infarction and Cardiogenic Shock. Intravenous infusions of sympathomimetic amines have been used in the treatment of cardiogenic shock associated with acute myocardial infarction. The mortality in this situation is extremely high. Since myocardial oxygen demand depends on ventricular wall tension, heart rate, and myocardial contractility, any drug which increases these parameters may exacerbate myocardial ischemia. Norepinephrine, epinephrine, isoproterenol, and dopamine all increase coronary blood flow in the intact animal by raising cardiac output and, hence, coronary perfusion pressure. However, when norepinephrine, epinephrine, and dopamine are infused directly into the coronary arteries in animal studies, they cause vasoconstriction; isoproterenol causes vasodilation. Catecholamines are therefore administered to patients with cardiogenic shock following myocardial infarction to raise cardiac output and increase coronary blood flow. However, these agents may cause a myocardial oxygen debt by increasing myocardial oxygen utilization. Epinephrine should not be administered to patients in cardiogenic shock resulting from myocardial infarction, because of the increase in heart rate, contractility, and wall tension that all combine to increase myocardial oxygen demand, as explained previously. Isoproterenol and epinephrine might also be disadvantageous in this situation due to their tendency to produce arrhythmias. In addition, isoproterenol can decrease coronary artery perfusion due to a reduction in diastolic blood pressure. Dopamine would thus seem to be a logical drug choice in this clinical situation. If coronary perfusion is low and diastolic arterial pressure is also low, norepinephrine is also a useful agent. Disadvantages include its powerful vasoconstrictor properties and reduction of blood flow to peripheral organs. Other newer inotropic agents such as amrinone have also been used.

Low Cardiac Output Syndrome following Cardiopulmonary Bypass. All the sympathomimetic amines have been used as inotropic agents to facilitate the emergence from cardiopulmonary bypass. Isoproterenol and epinephrine have both been used to increase myocardial contractility and heart rate. However, these two drugs have a potent chronotropic action and, in addition, often produce dysrhythmias, both disadvantageous in this situation. Dopamine has been shown to be a useful agent because, in addition to increasing cardiac output, it has less potential to cause tachycardia and arrhythmias and specifically increases renal blood flow and glomerular filtration rate. Clinical studies that compared the hemodynamic effects of isoproterenol and dopamine during open heart surgery have shown that several patients unresponsive to other sympathomimetic amines improved after the commencement of dopamine therapy. Dobutamine, a synthetic catecholamine with relatively cardioselective β_1-receptor stimulating properties and reduced chronotropic/inotropic ratio, has also proven effective. Amrinone, a phosphodiesterase inhibitor with inotropic and vasodilator properties described earlier in this chapter, has also been used in the management of termination from cardiopulmonary bypass.

Congestive Heart Failure. The use of catecholamines for the long-term treatment of intractable congestive heart failure has often been disappointing because, although there is an improvement in blood pressure and cardiac output, this is often accompanied by decreased peripheral tissue perfusion and reduced myocardial oxygenation. In addition, they increase peripheral resistance and afterload and, hence, have a detrimental effect on myocardial performance. However, dopamine has been used recently with encouraging results. The combined administration of dopamine and the vasodilator nitroprusside has resulted in significant improvement in patients who did not respond to either agent alone. Such use combines the beneficial effects on renal blood flow and cardiac output with the reduction of afterload achieved by nitroprusside.

Recently, new positive inotropic drugs with vasodilator and inotropic effects, such as amrinone, have been successfully used in the management of conges-

tive cardiac failure and are discussed earlier in the chapter. In addition, dopamine analogs and prodrugs have also been developed and are discussed previously in this chapter.

Respiratory Disorders. Epinephrine, isoproterenol, and selective β_2-receptor-stimulating agents cause bronchodilation and are effective agents in the treatment of bronchospasm due to allergic disorders and respiratory disease such as asthma and chronic obstructive airway disease. For a detailed consideration of their use, see Chapter 19, Drugs and the Respiratory System.

BIBLIOGRAPHY

General

Axelrod J, Weinshilboum R: Catecholamines. *N Engl J Med* 287:237–242, 1972.

Colucci WS, Wright RF, Braunwald E: New positive inotropic agents in the treatment of congestive heart failure. Mechanisms of action and recent clinical developments (part II). *N Engl J Med* 314:349–358, 1986.

Horrigan RW, Eger EI, Wilson C: Epinephrine-induced arrhythmias during enflurane anesthesia in man: a non-linear dose-response relationship and dose-dependent protection from lidocaine. *Anesth Analg* 57:547–550, 1978.

Johnston RR, Eger EI, Wilson C: A comparative interaction of epinephrine with enflurane, isoflurane, and halothane in man. *Anesth Analg* 55:709–712, 1976.

Katz RL, Bigger JT: Cardiac arrhythmias during anesthesia and operation. *Anesthesiology* 33:193–213, 1970.

Katz RL, Epstein RA: The interaction of anesthetic agents and adrenergic drugs to produce cardiac arrhythmias. *Anesthesiology* 29:763–784, 1968.

Katz RL, Matteo RS, Papper EM: The injection of epinephrine during general anesthesia. *Anesthesiology* 23:597–600, 1962.

Liu WS, Wong KC, Port JD, Andriano KP: Epinephrine-induced arrhythmias during halothane anesthesia with the addition of nitrous oxide, nitrogen, or helium in dogs. *Anesth Analg* 61:414–417, 1982.

Price JL, Ohnishi ST: Effects of anesthetics on the heart. *Fed Proc* 39:1575–1579, 1980.

Rocci ML, Wilson H: The pharmacokinetics and pharmacodynamics of newer inotropic agents. *Clin Pharmacokinet* 13:91–109, 1987.

Scallan MJH, Gothard JWW, Branthwaite MA: Inotropic agents. *Br J Anaesth* 51:649–658, 1979.

Smith LDR, Oldershaw PJ: Inotropic and vasopressor agents. *Br J Anaesth* 56:767–780, 1984.

Smith NT, Corbascio AN: The use and misuse of pressor agents. *Anesthesiology* 33:58–101, 1970.

Tucker WK, Rackstein AD, Munson ES: Comparison of arrhythmic doses of adrenaline, metaraminol, ephedrine, and phenylephrine during isoflurane and halothane anesthesia in dogs. *Br J Anaesth* 46:392–396, 1974.

Weber KT, Gill SK, Janicki JS, Maskin CS, Jain MC: New positive inotropic agents in the treatment of chronic cardiac failure. Current status and future directions. *Drugs* 33:503–519, 1987.

Zaimis E: Vasopressor drugs and catecholamines. *Anesthesiology* 29:732–762, 1968.

Adrenergic Receptors

Ahlquist RP: A study of adrenotropic receptors. *Am J Physiol* 153:586–600, 1948.

Ahlquist RP: Adrenergic receptors and others. *Anesth Analg* 58:510–515, 1979.

Bristow MR, Ginsburg R, Minobe W, Cubicciotti RS, Sageman WS, Lurie K, Billingham ME, Harrison DC, Stinson EB: Decreased catecholamine sensitivity and β-adrenergic-receptor density in failing human hearts. *N Engl J Med* 307:205–211, 1982.

Brodde O-E, Kretsch R, Ikezono K, Zerkowski H-R, Reidemeister JC: Human β-adrenoceptors: relation of myocardial and lymphocyte β-adrenoceptor density. *Science* 231:1584–1585, 1986.

Brown MJ, Brown DC, Murphy MB: Hypokalemia from beta₂-receptor stimulation by circulating epinephrine. *N Engl J Med* 309:1414–1419, 1983.

Hilditch A, Drew GM: Peripheral dopamine receptor subtypes—a closer look. *Trends Pharm Sci* 6:396–400, 1985.

Hoffman BB, Lefkowitz RJ: Alpha-adrenergic receptor subtypes. *N Engl J Med* 302:1390–1396, 1980.

Lands AM, Arnold A, McAuliff JP, Luduena FP, Brown TG Jr: Differentiation of receptor systems activated by sympathomimetic amines. *Nature* 214:597–598, 1967.

Lefkowitz RJ: Direct binding studies of adrenergic receptors: biochemical, physiologic, and clinical implications. *Ann Intern Med* 91:450–458, 1979.

Marty J, Nivoche Y, Nimier M, Rocchiccioli C, Luscombe F, Hanzel D, Loiseau A, Desmonts JM: The effects of halothane on the human beta-adrenergic receptor of lymphocyte membranes. *Anesthesiology* 67:974–978, 1987.

Motulsky HJ, Insel PA: Adrenergic receptors in man. Direct identification, physiologic regulation, and clinical alterations. *N Engl J Med* 307:18–29, 1982.

Schwinn DA, McIntyre RW, Hawkins ED, Kates RA, Reves JG: α₁-Adrenergic responsiveness during coronary artery bypass surgery: effect of preoperative ejection fraction. *Anesthesiology* 69:206–217, 1988.

Mechanism of Action of Inotropic Drugs

Colucci WS, Wright RF, Braunwald E: New positive inotropic agents in the treatment of congestive heart failure. Mechanisms of action and recent clinical developments (part I). *N Engl J Med* 314:290–299, 1986.

Scholz H: Inotropic drugs and their mechanisms of action. *J Am Coll Cardiol* 4:389–397, 1984.

Phosphodiesterase Inhibitors

Anderson JL, Askins JC, Gilbert EM, Menlove RL, Lutz JR: Occurrence of ventricular arrhythmias in patients receiving acute and chronic infusions of milrinone. *Am Heart J* 111:466–474, 1986.

Baim DS, McDowell AV, Cherniles J, Monrad ES, Parker JA, Edelson J, Braunwald E, Grossman W: Evaluation of a new bipyridine inotropic agent—milrinone—in patients with severe congestive heart failure. *N Engl J Med* 309:748–756, 1983.

Benotti JR, Grossman W, Braunwald E, Davolos DD, Alousis AA: Hemodynamic assessment of amrinone. A new inotropic agent. *N Engl J Med* 299:1373–1377, 1978.

Klein NA, Siskind SJ, Frishman WH, Sonnenblick ED, LeJemtel TH: Hemodynamic comparison of intravenous amrinone and dobutamine in patients with chronic congestive heart failure. *Am J Cardiol* 48:170–175, 1981.

Makela VHM, Kapur PA: Amrinone and verapamil-propranolol induced cardiac depression during isoflurane anesthesia in dogs. *Anesthesiology* 66:792–797, 1987.

Makela VHM, Kapur PA: Amrinone blunts cardiac depression caused by enflurane or isoflurane anesthesia in the dog. *Anesth Analg* 66:215–221, 1987.

Makela VHM, Kapur PA: Is milrinone equivalent to amrinone during enflurane anesthesia in the dog? *Anesth Analg* 67:349–355, 1988.

Siskind SJ, Sonnenblick EH, Forman R, Scheuer J, LeJemtel TH: Acute substantial benefit of inotropic therapy with amrinone on exercise hemodynamics and metabolism in severe congestive heart failure. *Circulation* 64:966–973, 1981.

Sonnenblick EH, Grose R, Strain J, Zelcer AA, LeJemtel TH: Effects of milrinone on left ventricular performance and myocardial contractility in patients with severe heart failure. *Circulation* 73 (Suppl III):162–167, 1986.

Other Inotropic Agents

Jennings G, Bobik A, Oddie C, Hargreaves M, Korner P: Cardioselectivity of prenalterol and isoproterenol. *Clin Pharmacol Ther* 34:749–757, 1983.

Malta E, McPherson GA, Raper C: Selective β₁-adrenoceptor agonists—fact or fiction? *Trends Pharm Sci* 6:400–403, 1985.

Rae AP, Tweddel AC, Hutton I: The clinical use of inotropes in cardiac failure: dopamine, dobutamine, prenalterol, and pirbuterol. *Herz* 8:23–33, 1983.

Roubin GS, Choong CYP, Devenish-Meares S, Sadick NN, Fletcher PJ, Kelly DT, Harris PJ: β-Adrenergic stimulation of the failing ventricle: a double-blind, randomized trial of sustained oral therapy with prenalterol. *Circulation* 69:955–962, 1984.

Sainsbury EJ, Fitzpatrick D, Ikram H, Nicholls MG, Espiner EA, Ashley JJ: Pharmacokinetics and plasma-concentration-effect relationships of prenalterol in cardiac failure. *Eur J Clin Pharmacol* 28:397–403, 1985.

Young RA, Ward A: Milrinone. A preliminary review of its pharmacological properties and therapeutic use. *Drugs* 36:158–192, 1988.

Therapeutic Uses

Goldberg LI: Use of sympathomimetic amines in heart failure. *Am J Cardiol* 22:177–182, 1968.

Pentel P, Benowitz N: Pharmacokinetic and pharmacodynamic considerations in drug therapy of cardiac emergencies. *Clin Pharmacokinet* 9:273–308, 1984.

Smith TE, Forgacs P: Haemodynamic interventions and therapy in septic shock. *Drugs* 24:75–82, 1982.

Physiology

Allwood MJ, Cobbold AF, Ginsburg J: Peripheral vascular effects of noradrenaline, isopropylnoradrenaline, and dopamine. *Br Med Bull* 19:132–136, 1963.

Aviado DM Jr: Cardiovascular effects of some commonly used pressor amines. *Anesthesiology* 20:71–97, 1959.

Cryer PE: Physiology and pathophysiology of the human sympathoadrenal neuroendocrine system. *N Engl J Med* 303:436–444, 1980.

Derbyshire DR, Smith G: Sympathoadrenal responses to anaesthesia and surgery. *Br J Anaesth* 56:725–739, 1984.

Eckstein JW, Abboud FM: Circulatory effects of sympathomimetic amines. *Am Heart J* 63:119–135, 1962.

Kopin IJ: Biosynthesis and metabolism of catecholamines. *Anesthesiology* 29:654–660, 1968.

Langer SZ, Hicks PE: Physiology of the sympathetic nerve ending. *Br J Anaesth* 56:689–700, 1984.

Dopamine

Goldberg LI: Cardiovascular and renal actions of dopamine: potential clinical applications. *Pharmacol Rev* 24:1–29, 1972.

Goldberg LI: Dopamine-clinical uses of an endogenous catecholamine. *N Engl J Med* 291:707–710, 1974.

Goldberg LI: Dopamine and new dopamine analogs: receptors and clinical applications. *J Clin Anesth* 1:66–74, 1988.

Goldberg LI, McDonald JH, Zimmerman, AM: Sodium diuresis produced by dopamine in patients with congestive heart failure. *N Engl J Med* 269:1060–1064, 1963.

Hilberman M, Maseda J, Stinson EB, Derby GC, Spencer RJ, Miller DC, Oyer PE, Myers BD: The diuretic properties of dopamine in patients after open-heart operations. *Anesthesiology* 61:489–494, 1984.

Holloway EL, Stinson EB, Derby GC, Harrison DC: Action of drugs in patients early after cardiac surgery. I. Comparison of isoproterenol and dopamine. *Am J Cardiol* 35:656–659, 1975.

Lorenzi M, Karam JH, Tsalikian E, Bohannon NV, Gerich JE, Forsham PH: Dopamine during α- or β-adrenergic blockade in man. Hormonal, metabolic, and cardiovascular effects. *J Clin Invest* 63:310–317, 1979.

MacCannell KL, McNay JL, Meyer MB, Goldberg LI: Dopamine in the treatment of hypotension and shock. *N Engl J Med* 275:1389–1398, 1966.

Miller ED: Editorial. Renal effects of dopamine. *Anesthesiology* 61:487–488, 1984.

Rosenblum R, Frieden J: Intravenous dopamine in the treatment of myocardial dysfunction after open heart surgery. *Am Heart J* 83:743–748, 1972.

Dobutamine

Berkowitz C, McKeever L, Croke RP, Jacobs WR, Loeb HS, Gunnar RM: Comparative responses to dobutamine and nitroprusside in patients with chronic low output cardiac failure. *Circulation* 56:918–924, 1977.

Leier CV, Unverferth DV: Dobutamine. *Ann Intern Med* 99:490–496, 1983.

Leier CV, Webel J, Bush CA: The cardiovascular effects of the continuous infusion of dobutamine in patients with severe cardiac failure. *Circulation* 56:468–472, 1977.

Sonnenblick EH, Frishman WH, LeJemtel TH: Dobutamine: a new synthetic cardioactive sympathetic amine. *N Engl J Med* 300:17–22, 1979.

Steen PA, Tinker JH, Pluth JR, Barnhorst DA, Tarhan S: Efficacy of dopamine, dobutamine, and epinephrine during emergence from cardiopulmonary bypass in man. *Circulation* 57:378–384, 1978.

Tinker JH, Tarhan S, White RD, Pluth JR, Barnhorst DA: Dobutamine for inotropic support during emergence from cardiopulmonary bypass. *Anesthesiology* 44:281–286, 1976.

β₂-Receptor Agonists

Mueller RA: Recent developments in the physiology of bronchomotor tone and the pharmacology of bronchodilators, in anesthesia and respiratory function. *Int Anesthesiol Clin* 15:137–167, 1977.

Drug Interactions

El-Ganzouri AR, Ivankovich Ad, Braverman B, McCarthy R: Monoamine oxidase inhibitors: should they be discontinued preoperatively? *Anesth Analg* 64:592–596, 1985.

Michaels I, Serrins M, Shier N-hQ, Barash PG: Anesthesia for cardiac surgery in patients receiving monoamine oxidase inhibitors. *Anesth Analg* 63:1041–1044, 1984.

Spiss CK, Smith CM, Maze M: Halothane-epinephrine arrhythmias and adrenergic responsiveness after chronic imipramine administration in dogs. *Anesth Analg* 63:825–828, 1984.

Stack CG, Rogers P, Linter SPK: Monoamine oxidase inhibitors and anaesthesia. *Br J Anaesth* 60:222–227, 1988.

14

Adrenoreceptor Blocking Agents

ALASTAIR J. J. WOOD

Adrenergic blockers are drugs which competitively antagonize the effects of the endogenous agonists epinephrine and norepinephrine at adrenergic receptors. These receptors were subdivided by Ahlquist into α- and β-receptors (see Chapter 13), and drugs have been developed which selectively block either α- or β-receptors in humans. The sympathetic nervous system and the effects of α- and β-agonists have been reviewed in Chapter 13. This chapter directs attention to antagonists which act at adrenergic receptors.

β-ADRENERGIC BLOCKING AGENTS

There are now a number of β-adrenoceptor blocking agents available. All of the currently available β-blockers are competitive antagonists of the naturally occurring β-receptor agonists. There are substantial differences, however, in their pharmacokinetic properties, i.e., in the way in which they are absorbed, metabolized, and excreted. In addition, the various β-blockers differ in some of their other properties, such as their ability to block β-receptors in different tissues (selectivity), their ability to stimulate the β-receptor, and their cardiac depressant activity, as well as in their membrane-stabilizing, local anesthetic, or "quinidine-like" activity. Rational choice of a β-blocker for an individual patient clearly depends on an understanding of the significance of these differences among the various agents.

PHARMACODYNAMIC PROPERTIES OF THE β-BLOCKERS

Much has been made of the differences in the actions of the various β-blockers. However, all of the β-blockers competitively block the effects of both endogenously and exogenously administered catecholamines at the β-adrenergic receptors. This means that a larger concentration of agonist is required to produce an effect in the presence of the antagonist, resulting in a parallel shift to the right in the dose-response curve (see Chapter 3).

Figure 14.1 shows the effect of increasing doses of isoproterenol on heart rate. A dose of 1.1 μg of isoproterenol was required to raise the heart rate by 25 beats/min prior to an infusion of propranolol. Following the propranolol infusion, there was a more than 40-fold increase in the dose of isoproterenol required to produce the same rise in heart rate. This emphasizes a common point of confusion surrounding the effects of β-blockers. Since they are competitive antagonists of sympathetic agonists, it is always possible to completely overcome their effects, provided enough β-agonist is administered to achieve an adequate concentration at the receptor. There is, therefore, no such thing as complete β-blockade. One can

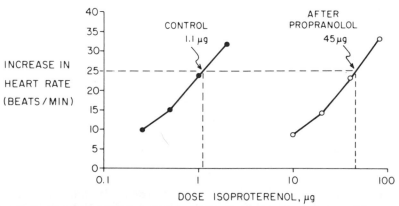

Figure 14.1.   Increase in heart rate in response to increasing doses of isoproterenol before (●) and following (○) propranolol.   Note the parallel shift in the dose-response curve.

only assess β-blockade in terms of the amount of an agonist or the strength of a stimulus required to overcome the blockade.

The dose of agonist required to raise the heart rate by a constant amount (25 beats/min) increases with advancing age, the elderly requiring around 5-fold more isoproterenol than the young (Fig. 14.2). Receptor theory (Chapter 3) would predict that, following the administration of an antagonist

$$DR - 1 = \frac{P}{K_d}$$

where *DR* is the ratio of the dose of isoproterenol required to raise the heart rate by a given amount (e.g., 25 beats/min) after propranolol administration to the dose of isoproterenol required to produce the same increase before propranolol. *P* is the unbound propranolol concentration in plasma; this is the concentration available for binding to receptor sites. K_d is the apparent dissociation constant for propranolol binding to the receptor and, hence, is a measure of propranolol resistance, since larger values imply less effect. Following the administration of pro-

pranolol, it was found that the elderly were 4 to 5 times more resistant to propranolol than the young (Fig. 14.3).

In addition to their ability to antagonize the effects of β-receptor agonists at the β-receptors, some of the β-blockers have additional effects that may or may not be of therapeutic importance (Table 14.1).

Membrane-stabilizing or "Quinidine-like" Activity

Early in the study of β-blocking drugs, it was found that propranolol had electrophysiological properties that were not related to its antagonism of β-adrenergic receptors. Specifically, it was shown that propranolol slowed the rate of rise of the intracardiac action potential, whereas resting potential and spike duration were unchanged, i.e., a membrane-stabilizing or quinidine effect. It has since been shown that a number of other β-blockers possess this effect, including oxprenolol and alprenolol.

It was initially suggested that propranolol concentrations as high as 10,000 ng/ml in vitro were required to produce this effect, but more recent studies have sug-

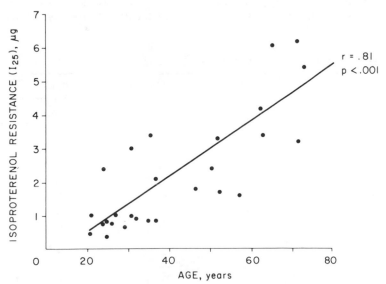

Figure 14.2.   Relationship between age and isoproterenol resistance as measured by the dose (I_{25}) of isoproterenol required to raise the heart rate by 25 beats/min.   (With permission from Vestal RE, Wood AJJ, Shand DG: Reduced beta-adrenoceptor sensitivity in the elderly. *Clin Pharmacol Ther* 26:181–186, 1979.)

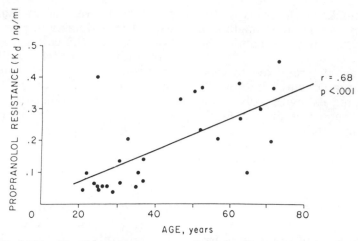

Figure 14.3.   Relationship between age and the resistance to propranolol (K_d—see text).   As age advances, greater concentrations of propranolol are required for β-blockade. (With permission from Vestal RE, Wood AJJ, Shand DG: Reduced beta-adrenoceptor sensitivity in the elderly. *Clin Pharmacol Ther* 26:181–186, 1979.)

gested that the in vitro concentrations required for membrane-stabilizing effects may be much lower than originally proposed. However, inhibition of exercise tachycardia and suppression of arrhythmias occur at plasma concentrations of only 100 ng/ml.

The D-isomer of propranolol is 60- to 100-fold less potent as a β-blocker than the L-isomer and does not have therapeutic activity. However, high doses of D-propranolol have recently been shown to have antiarrhythmic activity which appears to be due to properties other than β-blockade.

Selectivity

Following Ahlquist's original subdivision of adrenoreceptors into two types (α and β) according to the relative potency of different sympathomimetic amines, al-

Table 14.1.
Pharmacodynamic Properties of β-Blockers

	Potency* as β-blocker	Selectivity for β_1-receptors	Membrane-stabilizing activity	Intrinsic sympathomimetic activity	α-Blockade
Acebutolol	0.3	+	+	+	0
Alprenolol	0.3	0	+	+	0
Atenolol	1	+	0	0	0
Esmolol	0.01	+	0	0	0
Labetalol	0.3	0	+	0	+
Metoprolol	1	+	±	0	0
Nadolol	0.5	0	0	0	0
Oxprenolol	0.5–1	0	+	+	0
Penbutolol	4	0	+	+	0
Pindolol	6	0	±	+	0
Propranolol	1	0	+	0	0
Sotalol	0.3	0	0	0	0
Timolol	6	0	0	0	0

*Relative to propranolol = 1.

Table 14.2.
Site and Effect of Stimulating β_1- and β_2-Receptors

β_1-Receptors		β_2-Receptors	
Site	Effect of stimulation	Site	Effect of stimulation
Heart	Increased rate Increased contractility	Bronchi Blood vessels Uterus Insulin	Dilation Dilation Relaxation Production Increase

most two decades passed before these receptors were further subdivided into the so-called β_1- and β_2-receptors (Table 14.2). Stimulation of β_1-receptors produces positive inotropic and chronotropic effects on the heart, whereas β_2 stimulation dilates the bronchi and certain vascular beds. β-Blockers, such as propranolol, act at both the β_1- and β_2-receptors. However, the so-called selective β_1-receptor antagonists have a relatively greater potency for the β_1-receptor than the β_2-receptor. This means that these drugs will antagonize the effects of agonists on the cardiac receptors at concentrations that have little effect on the β_2-receptors. However, with increasing concentrations of drug, the β_2-receptors will also be blocked. Figure 14.4 shows that, as the concentration of a nonselective antagonist is increased, β_1- and β_2-receptors will be equally antagonized. However, for a selective β-blocker, lower doses, or concentrations, will antagonize β_1-receptors, whereas higher concentrations will be required to block β_2-receptors, reflecting the differing affinity of a selective drug for the β_1- and β_2-receptors. Provided the concentrations are raised high enough, however, even a β_1-selective agent will produce blockade of β_2-receptors.

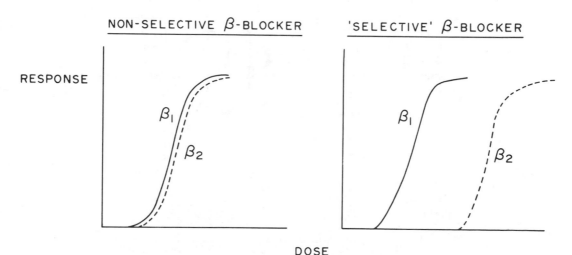

Figure 14.4.   Effects of increasing concentrations of a non-selective *(left panel)* and selective *(right panel)* β-blocker. As the concentration or dose of a nonselective drug is increased, β_1- and β_2-receptors are antagonized at equal concentrations. However, increasing the concentration of a β_1-selective drug produces antagonism of β_1-receptors at concentrations below those required to antagonize β_2-receptors, reflecting the drug's higher affinity for β_1-receptors.

In patients with bronchial asthma, selectivity may be a useful property, since the selective β-blockers are less likely to precipitate bronchospasm in such patients. However, it should be understood that even these selective agents may, in some patients at low doses and probably in many asthmatic patients at high doses, cause bronchial constriction, and today other drugs such as calcium blockers might be better choices for such patients.

Another situation in which the use of a selective β-blocker may be desirable is in the treatment of diabetic patients. Nonselective β-blockers may delay the blood glucose recovery from hypoglycemia, whereas selective β-blockers, such as metoprolol and atenolol, do not. In addition, severe bradycardia and raised diastolic blood pressure have occurred during hypoglycemia while taking propranolol. These effects were milder with a cardioselective β blocker.

Stimulation of β_2-receptors in muscle increases potassium entry into cells. This increase in intracellular potassium results in a fall in plasma potassium. Thus, stress-induced rise in catecholamines may result in a reduction in plasma potassium to hypokalemic levels, particularly in patients whose potassium is already reduced by administration of diuretics. Such rises in catecholamines may be seen in patients after a myocardial infarction and during surgical and postsurgical stress, and the resultant β_2-receptor stimulation may result in hypokalemia. Although the implications of this catecholamine-induced hypokalemia are not entirely clear, it has been suggested that an increased incidence of ventricular arrhythmias occurs in such patients. This effect of β_2-receptor stimulation is more effectively blocked by administration of a nonselective β-blocker, such as propranolol, than by β_1-selective agents, such as atenolol (Fig. 14.5).

In conclusion, therefore, cardioselectivity may be of value in some special situations, but these differences are not absolute, and antagonism of β_2-receptors does occur, particularly at higher doses. Conversely, nonselective drugs are required to prevent the stress-induced fall in plasma potassium.

Intrinsic Sympathomimetic Activity (ISA)

In noradrenaline-depleted animal models, it is possible to demonstrate that

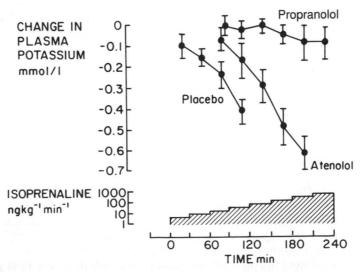

Figure 14.5. Blockade of β_2-receptor-mediated hypokalemia. Isoproterenol lowers serum potassium through stimulation of β_2-receptors. The hypokalemia is blocked more effectively by a nonselective drug, such as propranolol, than a selective drug, like atenolol. (With permission from Vincent HH, Int't Veld AJM, Boomsma F., Schalekamp MADH: Prevention of epinephrine-induced hypokalemia by nonselective beta blockers. *Am J Cardiol* 56:10D–14D, 1985.)

some of the β-blockers (Table 14.1) have slight agonist activity in addition to their predominant β-antagonist properties. The maximum stimulation of the receptors that these drugs can produce is clearly much less than full agonists, such as epinephrine or isoproterenol. The ability of partial agonists to act as competitive antagonists of full agonists is discussed in Chapter 3.

A partial agonist differs from a full agonist in that its maximal ability to stimulate the β-receptor is less than that produced by a full agonist (Fig. 14.6). When a partial agonist is administered in the presence of a full agonist, it acts as an an-

tagonist, reducing the effect of the full agonist to the maximal effect of the partial agonist. Conversely, in the absence of agonist stimulation, such as when sympathetic tone is low, the partial agonist will act as an agonist and raise heart rate, but again its maximal effect will be limited (Fig. 14.6).

It was initially suggested that the drugs lacking in ISA were more effective in the treatment of hyperthyroidism. However, this has now been challenged. It has also been suggested that drugs with intrinsic agonist activity would be less likely to precipitate cardiac failure in patients prone to this, and that drugs with less

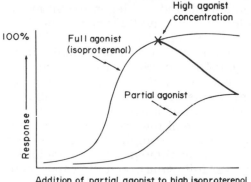

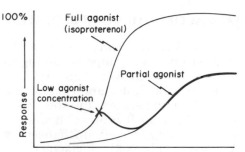

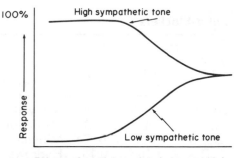

Figure 14.6. Effects of a partial agonist. A full agonist, such as isoproterenol, in high dose produces 100% of the maximal response as will a high level of sympathetic tone or igh catecholamine concentrations. On the other hand, the effect of the partial agonist is less than that produced by a full agonist. Increasing concentrations of a partial agonist will reduce the effect of the full agonist to the maximal effect of the partial agonist (*heavy line, left upper panel*). On the other hand, at low concentrations of the full agonist or when endogenous catecholamines (sympathetic tone) are low, the partial agonist will increase the response to its maximal effect (*heavy line, right upper panel*). The dose response to a partial agonist in the presence (high sympathetic tone) and absence of a full agonist (low sympathetic tone) is shown in the *lower panel*.

myocardial depressant action may be safer in this regard. However, it is likely that the principal reason for the precipitation of cardiac failure by β-blockers in patients already on the brink of cardiac failure is the removal of the increased sympathetic drive to the heart by β-blockade. Patients with compromised cardiac function attempt to maintain adequate cardiac output through increased sympathetic drive to the heart. Removal of this increased drive through the use of a β-blocker is likely to precipitate cardiac failure, whatever the drug's effect on the contraction of isolated cardiac tissue in vitro.

β-Blockers with ISA may be less effective than those without ISA in preventing death after myocardial infarction.

PHARMACOKINETICS OF β-BLOCKERS

The β-blockers currently available can be divided into two groups according to their route of elimination. Some, such as propranolol, metoprolol, and timolol, are extensively metabolized by the liver, whereas others, such as atenolol and nadolol, are excreted largely unchanged by the kidneys (Table 14.3). The factors controlling the excretion of the drugs in

these two groups are quite different. Propranolol, the first of this group of drugs to become available, has been studied extensively, partly because of its therapeutic importance but also because of its utility as a model compound.

PROPRANOLOL, METOPROLOL, AND TIMOLOL

These drugs are almost completely absorbed following an oral dose, and peak concentrations are achieved quickly. Food appears to enhance the systemic availability of both propranolol and metoprolol. Following oral administration and absorption, the drug passes to the liver where it is exposed to the liver's drug-metabolizing system. In the case of propranolol, and to a lesser extent metoprolol, the liver avidly removes the drug from the blood.

The avid removal of propranolol from the portal blood prior to its entry into the systemic circulation (first-pass elimination) results in a low systemic availability of the drug following oral administration, in spite of the excellent absorption. An additional complication is the fact that the avid removal of propranolol by the liver following oral dosing appears to be dose dependent. This has two impor-

Table 14.3.
Pharmacokinetic Properties of β-Blockers

	Absorption (%)	Systemic bioavailability (%)	Protein binding	Half-life (hr)	Metabolic Pathways	Urinary excretion unchanged* (%)
Acebutolol	>90	20–60	15–20	3–6	Acetylation	20
Alprenolol	>90	15	85	2–3	Oxidation	<1
Atenolol	46–62	55	<5	6–7	Minimal	85–100
Esmolol			56	0.15	Hydrolysis	<1%
Labetalol	>90	30–40	50	4	Conjugation	<5
Metoprolol	>95	50	12	3–4	Oxidation	<5
Nadolol	15–25	20	14	12–24	Minimal	70–100
Oxprenolol	70–95	20–60	80	1–2	Oxidation	2–5
Penbutolol	100	100	>95	26	Conjugation/oxidation	<10
Pindolol	>90	>90	46	2–5	Conjugation/oxidation	40
Propranolol	100	33	90	4–6	Oxidation	<1
Sotalol	100	>60	<1	5–13	Minimal	60
Timolol	>90	75	10	4–5	Oxidation	13–20

*Percentage of absorbed dose excreted unchanged in urine.

tant practical consequences. First, at low doses, less of the drug enters the systemic circulation than at higher doses, and second, it is impossible to predict the disposition characteristics of the drug at steady state from a single oral dose, because the bioavailability is higher during chronic oral dosing than after the first oral dose.

The high hepatic extraction of propranolol following oral administration, which is dependent on the liver's drug-metabolizing ability, also accounts for the large difference in dosage requirements following intravenous administration (where there is no presystemic elimination) and oral administration. The factors determining the clearance of propranolol, and hence, steady state levels, following oral and intravenous dosing are also different. The oral clearance of the drug is dependent solely on the liver's drug-metabolizing ability while, at steady state, the intravenous clearance is influenced mainly by liver blood flow in addition to the liver's drug-metabolizing ability (see Chapter 1). Liver blood flow is much less variable between individuals than is liver drug-metabolizing ability; thus, it is not surprising that the variability in propranolol concentrations is less following intravenous administration than after oral administration, when variations of up to 20-fold have been found. In a strictly controlled trial in which 24 normal volunteers, aged 21 to 73 years, received 80 mg of propranolol every 8 hours in the hospital, a more than 10-fold variation in plasma propranolol concentrations was found (Fig. 14.7). As pointed out previously, the clearance following oral administration reflects the drug-metabolizing ability of the liver, and since this varies widely and is affected by the patient's genetic makeup, the environment to which he is and has been ex-

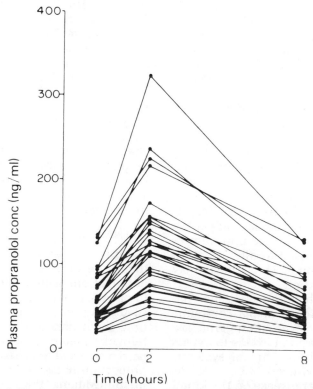

Figure 14.7.   Variability in propranolol concentraton at steady state in a group of normal hospitalized volunteers receiving 80 mg of propranolol every 8 hours.   (With permission from Routledge PA, Shand DG: *Clin Pharmacokinet* 4:73–90, 1979.)

posed, his age, and numerous other factors, it is not surprising that steady-state drug levels vary so widely. (Some of the factors responsible for this variation will be addressed in more detail later.)

Although most of the studies of the presystemically extracted β-blockers have used propranolol, it is likely that these findings can be extrapolated to the other β-blockers that are avidly removed by the liver.

ATENOLOL, NADOLOL, AND SOTALOL

These agents are mainly excreted by the kidneys as unchanged drug. Thus, their elimination is impaired in renal disease, but it is not dependent on the vagaries of drug metabolism. It has, therefore, been suggested that the steady-state plasma levels of these drugs will be subject to much less interindividual variation than the highly metabolized β-blockers. While that may well be true, it is important to note (Table 14.3) that both atenolol and nadolol are poorly absorbed. One must also remember that, because of the poor absorption of atenolol and nadolol following oral administration, they too require lower doses intravenously than orally.

Effects of Disease on the Kinetics of β-Blockers

LIVER DISEASE

For β-blockers such as propranolol and metoprolol and, to a lesser extent, timolol, all of which are highly metabolized by the liver, liver disease might be expected to have a significant effect on plasma clearance following oral administration. In addition, the alterations in plasma proteins found in cirrhosis may alter the disposition of propranolol, which is highly bound in plasma. Because of the existence of portosystemic shunts, some of the drug coming from the gut following absorption is able to bypass the liver, resulting in a higher systemic availability of the drug.

The effect of liver disease on the kinetics of propranolol has been carefully investigated using a technique that involves the simultaneous administration of native drug orally and labeled drug intravenously. This allows the measurement of all of the parameters controlling elimination, including systemic availability, oral or intrinsic clearance (which, as discussed earlier, is dependent on liver drug-metabolizing ability), and systemic or intravenous clearance, which is determined at steady state by both drug-metabolizing ability (intrinsic clearance) and liver blood flow. In addition, the plasma binding of the drug was measured and used to express the drug concentrations in terms of free or unbound drug in blood. Steady-state concentrations of propranolol were markedly higher in cirrhotic patients than in controls (Fig. 14.8). This was due to an increase in systemic availability—38% in the control group as compared to 54% in the cirrhotic group—and a decrease in systemic clearance. Because of the increased average total steady-state concentrations in blood, coupled with an elevation in the fraction of the drug free in plasma, there was a 3-fold increase in the average free drug concentration from 7.5 ng/ml to 22.3 ng/ml. The steady-state levels of β-blockers, such as nadolol and atenolol, which are largely excreted by renal routes, will be little affected by liver disease, while the drugs that are highly metabolized by the liver will be more susceptible to such changes. However, it should be remembered that changes in protein binding are less likely to be important for drugs such as metoprolol, which is only 12% bound in plasma.

RENAL DISEASE

It might be anticipated that β-blockers that have largely renal routes of elimination might accumulate in patients with impaired renal function; however, it is surprising that there have been suggestions that the excretion of some of the extenively metabolized drugs is also impaired in renal disease. Although a small proportion of timolol (13%) is eliminated unchanged in the urine, the overall clearance of timolol was not prolonged in patients with renal failure and, therefore,

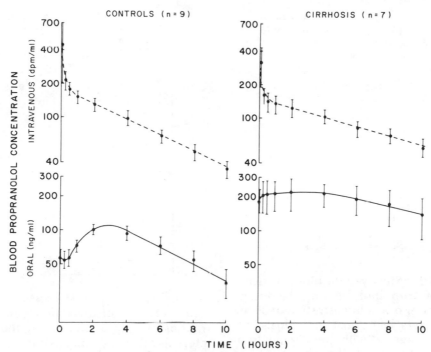

Figure 14.8.   The concentration of unlabeled propranolol (ng/ml) in whole blood after oral admistration (●————●) and the concentration of tritiated propranolol (dpm/ml) after intravenous administration (●– – –●) following simultaneous determination of intravenous and oral dose kinetics of propranolol at the seventh dosing interval in nine normal subjects and seven patients with cirrhosis (mean ± SEM). (With permission from Wood AJJ, Kornhauser DM, Wilkinson GR, Shand DG, Branch RA: The influence of cirrhosis on steady-state blood concentrations of unbound propranolol after oral administration. *Clin Pharmacokinet* 3:478–487, 1978.)

no change in the oral dosage is required.

However, since approximately 70% of nadolol is excreted in the urine, its elimination is impaired in patients with renal failure. In fact, the rate of elimination of nadolol correlated well with creatinine clearance and, in patients with the most severe degree of renal failure, the half-life of nadolol was prolonged to 45 hours from the half-life of 14 to 20 hours in patients with normal renal function.

The effect of renal disease on the elimination of propranolol has been the source of some confusion which may now be clarified following a study of patients with severe renal failure, whether on hemodialysis or not yet on dialysis. No impairment of propranolol elimination when compared to age-matched controls was found. Thus, it is unlikely that

any adjustment of propranolol dosage is required in patients with renal failure.

OTHER FACTORS: AGE

It is now widely appreciated that the elderly suffer a higher incidence of adverse drug reactions than the young. This higher incidence may be partly due to alteration in their ability to eliminate drugs.

It has recently been shown that, following 80 mg every 8 hours, blood levels of propranolol were 2-fold higher in normal subjects over the age of 35 compared to those under 35 (Fig. 14.9). In addition, when the effect ot smoking was examined, it was found that the smokers had significantly lower levels of propranolol throughout the dosing interval than nonsmokers (Fig. 14.10). These changes

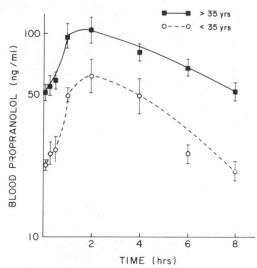

Figure 14.9. Steady-state blood concentrations of propranolol during the dosage intervals after oral administration of 80 mg every 8 hours in normal individuals, according to age. (With permission from Vestal RE, Wood AJJ, Branch RA, Shand DG, Wilkinson GR: Effects of age and cigarette smoking on propranolol disposition. *Clin Pharmacol Ther* 26:8–15, 1979.)

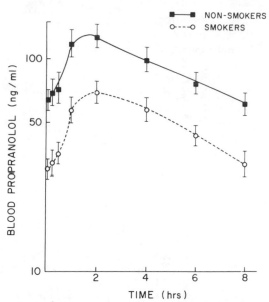

Figure 14.10. Steady-state blood concentrations of propranolol during the dosage intervals after oral administration of 80 mg every 8 hours in normal individuals—smokers vs nonsmokers. (With permission from Vestal RE, Wood AJJ, Branch RA, Shand DG, Wilkinson GR: Effects of age and cigarette smoking on propranolol disposition. *Clin Pharmacol Ther* 26:8–15, 1979.)

appeared to be due to an age-related effect of smoking. The oral or intrinsic clearance of propranolol fell significantly with age only in smokers, suggesting that smoking increased the ability to eliminate propranolol only in the young, the elderly being relatively resistant to this effect. Liver blood flow, on the other hand, fell significantly with age in both smokers and nonsmokers, and there appeared to be no effect of smoking on the age-related fall in liver blood flow. These changes resulted in a significant age-related fall in the systemic or intravenous clearance of propranolol in smokers alone.

The effects of age on the kinetics of nadolol and atenolol which are excreted largely by the kidneys can be predicted as their rate of excretion is known to be closely correlated with creatinine clearance, which falls with advancing age. Their stead-state levels will be higher in the elderly, due to their poor renal function. The plasma levels of metoprolol also tend to be higher in the elderly.

From this discussion, it is clear that a number of variables affect blood levels of β-blockers. As many of the effects of β-blockers have a clear relationship to drug concentration in the blood and, hence, at the β-adrenergic receptor site, changes in drug concentration will alter the intensity of the drug's effect.

Adverse Effects of β-Blockade

Most of the adverse effects of β-blockers are due to β-blockade and, therefore, are predictable from a knowledge of their pharmacological effects. The most dramatic effects usually occur following the first dose when β-blockade quickly demonstrates the patient's dependence on adrenergic stimulation. Further doses only produce relatively modest increases in the degree of β-blockade. For that reason, patients thought to be particularly at risk should be given a small starting dose and observed carefully.

Bronchospasm. Blockade of β_2-receptors in the bronchi can precipitate bronchospasm in patients with asthma or obstructive airway disease. This can also occur with relative β_1-selective drugs; however, higher concentrations are usually required before β_2-blockade and bronchospasm are produced.

Cardiac Failure. the administration of β-blockers to patients with impaired cardiac reserve may precipitate cardiac failure. Although the negative inotropic actions of some of the drugs may be responsible in some cases, it is likely that most cases of β-blocker-precipitated cardiac failure are due to reversal of the increased sympathetic drive to the heart which the patient requires to maintain adequate cardiac output. In such cases, reversal of this increased sympathetic drive will be produced equally effectively by all β-blockers, irrespective of their selectivity or intrinsic sympathetic activity.

Peripheral Vascular Disease and Raynaud's Phenomena. These may be caused by β_2-receptor blockade in the vasculature. The relatively selective β-blockers would be the preferred agents in such patients, if indeed β-blockade is justified at all.

Diabetes. In diabetics, β-blockers can mask the usual warning signs of hypoglycemia which are adrenergically mediated. Increased sweating is a characteristic symptom of hypoglycemia. Though the sweat glands are innervated by the sympathetic nervous system, the neurotransmitter is acetylcholine, not norepinephrine. It is therefore not surprising that β-blockade does not reduce and may increase the degree of sweating in response to hypoglycemia. In addition to masking the symptoms of hypoglycemia, the nonselective β-blockers may worsen the physiological effects of hypoglycemia by increasing the rise in blood pressure, prolonging the period of hypoglycemia, and increasing the bradycardia. Selective β_1-blockers such as metoprolol seem to produce less marked changes.

Bradycardia. This is a pharmacological manifestation of β-blockade which should only be considered an adverse effect when accompanied by signs of inadequate cardiac output. Bradycardia per se is almost never an indication for stopping or reducing the dose of β-blocker if cardiac output is maintained.

β-Blocker Withdrawal Syndrome. There have been a number of case reports describing the development of ventricular arrhythmias, severe angina, myocardial infarction, and even death soon after sudden cessation of propranolol therapy. It was at first thought that this might occur because of the progression of the underlying cardiovascular disease during the period the patient had received β-blockade and that uncovering of this progression by withdrawal of propranolol gave rise to the exacerbation of symptoms. However, this observation cannot be the total explanation as the withdrawal syndrome has been observed in patients crossed over from propranolol to placebo during 5- to 6-week-long clinical trials.

Many of the symptoms, such as tremulousness and tachycardia, suggest a hyperadrenergic state, perhaps due to rebound increase in sensitivity to circulating catecholamines. A hypersensitivity to isoproterenol has been shown by some in the period following propranolol therapy. However, others, using epinephrine, have failed to confirm this.

The suggestion has been made that the withdrawal syndrome could be due to the propranolol-induced increase in β-receptor number persisting after the propranolol had been eliminated (Fig. 14.11). Others have suggested that the withdrawal syndrome might be due to increased levels of the active thyroid hormone triiodothyronine.

Indications for β-Blockade

HYPERTENSION

There is now considerable experience with the use of β-blockers in hypertensive patients, but despite this, their mechanism of action remains unclear. Although the acute (intravenous) administration of propranolol produces an immediate fall in cardiac output and rate,

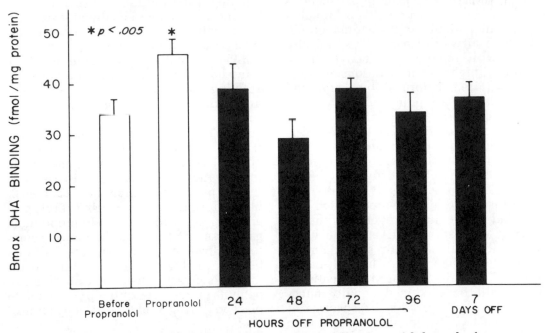

Figure 14.11. *β*-**Receptors on human lymphocytes following withdrawal of propranolol.** Although receptor density increases significantly during propranolol therapy, it is not significantly above baseline 24 hours after propranolol is stopped. (With permission from Fraser J, Nadeau J, Robertson D, Wood AJJ: Regulation of human leukocyte beta receptors by endogenous catecholamines. *J Clin Invest* 67:1777–1784, 1981.)

blood pressure does not fall until later because of an initial reflex rise in total peripheral resistance, which gradually wanes to produce a sustained fall in blood pressure.

A number of theories have been proposed to explain the hypotensive effect of *β*-blockers. It was initially suggested that the chronic reduction in cardiac output produced by long-term oral therapy resulted in resetting of the baroreceptors with a fall in blood pressure. A central hypotensive action and suppression of renin secretion have also been proposed as other possible mechanisms of action. It is likely that some of the confusion which still surrounds this area has resulted from the variation in dosage between studies and also because hypertension is multifactorial in its etiology.

The role of renin suppression in the hypotensive action of *β*-blockers which was first suggested by Buhler *et al.* has been

clarified by Hollifield and his colleagues, who showed that propranolol in low dosage (160 mg/day) lowered renin levels and blood pressure of hypertensives with high and normal renin levels, but did not affect the blood pressure of the low-renin group. However, increasing the dose of propranolol, to as much as 960 mg/day in some patients, produced a fall in blood pressure even in the low-renin group and a further fall in blood pressure in the high-renin group without further reduction in renin levels. They, therefore, postulated that the hypotensive effect of propranolol in low doses is associated with suppression of renin secretion in hypertensives with high and normal renin levels, while higher doses of propranolol lower blood pressure by a renin-independent mechanism. Others have proposed a central site for the hypotensive action of propranolol. It has been shown that propranolol exerts a hypotensive effect when injected into the cerebral ventricular system of the conscious cat. This effect does not occur with the D-isomer, which has no hypotensive effect, and it can be antagonized by isoprenaline similarly administered.

A reasonable plan for treating hypertension is to start the patient on a diuretic or β-blocker and then, if control remains unsatisfactory, to add the other. A vasodilator such as hydralazine can then be added if required. The combination of hydralazine and β-blocker has been shown to be more effective than β-blocker alone and to be adequate therapy for the control of severe hypertension. The combined use of a β-blocker and a vasodilator is particularly attractive because the β-blocker prevents the reflex increase in heart rate and cardiac output which would otherwise follow vasodilation.

CORONARY ARTERY DISEASE

Angina Pectoris. It was for the treatment of angina that β-blockers were originally developed, and their efficacy has now been shown in many clinical studies.

Angina pectoris is produced by an episode of exercise or emotional stress which increases the oxygen requirements of the left ventricle beyond the capacity of the diseased coronary arteries. β-Blockade produces a dose-dependent reduction in heart rate and the arterial pressure response to exercise. This is thought to reduce the oxygen requirements of the left ventricle and so prevent angina. Although it was suggested that the membrane-stabilizing action of propranolol might account for its antianginal effect, this has not been borne out experimentally because D-propranolol has the same membrane-stabilizing effect as the therapeutically active racemic mixture but has no antianginal activity, and other β-blockers which lack membrane-stabilizing ability are potent antianginal agents.

The other mainstay of antianginal therapy is the use of nitrates, such as nitroglycerin. It is likely that their principal beneficial effect is due to peripheral vasodilation and reduction in afterload.

However, this will result in a reflex increase in cardiac output and cardiac rate. These reflex changes which may increase left ventricular oxygen demands can be prevented by β-blockade so that the two drugs in combination provide complementary antianginal therapy.

Myocardial Infarction. The use of β-blockade in the acute and chronic treatment of patients with myocardial infarction is now established. It was initially suggested from studies using practolol (which was subsequently withdrawn because of adverse effects) and alprenolol that the number of cardiac deaths might be reduced after myocardial infarction by long-term β-blockade. This has been confirmed in a large study in which timolol or placebo was administered to patients after a myocardial infarct. The death rate was reduced by 45% in the timolol-treated group. Similar results have been obtained with propranolol. The reason for this beneficial effect of β-blockade following myocardial infarction is unknown but may be due to reduction in the incidence of life-threatening arrhythmias resulting in "sudden death." There is also evidence that β-blockers administered intravenously immediately following myocardial infarction can decrease infarct size and can even prevent some patients from progressing to actual infarction, perhaps by reducing myocardial oxygen demand.

β-Blockers with intrinsic sympathomimetic activity should not be used post myocardial infarction as they appear not to offer the protection of other β-blockers and, in fact, may increase mortality.

ARRHYTHMIAS (SEE CHAPTER 16)

At β-blocking concentrations, β-blockers reduce sinus rate, ectopic focal activity, and conduction velocity across the A-V node. All of these properties are useful in treating arrhythmias.

Sinus Tachycardia. It is important to determine the underlying cause for this condition before embarking on therapy. For example, reduction of the sympathetically induced tachycardia in patients with incipient cardiac failure will precipitate overt cardiac failure. On the other hand, β-blockade can usefully be employed to reduce the heart rate in thyrotoxicosis without affecting the underlying thyroid status of the patient. In treating patients whose sinus tachycardia is associated with an anxiety state, β-blockade may be useful not as an anxiolytic agent but purely to interrupt the sequence of events whereby the tachycardia is contributing to the maintenance of anxiety.

Paroxysmal Atrial Arrhythmias. Because β-blockers depress A-V conducting tissue including reentry pathways, they are very effective in both the prophylaxis and treatment of supraventricular arrhythmias. Many cases of supraventricular tachycardia will revert to sinus rhythm after β-blockade. Paroxysmal atrial tachycardia, including that associated with the Wolff-Parkinson-White syndrome, can be prevented by long-term β-blockade.

Atrial Fibrillation. Digitalis remains the drug of choice in slowing the ventricular response in atrial fibrillation. However, β-blockers also depress A-V conduction and, although sinus rhythm is seldom restored, the ventricular rate may be reduced. The place of β-blockade in the treatment of atrial fibrillation is probably as an adjunct to digoxin therapy. For example, if a satisfactory reduction in ventricular rate has not been obtained with digoxin and the dosage cannot be increased due to toxicity, the synergistic effect of β-blockade on the A-V conducting tissue can be used to further slow the ventricular rate.

Digitalis-induced Arrythmias. Although not necessarily the treatment of first choice in such cases, β-blockade has been shown to be effective in nearly all types of digitalis-induced arrhythmias. However, for the reasons outlined previously, the A-V block often seen in these arrhythmias may be worsened by β-blockade. Because of its anticholinergic activity, phenytoin facilitates A-V conduction and remains the drug of choice in this situation.

Ventricular Arrhythmias. The ability of propranolol to control ventricular arrhythmias in pheochromocytoma and during anesthesia results from its antagonism of circulating catecholamines (see Chapter 20). In addition, however, the drug may be very effective in controlling premature ventricular beats of other causes and is worthy of therapeutic trial in such patients.

Hypertrophic Obstruction Cardiomyopathy. It has been shown that positive inotropic agents worsen the functional obstruction of ventricular outflow in this condition. There is also evidence of increased levels of catecholamines in cardiac muscle from such patients. It was natural, therefore, that propranolol would be tried in therapy, and it has been found helpful in some patients, particularly those with a high resting and exercise heart rate but without evidence of fluid retention. It has also been used to treat the cyanotic attacks associated with Fallot's tetralogy.

DISSECTING ANEURYSM OF THE AORTA

The aim of therapy for this condition is to reduce blood pressure, cardiac impulse, and first derivative of maximal aortic pressure (dp/dt). Nitroprusside, which must be given intravenously, effectively lowers blood pressure, but can produce undesirable reflex sympathetic changes which are effectively blocked by propranolol. This combination has been successfully used in treating dissecting aneurysms.

GLAUCOMA

β-Blockers lower intraocular pressure in open angle glaucoma. Because of its lack of local anesthetic effects (membrane-stabilizing properties), timolol is used topically to lower intraocular pressure.

THYROID DISEASE

β-Blockade produces symptomatic relief in thyrotoxic patients and has been used to prepare such patients for surgery (see Chapter 20).

CARDIAC SURGERY

The safety of continuing β-blocker administration in patients undergoing cardiac surgery is now established. A double blind randomized study comparing propranolol to placebo showed that, when β-blockade was begun at least 24 to 48 hours prior to surgery and continued both during surgery and postoperatively, myocardial oxygen demand and the incidence of postoperative hypertension were significantly reduced in the propranolol-treated group. In addition, the incidence of arrhythmias was significantly lower in the propranolol-treated group (Fig. 14.12)

ESMOLOL

Esmolol is a β_1-selective β-blocker which differs from other available agents by being metabolized by blood esterases so that its half-life is extremely short (9 minutes), giving it an equally short duration of action. Because of its pharmacokinetic properties, it is only available for intravenous use when it can rapidly achieve therapeutic concentrations with rapid decline of plasma concentrations

and reversal of effect when the infusion is stopped (Fig. 14.13).

PHARMACOKINETICS

The pharmacokinetic properties of esmolol are outlined in Table 14.3. The principal feature that distinguishes esmolol from the other β-blockers is its extremely short elimination half-life of 9 minutes (Fig. 14.14). The structure of esmolol is shown in Figure 14.15. The ester linkage is rapidly hydrolyzed to yield methanol and an inactive metabolite which lacks pharmacological activity but has a relatively long elimination half-life of 3.7 hours. The esterase responsible for esmolol hydrolysis in humans is situated in the cytosol of red cells and is different from both acetyl cholinesterase and plasma cholinesterase (see Chapter 5). Because of its extensive metabolism in the blood itself, esmolol has a very high clearance of 17.1 L/kg/hour which far exceeds cardiac output, demonstrating that metabolism must be extrahepatic.

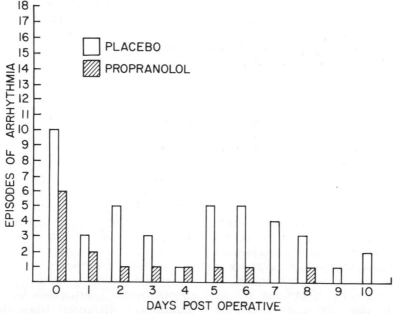

Figure 14.12. Effect of propranolol on postoperative arrhythmias. Propranolol reduces the frequency of arrhythmias in patients undergoing coronary artery bypass grafting compared to placebo. (With permission from Hammon JW, Wood AJJ, Prager RL, Wood M, Muirhead J, Bender HW: Perioperative beta blockade with propranolol: reduction in myocardial oxygen demands and the incidence of atrial and ventricular arrhythmias. *Ann Thoracic Surg* 38:363–367, 1984.)

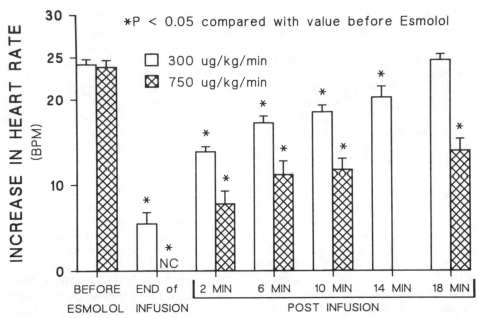

Figure 14.13.   Rapid reversal of β-blockade following discontinuation of esmolol infusion.   The dose of isoproterenol which had produced an approximately 25 beat/min, rise in heart rate prior to esmolol was readministered on multiple occasions after infusion of 300 or 750 μg/kg/min of esmolol was stopped. During the 750-μg/kg/min infusion, this dose of isoproterenol failed to produce any response and produced only a minimal response during the 300-μg/kg/min infusion. However, full recovery occurred within 18 minutes following 300 μg/kg/min, and more than 50% recovery had occurred by 18 minutes following the higher dose. (With permission from Reilly CS, Wood M, Koshakji RP, Wood AJJ: Ultra short acting beta-blockade: a comparison with conventional beta blockade. *Clin Pharmacol Ther* 38:579–585, 1985.)

Plasma cholinesterase activity is unaltered in the plasma of patients who received an esmolol infusion of 500 mg/kg/min for 4 minutes.

SUGGESTED DOSAGE AND ADMINISTRATION

Esmolol is only available for intravenous use when its short half-life makes it an attractive choice for the management of acute therapy. Its effects are similar to those of other β_1-adrenergic blockers. It has been shown to be effective in reducing the ventricular rate in patients with supraventricular tachyarrhythmias. The principal dose-limiting side effect from esmolol has been the development of hypotension. The mechanism for the hypotensive action of esmolol is not clear.

However, the combination of β-blockade and blood pressure reduction produced by esmolol has proven useful in the perioperative period. Esmolol may be a useful agent in the perioperative management of hypertension and tachycardia. Stressful surgical stimuli, such as laryngoscopy and endotracheal intubation, surgical incision, and emergence elicit adrenergic responses which may result in short-lived but large increases in heart rate and blood pressure. Esmolol has been shown to attenuate but not always completely eliminate the cardiovascular response to endotracheal intubation and other stressful incidents, such as sternotomy, during cardiac surgery (Fig. 14.16). Although other β-blockers also have this effect, the hemodynamic effects of es-

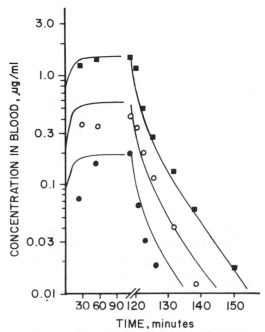

Figure 14.14. Pharmacokinetics of esmolol. Esmolol concentrations during and after a 120-min infusion of 50, 150, and 400 μg/kg/min of esmolol. Note the rapid decline in esmolol concentrations after discontinuation of esmolol infusion. (With permission from Sum CY, Yacobi A, Kartzinel R, Stampfli H, Davis CS, Lai CM: Kinetics of esmolol, an ultra-short-acting beta blocker, and of its major metabolite. *Clin Pharmacol Ther* 34:427–434, 1983.)

molol dissipate rapidly after the infusion and, thus, do not persist after the therapeutic effect is no longer required.

Esmolol has been used to control postoperative hypertension, for example, following coronary artery bypass. In addition to its use as a single agent for blood pressure reduction either intra- or postoperatively, esmolol can also be used to increase the effects of vasodilators such as nitroprusside. By blocking the sympathetic response that occurs during vasodilator therapy (see Fig. 15.5, page 445), the compensatory increase in heart rate and cardiac output is decreased and, hence, the hypotensive effect is increased, allowing a lower dose of nitroprusside to be used.

Esmolol may also be useful in providing rapidly reversible β-blockade for patients in the hemodynamically unstable period following a myocardial infarction.

The recommended dose of esmolol intravenously ranges from 100 to 300 μg/kg/min. Although a loading dose has usually preceded the continuous infusion, in many settings it may be simpler just to administer the continuous infusion as steady state will be reached very rapidly. To minimize the risk of irritation at the injection site, the infusion concentration should not exceed 10 mg/ml. In large patients at the higher dosage levels,

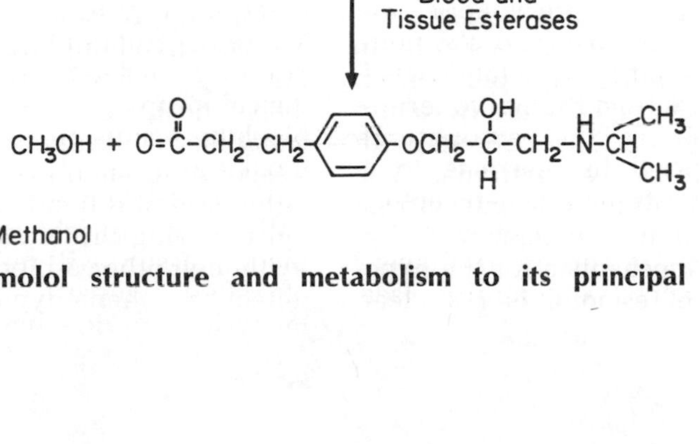

$$H_3C-O-\overset{\overset{O}{\|}}{C}-CH_2-CH_2-\underset{}{\bigcirc}-O-CH_2-\overset{\overset{OH}{|}}{\underset{\underset{H}{|}}{C}}-CH_2-\overset{H}{\underset{}{N}}-CH\overset{CH_3}{\underset{CH_3}{}}$$

ESMOLOL

↓ Blood and Tissue Esterases

$$CH_3OH + O=\overset{\overset{O}{\|}}{C}-CH_2-CH_2-\underset{}{\bigcirc}-OCH_2-\overset{\overset{OH}{|}}{\underset{\underset{H}{|}}{C}}-CH_2-\overset{H}{\underset{}{N}}-CH\overset{CH_3}{\underset{CH_3}{}}$$

Methanol

Figure 14.15. Esmolol structure and metabolism to its principal metabolite and methanol.

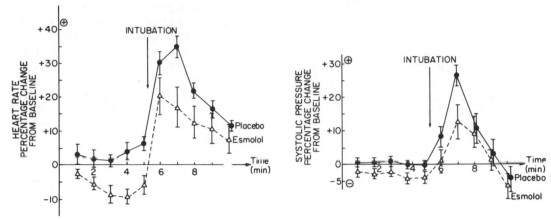

Figure 14.16. Effects of esmolol on the stress of intubation.   The rise in heart rate and blood pressure was attenuated but not completely blocked by the administration of esmolol. (Modified from Liu PL, Gatt S, Gugino LD, Mallamptai SR, Covino BG: Esmolol for control of increase in heart rate and blood pressure during tracheal intubation after thiopentone and succinylcholine. *Can Anaesth Soc J* 33:556–562, 1986.)

the total volume of fluid administered during an esmolol infusion may be substantial, and care should be taken to avoid fluid overload.

α-ADRENERGIC BLOCKING AGENTS

α-Adrenergic blocking agents bind preferentially to α-adrenergic receptors and, hence, antagonize the effects of sympathomimetics at these sites. The effects of stimulating α-receptors were reviewed in the preceding chapter. It is now recognized that α-adrenoceptors, like β-receptors, can be subdivided into two classes (see Chapter 15): α_1-*receptors*, which are postsynaptic and are found mainly on smooth muscle and glands; and α_2-*receptors*, which in the periphery are presynaptic and exist on nerve terminals.

Stimulation of the presynaptic α_2-receptors inhibits the release of the neurotransmitter norepinephrine (and possibly, acetylcholine) from the nerve terminal, thus reducing the amount of transmitter released in response to a nerve impulse. Postsynaptic α_2-receptors in the brain may have importance in mediating the effects of certain antihypertensive agents such as clonidine (see Chapter 15.)

Pharmacological Effects of α-Adrenergic Receptor Blockers

Phentolamine, phenoxybenzamine, prazosin, and terazosin all antagonize the effects of sympathomimetics at α-receptors. However, there are important differences in their actions. Phenoxybenzamine binds covalently to the α-receptor, resulting in a noncompetitive and irreversible blockade (see Chapter 3). Phentolamine and prazosin, on the other hand, bind competitively and reversibly to the α-receptors. These drugs also differ in their relative potencies at α_1-and α_2-receptors. Phenoxybenzamine is a more potent blocker of α_1- than α_2-receptors (100-fold). Phentolamine is much less selective, being only 3 to 5 times more potent at α_1-receptors. Prazosin, on the other hand, is a highly selective α_1 antagonist having little α_2-blocking effects. These differences have considerable importance in determining the pharmacological properties of the individual α-blocking agents. All of these agents by blocking α_1-receptors will cause vasodilation and lower blood pressure, principally in the upright posture. This fall in blood pressure will result in some degree of reflex sympathetic stimulation and tachycardia. However, phenoxybenzamine and, to an even greater extent, phentolamine block presynaptic α_2-receptors and, hence, increase the norepinephrine produced from the adrenergic nerve ending in response to sympathetic stimulation, so that marked tachycardia can result. This is most obvious with phentolamine, the least α_1-selective and least apparent with the highly selective α_1-antagonist, prazosin.

Phenoxybenzamine

Phenoxybenzamine irreversibly blocks α-receptors by covalently binding to them. It is probably a highly reactive metabolite of phenoxybenzamine and not the drug itself which actually binds to the receptors, resulting in a relatively slow onset of action, reflecting the time taken for the production of the metabolite. Its effects are predictable from a knowledge of its pharmacology. By antagonizing the α-adrenergic effects of norepinephrine and epinephrine, it lowers blood pressure. However, in the supine patient, sympathetic tone is relatively low, so that α-blockade produces little, if any, fall in blood pressure, but when sympathetic tone is increased in order to maintain blood pressure, such as is seen following hemorrhage, hypovolemia, or assumption of the upright posture, α-blockade will produce profound blood pressure falls. The effect of α-blockers is also enhanced by anesthetic agents and strong analgesics, such as morphine and meperidine. Phenoxybenzamine is poorly absorbed following oral administration (20 to 30%). Its effects pass off slowly with a half-life of 24 hours. Thus, it takes some days to accumulate to steady state unless a loading dose is used.

INDICATIONS

The principal indications for phenoxybenzamine are the preoperative preparation of patients with pheochromocytoma or in the long-term management of inoperable malignant pheochromocytoma (see Chapter 20). Because of the excess vasoconstrictor tone in such patients, their intravascular volume is contracted. Preoperative α-blockade allows expansion of the intravascular volume and, hence, reduces the hypotension that otherwise would follow tumor removal and relief from the excess vasoconstrictor tone that had been produced by catecholamine excess. In addition, α-blockade reduces the pheochromocytoma-associated hypertension.

DOSAGE

It is usual to start phenoxybenzamine in patients with pheochromocytoma at a dose of 10 mg/day and to increase this gradually until evidence of mild postural hypotension develops. Most patients require between 40 and 60 mg/day. Accumulation will occur because of the long half-life of effect (24 hours), and this should be taken into account when altering the dose.

Phentolamine

In addition to its activity as an α-blocker where it is less selective for the α_1-receptor than is phenoxybenzamine, phentolamine has actions at acetylcholine and histamine receptors so that it is difficult to be certain which of phentolamine's pharmacological actions is responsible for an observed effect.

Phentolamine used to be adminstered intravenously as a diagnostic test for pheochromocytoma, a drop of 35/25 mm Hg in the blood pressure following a dose of 5 mg intravenously being interpreted as highly suggestive of the presence of a pheochromocytoma. However, this test is seldom used today because of both the ready availability of chemical tests for pheochromocytoma and the severe cardiovascular collapse and death that have followed phentolamine tests.

Phentolamine may be administered intravenously during surgical removal of a pheochromocytoma to control hypertension; 0.5 mg should be administered as an intravenous bolus and the effects observed prior to further administration. Double the dose can be administered 3 minutes later until the blood pressure is controlled.

Prazosin is discussed in detail in Chapter 15.

Labetalol

Labetalol is a nonselective β-blocker which also possesses α_1-adrenergic blocking activity. It is less potent at β-receptors than propranolol and less potent at α_1-receptors than the selective α_1-receptor blocker prazosin (Table 14.4). As the labetalol molecule contains two optical centers, if forms four optical isomers, RR, SS, RS, and SR), and the commercial preparation contains equal amounts of all four isomers. These isomers differ in both their pharmacokinetic and pharmacodynamic properties. The RR isomer has greater β-blocking activity and less α-blocking effects than total labetalol and also produces direct vasodilation which may be due to partial agonist activity at vascular β_2-receptors. Thus, the effects at α-receptors differ substantially between the isomers, the SR isomer being the most potent and the RR isomer the least potent α-blocker, while at β-receptors, the reverse is true with the RR isomer being the most potent and the SR isomer the least potent β-antagonist.

PHARMACOKINETICS

Labetalol, like propranolol, is highly metabolized in the liver with very little (less than 5%) of the drug being excreted unchanged (Table 14.3). The rapid removal of labetalol (first-pass metabolism)

Table 14.4.
Dose Required to Produce 50% Inhibition of α_1- and β-Adrenergic Receptor Stimulation (ID_{50})

	ID_{50} (μg/kg)*	
	α_1	β
Propranolol	>3000	20
Labetalol	1000	200
Prazosin	2.6	>1000

(With permission from Louis WJ, McNeil JJ, Drummer OH: Pharmacology of combined α, β-blockade. *Drugs* 28 (Suppl 2):16–34, 1984.
*The higher the ID_{50}, the less potent the drug. Thus, propranolol was more potent as a β-blocker than labetalol, while prazosin was considerably more potent than labetalol at α_1-receptors in pithed rats.

results in only 30 to 40% of an oral dose entering the systemic circulation. The principal pathway of metabolism is by conjugation to the inactive glucuronide in contrast to many of the other lipid-soluble β-blockers whose principal route of metablism is by oxidation. The pharmacokinetic properties of labetalol are outlined in Table 14.3. Labetalol has been used in the management of pregnancy-induced hypertension, and there have been a number of studies describing the pharmacokinetics of labetalol in pregnancy which suggest that labetalol pharmacokinetics in pregnancy does not differ significantly from that in nonpregnant patients. The concentration in both cord blood at delivery and breast milk appears to be substantially lower than that in the mother's plasma.

In patients with liver disease, the first-pass hepatic extraction of labetalol is substantially reduced so that plasma labetalol concentrations following the usual dose are higher in patients with cirrhosis. Renal disease does not alter the pharmacokinetics of labetalol, reflecting the minimal amount which is excreted unchanged (Table 14.3).

SUGGESTED DOSAGE AND ADMINISTRATION

Oral labetalol is used in the chronic management of hypertension in doses of 100 to 400 mg twice per day when it is effective either as sole therapy or when combined with a diuretic. It causes postural hypotension more frequently than the pure β-blockers, presumably due to its α-blocking activity. However, labetalol is also a β-blocker and therefore produces the classic adverse effects of a nonselective β-blocker.

Intravenous labetalol has been used in the management of severe hypertension, postoperative hypertension, and to induce hypotension during anesthesia. It is best given as either multiple bolus injections or as a continuous infusion (Fig. 14.17). When given by bolus injections, 20 to 40 mg should be given i.v. every 10 to 15 minutes up to a total dose of 300 mg or until the blood pressure has fallen to a satisfactory level. Labetalol has also been

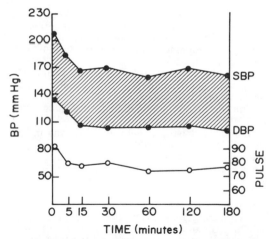

Figure 14.17.   Effect of labetalol on blood pressure and heart rate.   Twenty mg of labetalol were given intravenously followed by 40- to 80-mg intravenous injections at 10-minute intervals until the blood pressure was reduced by 30 mm Hg. (With permission from Cressman MD, Vidt DG, Gifford   RW,   Moore   WS,   Wilson   DJ: Intravenous labetalol in the management of severe hypertension and hypertensive emergencies. *Am Heart J* 107:980–985, 1984.)

administered as a continuous infusion, when 2 mg/min up to a total dose of 150 mg have been given. The use of either the multiple bolus technique or the continuous infusion appears to be safer than the use of a single large injection. In contrast to other acute therapy for hypertension such as nitroprusside, the fall in blood pressure produced by labetalol is not accompanied by tachycardia but, rather, a small reduction in heart rate may occur (Fig. 14.17). Cardiac output may also fall slightly during acute blood pressure reduction by labetalol; however, the fall in cardiac output appears less than that associated with β-blockers such as propranolol, which lack the α-blocking properties of labetalol.

Labetalol has been used to manage postoperative hypertension, when lower starting doses of 5 to 10 mg should be administered intravenously and the dosage cautiously increased and titrated to clinical effect. Similarly, dose titration beginning with doses of 5 to 10 mg is recom-

mended to induce hypotension during inhalational anesthesia.

The hypotensive effect of intravenous labetalol is long lasting and persists for 12 hours or more. Because of its α-blocking effects, upright blood pressure falls more than supine, and when used to lower blood pressure acutely, the hypotensive effect of labetalol can be magnified by placing the patient in the head-up position.

A metabolite of labetalol interferes with the fluorimetric assay for catecholamines and gives falsely high measurements for catecholamines.

DILEVALOL is the *RR* isomer of labetalol and is currently undergoing study for intravenous use in hypertension.

BIBLIOGRAPHY

General

Ahlquist RP: Study of the adrenotropic receptors. *Am J Physiol* 153:586–600, 1948.

Coltart DJ, Shand DG: Plasma propranolol levels in the quantitative assessment of beta adrenergic blockade in man. *Br Med J* 3:731–734, 1970.

Prichard BNC: Beta-adrenergic receptor blockade in hypertension, past, present, and future. *Br J Clin Pharmacol* 5:379–399, 1978.

Singh BN, Jewitt DE: Beta-adrenergic receptor blocking drugs in cardiac arrhythmias. *Drugs* 7:426–461, 1974.

Thandani U, Davidson C, Singleton W, Taylor SH: Comparison of the immediate effects of five beta-adrenoreceptor blocking drugs with different ancillary properties in angina pectoris. *N Engl J Med* 300:750–755, 1979.

Vestal RE, Wood AJJ, Shand DG: Reduced beta-adrenoceptor sensitivity in the elderly. *Clin Pharmacol Ther* 26:181–186, 1979.

Zonszein J, Santangelo RP, Mackin JF, Lee TC, Coffey RJ, Canary JJ: Propranolol therapy in thyrotoxicosis. *Am J Med* 66:411–416, 1979.

Cardioselectivity

Brodde O-E, O'Hara N, Zerkowski H-R, Rohm N: Human cardiac β-adrenoceptors: both β_1-and β_2-adrenoceptors are functionally coupled to the adenylate cyclase in right atrium. *J Cardiovasc Pharmacol* 6:1184–1191, 1984.

Brown MJ, Brown DC, Murphy MB: Hypokalemia from beta$_2$-receptor stimulation by circulating epinephrine. *N Engl J Med* 309:1414–1419, 1983.

Cruickshank JM: The clinical importance of cardiovascular and liphophilicity in beta blockers. *Am Heart J* 100:160–178, 1980.

Decalmer PBS, Chatterjee SS, Cruickshank JM, Benson MK, Sterling GM: Beta-blockers and asthma. *Br Heart J* 40:184–189, 1978.

Hiatt WR, Wolfel EE, Stoll S, Nies AS, Zerbe GO, Brammell HL, Horwitz LD: Beta-2 adrenergic blockade evaluated with epinephrine after placebo, atenolol, and nadolol. *Clin Pharmacol Ther* 37:2–6, 1985.

Lands AM, Luduena FP, Buzzo HJ: Differentiation of receptors responsive to isoproterenol. *Life Sci* 6:2241–2249, 1967.

Leenen FHH, Coenen CHM, Zonderland M, Maas AHJ: Effects of cardioselective and nonselective beta-blockade on dynamic exercise performance in mildly hypertensive men. *Clin Pharmacol Ther* 28:12–21, 1980.

Pringle TH, Riddell JG, Shanks RG: A comparison of the cardioselectivity of five β-adrenoceptor blocking drugs. *J Cardiovasc Pharmacol* 10:228–237, 1987.

Struthers AD, Whitesmith R, Reid JL: Prior thiazide diuretic treatment increases adrenaline-induced hypokalemia. *Lancet* 1:1358–1360, 1983.

Vincent HH, Boomsma F, Man in't Veld AJ, Derkx FHM, Wenting GJ, Schalekamp MADH: Effects of selective and nonselective β-agonists on plasma potassium and norepinephrine. *J Cardiovasc Pharmacol* 6:107–114, 1984.

Vincent HH, Man in't Veld AJ, Boomsma F, Schalekamp MADH: Prevention of epinephrine-induced hypokalemia by nonselective beta blockers. *Am J Cardiol* 56:10D-14D, 1985.

Beta Blockers in Diabetes

Barnett AH, Leslie D, Watkins RJ: Can insulin-treated diabetics be given beta-adrenergic blocking drugs? *Br Med J* 280:976–978, 1980.

Deacon SP, Karunanayake A, Barnett D: Acebutolol, atenolol, and propranolol and metabolic responses to acute hypoglycaemia in diabetics. *Br Med J* 2:1255–1257, 1977.

Lager I, Blohme G, Smith U: Effect of cardioselective and non-selective beta-blockade on the hypoglycaemic response in insulin-dependent diabetics. *Lancet* 1:458–462, 1979.

Molnar GW, Read RC: Propranolol enhancement of hypoglycemic sweating. *Clin Pharmacol Ther* 15:490–496, 1974.

Woods KL, Wright AD, Kendall MJ, Black E: Lack of effect of propranolol and metoprolol on glucose tolerance in maturity onset diabetics. *Br Med J* 281:1321, 1980.

Beta Blockers: Anesthesia and Surgery

Chung DC: Anaesthetic problems associated with the treatment of cardiovascular disease. II. Beta-adrenergic antagonists. *Can Anaesth Soc J* 28:105–113, 1981.

Coltart DJ, Cayen MN, Stinson EB, Goldman RH, Davies RO, Harrison DC: Investigation of the safe withdrawal period for propranolol in patients scheduled for open heart surgery. *Br Heart J* 37:1228–1234, 1975.

Faulkner SL, Hopkins JT, Boerth RC, Young JL, Jellett LB, Nies AS, Bender HW, Shand DG: Time required for complete recovery from chronic propranolol therapy. *N Engl J Med* 289:607–609, 1973.

Hammon JW, Jr, Wood AJJ, Prager RL, Wood M, Muirhead J, Bender HW Jr: Perioperative beta blockade with propranolol: reduction in myocardial oxygen demands and the incidence of atrial and ventricular arrhythmias. *Ann Thorac Surg* 38:363–367, 1984.

Horan BF, Prys-Roberts C, Hamilton WK, Roberts JG: Haemodynamic responses to enflurane anaesthesia and hypovolaemia in the dog, and their modification by propranolol. *Br J Anaesth* 49:1189–1197, 1977.

Horan BF, Prys-Roberts C, Roberts JG, Bennet MJ, Foex P: Haemodynamic responses to isoflurane anaesthesia and hypovolaemia in the dog, and their modification by propranolol. *Br J Anaesth* 49:1179–1187, 1977.

Hunter JM: Synergism between halothane and labetalol. *Anaesthesia* 34:257–259, 1979.

Kaplan JA, Dunbar RW, Bland JW, Sumpter R, Jones EL: Propranolol and cardiac surgery: a problem for the anesthesiologist? *Anesth Analg* 54.571– 578, 1975.

Kopriva CJ, Brown ACD, Pappas G: Hemodynamics during general anesthesia in patients receiving propranolol. *Anesthesiology* 48:28–33, 1978.

Kopriva CJ, Guinazu A, Barash PG: Massive propranolol therapy and uncomplicated cardiac surgery. *JAMA* 239:1157, 1978.

Magnusson J, Thulin T, Werner O, Jarhult J, Thomson D: Haemodynamic effects of pretreatment with metoprolol in hypertensive patients undergoing surgery. *Br J Anaesth* 58:251–260, 1986.

McAllister RG, Bourne DW, Tan TG, Erickson JL, Wachtel CC, Todd EP: Effects of hypothermia on propranolol kinetics. *Clin Pharmacol Ther* 25:1–7, 1979.

McCammon RL, Hilgenberg JC, Stoelting RK: Effect of propranolol on circulatory responses to induction of diazepam-nitrous oxide anesthesia and to endotracheal intubation. *Anesth Analg* 60:579–583, 1981.

Moran JM, Mulet J, Caralps JM, Pifarre R: Coronary revascularization in patients receiving propranolol. *Circulation* 50 (Suppl 2):II-116–II-121, 1974.

Oka Y, Frishman W, Becker RM, Kadish A, Strom J, Matsumoto M, Orkin L, Frater R: Clinical pharmacology of the new beta-adrenergic blocking drugs. Part 10. Beta-adrenoceptor blockade and coronary artery surgery. *Am Heart J* 99:255–269, 1980.

Prys-Roberts C, Foex P, Biro GP, Roberts JG: Studies of anaesthesia in relation to hypertension. V. Adrenergic beta-receptor blockade. *Br J Anaesth* 45:671–680, 1973.

Roberts JG: Beta-adrenergic blockade and anaesthesia with reference to interactions with anaesthetic drugs and techniques. *Anaesth Intensive Care* 8:318–335, 1980.

Roberts JG, Foex P, Clarke TNS, Bennett MJ: Haemodynamic interactions of high-dose propranolol pretreatment and anesthesia in the dog. I. Halothane dose-response studies. *Br J Anaesth* 48:315–325, 1976.

Roberts JG, Foex P, Clarke TNS, Bennett MJ, Saner CA: Haemodynamic interactions of high-dose propranolol pretreatment and anaesthesia in the dog. III. The effects of haemorrhage during halothane and trichloroethylene anaesthesia. *Br J Anaesth* 48:411–418, 1976.

Roberts JG, Foex P, Clarke TNS, Prys-Roberts C, Bennett MJ: Haemodynamic interactions of high-dose propranolol pretreatment and anaesthesia in the dog. II. The effects of acute arterial hypoxaemia at increasing depths of halothane anaesthesia. *Br J Anaesth* 48:403–410, 1976.

Safwat AM, Reitan JA, Misle GR, Hurley EJ: Use of propranolol to control rate-pressure product during cardic anesthesia. *Anesth Analg* 60:732–735, 1981.

Shand DG, Wood AJJ: Editorial: propranolol withdrawal syndrome—why? *Circulation* 58:202–203, 1978.

Slogoff S, Keats AS, Hibbs CW, Edmonds CH, Bragg DA: Failure of general anesthesia to potentiate propranolol activity. *Anesthesiology* 47:504–508, 1977.

Slogoff S, Keats AS, Ott E: Preoperative propranolol therapy and aortocoronary bypass operation. *JAMA* 240:1487–1490, 1978.

Stanley TH, de Lange S, Boscoe MJ, de Bruijn N: The influence of chronic preoperative propranolol therapy on cardiovascular dynamics and narcotic requirements during operation in patients with coronary artery disease. *Can Anaesth Soc J* 29:319–324, 1982.

Viljoen JF, Estafanous FG, Kellner GA: Propranolol and cardiac surgery. *J Thorac Cardiovasc Surg* 64:826–830, 1972.

White HD, Antamn EM, Glynn MA, Collins JJ, Cohn LH, Shemin RJ, Friedman PL: Efficacy and safety of timolol for prevention of supraventricular tachyarrhythmias after coronary artery bypass surgery. *Circulation* 70:479–484, 1984.

Wood AJJ: β-blocker withdrawal. *Drugs* 25:318–321, 1983.

Wood M, Shand DG, Wood AJJ: Propranolol binding in plasma during cardiopulmonary bypass. *Anesthesiology* 51:512–516, 1979.

Beta Blockers after Myocardial Infarction

β-Blocker Heart Attack Trial Research Group: A randomized trial of propranolol in patients with acute myocardial infarction. I. Mortality results. *JAMA* 247:1707–1714, 1982.

β-Blocker Heart Attack Trial Research Group: A randomized trial of propranolol in patients with acute myocardial infarction. II. Morbidity results. *JAMA* 250:2814–2819, 1983.

Frishman WH, Furberg CD, Friedewald WT: β-Adrenergic blockade for survivors of actue myocardial infarction. *N Engl J Med* 310:830–837, 1984.

Norris RM, Brown MA, Clarke ED, Barnaby PF, Geary GG, Logan RL, Sharpe DN: Prevention of ventricular fibrillation during acute myocardial infarction by intravenous propranolol. *Lancet* 2:883–886, 1984.

Sleight P: Editorial: beta-adrenergic blockade after myocardial infarction. *N Engl J Med* 304:837–838, 1981.

The European Infarction Study Group: European infarction study (EIS): a secondary prevention study with slow release oxprenolol after myocardial infarction: morbidity and mortality. *Eur Heart J* 5:189–202, 1984.

The Norwegian Multicenter Study Group: Timolol-induced reduction in mortality and reinfarction in patients surviving acute myocardial infarction. *N Engl J Med* 304:801–807, 1981.

Pharmacokinetics

Riddell JG, Harron DWG, Shanks RG: Clinical pharmacokinetics of β-adrenoceptor antagonists: an update. *Clin Pharmacol* 12:305–320, 1987.

β-Blocker Withdrawal

Alderman EL, Coltart DJ, Wettach GE, Harrison DC: Coronary artery syndromes after sudden propranolol withdrawal. *Ann Intern Med* 81:625–627, 1974.

Boudoulas H, Lewis RP, Kates RE, Dalamangas G: Hypersensitivity to adrenergic stimulation after propranolol withdrawal in normal subjects. *Ann Intern Med* 87:433–436, 1977.

Fraser J, Nadeau J, Robertson D, Wood AJJ: Regulation of human leukocyte beta receptors by endogenous catecholamines. *J Clin Invest* 67:1777–1784, 1981.

Kristensen BO, Steiness E, Weeke J: Propranolol withdrawal and thyroid hormones in patients with essential hypertension. *J Clin Pharmacol Ther* 23:624–629, 1978.

Lindenfeld JA, Crawford MH, O'Rourke RA, Levine SP, Monteil MM, Horwitz LD: Adrenergic responsiveness after abrupt propranolol withdrawal in normal subjects and in patients with angina pectoris. *Circulation* 62:704–711, 1980.

Miller RR, Olson HG, Amsterdam EA, Mason DT: Propranolol-withdrawal rebound phenomenon. *N Engl J Med* 293:416–418, 1975.

Myers MG, Freeman MR, Juma ZA, Wisenberg G: Propranolol withdrawal in angina pectoris: a prospective study. *Am Heart J* 97:298–302, 1979.

Nattel S, Rangno RE, Loon GV: Mechanism of propranolol withdrawal phenomena. *Circulation* 59:1158–1164, 1979.

Shand DG, Wood AJJ: Editorial: propranolol withdrawal syndrome—why? *Circulation* 58:202–203, 1978.

Acebutalol

Thomas MS, Tattersfield AE: Comparison of beta-adrenoceptor selectivity of acebutolol and its metabolite diacetolol with metoprolol and propranolol in normal man. *Eur J Clin Pharmacol* 29:679–683, 1986.

Atenolol

Heel RC, Brogden RN, Speight TM, Avery GS: Atenolol: a review of its pharmacological properties and therapeutic efficacy in angina pectoris and hypertension. *Drugs* 17:425–460, 1979.

Kirch W, Kohler H, Mutschler E, Schafer M: Pharmacokinetics of atenolol in relation to renal function. *Eur J Clin Pharmacol* 19:65–71, 1981.

Mason WD, Winer N, Kochak G, Cohen I, Bell R: Kinetics and absolute bioavailability of atenolol. *Clin Pharmacol Ther* 25:408–415, 1979.

Waal-Manning HJ: Atenolol and three nonselective β-blockers in hypertension. *Clin Pharmacol Ther* 25:8–18, 1979.

Esmolol

Barabas E, Zsigmond EK, Kirkpatrick AF: The inhibitory effect of esmolol on human plasmacholinesterase. *Can Anaesth Soc J* 33:332–335, 1986.

Benfield P, Sorkin EM: Esmolol: a preliminary review of its pharmacodynamic and pharmacokinetic properties, and therapeutic efficacy. *Drugs* 33:392–412, 1987.

de Bruijn NP, Croughwell N, Reves JG: Hemodynamic effects of esmolol in chronically β-blocked patients undergoing aortocoronary bypass surgery. *Anesth Analg* 66:137–141, 1987.

de Bruijn NP, Reves JG, Croughwell N, Clements F, Drissel DA: Pharmacokinetics of esmolol in anesthetized patients receiving chronic beta blocker therapy. *Anesthesiology* 66:323–326, 1987.

Cucchiara RF, Benefiel DJ, Matteo RS, DeWood M, Albin MS: Evaluation of esmolol in controlling increases in heart rate and blood pressure during endotracheal intubation in patients undergoing carotid endarterectomy. *Anesthesiology* 65:528–531, 1986.

Girard D, Shulman BJ, Thys DM, Mindich BP, MIkula SK, Kaplan JA: The safety and efficacy of esmolol during myocardial revascularization. *Anesthesiology* 65: 157–164, 1986.

Gold MI, Brown M, Coverman S, Herrington C: Heart rate and blood pressure effects of esmolol after ketamine induction and intubation. *Anesthesiology* 64:718–725, 1986.

Harrison L, Ralley FE, Wynands JE, Robbins GR, Sami M, Ripley R, Fullerton HA: The role of an ultra short-acting adrenergic blocker (esmolol) in patients undergoing coronary artery bypass surgery. *Anesthesiology* 66:413–418, 1987.

Liu PL, Gatt S, Gugino LD, Mallampati SR, Covino BG: Esmolol for control of increases in heart rate and blood pressure during tracheal intubation after thiopentone and succinylcholine. *Can Anaesth Soc J* 33:556–562, 1986.

Menkhaus PG, Reves JG, Kissin I, Alvis JM, Govier AV, Samuelson PN, Lell WA, Henling CE, Bradley E: Cardiovascular effects of esmolol in anesthetized humans. *Anesth Analg* 64:327–334, 1985.

Newsome LR, Roth JV, Hug CC, Nagle D: Esmolol attenuates hemodynamic responses during fentanyl-pancuronium anesthesia for aortocoronary bypass surgery. *Anesth Analg* 65:451–456, 1986.

Reilly CS, Wood M, Koshakji RP, Wood AJJ: Ultra-short-acting beta-blockade: a comparison with conventional beta-blockade. *Clin Pharmacol Ther* 38:579–585, 1985.

Reves JG, Flezzani P: Perioperative use of esmolol. *Am J Cardiol* 56:57F–62F, 1985.

Sidi A, Davis RF: Esmolol decreases the adverse effects of acute coronary artery occlusion on myocardial metabolism and regional myocardial blood flow in dogs. *Anesth Analg* 67:124–130, 1988.

Sum CY, Yacobi A, Kartzinel R, Stampfli H, Davis CS, Lai C-M: Kinetics of esmolol, an ultra-short-acting beta blocker, and of its major metabolite. *Clin Pharmacol Ther* 34:427–434, 1983.

Turlapaty P, Laddu A, Murthy VS, Singh B, Lee R: Esmolol: a titratable short-acting intravenous beta blocker for acute critical care settings. *Am Heart J* 114:866–885, 1987.

Labetalol

Baum T, Sybertz EJ: Antihypertensive actions of an isomer of labetalol and other vasodilator-β-adrenoceptor blockers. *Fed Proc* 42:176–181, 1983.

Baum T, Watkins RW, Sybertz EJ, Vemulapalli S, Pula KK, Eynon E, Nelson S, Vliet GV, Glennon J, Moran RM: Antihypertensive and hemodynamic actions of SCH 19927, the R,R-isomer of labetalol. *J Pharmacol Exp Ther* 218:444–452, 1981.

Chauvin M, Deriaz H, Viars P: Continuous i.v. infusion of labetalol for postoperative hypertension. *Br J Anaesth* 59:1250–1256, 1987.

Cope DHP: Use of labetalol during halothane anaesthesia. *Br J Clin Pharmacol* 8:223S–227S, 1979.

Cressman MD, Vidt DG, Gifford RW, Moore WS, Wilson DJ: Intravenous labetalol in the management of severe hypertension and hypertensive emergencies. *Am Heart J* 107:980–985, 1984.

Gustafson C, Ahlgren I, Aronsen K-F, Rosberg B: Haemodynamic effects of labetalol-induced hypotension in the anaesthetized dog. *Br J Anaesth* 53:585–590, 1981.

Halperin JL, Mindich BP, Rothlauf EB, Reder RF, Litwak RS, Kupersmith J: Effect of labetalol on limb haemodynamics in patients following coronary artery bypass graft surgery. *Br J Clin Pharmacol* 21:537–542, 1986.

Kaufman L: Use of labetalol during hypotensive anaesthesia and in the management of phaeochromocytoma. *Br J Clin Pharmcol* 8:229S–232S, 1979.

Lebel M, Langlois S, Belleau LJ, Grose JH: Labetalol infusion in hypertensive emergencies. *Clin Pharmacol Ther* 37:615–618, 1985.

Leslie JB, Kalayjian RW, Sirgo MA, Plachetka JR, Watkins WD: Intravenous labetalol for treatment of postoperative hypertension. *Anesthesiology* 67:413–416, 1987.

Louis WJ, McNeil JJ, Drummer OH: Pharmacology of combined α-β-blockade. I. *Drugs* 28 (Suppl 2):16–34, 1984.

Lund-Johansen P: Pharmacology of combined α-β-blockade. II. Haemodynamic effects of labetalol. *Drugs* 28 (Suppl 2):35–50, 1984.

McNeil JJ, Louis WJ: Clinical pharmacokinetics of labetalol. *Clin Pharmacokinet* 9:157–167, 1984.

Scott DB: The use of labetalol in anaesthesia. *Br J Clin Pharmacol* 13:133S–135S, 1982.

Sybertz EJ, Sabin CS, Pula KK, Vliet GV, Glennon J, Gold EH, Baum T: Alpha and beta adrenoceptor blocking properties of labetalol and its R,R-isomer, SCH 19927. *J Pharmacol Exp Ther* 218:435–443, 1981.

Vlachakis ND, Maronde RF, Maloy JW, Medakovic M, Kassem N: Pharmacodynamics of intravenous labetalol and follow-up therapy with oral labetalol. *Clin Pharmacol Ther* 38:503–508, 1985.

Metoprolol

Abraham TA, Hasan FM, Fenster PE, Marcus FI: Effect of intravenous metoprolol on reversible obstructive airways disease. *Clin Pharmacol Ther* 29:582–587, 1981.

Benfield P, Clissold SP, Brogden RN: Metoprolol: an updated review of its pharmacodynamic and pharmacokinetic properties, and therapeutic efficacy, in hypertension, ischaemic heart disease, and related cardiovascular disorders. *Drugs* 31:376–429, 1986.

Regardh CG, Johnsson G: Clinical pharmacokinetics of metoprolol. *Clin Pharmacokinet* 5:557–569, 1980.

Nadolol

Frishman WH: Clinical pharmacology of the new beta-adrenergic blocking drugs. Part 9. Nadolol: a new long-acting beta-adrenoceptor blocking drug. *Am Heart J* 99:124–128, 1980.

Herrera J, Vukovich RA, Griffith DL: Elimination of nadolol by patients with renal impairment. *Br J Clin Pharmacol* 7 (Suppl 2):227S–231S, 1979.

Lee RJ, Evans DB, Baky SH, Laffan RJ: Pharmacology of nadolol (SQ 11725), a β-adrenergic antagonist lacking direct myocardial depression. *Eur J Pharmacol* 33:371–382, 1975.

Pindolol

Frishman WH: Pindolol: a new β-adrenoceptor antagonist with partial agonist activity. *N Engl J Med* 308:940–944, 1983.

Propranolol

Buhler FR, Laragh JH, Vauchan ED, Brunner HR, Gavras H, Baer L: Antihypertensive action of propranolol. *Am J Cardiol* 32:511–522, 1973.

Feely J, Wilkinson GR, Wood AJJ: Reduction of liver blood flow and propranolol metabolism by cimetidine. *N Engl J Med* 304:692–695, 1981.

Hollifield JW, Sherman K, Zwagg RV, Shand DG: Proposed mechanisms of propranolol's antihypertensive effect in essential hypertension. *N Engl J Med* 295:68–73, 1976.

Kornhauser DM, Wood AJJ, Vestal RE, Wilkinson GR, Branch RA, Shand DG: Biological determinants of propranolol disposition in man. *Clin Pharmacol Ther* 23:165–174, 1978.

Palmer RF, Lasseter KC: Sodium nitroprusside. *N Engl J Med* 292:294–297, 1975.

Reid JL, Lewis PJ, Myers MG, Dollery CT: Cardiovascular effects of intracerebroventricular D, L, and DL-propranolol in the conscious rabbit. *J Pharmacol Exp Ther* 188:394–399, 1974.

Vestal RF, Wood AJJ: Influence of age and smoking on drug kinetics in man. *Clin Pharmacokinet* 5:309–319, 1980.

Vestal RE, Wood AJJ, Branch RA, Shand DG, Wilkinson GR: Effects of age and cigarette smoking on propranolol disposition. *Clin Pharmacol Ther* 26:8–15, 1979.

Wood AJJ, Carr K, Vestal RE, Belcher S, Wilkinson GR, Shand DG: Direct measurement of propranolol bioavailability during accumulation to steadystate. *Br J Clin Pharmacol* 6:345–350, 1978.

Wood AJJ, Kornhauser DM, Wilkinson GR, Shand DG, Branch RA: The influence of cirrhosis on steady-state blood concentrations of unbound propranolol after oral administration. *Clin Pharmacokinet* 2:478–487, 1978.

Wood AJJ, Vestal RE, Spannuth CL, Stone WJ, Wilkinson GR, Shand DG: Propranolol disposition in renal failure. *Br J Clin Pharmacol* 10:561–566, 1980.

Timolol

Batchelor ED, O'Day DM, Shand DG, Wood AJJ: Interaction of topical and oral timolol in glaucoma. *Ophthalmology* 86:60–65, 1979.

Firshman WH: Atenolol and timolol, two new systemic β-adrenoceptor antagonists. *N Engl J Med* 306:1456–1462, 1982.

15

Hypotensive and Vasodilator Drugs

ALASTAIR J. J. WOOD

ARTERIOLAR AND VENOUS DILATORS
Sodium Nitroprusside
Hypotensive Surgery
Congestive Cardiac Failure
Suggested Dosage and Administration
Toxicity
Nitroglycerin
Mechanism of Action
Angina
Cardiac Failure
Myocardial Infarction

SEROTONIN ANTAGONISTS
Ketanserin

ANGIOTENSIN CONVERTING ENZYME INHIBITORS
Captopril
Enalapril
Lisinopril

The treatment of hypertension has been considerably advanced recent years by the introduction of a variety of new drugs, some with novel actions. A better understanding of the mechanism and sites of action (Table 15.1) of the older drugs has allowed drugs to be used more rationally to produce greater blood pressure reduction with fewer side effects. In addition, by combining drugs with different sites of action, it is often possible to gain greater therapeutic effect. Some of these advances have occurred because of improved knowledge of the factors responsible for blood pressure control and, in some cases, the use of these new drugs has in itself provided considerable information about normal physiological function.

PHYSIOLOGY OF ADRENERGIC FUNCTION

Many of the drugs which are used to lower blood pressure act by altering the function of the sympathetic nervous system. A clear understanding of this system is therefore central to the understanding of the action of antihypertensives. The function of the sympathetic nervous system is reviewed in Chapter 13, and only a brief outline of the key factors of relevance to blood pressure control will be given here.

Norepinephrine and epinephrine are synthesized by the biosynthetic pathways outlined in Chapter 13 and are then taken up into storage vesicles which exist in large numbers within the adrenergic varicosities (Fig. 15.1). During nerve stimulation the vesicles liberate their catecholamine contents into the synaptic cleft by the process of exocytosis. The liberated catecholamines cross the synaptic cleft to bind to receptors on the effector cell (postsynaptic) to produce their effect. The action of catecholamines is terminated by both reuptake of the catecholamines into the adrenergic neuron and to a lesser extent by uptake into the effector cells.

The catecholamines produce their effect by binding to specific adrenergic receptors on the cell surface (see Chapter

Table 15.1.
Site of Action of the Hypotensive and Vasodilator Drugs

Decreased central sympathetic activity
  Central α_2-receptor agonists
    Clonidine
    Methyldopa (through metabolite methylnorepinephrine)
    Guanfacine
    Guanabenz
  β Receptor antagonists (see Chapter 14)
Peripheral α-adrenergic receptor antagonists
  Prazosin
  Terazosin
  Indoramin
Adrenergic neuron blockers
  Guanethidine
  Guanadrel
  Debrisoquine
  Bethanidine
  Reserpine
Vasodilators
  Arteriolar vasodilators
    Hydralazine
    Minoxidil
    Diazoxide
    Pinacidil
  Arteriolar and venodilators
    Nitroprusside
    Organic nitrates
Serotonin antagonists
  Ketanserin
Angiotensin converting enzyme inhibitors
  Captopril
  Enalapril
  Lisinopril
Diuretics

3). These receptors can be subdivided according to both their site (presynaptic being on the adrenergic neurons, postsynaptic being on the effector cell) and their relative affinity for a series of adrenergic agonists. Ahlquist originally divided adrenergic receptors into α and β; however, this has now been expanded to further subdivide the receptors into α_1, α_2 and β_1, β_2. The receptors were originally subdivided into α and β on the basis that β-receptors had a greater affinity for isoproterenol than norepinephrine,

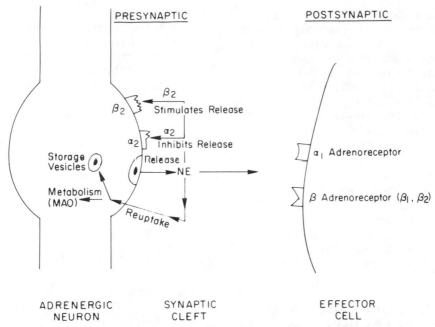

Figure 15.1.   Release of norepinephrine (*NE*), its reuptake, and action at presynaptic and postsynaptic receptors.   Norepinephrine is released from the storage vesicles in the terminal varicosities by exocytosis and then binds to postsynaptic α_1 or β) receptors or to presynaptic (α_2-receptors or presynaptic β_2-receptors to inhibit or stimulate, respectively, further norepinephrine release. Its action is terminated by reuptake into the adrenergic neuron.

while the reverse was true of α-receptors. The subdivision of β-receptors into β_1 (similar affinity for epinephrine and norepinephrine) and β_2 (greater affinity for epinephrine than norepinephrine) has been further strengthened by the development of relatively selective β-blocking drugs (see Chapter 14).

α-Receptors are found postsynaptically (α_1) on effector cells such as vascular smooth muscle, where their stimulation causes contraction, vasoconstriction, and a rise in blood pressure. Stimulation of presynaptic α-receptors (α_2) causes inhibition of further transmitter release following nerve stimulation. α_2-Receptors have been identified postsynaptically in the central nervous system. Stimulation of these central postynaptic α_2-receptors situated in the nucleus tractus solitarius and medulla oblongata lowers sympathetic outflow from the central nervous system, reduces catecholamines, and re-

sults in a fall in blood pressure (Fig. 15.2). Central β-receptors have also been identified, stimulation of which increases blood pressure while blockade (for example, by β-blockers) lowers blood pressure. Presynaptic β-receptors have also been identified which appear to be the β_2 type. Stimulation of these presynaptic β-receptors situated on the adrenergic neuron facilitates catecholamine release. Presynaptic dopamine receptors have also been described, stimulation of which appears to inhibit transmitter release. These presynaptic inhibitory dopamine receptors may account for some of the renal vasodilation and blood pressure-lowering effects of dopamine agonists (see Chapter 13). The effects of stimulation and blockade of the presynaptic receptors are outlined in Table 15.2, and the site of action of some of the antihypertensives which act through adrenergic receptors is contrasted in Table 15.3.

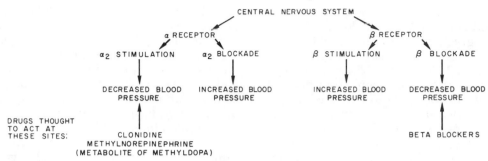

Figure 15.2. Effects of stimulation and blockade of α- and β-receptors in the central nervous system.

Table 15.2.
Effects of Presynaptic Receptors on Catecholamine Release

Presynaptic receptor subtype	Effects on catecholamine release of	
	Stimulation	Blockade
α_2	Decreased	Increased
β_2	Increased	Decreased

CENTRALLY ACTING HYPOTENSIVE AGENTS

Clonidine

Clonidine was originally developed as an α-agonist to be used as a nasal decongestant. However, it is a relatively selective α_2-agonist, and by stimulating α_2-receptors in the central nervous system, sympathetic outflow from the central nervous system is reduced, catecholamine levels fall, and a reduction in blood pressure occurs. In addition, plasma renin activity falls, probably as a result of reduced sympathetic stimulation at the renal adrenergic receptors. Stimulation of the presynaptic receptors on the adrenergic neurons, which inhibit catecholamine release, may also contribute to the observed reduction in catecholamines following clonidine administration.

Dry mouth and sedation may occur during therapy, particulary at high doses; however, these effects usually wear off to some extent with time. Impotence and postural hypotension are less of a prob-

Table 15.3.
Site of Action of Antihypertensives

	Peripheral		Central nervous system	
	α_1 postsynaptic	α_2 presynaptic	α_2 postsynaptic	β
Clonidine, guanfacine, guanabenz		Agonist	Agonist	
Methyldopa (through metabolite α-methyl-norepinephrine)			Agonist	
Prazosin, terazosin indoramin	Antagonist			
β-Blockers				Antagonist
Phentolamine	Antagonist	Antagonist		
Phenoxybenzamine	Antagonist	Antagonist		

lem than with some other hypotensive agents. The side effect of clonidine which has received most attention and is of particular concern to anesthesiologists is the so-called "clonidine withdrawal syndrome" which has been described following abrupt cessation of the drug. It has the features of a "hyperadrenergic state," resembling pheochromocytoma with increased blood pressures, pulse rate, and catecholamine concentrations. The best treatment is to reinstitute clonidine therapy. α-Blockers such as phentolamine are also effective. Care should be taken if clonidine is discontinued abruptly prior to anesthesia, when the dose should be slowly tapered while other antihypertensives are substituted.

Clonidine is given orally in a total dose of 0.2 to 0.8 mg/day. The terminal half-life is around 8 to 12 hours and the drug is usually administered twice daily.

CLONIDINE SUPPRESSION TEST

Clonidine's ability to suppress catecholamine secretion in both normal individuals and patients with essential hypertension has been made use of as a diagnostic test to distinguish between autonomous production of catecholamines in pheochromocytoma and normal individuals with other causes of increased plasma catecholamine concentrations. In patients with elevated plasma catecholamine levels, the administration of 0.3 mg of clonidine orally suppresses plasma norepinephrine into the normal range 3 hours after clonidine in normal patients but not in patients with pheochromocytoma (Fig. 15.3).

OTHER CENTRAL α_2-ADRENERGIC RECEPTOR AGONISTS

Guanfacine

Like clonidine, guanfacine is a centrally acting α_2-adrenergic receptor agonist. It is 12 times more selective than clonidine for α_2-receptors. Guanfacine is well absorbed orally and is both metabolized by the liver and excreted unchanged (30 to 40%) in the urine. Its half-life is 15 to 20 hours which is considerably longer than clonidine. Guanfacine produces similar adverse effects to those seen with clonidine, namely, sleepiness, fatigue, dry mouth, postural hypotension, and impotence, but these may be less common than with clonidine or guanabenz. Rebound hypertension occurs less commonly and, in addition, is less severe than with clonidine. Dosage regimens range from 0.5 to 3 mg, usually given once daily at bedtime.

Guanabenz

Another centrally acting α_2-adrenergic agonist, guanabenz, seems similar to clonidine in both its therapeutic effects and adverse effects, except that it may produce dry mouth, drowsiness, and weakness more often. It is administered twice daily in doses of 4 to 32 mg.

Methyldopa

Methyldopa, which structurally differs from DOPA only by the presence of an extra methyl group, is metabolized by the same pathway as is used to synthesize norepinephrine (Fig. 15.4; see also Chapter 13). It is decarboxylated by the enzyme L-amino acid decarboxylase to yield α-methyldopamine and further metabolized by dopamine hydroxylase to α-methylnorepinephrine. It was initially thought that methyldopa's hypotensive action was due to its ability to inhibit the decarboxylase enzyme. However, it has subsequently become clear that other decarboxylase inhibitors are not hypotensive. It is now thought that the drug's hypotensive action is due to the production of the relatively selective α_2-receptor agonist, α-methylnorepinephrine or perhaps α-methylepinephrine, in the brain which by stimulating postsynaptic α_2-receptors reduces sympathetic outflow from the brain.

Methyldopa is administered in doses of 250 to 2000 mg/day, usually divided into two daily doses. Absorption of methyldopa is both incomplete (around 50%) and variable following oral administra-

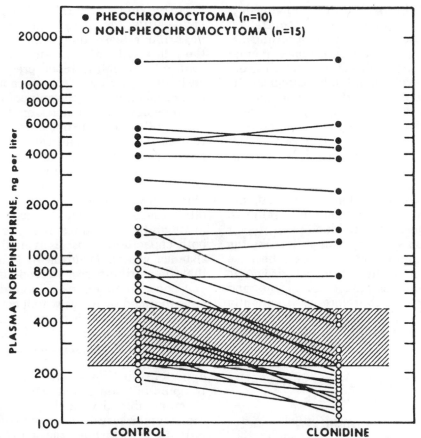

Figure 15.3.   Plasma norepinephrine concentrations before and 3 hours after 0.3 mg of clonidine orally.   The normal individuals (○) suppressed to within or below the normal range (▨), whereas the patients with pheochromocytoma (●) did not. (With permission from Bravo EL, Tarazi RC, Fouad FM, Vidt DG, Gifford RW: Clonidine suppression test: a useful aid to the diagnosis of pheochromocytoma. *N Engl J Med* 305:623–626, 1981.)

tion. Protein binding is low at 15%. The maximum hypotensive effect develops 6 to 8 hours after the dose and may persist for as long as 24 hours, leading some to suggest the use of once daily methyldopa administered just before bedtime to achieve maximum sedative effects during the night while hypotensive effects

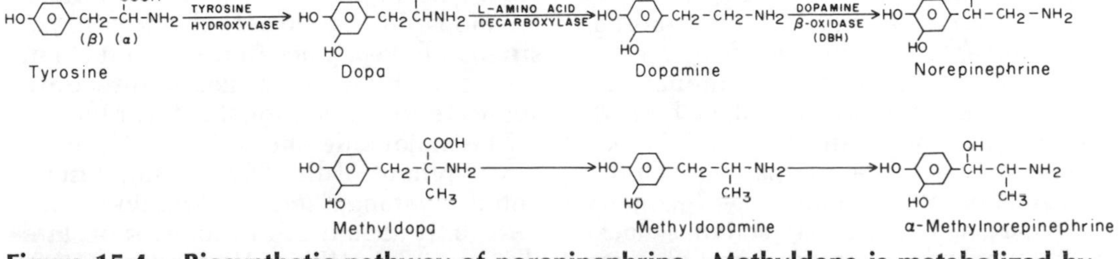

Figure 15.4.   Biosynthetic pathway of norepinephrine   Methyldopa is metabolized by the same pathway to methylnorepinephrine.

would last throughout the following day. Particularly at high doses, its central actions are associated with sedation and difficulty in performing complex mental tasks. A more serious side effect is the occasional development of hepatic necrosis which, if not detected early enough and the drug discontinued, may be fatal. About 20% of patients on long-term methyldopa develop a positive Coomb's test, but hemolytic anemia only develops in less than 1%.

The centrally acting hypotensive agents, clonidine and methyldopa, do not interfere with the sympathetic reflexes, and therefore a fall in blood pressure, for example on standing, can still evoke the required compensatory reflexes because the function of the peripheral adrenergic nerves remains intact. Clonidine and methyldopa are therefore less frequently associated with troublesome postural hypotension than are some of the other hypotensive agents.

α_1-ADRENERGIC RECEPTOR ANTAGONISTS

Prazosin

Prazosin is a *selective* blocker of α_1-adrenergic receptors, having 5000 times higher affinity for α_1- than α_2-receptors. Thus, by blocking norepinephrine's action on the postsynaptic α_1-receptors, a fall in peripheral resistance and blood pressure occurs. Prazosin was introduced as a direct acting vasodilator thought to act through phosphodiesterase inhibition. However, it is now clear that the concentrations required for this action are in excess of those actually achieved clinically and are much in excess of those required for blockade of α_1-adrenergic receptors. The nonselective α-blockers, such as phentolamine and phenoxybenzamine which block both α_1- and α_2-receptors, cause a fall in blood pressure, which is accompanied by a rise in catecholamines and a compensatory tachycardia. These nonselective α-blockers by blocking α_2-receptors and blocking the normal negative feedback of norepi-

nephrine on its own release magnify the tachycardia by increasing the norepinephrine release that occurs following the reflex sympathetic stimulation in response to the fall in blood pressure. Prazosin, by leaving the α_2-receptors unblocked, allows norepinephrine to produce negative feedback on its own release, so limiting further norepinephrine release. Thus, the fall in blood pressure produced by prazosin is not accompanied by the tachycardia seen with the nonselective α-blockers. The lack of tachycardia following prazosin, in contrast to other vasodilators, may be partially due to its ability to reduce vascular tone in both capacitance vessels (veins) and resistance vessels (arterioles). This means that the striking rise in venous return and consequent increase in cardiac output produced by drugs which act only on the resistance vessels do not occur.

Prazosin is administered orally in doses of 2 to 40 mg/day, usually divided into two daily doses for the treatment of hypertension. The absorption of prazosin is poor and somewhat variable which, when combined with the high first-pass metabolism, results in a bioavailability of only 44 to 69%. Peak plasma concentrations are achieved 2 to 3 hours after administration, and the half-life is 3 to 4 hours. The drug is avidly removed by the liver and is more than 90% protein bound in plasma.

Prazosin has also been used in the treatment of severe congestive cardiac failure, where its ability to cause a reduction in arteriolar resistance (afterload reduction), increased venous pooling, and a reduction in filling pressures (reduced venous tone, preload reduction) is valuable. Although some degree of tolerance develops during chronic therapy, prazosin may have a place in the chronic management of severe cardiac failure unresponsive to conventional measures.

The major side effect of prazosin is the development of the "first dose phenomenon" characterized by dizziness, faintness, and sometimes syncope soon after the administration of the first dose. It is thought that most of the cases have been due to a hypotensive episode and that patients who are sodium depleted or on diuretics are more likely to develop this problem. It can be avoided by instructing the patient to take the first dose once he is in bed for the night.

Terazosin

A selective α_1-adrenergic blocker whose structure is very similar to that of prazosin, terazosin, is about 3-fold less potent than prazosin in binding to α_1-adrenergic receptors while its affinity for α_2-receptors is similar to that of prazosin.

The principal differences between terazosin and prazosin are their pharmacokinetic properties. The structural differences between prazosin and terazosin result in terazosin being much more water soluble so that it can be administered intravenously. Terazosin also has a longer half-life of 12 hours, so that terazosin can be given once daily. Terazosin is excreted mainly by hepatic metabolism and biliary excretion. Unlike prazosin, it is well absorbed with a bioavailability of approximately 90%. Its binding in plasma is similar to prazosin (90 to 94%). Thus, terazosin differs from prazosin mainly in its more reliable absorption and longer half-life. The usual dose ranges from 1 to 40 mg/day.

Indoramin

Like prazosin and terazosin, indoramin is a selective α_1-adrenergic antagonist which is an effective antihypertensive. It is given in starting doses of 25 mg 2 to 3 times daily up to a total dose of 200 mg/day.

ADRENERGIC NEURON BLOCKERS

Reserpine

Following uptake into the adrenergic neuron, catecholamines are taken up into storage vesicles within the terminal varicosities (Fig. 15.1). Reserpine interferes with uptake into the storage vesicles so that catecholamines leak out from these vesicles and are degraded by the enzyme

monoamine oxidase within the axoplasm. Thus, reserpine's action is to deplete the adrenergic neuron of catecholamines so that the amount of catecholamine released in response to nerve stimulation is reduced and blood pressure falls. Although reserpine disappears relatively rapidly from plasma, the drug has a prolonged effect probably because of its persistence on the vesicular membrane.

Reserpine readily enters the brain where its presence is associated with central nervous system side effects such as sedation and drowsiness. More serious, however, is the production of depression which in some cases has resulted in suicide. For this reason, reserpine's use has decreased dramatically over recent years and probably should be limited to low-dose administration.

Guanethidine

Guanethidine is actively taken up into the adrenergic neuron via the norepinephrine reuptake pump. The drug is taken up into the storage vesicles where it displaces norepinephrine, resulting in reduced catecholamine release in response to adrenergic nerve stimulation, which results in a drop in blood pressure. Because sympathetic tone is particularly important in the maintenance of blood pressure and the increase in peripheral resistance in response to assumption of the upright posture, the effects of guanethidine are much more obvious on standing than when the patient is supine, resulting in a pronounced postural drop in blood pressure. Postural hypotension is thus a limiting side effect of this drug. Guanethidine causes sodium and fluid retention, resulting in loss of hypotensive control unless a diuretic is administered concurrently. The terminal half-life is very long (5 days), so that dosage adjustments should be made no more frequently than every 2 weeks.

To produce its therapeutic effect, guanethidine must enter the adrenergic neuron via the norepinephrine pump. Inhibitors of this pump such as the tricyclic antidepressants, chlorpromazine and ephedrine, will block guanethidine's access to its site of action and hence prevent its hypotensive effect. This is an extremely important drug interaction and is not infrequently the explanation for loss of blood pressure control in a previously well-controlled patient on guanethidine or for "guanethidine resistance." In addition to postural hypotension, guanethidine's main side effects are fluid retention, delayed or retrograde ejaculation, and diarrhea.

Guanadrel

Guanadrel is an adrenergic nerve-blocking agent whose mechanism of action is similar to guanethidine. In contrast to guanethidine, however, its half-life is only 10 hours, which means that dosage adjustments can be made rapidly, but it must be administered twice daily. Dosage ranges from 10 to 40 mg twice daily.

Debrisoquine and Bethanidine

These are other adrenergic nerve-blocking agents with shorter half-lives than guanethidine available in some countries. All of these drugs would be

expected to interact with drugs such as tricyclic antidepressants as described earlier for guanethidine.

ARTERIOLAR VASODILATORS

Drugs of this group, examples of which include hydralazine, diazoxide, minoxidil, and pinacidil, reduce peripheral resistance by a direct vasodilating action on the arterioles, without significantly affecting the venous capacitance vessels. The reduction in afterload (arteriolar dilation) and the absence of effect on the capacitance vessels (veins) result in an increased venous return, increased preload, and reflex increase in cardiac output. In addition to the direct mechanical effects of increased venous return resulting in increased cardiac output, the reduction in arterial pressure activates the baroreceptor reflex and results in increased sympathetic activity (Fig. 15.5). An understanding of the compensatory reflex brought into play by the vasodilators is essential to their rational use in therapy. Increased sympathetic activity (Fig. 15.5) results in increased catecholamines, increase in heart rate, myocardial contractility, and cardiac output, which in turn increases myocardial work, and hence myocardial oxygen demand. In patients with coronary artery disease, this

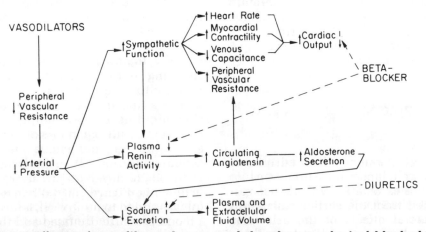

Figure 15.5. Effects of vasodilator therapy and the pharmacological blockade of these effects. (Modified with permission from Koch-Weser J: Vasodilator drugs in the treatment of hypertension. *Arch Intern Med* 103:1017–1027, 1974.)

increase in myocardial oxygen demand may precipitate angina or even myocardial infarction. Plasma renin activity is also increased by the increased sympathetic activity (Fig. 15.5) resulting in increased aldosterone secretion and sodium retention. The sodium retention is probably also due to direct hemodynamic changes within the kidney. The net result of the increased sympathetic activity, hyperaldosteronism and fluid retention, is to cause reflex vasocontriction, expanded intravascular fluid volume, and increased cardiac output. If these effects are unchecked, they will overcome the reduction in blood pressure produced by the vasodilator and may precipitate angina, edema, or cardiac failure in patients with impaired cardiac function. These reflex changes account for many of the side effects seen during vasodilator therapy. The deleterious reflex changes associated with vasodilator administration can be overcome by the simultaneous administration of a sympatholytic agent, such as a β-blocker, which blocks the effects of the increase in sympathetic activity, and a diuretic to prevent sodium retention (Fig. 15.5).

Hydralazine

When hydralazine was first introduced in the 1950s, it was found that its hypotensive effect tended to be lost during chronic administration and that by today's standards, relatively large doses were required, which were frequently associated with toxicity. However, with the improved understanding of the reflex changes produced by vasodilators and the development of pharmacological approaches to overcome them, hydralazine has developed into a useful and effective antihypertensive agent. Hydralazine acts directly to produce arterial muscle relaxation with consequent fall in peripheral resistance and blood pressure. Most of the problems associated with its use can be predicted from the earlier discussion of the general effects of the arteriolar vasodilators (Fig. 15.5) and include headache, cutaneous flushing, increased cardiac output, and myocardial work, re-

sulting in angina in patients with myocardial ischemia.

A drug-induced lupus syndrome is produced by prolonged high-dose hydralazine therapy. This side effect occurs more commonly at high hydralazine concentrations, being seen in 10 to 20% of patients receiving 400 mg/day. Hydralazine is metabolized partially by acetylation, the rate of which is bimodally distributed in the population, resulting in both slow and fast acetylators (see Chapter 2). Slow acetylators, because they eliminate the drug more slowly and achieve higher plasma concentrations, develop drug-induced lupus at lower hydralazine doses than do fast acetylators.

The dose of hydralazine should be limited to 200 mg/day except in fast acetylators or blacks who seldom develop lupus associated with hydralazine therapy. Hydralazine should be administered only to patients already receiving a diuretic and β-blocker or other sympathetic antagonist. In such patients, vasodilators are very effective and do not have the central depressive effect seen with the centrally acting antihypertensives.

Minoxidil

Minoxidil is a potent arteriolar vasodilator which is extremely effective even in patients who have proved refractory to other drug regimens. Because of its potency, it produces even more profound reflex increase in sympathetic activity and sodium retention than hydralazine and therefore should only be administered along with both a diuretic and sympathetic blocker such as propranolol. Large doses of diuretic may be required to prevent sodium retention, particulary in patients with renal impairment. The rise in heart rate and plasma renin activity following the fall in blood pressure produced by minoxidil treatment alone is shown in Figure 15.6. When propranolol was added to minoxidil, a further fall in blood pressure occurred and the heart rate and plasma renin levels were restored to pretreatment values. The usual dose of minoxidil ranges from 5 to 40

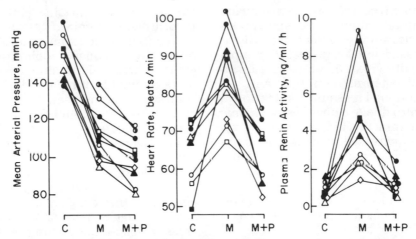

Figure 15.6.   Mean arterial pressure, heart rate and plasma renin activity on no treatment (C), minoxidil (M), and minoxidil and propranolol (M + P).   (Modified with permission from O'Malley K, Velasco M, Wells J, McNay J: Mechanism of the interaction of propranolol and a potent vasodilator antihypertensive agent—minoxidil. *Eur J Clin Pharmacol* 9:355–360, 1976.)

mg/day. The plasma half-life is around 4 hours, but its half-life of effect appears to be much longer so that the drug can usually be given twice daily.

Side effects include all those previously described which are associated with other arteriolar vasodilators as well as occasional development of pericardial effusion. Increased hair growth (hypertrichosis) develops within 5 to 8 weeks of starting treatment and is characteristically over the forehead and temple areas. This can sometimes be very distressing in women but can be controlled by the use of dipilatory creams. Minoxidil can be lifesaving in patients with hypertension resistant to other drugs, and because of minoxidil's freedom from central nervous system effects, it is particularly valuable in patients who develop such side effects from other agents.

Diazoxide

Diazoxide is a thiazide devoid of diuretic activity, which produces predominantly arteriolar dilation. It is only available for intravenous administration and is usually used in the emergency treatment of hypertension. It produces similar reflex changes to those described earlier for the other arteriolar vasodilators. It

has a prolonged action, often up to 24 hours. Diazoxide should be administered intravenously in small bolus doses of 75 to 150 mg repeated every 5 minutes until the blood pressure is controlled. Earlier claims that the drug had to be administered in a single rapid intravenous bolus have proved incorrect.

Pinacidil

Pinacidil is a new potent direct acting vasodilator which acts as a potassium channel opener in vascular smooth muscle. Pinacidil's antihypertensive action is mediated through vasodilation and reduction in peripheral resistance. These changes are associated with the expected reflex increase in heart rate and cardiac output described earlier and with fluid retention. Thus, pinacidil will increase myocardial oxygen demand when administered without a β-blocker and therefore may precipitate myocardial ischemia. In addition, because of its propensity to cause fluid retention, administration of a diuretic is usually required.

Pinacidil has a relatively short elimination half-life of approximately 2 hours and is only 40% bound to plasma proteins. It is usually administered as retarded release tablets which prolong the drug's duration of action. The use of the retarded release preparation allows pinacidil to be administered twice daily, usually in doses of up to 37.5 mg twice daily. The principal route of excretion is by metabolism to pinacidil-N-oxide.

The side effects seen with the drug are those predicted for a direct acting vasodilator, namely, dizziness, headache flushing, and the reflex cardiac stimulation and sodium-retaining effects discussed above.

Adenosine

The cardiovascular effects of adenosine have recently been recognized, and some of these have been utilized therapeutically. Adenosine produces peripheral vasodilation and lowers blood pressure when infused intravenously. The peripheral vasodilation in response to adenosine is probably part of a homeostatic mechanism to restore normal energy balance. When increased energy demands result in ATP breakdown to adenosine, then the vasodilation produced by adenosine increases blood flow and hence increases energy supply to the affected tissues.

The vasodilating effects of adenosine infusions have been used therapeutically to produce deliberate hypotension during cerebral aneurysm surgery in doses ranging from 80 to 500 μg/kg/min starting at 40 μg/kg/min. Adenosine produces rapid reduction in blood pressure which returns to normal within 3 minutes of stopping the infusion.

Adenosine also slows cardiac rate and impairs conduction through the A-V node. This action has been made use of in the treatment of supraventricular tachycardia. The development of an A-V block progressing from first degree to complete A-V block in some cases may be detrimental during the induction of deliberate hypotension with adenosine during surgery.

ARTERIOLAR AND VENOUS DILATORS

Vasodilators such as hydralazine, minoxidil, and diazoxide which act predominantly on the arterial side of the circulation produce a fall in afterload without increasing venous capacitance. This results in increased venous return, increased filling pressure, increased cardiac output, and increased pulmonary artery pressure (Fig. 15.7). In contrast, nitroprusside produces both arteriolar and venous dilation while the organic nitrates produce predominantly venous dilation. This increase in venous capacitance reduces preload and in patients without cardiac failure reduces pulmonary artery pressure (Fig. 15.7). The degree of afterload reduction is greater with nitroprusside because of its greater effect on the arterial side of the circulation than nitroglycerin.

Sodium Nitroprusside

Although the hypotensive effect of nitroprusside was demonstrated in laboratory animals over 100 years ago and was described in humans in 1929, sodium nitroprusside has only recently been widely used by clinicians. Nitroprusside (Fig. 15.8) acts directly on vascular smooth muscle (both venous and arterial) to produce relaxation. It therefore produces dilation in both arteriolar and venous beds resulting in both preload and afterload reduction. The particular characteristic which has made it so useful clinically is its rapid onset of action (within seconds) and its short duration of effect (1 to 3 minutes). It is administered by continuous intravenous infusion but, because of its potency and rapidity of action, it is important that some kind of automated infusion device be used to ensure a constant and controlled rate of administration. Obviously careful and frequent blood pressure monitoring with appropriate dosage adjustments is a prerequisite to the safe clinical use of this agent.

THERAPEUTIC USES

Hypertensive Emergencies. It is an ideal agent for treating hypertensive emergencies including accelerated or malignant hypertension when it is usual to start with a dose of 0.5 to 1.5 μg/kg/min (30 to

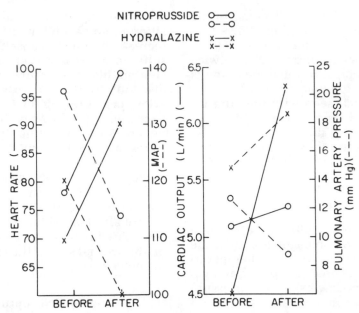

Figure 15.7.   Contrasting hemodynamic effects of nitroprusside and hydralazine. *Left panel* shows that, for a similar fall in blood pressure, a similar rise in heart rate is produced. However, cardiac output rises more with hydralazine *(right panel)* accompanied by a rise in pulmonary artery pressure. In contrast, following nitroprusside, pulmonary artery pressure falls. (Data derived with permission from Tarazi RC, Dustan HP, Bravo EL, Niarchos AP: Vasodilating drugs: contrasting hemodynamic effects. *Clin Sci Mol Med* 51:575s–578s, 1976.)

90 μg/kg/hour). Most patients are controlled wtih doses of less than 5 μg/kg/min (0.3 mg/kg/hour), although occasionally patients will require more. It has also been used successfully to lower blood pressure and stabilize patients

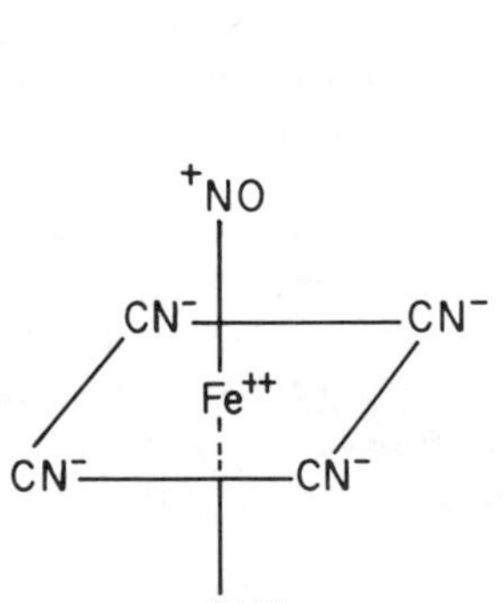

Figure 15.8.   Structural formula for the nitroprusside complex. There is an overall net negative charge which results in association with cations such as sodium in sodium nitroprusside.

prior to surgery for aortic dissection. By lowering blood pressure, the tearing force on the aortic wall is reduced. This shearing force is dependent on the rate of rise of aortic pressure, dp/dt. Activation of the sympathetic reflexes due to the fall in blood pressure tends to increase dp/dt so that propranolol should be administered along with nitroprusside in patients with aortic dissection to block any tachycardia or increased cardiac output produced by the nitroprusside.

Deliberate or Induced Hypotension during Surgery. Induced hypotension is sometimes used to decrease blood loss and maintain a bloodless field during certain neurosurgical, major orthopedic, and middle ear procedures. Because of its rapid onset and short duration of action, nitroprusside is an ideal agent to induce hypotension. In addition, tachyphylaxis does not usually occur. However, larger doses of nitroprusside are often required to lower the blood pressure in normoten-

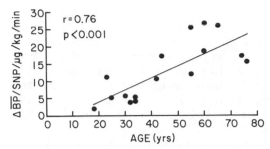

Figure 15.9. Effect of age on the drop in blood pressure per $\mu g/kg/min$ of sodium nitroprusside. The elderly have a greater drop in blood pressure *(BP)* than the young for the same dose of sodium nitroprusside *(SNP)*. (With permission from Wood M, Hyman S, Wood AJJ: A clinical study of sensitivity to sodium nitroprusside during controlled hypotensive anesthesia in young and elderly patients. *Anesth Analg* 66:132–136, 1987.)

sive patients than in the hypertensive patients discussed previously.

Factors affecting nitroprusside response have recently been the subject of investigation. The elderly have been found to be more sensitive to nitroprusside-induced blood pressure reduction during anesthesia (Fig. 15.9) so that to produce the same reduction in blood pressure they require a smaller dose of nitroprusside. The explanation for this appears to be that the impaired β-recep-

tor responsiveness in the elderly (see Chapter 3) limits the cardiac reflex changes produced in response to hypotension. In young patients, reflex sympathetic stimulation increases cardiac rate substantially in an attempt to overcome the nitroprusside-induced hypotension. However, in elderly patients similar increases in sympathetic activity do not increase heart rate to the same extent as in the young because of impaired β-receptor response. Therefore their ability to compensate for the nitroprusside-induced hypotension is reduced.

Congestive Cardiac Failure. The value of blood pressure reduction in hypertensive patients with left ventricular failure and pulmonary edema has long been recognized. However, recently, vasodilator therapy has been used to treat normotensive patients with left ventricular failure. In patients with impaired cardiac function, the arteriolar dilation reduces afterload and, therefore, because of the fall in the pressure against which the left ventricle is pumping, ejection fraction and cardiac output increase, resulting in a reduction in left ventricular size. This reduction in left ventricular volume reduces myocardial wall tension which, because it is a major determinant of myocardial oxygen demand, may be beneficial to patients with myocardial ischemia (Fig. 15.10). The venodilation produced by nitroprusside expands venous capaci-

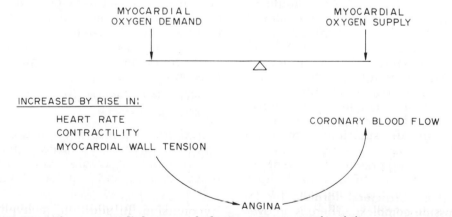

Figure 15.10. The myocardial oxygen balance. Because of inability to increase coronary blood flow angina will result, if myocardial oxygen demand exceeds myocardial oxygen supply.

tance so that the intravascular volume is shifted from the central to the peripheral compartment with a consequent reduction in filling pressure. The net result is both a decrease in end systolic volume, end diastolic volume, and pulmonary artery pressure and an increase in stroke volume and cardiac output. Because the improved cardiac output reduces the sympathetic drive to the heart, the heart rate falls. During intravenous vasodilator treatment of cardiac failure, arterial pressure (preferably measured invasively) and pulmonary artery pressure or wedge pressure should be monitored. If systemic hypotension develops prior to adequate increase in cardiac output during vasodilator therapy with nitroprusside, the administration of an inotropic agent, such as dobutamine or dopamine, may be appropriate; however, care must be taken to ensure that the possibility of increased myocardial oxygen demand does not worsen myocardial ischemia.

SUGGESTED DOSAGE AND ADMINISTRATION

Nitroprusside should be dissolved in 5% dextrose/water immediately prior to use, when it forms a light brown solution. It decomposes when exposed to light and, for that reason, it is usual to protect the infusion bag and, in the case of slow rates of infusion the tubing, from light by wrapping in aluminum foil. If the solution turns dark brown, this indicates decomposition and the solution should be discarded. Sodium nitroprusside, 50 mg, is dissolved in either 250 ml (0.02% solution; 200 μg/ml) or 500 ml (0.01% solution; 100 μg/ml) and is administered with an automatic infusion device starting at a dose of 0.5 μg/kg/min and increased until adequate therapeutic effect is achieved. The average dose of 3 μg/kg/min is usually sufficient to maintain the systolic blood pressure at about 80 mm Hg. If arterial pressure is to be deliberately lowered, it is important to have an accurate and reliable method of measuring blood pressure, and it is mandatory to use an indwelling arterial catheter whenever controlled hypotension with

sodium nitroprusside is required. In addition, easy access to arterial blood allows the frequent determination of arterial blood gases and acid-base status. It is important to maintain intravascular volume within the normal range, and a reflex tachycardia that sometimes occurs can usually be corrected by fluid administration and/or β-blockade.

The dangers of sodium nitroprusside administration include the dangers inherent in the technique of induced hypotension but, in addition, cyanide toxicity may occur (see later in this section). The capacity of the body to detoxify sodium nitroprusside is limited and, thus, dosage recommendations should not be exceeded. For *acute short-term* use, as during hypotensive surgery, the total intraoperative dose should be limited to 1.0 to 1.5 mg/kg administered over a 1- to 3-hour period. A total intraoperative dose of 1.5 mg/kg should not be exceeded and, if the initial dose requirements are such that it seems likely this figure will be exceeded, alternate methods of inducing hypotension should be used. The rate of infusion should be limited to 8.0 μg/kg/min. For chronic use, a maximum recommended dosage of 0.5 mg/kg/hour or 8 μg/kg/min should not be exceeded. The development of a metabolic acidosis or "resistance" (increasing dosage requirements) to sodium nitroprusside mandates cessation of therapy. Cyanide toxicity is manifest early by the development of a metabolic acidosis and an increased mixed venous oxygen content. Pretreatment of patients with captopril (see later) allows lower doses of nitroprusside to be used to produce hypotension.

TOXICITY, PRECAUTIONS, AND CONTRAINDICATIONS

Toxicity from nitroprusside may occur due to excessive hypotension which can be avoided by careful monitoring of blood pressure and judicious dosage adjustments. In addition, toxicity may occur due to nitroprusside's metabolism. Nitroprusside contains five cyanide groups and breaks down in the body to yield cyanide ions which, when reacted with sulfur, yield *thiocyanate*. Toxicity may occur from excessive accumulation of either cyanide or thiocyanate. Thiocyanate is renally excreted and has a half-life of 4 to 7 days in patients with normal renal function and even longer in patients with impaired renal function. When thiocyanate levels rise above 10 mg/100 ml (100 μg/ml). Toxicity may appear as drowsiness, fatigue, slurred speech, nausea, tinnitus, muscle twitching and spasm, disorientation, and psychosis, all of which may progress to stupor or convulsions. Nitroprusside reacts with hemoglobin to produce cyanomethemoglobin and the liberation of cyanide ions, which are then further converted to thiocyanate. During high infusion rates of nitroprusside, cyanide accumulation may occur resulting in cyanide toxicity. This appears to be a particular problem during the use of high nitroprusside doses of greater than 10 μg/kg/min (0.6 mg/kg/hour) during hypotensive anesthesia. Cyanide ion combines with cytochrome *c*, an enzyme required for aerobic metabolism. The impairment of aerobic metabolism results in a shift to anaerobic metabolism which is manifested as metabolic acidosis, with elevated plasma lactate concentrations. Hydroxycobalamin combines with cyanide ions to yield cyanocobalamin (vitamin B_{12}). Cottrell demonstrated in a controlled study that hydroxycobalamin infusion (25 mg/hour) resulted in lower cyanide concentrations and less evidence of tissue hypoxia during hypotensive anesthesia with nitroprusside. It is unfortunate that hydroxycobalamin, which appears safe and effective, has not been more widely used as an adjunct to nitroprusside therapy.

Nitroglycerin

Nitroglycerin was described as a remedy for angina pectoris in 1879. Since then, it has remained the mainstay of symptomatic treatment for this condition. However, recently it has found new uses in the treatment of congestive heart failure, limitation of infarct size, and acute treatment of ischemia.

MECHANISM OF ACTION OF NITRATES

Although nitrates have been used for many years, it is only very recently that their mechanism of action at the tissue level has been understood. An increased understanding of the mechanism of nitroglycerin's action has also helped explain the action of other vasodilators.

The nitrate vasodilators act through the production of nitric oxide (NO) in tissues (Fig. 15.11). A number of "nitrovasodilators" act through this mechanism, including the organic and inorganic nitrates and nitroprusside. The nitric oxide production may occur either through enzymatic or nonenzymatic mechanisms. The ability to produce NO is dependent on both pH and Po_2, and, thus, variability in tissue pH or Po_2 may explain the differences in the relative tissue specificity of the various nitrovasodilators. Nitric oxide formation activates the soluble guanylate cyclase present in the cytosol of smooth muscle cells which results in increased cyclic GMP production, activation of a cyclic GMP-dependent protein kinase, and eventually *dephosphorylation* of myosin light chains causing smooth muscle relaxation.

Certain other vasodilators appear to act through the same final common pathway. In the case of the so-called *entothelium-dependent vasodilators*, they require the presence of vascular endothelium to produce vasodilation (Fig. 15.11). These vasodilators include histamine, acetylcholine, thrombin, ATP, and bradykinin. When these vasodilators interact with receptors on endothelial cells, a transmitter is produced which has been called *endothelial-derived relaxant factor* (EDRF). EDRF is probably nitric oxide which then stimulates guanylate cyclase in the same fashion as the nitrovasodilators with the eventual dephosphorylation of myosin light chains and smooth muscle relaxation.

Atriopeptins such as atrial natriuretic factor (ANF) (Chapter 17) stimulate membrane-bound guanylate cyclase (in

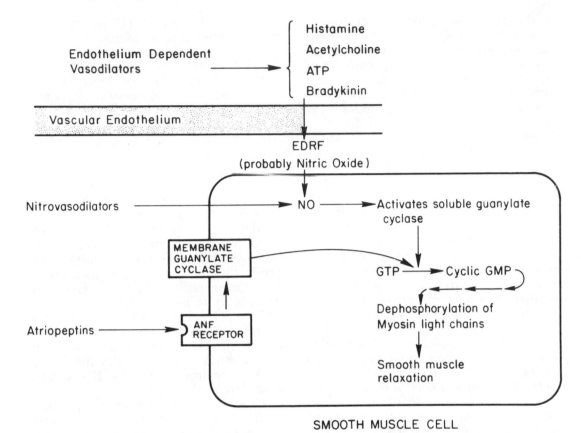

Figure 15.11.   Mechanism of action of nitrate and other vasodilators.   The *endothelium-dependent vasodilators* such as histamine require the presence of vascular endothelium to produce *endothelial-derived relaxing factor* (EDRF) which is probably nitric oxide (NO) to activate the cytosolic, soluble guanylate cyclase. *Nitrovasodilators,* on the other hand, produce nitric oxide directly to activate guanylate cyclase. *Atriopeptins* interact with a cell surface receptor and membrane-bound guanylate cyclase to increase cyclic GMP which, after a series of steps results in dephosphorylation of myosin light chains and smooth muscle relaxation.

contrast to the soluble cytosolic guanylate cyclase stimulated by EDRF and the nitrovasodilators) resulting in increased cyclic GMP production and vascular relaxation.

CLINICAL EFFECTS

As discussed earlier, nitroglycerin is a potent vasodilator producing relaxation of both arterial and venous smooth muscle. Its effects, however, are mainly on the venous side of the circulation where it produces an increase in venous capacitance resulting in a fall in venous return

and right atrial and pulmonary capillary wedge pressures. Ventricular systolic and diastolic volumes also fall, resulting in a fall in myocardial wall tension which results in decreased myocardial oxygen demand.

Although it was initially thought that nitroglycerin's ability to relieve angina was due to coronary artery dilation and increased coronary blood flow, it is now recognized that this is not so and that, in fact, total coronary blood flow may fall during nitroglycerin therapy. However, because myocardial work is decreased, resulting in a decrease in myocardial oxygen demand, the oxygen supply and demand are brought back into balance (Fig. 15.10). Angina occurs when myocardial oxygen demand exceeds myocardial oxygen supply. This imbalance can occur either because of excess demand such as in hypertension, thyrotoxicosis, aortic stenosis, or more commonly because of inadequate supply as in coronary atherosclerosis. Usually little can be done without surgery to increase myocardial oxygen supply; therefore, attention has to be directed to reducing demand. Patients themselves will usually have found that, by stopping the exercise which precipitated the angina attack, they are able to reduce myocardial oxygen demand sufficiently to terminate the attack. However, in more serious cases, nitroglycerin acts to reduce left ventricular systolic and diastolic wall tension, both of which are major determinants of myocardial oxygen demand (Fig. 15.10). Diastolic wall tension which is related to "preload" can be conceptualized as the pressure during diastole which is dilating the relaxed ventricular muscle. Increase in venous capacitance reduces this pressure. Systolic wall tension is the tension generated in the ventricular muscle during ejection and is determined by the pressure against which the ventricle is contracting, that is, aortic blood pressure.

Patients should be instructed to take nitroglycerin sublingually at the first sign of pain and should expect rapid relief (in 1 to 2 minutes). Nitroglycerin is highly extracted from blood by the liver, so that if swallowed, very little nitroglycerin reaches the systemic circulation. However, this presystemic removal can be bypassed by sublingual administration. Nitroglycerin is rapidly metabolized in the body by both the liver and perhaps peripheral tissues. The half-life is extremely short at 2.8 minutes. Extensive distribution occurs to tissues resulting in a volume of distribution of around 3 L/kg. Nitroglycerin can also be used prophylactically prior to beginning a task known to precipitate angina. Nitroglycerin is volatile and relatively unstable, so

that tablets will lose their effectiveness over a period of 4 to 6 months. Patients should be instructed to keep their tablets in a light-proof, air-tight container and replace them every 4 to 6 months.

Nitroglycerin has been used in the treatment of patients with cardiac failure. It is particularly useful in patients with elevated pulmonary wedge pressures (greater than 15 mm Hg) where reduction in wedge pressure has been associated with venous and arteriolar dilation, increased stroke volume, and beneficial therapeutic effects.

In patients with cardiac failure, the aim of therapy is to both improve cardiac output and reduce left ventricular filling pressure. Hydralazine because of its predominantly arteriolar effects increases cardiac output by afterload reduction, which results in an increase in venous return to the heart and an increase in filling pressure and reflex increase in cardiac output. Nitroglycerin, on the other hand, has predominantly venodilator effects resulting in reduction in preload and fall in filling pressures. Attempts have, therefore, been made to gain the benefits of both afterload and preload reduction by combining chronic nitrate and hydralazine therapy (Table 15.4). Chatterjee and his colleagues found that left ventricular filling pressure fell when nitrates were administered, while cardiac output rose in response to hydralazine (Table 15.4). The combination of hydralazine and nitrates resulted in both a fall in left ventricular filling pressure and a rise in cardiac output without any additional fall in blood pressure (Table 15.4).

Intravenous nitroglycerin has recently been advocated in the management of myocardial ischemia during coronary revascularization surgery, to control perioperative hypertension, in the treatment of angina pectoris in the coronary care unit and cardiac catheterization laboratory, as a vasodilator in severe congestive cardiac failure, and finally, as a deliberate hypotensive agent during anesthesia. Until recently, nitroglycerin for intravenous use usually had to be prepared by

Table 15.4.
Additive Hemodynamic Effects of Nitrates and Hydralazine in Patients with Chronic Heart Failure

	Control	Nitrates	Hydralazine	Hydralazine + nitrates
Left ventricular filling pressure (mm Hg)	28	17	25	18
Cardiac output (L/min/m^2)	2.1	2.1	3.2	3.3
Mean blood pressure (mm Hg)	87	85	83	85

Data with permission from Chatterjee J, Massie B, Rubin S, Gelberg H, Brundage BH, Ports TA: Long-term outpatient vasodilator therapy of congestive heart failure. Consideration of agents at rest and during exercise. *Am J Med* 65:134–145, 1978.

the hospital pharmacy immediately prior to use and added to 5% dextrose in water to attain a concentration of 100 μg/ml. Recently, commercially prepared intravenous nitroglycerin has become available. Nitroglycerin should be administered using an automated infusion pump and the dose titrated to achieve clinical effect; the dose required to reduce preload, control hypertension, and relieve ischemia in patients undergoing general anesthesia for coronary bypass surgery is usually in the range of 0.5 to 1.5 μg/kg/min. Hypotension may be treated by the administration of an α-agonist such as methoxamine to ensure that coronary perfusion pressure is maintained. Nitroglycerin readily migrates into plastic and, thus, it is important to use glass bottles for dilution. In addition, nitroglycerin is adsorbed by many of the intravenous administration sets used for automated infusion, and thus, the dose may vary with time of administration.

TOPICAL NITROGLYCERIN AND NITRATE TOLERANCE

To facilitate the chronic administration of nitroglycerin, topical administration has been developed starting with nitroglycerin ointment. More recently, nitroglycerin patches have become available and have received widespread use. These patches release nitroglycerin at a constant rate which is absorbed through the skin and produce sustained nitroglycerin plasma concentrations. However, although a good hemodynamic response is obtained to a single patch application, it appears that continuous topical use rapidly results in tolerance to nitroglycerin's hemodynamic effects. This tolerance results in total loss of nitroglycerin's hemodynamic effects. It appears that, by avoiding continuous administration and, for example, removing the patch during the night, the development of tolerance can be prevented.

Isosorbide Dinitrate

Isosorbide dinitrate differs from nitroglycerin in its longer terminal half-life of 20 minutes following intravenous administration or 64 minutes following sublingual administration. It undergoes extensive first-pass metabolism by the liver to isosorbide-5-mononitrate and isosorbide-2-mononitrate which have greater activity than isosorbide dinitrate. In addition, the half-life of the 5- and 2-mononitrate metabolites is longer than that of the parent drug (4.2 h for the 5-mononitrate and 1.9 h for the 2-mononitrate). The longer half-life of both isosorbide dinitrate and its metabolites gives this agent some advantage during chronic oral therapy, but the longer half-life may also increase the likelihood of nitrate tolerance developing as has been seen with nitrate patches.

Although isosorbide dinitrate has been used intravenously, its longer half-life and that of its metabolite will make its duration of action longer than that of nitroglycerin; however, it is stable in solution and does not require special preparation. A continuous infusion of 1.5 to 6.0 μg/kg/min has been used postoperatively to control hypertension.

SEROTONIN ANTAGONISTS: KETANSERIN

Ketanserin is a serotonin antagonist which selectively binds to the serotonin S_2-receptors. Stimulation of this receptor mediates the vasoconstrictive effects of serotonin, while stimulation of the S_1-receptor type causes vasodilation. Although the role of serotonin in hypertension has not been well defined, it appears that ketanserin by antagonizing the vasoconstrictor effect of serotonin is an effective antihypertensive. Ketanserin also binds to α_1-adrenergic receptors, and it was speculated that this action might account for ketanserin's hypotensive actions. However, at therapeutic doses, its α-blocking activity is not sufficient to account for the reduction in blood pressure produced.

Ketanserin has a relatively long half-life of 15 hours and is excreted principally by metabolism. Its major side effects are on the central nervous system and include headache, drowsiness, and lack of concentration. A more serious problem has been the description of prolongation of the QT interval on the electrocardiogram and the production of torsade de pointes ventricular tachycardia in a few patients.

ANGIOTENSIN CONVERTING ENZYME INHIBITORS

Captopril

The renin-angiotensin system is now recognized to have an important physiological role in the control of blood pressure (Fig. 15.12). Renin is secreted by cells in the juxta glomerular apparatus in the kidney in response to a fall in blood pressure. Renin then generates the decapeptide angiotensin I from angiotensinogen in blood by a proteolytic action. Angiotensin I (AI) is, in turn, converted into the octapeptide angiotensin II (AII) by the angiotensin-converting enzyme present in blood vessel walls. Angiotensin II then acts to raise blood pressure through both its potent vasoconstrictor effect and by stimulating the secretion of aldosterone which, acting through the kidney, causes sodium retention and expands intravascular fluid volume.

Captopril is an inhibitor of angiotensin

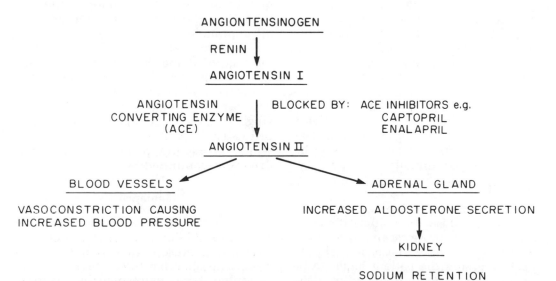

Figure 15.12.   The renin-angiotensin system and its control of blood pressure.

converting enzyme and therefore prevents the generation of angiotensin II. It acts by binding to the active site on the angiotensin converting enzyme where angiotensin I is bound. As captopril has 30,000 times greater affinity for this site than the natural substrate angiotensin I, it effectively excludes angiotensin I from the binding site. Angiotensin converting enzyme, however, is also responsible for the metabolism of bradykinin which is a potent vasodilator. It is therefore possible that captopril's ability to inhibit the breakdown of bradykinin may contribute to its hypotensive effect.

PHARMACOKINETICS

Approximately 60 to 70% of an oral dose of captopril is absorbed. Following absorption, captopril is excreted both through metabolism and by urinary excretion of unchanged drug. Tubular secretion is the primary route of renal excretion. The tubular secretion can be antagonized by probenecid, resulting in increased captopril concentrations.

The plasma protein binding of captopril is low (20 to 30%). Captopril's half life in patients with normal renal function is 1.7 hours but is increased in patients with impaired renal function, so that in patients whose creatinine clearance is less than 20 ml/min, the half-life is prolonged to 20 to 40 hours. Thus, captopril dosage should be reduced in patients with renal dysfunction. Early therapeutic studies with captopril included a large number of patients with renal dysfunction who received relatively high doses of captopril, and this probably accounts for the high incidence of side effects seen in such patients. In patients with normal renal function the frequency of adverse effects appears to be much lower than initially reported.

DOSAGE

Patients should receive 12.5 mg as an initial single dose. In volume-depleted patients such as those receiving concomitant diuretics, the initial dosage should be 6.25 mg, and the patient ought to be observed for 2 to 3 hours after drug admninstration in case hypotension develops. Initial chronic dosing of 6.25 to 12.5 mg 3 times daily can then be initiated. The effects of angiotensin converting enzyme inhibitors are increased by concurrent administration of diuretics, vasodilators, and calcium channel-blocking agents. The preoperative treatment of patients with captopril reduces the dose of nitroprusside required to produce deliberate hypotension during anesthesia.

ADVERSE EFFECTS

Adverse effects produced by captopril include some effects that appear to be common to other angiotensin-converting enzyme (ACE) inhibitors such as enalapril and some that appear to be more frequent with captopril. Both enalapril and captopril are associated with the production of cough, renal impairment, hypotension, and angioedema. However, skin rash, taste loss, and blood dyscrasias appear to be more common during captopril than enalapril therapy. On the other hand, ACE inhibitors do not produce many of the troublesome adverse effects seen with the older antihypertensives. For example, sedation, depression, sexual dysfunction, or reflex cardiac effects are not seen with ACE inhibitors. Probably because of their better side effect profile, patients report a significantly higher quality of life during captopril therapy than while receiving either methyldopa or propranolol.

Angiotensin II is important in maintaining adequate glomerular filtration when renal perfusion is reduced. In patients with bilateral renal artery stenosis or those with renal artery stenosis in a single kidney, both captopril and enalapril cause impairment of renal function which is usually reversible when the drug is discontinued.

Enalapril

Enalapril is an angiotensin converting enzyme inhibitor that lacks the sulfhydryl group present in captopril. It has been suggested that the sulfhydryl group of captopril may be responsible for some of captopril's adverse effects including the rash, taste disturbance, proteinuria, and leukopenia. Thus, enalapril would be expected to produce such side effects less often.

Enalapril is a prodrug and must be converted in vivo to the biologically active diacid moiety enalaprilat. Enalaprilat has been successfully used intravenously to lower blood pressure. However, because enalaprilat is poorly absorbed after oral administration (less than 10%), enalapril which is 60 to 70% absorbed by mouth is given orally. The principal site of conversion of enalapril to enalaprilat is in the liver, while the kidney is the principal site of excretion of both unchanged enalapril and enalaprilat.

After absorption, enalapril is rapidly metabolized to the active form, enalaprilat, resulting in enalapril itself having a relatively short half-life of less than 2 hours, while the half-life of the active form, endoprilat, is approximately 5 hours. After a single 10-mg dose, plasma angiotensin converting enzyme activity is 100% inhibited for 10 hours and more than 80% inhibited for at least 24 hours. Thus, enalapril can be given once daily, although at low doses, it may be wiser to use a twice daily regimen to ensure adequate blood pressure control throughout the day.

Enalapril's adverse effects include those that appear to be common to all ACE inhibitors including cough, hypotension, renal impairment, and angioedema. However, neutropenia, skin rash, taste loss (dysgeusia), and proteinuria occur less frequently than with captopril.

In addition to their use in the treatment of hypertension, ACE inhibitors have been shown by recent studies to be effective therapy for congestive heart failure, and they appear to reduce both symptoms and possibly mortality.

Lisinopril

Lisinopril is a long acting angiotensin converting enzyme inhibitor which is the lysine analogue of the active metabolite of enalapril (enalaprilate—see above). It has a half life of more than 12 hours and seems to be effective when given once daily. The usual daily dose is 10-40 mg/day but this should be reduced in patients with renal impairment as the drug is excreted only by the kidneys.

BIBLIOGRAPHY

Clonidine

Bousquet P, Schwartz J: Alpha-adrenergic drugs: pharmacological tools for the study of the central vasomotor control. *Biochem Pharmacol* 32:1459–1465, 1983.

Houston MC: Treatment of hypertensive emergencies and urgencies with oral clonidine loading and titration. *Arch Intern Med* 146:586–589, 1986.

Lowenstein J: Clonidine. *Ann Intern Med* 92:74–77, 1980.

Peters RW, Hamilton BP, Hamilton J, Kuzbida G, Pavlis R: Cardiac arrhythmias after abrupt clonidine withdrawal. *Clin Pharmacol Ther* 34:435–439, 1983.

Pettinger WA: Clonidine, a new antihypertensive drug. *N Engl J Med* 293:1179–1180, 1975.

Van Zwieten PA: Overview of alpha$_2$-adrenoceptor angonists with a central action. *Am J Cardiol* 57:3E–5E, 1986.

Van Zwieten PA, Timmermans P, Van Brummelen P: Role of alpha adrenoceptors in hypertension and in antihypertensive drug treatment. *Am J Med* 17–25, 1984.

Guanfacine

Sorkin EM, Heel RC: Guanfacine: a review of its pharmacodynamic and pharmacokinetic properties, and therapeutic efficacy in the treatment of hypertension. *Drugs* 31:301–336, 1986.

Methyldopa

Bobik A, Jennings G, Jackman G, Oddie C, Korner P: Evidence for a predominantly central hypotensive effect of α-methyldopa in humans. *Hypertension* 8:16–23, 1986.

Myhre E, Rugstad HE, Hansen T: Clinical pharmacokinetics of methyldopa. *Clin Pharmacokinet* 7:221–233, 1982.

White WB, Andreoli JW, Cohn RD: Alpha-methyldopa disposition in mothers with hypertension and in their breast-fed infants. *Clin Pharmacol Ther* 37:387–390, 1986.

Prazosin

Colucci WS: Alpha-adrenergic receptor blockade with prazosin. *Ann Intern Med* 97:67–77, 1982.

Graham RM, Pettinger WA: Prazosin. *N Engl J Med* 300:232–236, 1979.

Leenen FHH, Smith DL, Farkas RM, Reeves RA, Marquez-Julio A: Vasodilators and regression of left ventricular hypertrophy: hydralazine versus prazosin in hypertensive humans. *Am J Med* 82:969–978, 1987.

Stanaszek WF, Kellerman D, Brogden RN, Rumankiewicz JA: Prazosin update: a review of its pharmacological properties and therapeutic use in hypertension and congestive heart failure. *Drugs* 25:339–384, 1983.

Vincent J, Meredith PA, Reid JL, Elliott HL, Rubin PC: Clinical pharmacokinetics of prazosin—1985. *Clin Pharmacokinet* 10:144–154, 1985.

Terazosin

Kyncl JJ: Pharmacology of terazosin. *Am J Med* 80:12–19, 1986.

Sonders RC: Pharmacokinetics of terazosin. *Am J Med* 80:20–24, 1986.

Indoramin

Holmes B, Sorkin EM: Indoramin: a review of its pharmacodynamic and pharmacokinetic properties, and therapeutic efficacy in hypertension and related vascular, cardiovascular, and airway diseases. *Drugs* 31:467–499, 1986.

Shanks RG: The clinical pharmacology of indoramin. *J Cardiovasc Pharmacol* 8:S8–S15, 1986.

Guanethidine

Mitchell JR, Cavanaugh JH, Arias L, Oates JA: Guanethidine and related agents. III. Antagonism by drugs which inhibit the norepinephrine pump in man. *J Clin Invest* 49:1596–1604, 1970.

Woosley RL, Nies AS: Guanethidine. *N Engl J Med* 295:1053–1057, 1976.

Guanadrel

Finnerty FA Jr, Brogden RN: Guanadrel: a review of its pharmacodynamic and pharmacokinetic properties and therapeutic use in hypertension. *Drugs* 30:22–31, 1985.

Vasodilators

Koch-Weser J: Vasodilator drugs in the treatment of hypertension. *Arch intern Med* 133:1017–1027, 1974.

Tarazi RC, Dustan HP, Bravo EL, Niarchos AP: Vasodilating drugs: contrasting haemodynamic effects. *Clin Sci Mol Med* 51:575s–578s, 1976.

Hydralazine

Koch-Weser J: Hydralazine. *N Engl J Med* 295:320–323, 1978.

Ludden TM, McNay JL Jr, Shepherd AMM, Lin MS: Clinical pharmacokinetics of hydralazine. *Clin Pharmacokinet* 7:185–205, 1982.

Minoxidil

Bryan RK, Hoobler SW, Rosenzweig J, Weller JM: Effect of minoxidil on blood pressure and hemodynamics in severe hypertension. *Am J Cardiol* 39:796–801, 1977.

Mitchell HC, Pettinger WA: Long term treatment of refractory hypertensive patients with minoxidil. *JAMA* 239:2131–2138, 1978.

Diazoxide

McDonald AJ, Smith G, Woods JW, Perry M, Danielson BD: Intravenous diazoxide therapy in hypertensive crisis. *Am J Cardiol* 40:409–415, 1977.

Ram CVS, Kaplan NM: Individual titration of diazoxide dosage in the treatment of severe hypertension. *Am J Cardiol* 43:627–630, 1979.

Thien TA, Huysmans FTM, Gerlag PGG, Koene RAP, Wijdeveld PGAB: Diazoxide infusion in severe hypertension and hypertensive crisis. *Clin Pharmacol Ther* 25:795–799, 1979.

Pinacidil

Carlsen JE, Kardel T, Jensen H, Tango M, Trap-Jensen J: Pinacidil, a new vasodilator: pharmacokinetics and pharmacodynamics of a new retarded release tablet in essential hypertension. *Eur J Clin Pharmacol* 25:557–561, 1983.

Carlsen JE, Kardel T, Lund JO, McNair A, Trap-Jensen J: Acute hemodynamic effects of pinacidil and hydralazine in essential hypertension. *Clin Pharmacol Ther* 37:253–259, 1985.

Shahenn O, Patel J, Avant GR, Wood AJJ: Effect of cirrhosis and debrisoquin phenotype on the disposition and effects of pinacidil. *Clin Pharmacol Ther* 40:650–655, 1986.

Adenosine

Gonzalez-Miranda F, Juarez JB, Santos ML, Feria M: Adenosine/ATP and induced hypotension. *Anesth Analg* 63:538–546, 1984.

Owall A, Gordon E, Lagerkranser M, Lindquist C, Rudehill A, Sollevi A: Clinical experience with adenosine for controlled hypotension during cerebral aneurysm surgery. *Anesth Analg* 66:229–234, 1987.

Sollevi A, Lagerkranser M, Irestedt L, Gordon E, Lindquist C: Controlled hypotension with adenosine in cerebral aneurysm surgery. *Anesthesiology* 61:400–405, 1984.

Watt AH, Routledge PA: Adenosine: an importance beyond ATP. *Br Med J* 293:1455–1456, 1986.

Ketanserin

Aldariz AE, Romero H, Baroni M, Baglivo H, Esper RJ: QT prolongation and torsade de pointes ventricular tachycardia produced by ketanserin. *PACE* 9:836–841, 1986.

Heykants J, Van Peer A, Woestenborghs R, Gould S, Mills J: Pharmacokinetics of ketanserin and its metabolite ketanserin-ol in man after intravenous, intramuscular, and oral administration. *Eur J Clin Pharmacol* 31:343–350, 1986.

Janssen PAJ: Pharmacology of potent and selective S_2-serotonergic antagonists. *Cardiovasc Pharmacol* 7:S2–S11, 1985.

Nitroprusside

Beford RF. Sodium nitroprusside: hemodynamic dose-response during enflurane and morphine anesthesia. *Anesth Analg* 58:174–178, 1979.

Bedford RF, Berry FA Jr, Longnecker DE: Impact of propranolol on hemodynamic response and blood cyanide levels during nitroprusside infusion: prospective study in anesthetized man. *Anesth Analg* 58:466–469, 1979.

Cohn JN, Burke LP: Nitroprusside. *Ann Intern Med* 91:752–757, 1979.

Cottrell JE, Casthely P, Brodie JD, Patel K, Lkein A, Turndorf H: Prevention of nitroprusside-induced cyanide toxicity with hydroxocobalamin. *N Engl J. Med* 298: 809–811, 1978.

Cottrell JE, Illner P, Kittay ML, Steele JM, Lowenstein J, Turndorf H: Rebound hypertension after sodium nitroprusside-induced hypotension. Clin Pharmacol Ther 27:32–36, 1980.

Dean CR, Maling T, Dargie HJ, Reid JL, Dollery CT: Effect of propranolol on plasma norepinephrine during sodium nitroprusside-induced hypotension. Clin Pharmacol Ther 27:156–164, 1980.

Durrer JD, Lie KI, Van Capelle FJL, Durrer D: Effect of sodium nitroprusside on mortality in acute myocardial infarction. N Engl J Med 306:1121–1128, 1982.

Khambatta HJ, Stone JG, Khan E: Propranolol alters renin release during nitroprusside induced hypotension and prevents hypertension on discontinuation of nitroprusside. Anesth Analg 60:569–573, 1981.

Lagerkranser M, Gordon E, Rudehill A: Cardiovascular effects of sodium nitroprusside in cerebral aneurysm surgery. Acta Anaesth Scand 24:426–432, 1980.

Lawson NW, Thompson DS, Nelson CL, Flacke JW, Seifen AB: A dosage nomogram for sodium nitroprusside-induced hypotension under anesthesia. Anesth Analg 55:574–581, 1976.

Lin MS, McNay JL, Shepherd AMM, Keeton TK: Effects of hydralazine and sodium nitroprusside on plasma catecholamines and heart rate. Clin Pharmacol Ther 34:474–480, 1983.

McDowall DG, Keaney NP, Turner JM, Lane JR, Okuda Y: The toxicity of sodium nitroprusside. Br J Anaesth 46:327–332, 1974.

Palmer RF, Lasseter KC: Sodium nitroprusside. N Engl J Med 292:294–297, 1975.

Schulz V: Clinical pharmacokinetics of nitroprussides, cyanide, thiosulphate, and thiocyanate. Clin Pharmacol 9:239–251 1984.

Tinker JH, Michenfelder JD: sodium nitroprusside: pharmacology, toxicology, and therapeutics. Anesthesiology 45:340–354, 1976.

Wildsmith JAW, Drummond GB, MacRae WR: Blood-gas changes during induced hypotension with sodium nitroprusside. Br J Anaesth 47:1205–1211, 1975.

Will RJ, Walker OM, Traugott RC, Treasure RL: Sodium nitroprusside and propranolol therapy for management of postcoarctectomy hypertension. J Thorac Cardiovasc Surg 75:722–724, 1978.

Wood M, Hyman S, Wood AJJ: A clinical study of sensitivity to sodium nitroprusside during controlled hypotensive anesthesia in young and elderly patients. Anesth Analg 66:132–136, 1987.

Nitroglycerin

Bogaert MG: Clinical pharmacokinetics of glyceryl trinitrate following the use of systemic and topical preparations. Clin Pharmacokinet 12:1–11, 1987.

Chestnut JS, Albin MS, Gonzales-Abola E, Newfield P, Marroon JC: Clinical evaluation of intravenous nitroglycerin for neurosurgery. J Neurosurg 48:704–711, 1978.

Cossum PA, Galbraith AJ, Roberts MS, Boyd GW: Loss of nitroglycerin from intravenous infusion sets. Lancet 2:349–350, 1978.

Herling IM: Intravenous nitroglycerin: clinical pharmacology and therapeutic considerations. Am Heart J 108:141–149, 1984.

Kaplan JA, Dunbar RW, Jones EL: Nitroglycerin infusion during coronary-artery surgery. Anesthesiology 45:14–21, 1976.

Ludbrook PA, Byrne JD, Kurnik PB, McKnight RC: Influence of reduction of preload and afterload by nitroglycerin on left ventricular diastolic pressure-volume relations and relaxation in man. Circulation 56:937–943, 1977.

McNiff EF, Yacobi A, Young-Chang FM, Golden LH, Goldfarb A, Fung HL: Nitroglycerin pharmacokinetics after intravenous infusion in normal subjects. J Pharm Sci 70:1054–1058, 1981.

Meretoja OA: Haemodynamic effects of combined nitroglycerin and dobutamine infusions after coronary by-pass surgery. Acta Anaesth Scand 24:211–215, 1980.

Murad F: Cyclic guanosine monophosphate as a mediator of vasodilation. J Clin Invest 78:1–5, 1986.

Parker JO: Nitrate therapy in stable angina pectoris. N Engl J Med in press, 1987.

Sorkin EM, Brogden RN, Romankiewicz JA: Intravenous glyceryl trinitrate (nitroglycerin), a review of its pharmacological properties and therapeutic efficacy. Drugs 27: 45–80, 1984.

Tobias MA: Comparison of nitroprusside and nitroglycerine for controlling hypertension during coronary artery surgery. Br J Anaesth 53:891–897, 1981

Isosorbide Dinitrate

Cattaneo SM, Leier CV: Intravenous isosorbide dinitrate in the management of acute hypertension following cardiopulmonary bypass. Soc Thorac Surg 33:345–353, 1982.

Morrison RA, Wiegand UW, Jahnchen E, Hohmann D, Bechtold H, Meinertz T, Fung HL: Isosorbide dinitrate kinetics and dynamics after intravenous sublingual, and percutaneous dosing in angina. Clin Pharmacol Ther 33:747–756, 1983.

Parker JO, Farrell B, Lahey KA, Moe G: Effect of intervals between doses on the development of tolerance to isosorbide dinitrate. N Engl J Med 316: 1440–1444, 1987.

Straehl P, Galeazzi RL, Soliva M: Isosorbide 5-mononitrate and isosorbide 2-mononitrate kinetics after intravenous and oral dosing. Clin Pharmacol Ther 36:485–492, 1984.

Captopril

Cooper RA: Captopril-associated neutropenia: who is at risk? Arch intern Med 143:659–660, 1983.

Duchin KL, Singhvi SM, Willard DA, Migdalof BH, McKinstry DN: Captopril kinetics. Clin Pharmacol Ther 31:452–458, 1982.

Johnston CI, Arnolda L, Hiwatari M: Angiotensin-converting enzyme inhibitors in the treatment of hypertension. Drugs 27:271–277, 1984.

Singhvi SM, Duchin LK, Willard DA, McKinstry DN, Migdalof BH: Renal handling of captopril: effect of probenecid. Clin Pharmacol Ther 32:182–189, 1982.

Suarez M, Ho PWL, Johnson ES, Perez G: Angioneurotic edema, agranulocytosis, and fatal septicemia following captopril therapy. *Am J Med* 81:336–338, 1986.

Taguma Y, Kitamoto Y, Futaki G, Ueda H, Monma H, Ishizaki M, Takahashi H, Sekino H, Sasaki Y: Effect of captopril on heavy proteinuria in azotemic diabetics. *N Engl J Med* 313:1617–1620, 1985.

Vidt DG, Bravo EL, Fouad FM: Captopril. *N Engl J Med* 306:214–219, 1982.

Woodside J, Garner L, Bedfor RF, Sussman MD, Miller ED, Longnecker DE, Epstein RM: Captopril reduces the dose requirement for sodium nitroprusside induced hypotension. *Anesthesiology* 60:413–417, 1984.

Enalapril

Cleland JGF, Dargie HJ, McAlpine H, Ball SG, Morton JJ, Robertson JIS, Ford I: Severe hypotension after first dose of enalapril in heart failure. *Br Med J* 291:1309–1312, 1985.

Dipette DJ, Ferraro JC, Evans RR, Martin M: Enalaprilat, an intravenous angiotensin-converting enzyme inhibitor, in hypertensive crises. *Clin Pharmacol Ther* 38:199–204, 1985.

Johnston CI, Arnolda L, Hiwatari M: Angiotensin-converting enzyme inhibitors in the treatment of hypertension. *Drugs* 27:271–277, 1984.

Kubo SH, Cody RJ: Clinical pharmacokinetics of the angiotensin converting enzyme inhibitors. *Clin Pharmacokinet* 10:377–391, 1985.

Marre M, Leblanc H, Suarez L, Guyenne T, Menard J, Passa P: Converting enzyme inhibition and kidney function in normotensive diabetic patients with persistent microalbuminuria. *Br Med J* 294:1448–1452, 1987.

Packer M, Lee WH, Yushak M, Medina N: Comparison of captopril and enalapril in patients with severe chronic heart failure. *N Engl J Med* 315:847–853, 1986.

Todd PA, Heel RC: Enalapril: a review of its pharmacodynamic and pharmacokinetic properties, and therapeutic use in hypertension and congestive heart failure. *Drugs* 31:198–248, 1986.

Miscellaneous

Langer SZ, Cavero I, Massingham R: Recent developments in noradrenergic neurotransmission and its relevance to the mechanism of action of certain antihypertensive agents. *Hypertension* 2:372–382, 1980.

Prys-Roberts C, Meloche R, Foex P: Studies of anaesthesia in relation to hypertension. I. Cardiovascular responses of treated and untreated patients. *Br J Anaesth* 43:122–137, 1971.

16

Antiarrhythmic Drugs

DAN M. RODEN
RAYMOND L. WOOSLEY

Abnormalities of cardiac rhythm are a common occurrence in patients undergoing anesthesia; with sophisticated monitoring techniques, arrhythmias can be detected in over 60% of patients. Most are generally benign supraventricular arrhythmias, but catastrophic events such as unheralded ventricular fibrillation in an otherwise healthy patient can occur. The basic mechanisms responsible for the genesis of most arrhythmias remain conjectural and, thus, the mode of action of antiarrhythmic drugs is unclear. Table 16.1 groups these agents largely according to their effects on single cells or Purkinje fibers. In general, these drugs block specific transmembrane ion currents to produce their effects. Despite such widely used classifications, treatment remains empiric. The most important prin-

Table 16.1.
Electrophysiologic Properties of Antiarrhythmic Drugs*

Electrophysiologic property	Speed of dissociation from sodium channels	Effects on repolarization in vitro	Electrocardiographic effects
Fast sodium channel blockade (class I)			
Quinidine like (Ia)	Intermediate		
Quinidine		↑APD†	↑QT
Procainamide		↑ERP	Slight ↑QRS
Disopyramide		↑ERP/APD	
Lidocaine like (Ib)	Rapid		
Lidocaine		↑APD	Slight ↓QT
Tocainide		↑ERP	QRS unchanged
Mexiletine		↑ERP/APD	
Flecainide like (Ic)	Very slow		
Flecainide		↑ERP	↑PR
Encainide		APD unchanged‡	↑QRS
Lorcainide		↑ERP/APD	± ↑QT (2° ↑QRS)
Propafenone			
Indecainide			
β-Blockade (class II)			↓Heart Rate ↑PR
Primary repolarization-prolonging action (class III)			
Amiodarone		↑APD‡	↑QT
Bretylium		↑ERP	(↓Heart rate§)
Sotalol			
N-Acetylprocainamide			
Clofilium			
Calcium channel blockade (class IV)			↓Heart rate ↑PR

*Many agents on this list have multiple actions (e.g., amiodarone also blocks sodium channels, and sotalol is a β-blocker).
†APD, action-potential duration; ERP, effective refractory period; ERP/APD, ratio of ERP to APD.
‡Some studies have indicated discordance between effects on repolarization in Purkinje and ventricular muscle tissue: class Ic drugs may actually prolong APD in muscle, while amiodarone may shorten APD in Purkinje tissue.
§Amiodarone and sotalol both also slow sinus rate; amiodarone prolongs PR and QRS.

Table 16.2.
Factors Associated with the Occurrence of Arrhythmias

Acute (reversible)
  Myocardial ischemia
  Hypoxemia
  Acidosis
  Alkalosis
  Hypokalemia
  Hyperkalemia
  Hypercarbia
  Hypocalcemia
  Hypothermia/hyperthermia
  Tracheal intubation
  Prsence of intracardiac catheters
  Chest trauma
  Thoracic, cardiac, adrenal, neurosurgical procedures
  Psychic stress
Drugs
  Digitalis intoxication
  Antiarrhythmic agents (not necessarily in excess)
  Theophylline
  Catecholamines (including topical pressors and over-the-counter decongestants)
  Anesthetic agents
  Succinylcholine
  Tricyclic antidepressants
  Phenothiazines
  Anorexiants
Chronic (disease related)
  Myocardial disease, especially ischemic heart disease
  Congestive heart failure of any etiology
  Other types of heart disease (Wolff-Parkinson-White syndrome, long QT syndromes, mitral valve prolapse)
  Chronic lung disease (usually atrial arrhythmias)
  Thyrotoxicosis
  Tetanus
  Cerebrovascular injury

ciples of antiarrhythmic therapy are, first, to identify and correct any precipitating factor and, second, to use antiarrhythmic drugs with a clear understanding of their indications, toxicity, and clinical pharmacokinetics.

FACTORS ASSOCIATED WITH THE DEVELOPMENT OF ARRHYTHMIAS

Factors that can be associated with the development of arrhythmias are listed in Table 16.2. Changes in normal homeostasis, particularly myocardial ischemia, hypoxemia, and respiratory acidosis, must always be considered when arrhythmias occur intraoperatively. In addition, certain drugs, including inhalational anesthetic agents, may precipitate arrhythmias. Modern anesthetic agents can be administered in concentrations that usually do not produce arrhythmias. However, the concomitant use of catecholamines and the halogenated hydrocarbons such as halothane can produce ventricular arrhythmias. Figure 16.1 shows the comparative interaction of epinephrine with enflurane, isoflurane, and

Figure 16.1. The interaction of epinephrine with enflurane, isoflurane and halothane in humans. Approximately 3 times as much epinephrine is required to produce three or more premature ventricular contractions in 50% of patients during isoflurane as during halothane anesthesia, with enflurane probably comparable to isoflurane in this regard. However, lidocaine given with epinephrine seems to protect against ventricular arrhythmias. With permission from Johnston R R, Eger EI, Wilson C. The interaction of epinephrine with enflurane, isoflurane and halothane in man. *Anesth Analg* 55:709–712, 1976.)

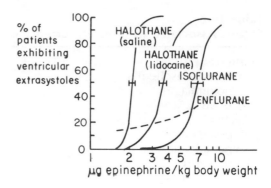

halothane in humans (see Chapter 9 and 13). Halothane may also potentiate theophylline-induced ventricular arrhythmias, but the most common rhythm disturbance seen with halothane is an accelerated A-V nodal rhythm due to sinus node depression and enhancement of A-V nodal pacemakers.

Excessive dosages of antiarrhythmic agents and the accidental intravascular injection of local anesthetics (with or without epinephrine) can cause serious myocardial depression and arrhythmias. In addition, most antiarrhythmic agents depress myocardial function; this effect can be potentiated by other perioperative factors and disturbances of cardiac rhythm may ensue. Combinations of antiarrhythmic agents may occasionally be effective, but should only be tried if single agents fail. The risk of additive toxicity without additional efficacy appears to be highest with concomitant use of agents with similar electrophysiological properties (see Table 16.1). An usual and potentially important exception is in vitro interaction of lidocaine and bupivacaine. Although it has long been recognized that accidental intravascular injection of bupivacaine may be associated with cardiovascular collapse, there has been renewed interest in the cardiotoxicity of bupivacaine (see Chapters 11 and 12). In in vitro studies, the drug is a potent sodium channel blocker and, interestingly, its effects are partially revers-

ible by the addition of lidocaine, another sodium channel blocker. No data are yet available to indicate whether lidocaine might be an antidote to clinical bupivacaine toxicity, but these experimental data do indicate the potential practical utility of a detailed understanding of the interactions of drugs and ion channels at the most basic level.

TREATMENT OF ABNORMALITIES OF CARDIAC RATE AND RHYTHM

General Considerations

The first step in antiarrhythmic therapy is the identification of the type of rhythm disturbance present and the removal, if possible, of any precipitating cause. Only then should drug therapy proceed. Table 16.3 describes the drug treatment of common abnormalities of cardiac rate and rhythm.

Sinus Bradycardia

Sinus bradycardia is usually benign, although treatment with atropine or pacing may occasionally be required if there is associated hypotension. However, it is important to understand that sinus bradycardia occurring suddenly during surgery is abnormal and may be due to hypoxia and improper ventilation, and the appropriate means should be taken to correct this situation.

Sinus Tachycardia

Sinus tachycardia (sinus rate > 100/ min in an adult) may be caused by a spectrum of underlying disorders, including congestive heart failure, hypovolemia, hypoxemia, thyrotoxicosis, sepsis, and anxiety. Therapy should be directed at the underlying cause, and agents to slow heart rate should not be used unless a diagnosis is established and it is clear that treatment is unlikely to be detrimental. If, for example, sinus tachycardia is present because of congestive heart failure, β-blockade could be disastrous by withdrawing the sympathetic drive required to maintain cardiac output.

Atrial Ectopic Beats

Atrial ectopic beats occur when the pacemaker of the heart arises in the atrium but outside the sinus node. Isolated premature atrial contractions usually do not require specific therapy. The nodal rhythm that may occur with halothane administration is similarly benign. Chaotic atrial rhythms are often associated with poor oxygenation, especially in patients with chronic lung disease. No specific antiarrhythmic therapy is indicated, and digitalis administration may actually be harmful. Limited reports have recently suggested a role for verapamil in multifocal atrial tachycardia, but

Table 16.3.
Treatment of Abnormalities of Cardiac Rate and Rhythm

Abnormality	Acute therapy (if hemodynamically compromising)	Maintenance therapy
Sinus bradycardia	Pacemmaker (atropine) (isoproterenol)	
Sinus tachycardia	Treat underlying cause	
Paroxysmal supraventricular tachycardia (A-V nodal reentry)	DC countershock, verapamil, vagomimetics, digitalis, propranolol, esmolol pacing	Propranolol, verapamil, digitalis
Wolff-Parkinson-White-associated supraventricular arrhythmias	DC countershock, verapamil; consider lidocaine or procainamide to slow accessory pathway conduction	Encainide, flecainide, sotalol, amiodarone(digitalis, verapamil, β-blockers may be contraindicated)
Atrial flutter, fibrillation	DC countershock, digitalis, verapamil, propranolol, esmolol, pacing (atrial flutter)	To control rate: digitalis, verapamil, propranolol. To maintain sinus rhythm: quinidine, disopyramide, procainamide, amiodarone
Ventricular ectopic depolarizations (VEDS, PVCs)		Quinidine, procainamide, disopyramide, phenytoin, mexiletine, tocainide, encainide, flecainide, sotalol, propranolol, acebutolol
Ventricular tachycardia/ fibrillation	DC countershock, lidocaine, bretylium, procainamide, amiodarone	As for VEDs plus amiodarone
Digitalis-induced ventricular arrhythmias	Lidocaine, phenytoin, potassium (see text); avoid countershock, bretylium	

this agent is contraindicated in the face of coexisting severe heart failure, a common clinical situation.

Supraventricular Tachycardia

Supraventricular tachycardia is present when the atrial rate suddenly increases to a regular rate between 150 and 250 beats/min usually with normal intraventricular conduction. If this arrhythmia occurs in episodes, it is often termed paroxysmal atrial tachycardia (PAT). Detailed electrophysiologic studies have indicated that, in the vast majority of patients, this arrhythmia has one of two etiologies: reentry within the A-V node (60 to 70%) or reentry using an accessory pathway for ventriculo-atrial conduction (25%). Thus, the term PAT is now outdated, and these arrhythmias should be termed paroxysmal supraventricular tachycardias (PSVT). Patients with accessory pathways usually will have typical preexcited QRS complexes (Wolff-Parksinson-White syndrome) during sinus rhythm but not during PSVT. However, about one-third will not have preexcited QRS complexes even in sinus rhythm. In a small number of patients, enhanced automaticity within the atrium will result in an arrhythmia superficially resembling typical PSVT. These patients will frequently show intermittent A-V block (extremely unusual in PSVT), abnormal P wave morphology and vector, and variable atrial rates, especially during the onset of the tachycardia. The commonest cause of this true paroxysmal atrial tachycardia is digitalis intoxication, although it can occur in patients with no other evidence of cardiac disease.

The primary consideration for treatment of these arrhythmias is the patient's hemodynamic status: carotid sinus massage should be tried but if hypotension, pulmonary edema, or myocardial ischemia develops, direct current (DC) countershock (at initially low energy) is the treatment of choice. Pressors (such as phenylephrine) and parasympathomimetic agents (edrophonium) may also be tried. Verapamil can convert PSVT to sinus rhythm in 75 to 95% of patients. Digitalis and/or propranolol may also be tried, but it should be recognized that intravenous propranolol plus verapamil can result in cardiac standstill. If the underlying mechanism is known or suspected to be dependent on an accessory A-V pathway, the treating physician must be aware that A-V blockers, such as verapamil, propranolol, or digitalis, while they do constitute the emergency drug treatment of choice, carry a risk: if atrial fibrillation develops, the ventricular rate can actually be increased by these drugs in patients with accessory pathways. Thus, continued cardiac monitoring is mandatory after treatment of PSVT. The automatic atrial tachycardia described above is generally best managed acutely by drugs which control the ventricular rate [digitalis (unless intoxication is suspected), propranolol, verapamil]; these agents do not usually convert the rhythm to normal, and sodium channel blockers (quinidine, encainide, flecainide), amiodarone, or surgical ablation is used if the arrhythmia is a chronic problem.

Atrial Flutter and Fibrillation

In *atrial flutter*, the atrial rate is regular at 250 to 350 beats/min, and there is usually some degree of atrioventricular block, so the ventricular rate is 100 to 180/min. The arrhythmia may be paroxysmal or sustained. DC countershock is the treatment of choice for atrial flutter causing hemodynamic compromise, while digitalis, propranolol, or verapamil may be used to slow ventricular response in less urgent cases. Specialized pacing techniques are useful in atrial flutter or PSVT but not in atrial fibriallation.

Atrial fibrillation is commonly due to underlying heart disease of rheumatic, thyrotoxic, ischemic, or alcholic etiology. Digitalis, propranolol, and verapamil have all been used to control the ventricular rate. DC countershock is also effective and should be used in atrial fibrillation producing hemodynamic compromise. Agents with vagolytic properties (Quinidine, disopyramide, and to a lesser extent procainamide) may enhance atrioventricular conduction and, thus, accelerate the ventricular response during atrial flutter or fibrillation; they should not be used in this setting prior to increasing A-V block with digitalization. However, these drugs, along with encainide, flecainide, and amiodarone, are often used to prevent recurrent atrial flutter or fibrillation. Patients with the Wolff-Parkinson-White syndrome and atrial fibrillation may develop extraordinarily rapid ventricular rates (e.g., >300/min). In this unusual situation, the treatments of choice are drugs which increase accessory pathway refractoriness (procainamide) or cardioversion, while A-V blockers are contraindicated since they may actually increase the ventricular rate and precipitate ventricular fibrillation.

Ventricular Arrhythmias

The primary aim in the treatment of ventricular arrhythmias is to remove or correct any underlying precipitating cause. Specific antiarrhythmic therapy may also be required while associated conditions are corrected. Occasionally, antiarrhythmic drug treatment can actually precipitate ventricular arrhythmias. Treatment is then critically dependent on recognition and withdrawal of the offending agents; further details of specific clinical syndromes are discussed below (long QT-associated arrhythmias: quinidine; increasing frequency of ventricular tachycardia: flecainide/encainide).

Isolated ventricular ectopic depolarizations (often termed VEDs, PVCs, or PVBs) are an extremely common finding in patients both with and without other underlying heart disease. Epidemiologic data suggest that VEDs in advanced ischemic heart disease identify the patient at risk for sudden death (presumably arrhythmia related). However, no data are available to suggest that chronic antiarrhythmic drug treatment reduces this risk. In fact, recently available data from a large multicenter, multinational trial have shown that suppression of VEDs by encainide or flecainide in patients with a history of myocardial infarction was associated with a 2- to 3-fold increased risk of sudden death in 1 year. On the other hand, VEDs arising *de novo* during surgery are a warning to search for underlying precipitating causes. This rhythm disturbance cannot be taken lightly, as progression to ventricular tachycardia and ventricular fibrillation may occur, particularly in the setting of myocardia ischemia. The proximity of the VED to the previous T wave and its morphology are not reliable indicators of malignancy.

Ventricular tachycardia is a life-threatening abnormality and requires immediate treatment. The ventricular rate is usually between 150 and 250 beats/min and may be paroxysmal or sustained. The vast majority of patients with ventricular tachycardia and all with ventricular fibrillation require DC countershock; when sinus rhythm is reestablished, such patients should be maintained on antiarrhythmic therapy, usually lidocaine, until their clinical condition stabilizes. Other parenteral agents which may prove useful in this setting are procainamide, bretylium, phenytoin, and amiodarone. An occasional patient may develop hemodynamically stable ventricular tachycardia; the response of such patients to pacing or antiarrhythmic drugs should be aggressively evaluated because this rhythm can rapidly degenerate to ventricular fibrillation. A distressingly common clinical error is to ascribe a wide complex tachycardia to a supraventricular mechanism if the patient is hemodynamically stable. The use of verapamil in patients with hemodynamically stable ventricular tachycardia almost inevitably results in cardiovascular collapse. A good clinical maxim is that wide complex tachycardia in older patients, particularly those with coronary artery disease, should be treated as ventricular tachycardia and not PSVT.

Anesthetic Considerations

Although arrhythmias during anesthesia and surgery are common, they are generally benign, well tolerated, and often do not require drug treatment. Arrhythmias occurring during anesthesia may be caused by mechanical stimulation (e.g., intubation), abnormalities of ventilation leading to hypercapnia or hypoxia, and the anesthetic agent itself. Thus, correction of these factors may control the arrhythmia and drug treatment will, therefore, be unnecessary.

Patients receiving chronic antiarrhythmic therapy who come to surgery should be evaluated on an individual basis, taking into account the type and severity of the arrhythmia and the agent(s) used to treat it. Some drugs (digitalis, procainamide, phenytoin, propranolol) can be continued parenterally, provided dose adjustments are made for differences in bioavailability. Others (quinidine, disopyramide) should not be used parenterally because of the risk of myocardial depression.

Digitalis should usually be continued in patients being treated for supraventricular arrhythmias. The patient with chronic ventricular arrhythmias preoperatively presents an unresolved problem. One approach is to continue effective therapy, bearing in mind the potential for increased adverse drug reactions in the perioperative period. In the patient not already on oral therapy, lidocaine can be used if necessary. However, as outlined above, in the absence of acute ischemia, such patients only require urgent treatment if arrhythmia frequency rises or more serious arrhythmias occur during surgery.

While the maintenance or institution of antiarrhythmic therapy is fairly common in the perioperative period, few data are available on changes in pharmacokinetics that may occur in this setting. Changes in cardiac output or liver blood flow might influence clearance, volume of distribution, or both. Concomitant drug therapy can profoundly alter response to drug therapy, for example, the enhanced neuromuscular blockade that results when d-tubocurarine is administered with most antiarrhythmic agents. Thus, the guidelines set forth below must be tempered by the knowledge that the perioperative period may be accompanied by recognized and unrecognized

changes in the drug pharmacokinetcs (see Chapter 1).

INDIVIDUAL ANTIARRHYTHMIC AGENTS

Lidocaine

Pharmacology. Lidocaine is the agent of choice for the acute suppression of most ventricular arrhythmias. Plasma concentrations required to produce an antiarrhythmic effect are generally greater than 1.5 μg/ml, and side effects occur more commonly once this concentration rises above 5 μg/ml. In conscious patients, these side effects include dysarthria, tremor, dysesthesia, and nonspecific mental disturbances. These symptoms may be useful in assessing adequacy of therapy in the absence of plasma concentration data. Similarly, the occurrence of such symptoms during local anesthesia with lidocaine is a warning that more serious toxicity (as a result of systemic absorption) may be imminent. *Higher concentrations* produce more serious adverse effects, primarily grand mal seizures and abnormalities of cardiac conduction, including asystole. Lidocaine should be administered with caution to patients in atrial flutter or fibrillation, since it occasionally accelerates the ventricular response; however, lidocaine may be very useful in decreasing the ventricular response during atrial fibrillation in patients whose A-V conduction is down an accessory pathway. Lidocaine decreases myocardial contractility, especially in excessive concentrations in patients with poor myocardial function.

Pharmacokinetics. Lidocaine should be used only intravenously in the therapy of arrhythmias. Its pharmacokinetc parameters are well described by a two-compartment open kinetic model following a single intravenous dose (see Chapter 11). The distribution half-life of lidocaine $(t_{1/2\alpha})$ is 8 minutes, while the elimination half-life $(t_{1/2\beta})$ is 90 to 110 minutes in normal humans and corresponds to the systemic elimination of lidocaine. This process is primarily by hepatic metabolism to the deethylated forms monoethylglycinexylidide (MEGX) and glycinexylidide (GX) which are subsequently excreted by the kidneys. There is some evidence that these metabolites may have pharmacological activity and, in particular, may be associated with the central nervous system side effects seen with lidocaine.

Suggested Dosage and Administration. Lidocaine is avidly removed from the blood as it passes through the liver, so that its clearance following intravenous administration is dependent on the amount of drug delivered to the liver; i.e., its clearance approximates liver blood flow. Reduction in liver blood flow will reduce lidocaine clearance and increase steady-state concentrations. Once the decision to use lidocaine has been made, therapy should be aimed at achieving therapeutic plasma concentrations rapidly and safely. This is generally done with a combination of doses designed to load the central and peripheral tissue compartments and the simultaneous institution of a maintenance regimen designed to replace losses due to drug metabolism by the liver (Fig. 16.2). The usual practice of administering a single loading dose of 100 mg may produce therapeutic plasma and myocardial concentrations transiently, but as distribution takes place, these concentrations fall rapidly into the subtherapeutic range in most patients. One possible solution to this problem is to simply use a larger single loading dose, but then unacceptably high initial plasma concentrations will result (Fig. 16.2B). The optimal way to administer the loading dose is by a series of loading boluses, each separated by 8 minutes (one $t_{1/2\alpha}$) from the preceding one, thus allowing distribution to take place. For patients without heart failure, an initial bolus of 100 mg should be administered, followed by three 50-mg boluses at 8-minute intervals for a total loading dose of 250 mg or 3 to 4 mg/kg. Each bolus should itself be administered over 2 to 3 minutes to prevent predistribution side effects. This approach rapidly provides an adequate loading dose and yet avoids the problem of ex-

cess dosing. Should side effects occur during loading, further boluses should not be administered.

Maintenance therapy should be instituted simultaneously with the first loading dose. The usual maintenance dosage for a normal individual is 20 to 60 μg/kg/min (1 to 4 mg/min) administered as a continuous intravenous infusion. Steady-state conditions will not be reached until four to five elimination half-lives have elapsed (see Chapter 1); similarly, any changes in maintenance infusion rates will attain new steady-state conditions four to five elimination half-lives later. It is important to recall that lidocaine elimination half-life is approximately 2 hours in normal individuals (and longer in certain disease states; see later in this chapter), and so steady-state conditions will not be reached for at least 8 to 10 hours. A loading dose will not alter the time required to reach steady state.

Precautions   and   Contraindications. Steady-state concentration (C_{ss}) is dependent only on the ratio of the rate of infusion to the drug's clearance (Cl), because

$$C_{ss} = \frac{\text{Rate of infusion}}{Cl}$$

However, the size of the loading dose is determined primarily by the volume of distribution (V_d) [loading dose = $V_d \times$ plasma concentration (C); see Chapter 1]. Volume of distribution is decreased in the presence of congestive heart failure, so that the loading dose should be halved. Clearance is determined primarily by liver blood flow, which is decreased in both congestive heart failure and liver disease. Thus, lidocaine maintenance infusion rates should be decreased in the presence of these disease states. Since half-life = $V_d \times 0.693/$ clearance, patients with liver disease tend to have the longest half-lives and so take the longest time to reach steady state. Conversely, patients with heart failure may have near normal elimination half-lives because of the reduction in both V_d and clearance. The ultimate

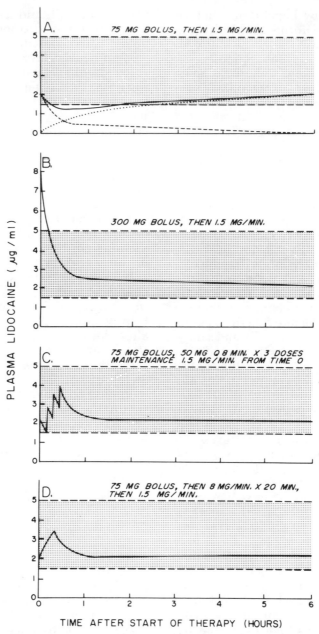

Figure 16.2. Plasma concentrations of lidocaine following various loading regimens. The *shaded area* represents the therapeutic range. *A* shows an inadequate single loading dose (– –, concentration due to bolus; ....., concentration due to infusion; ———; total concentration). Note that plasma concentrations fall into the usually ineffective range 10 minutes after the dose, and the maintenance infusion does not raise these levels into low therapeutic range until 1.5 hours later. A larger single bolus (*B*) avoids this dip, but produces toxic initial concentrations. *C* and *D* demonstrate multidose regimens which will provide adequate therapy from the first dose and avoid inadequate or excesssive concentrations. In any of the four cases, true steady state is only achieved after approximately 8 hours, a function of the half-life of elimination alone, and unaffected by the loading regimen.

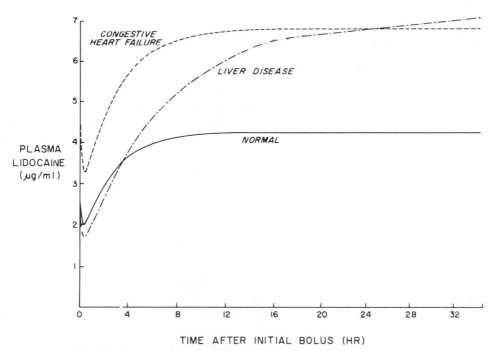

Figure 16.3. The effects of disease on lidocaine plasma levels. Heart failure is accompanied by reduced clearance and volume of distribution. Thus, the initial plasma concentrations are higher than normal (reduced V_d), and the steady-state concentration is higher than normal (reduced clearance). The half-life, dependent on both, may be only marginally prolonged so the time required to reach steady state is essentially unchanged (8 to 10 hours). Conversely, V_d is unchanged in liver disease (so the initial levels are normal), but clearance is reduced, leading to a higher steady-state concentration. In addition, elimination half-life (unlike in heart failure) is markedly prolonged, so well over 24 hours elapse before steady state is achieved.

steady-state concentration achieved (a function of clearance previously discussed) will be higher than desired in both disease states unless the maintenance dose is reduced (Fig. 16.3). It is important to note that lidocaine, like all antiarrhythmic agents, can exert a negative inotropic effect. Should the maintenance rate be excessive, this negative inotropic effect can decrease liver blood flow which, in turn, will decrease lidocaine clearance even further.

Lidocaine clearance is lower during chronic administration for greater than 24 hours than after a single dose. The reasons for this change are not clear, but possible explanations are inhibition of lidocaine metabolism by monoethylglycinexylidide and glycinexylidide or changes in protein binding. After 24 hours of therapy, plasma concentrations and symptoms should be monitored for lidocaine toxicity, and consideration should be given to decreasing the maintenance infusion rates. Renal disease does not significantly affect the clinical use of lidocaine. Table 16.4 lists situations where dosage adjustments of antiarrhythmic therapy may be required.

Drug Interactions. The negative inotropic effect that can occur during lidocaine therapy may be potentiated by other factors such as acid-base, electrolyte, or blood gas abnormalities; concomitant use of other myocardial depressant agents (including other antiarrhythmics and certain anesthetic agents); and preexisting myocardial disease. The combination of propranolol and lidocaine may be particularly dangerous in this regard since,

Table 16.4.
Situations Where Dosage Adjustment of Antiarrhythmic Drugs Are Required*

Lidocaine	Reduce dose	Congestive heart failure: reduce both loading and maintenance dose
		Liver disease: reduce maintenance dose
		Prolonged infusion: reduce maintenance dose
Procainamide	Reduce dose	Renal disease: monitor plasma procainamide and N-acetylprocainamide
		Congestive heart failure: reduce loading dose
Bretylium	Avoid in	Aortic stenosis, carotid obstruction, pulmonary hypertension, pheochromocytoma
	Reduce dose	Renal disease
Phenytoin	Reduce dose	Severe liver disease, therapy with barbiturates, carbamazepine, disulfiram, isoniazid, sulfonamides
Digitalis	Reduce dose	Quinidine therapy, advancing age, renal disease (digoxin), liver disease (digitoxin)
	Increase dose	Phenytoin therapy (digitoxin)
	Avoid in	Wolff-Parkinson-White-syndrome
Quinidine	Reduce dose	Advancing age
	Increase dose	Phenobarbital therapy, phenytoin therapy
	Avoid in	Long QT syndrome
Disopyramide	Reduce dose	Renal disease, liver disease
	Avoid in	Long QT syndrome, congestive heart failure, prostatism, glaucoma
Propanolol and other β-blockers	Reduce dose	Liver disease (propranolol); renal disease (sotalol)
	Avoid in	Congestive heart failure, bronchospasm, sinus node disease, clonidine withdrawal, pheochromocytoma, epinephrine administration, antidiabetic therapy, verapamil therapy, depression (all β-blockers)
		Long QT syndrome (sotalol)
Verapamil	Avoid in	Sinus or A-V node dysfunction, digitalis (use with caution), congestive heart failure
Mexiletine	Reduce dose	Liver disease
Tocainide	Reduce dose	Renal disease
Encainide	Reduce dose	Renal disease
Flecainide	Reduce dose	Renal disease
	Avoid in	Congestive heart failure

*All antiarrhythmic agents can reduce cardiac output, Bretylium and amiodarone are exceptions. Most antiarrhythmic agents will increase the duration of neuromuscular blockade induced by d-tubocurarine (see text). Other clinical states dictating caution (but not necessarily adjustment of antiarrhythmic dosing) are:

Lidocaine	N_2O, halothane requirements reduced
Procainamide	Increased risk of neuromuscular blockade in myasthenia gravis (also quinidine and propranolol)
Bretylium	Supersensitivity to infused catecholamines; tricyclic antidepressants block adrenergic effects
Phenytoin	Marked changes in plasma protein binding accompany renal disease and hyperbilirubinemia: monitor free plasma concentration of phenytoin. Warfarin requirements may rise—monitor prothrombin time

in addition to its negative inotropic properties, propranolol administration decreases liver blood and hence lidocaine clearance as well.

In therapeutic concentrations, lidocaine decreases nitrous oxide and halothane requirements by 10 to 28%. The probable mechanism is by additive central nervous system sedation. The clinical implications are 2-fold. (a) The physician can take advantage of this observation to decrease the amount of anesthetic administered. (b) Patients who have received lidocaine for local anesthesia (and attain therapeutic plasma concentrations) followed by general anesthesia (for example, during parturition) may run the risk of increased anesthetic effect if this potential interaction is not recognized.

Pretreatment with barbiturates in dogs increases lidocaine metabolism by the liver; in addition, dogs treated with lidocaine and pentobarbital had a higher incidence of apnea than dogs treated with lidocaine alone. The clinical implications of these observations are unclear. Similarly, diazepam can prevent lidocaine-induced seizures in cats without altering antiarrhythmic efficacy or cardiovascular performance, but the dosage of lidocaine used was much higher than that used therapeutically. The duration of neuromuscular blockade induced by d-tubocurarine can be prolonged by as much as 25% in the presence of a number of antiarrhythmic agents, including lidocaine, procainamide, propranolol, and phenytoin (diphenylhydantoin).

Lidocaine Resistance. Lidocaine therapy should be declared ineffective if arrhythmia continues in the face of adequate dosing, as assessed by symptoms or plasma concentrations. Cookbook therapy will be associated with a greater incidence of "lidocaine resistance" and "lidocaine toxicity" than therapy based on a sound knowledge of its pharmacokinetics. Guidelines to avoid problems during lidocaine therapy include:

1. Therapy should not be abandoned because no response or only a transient reponse is seen after an initial bolus.
2. It is important to appreciate that accumulation in plasma occurs for four to five elimination half-lives after the institution of maintenance therapy. This can result in toxicity many hours after the start of therapy, and may only manifest itself as nonspecific mental changes such as confusion or lethargy and, if unrecognized, can be misdiagnosed as "ICU psychosis" or even structural central nervous system disease.
3. Conversely, should the eventual steady state achieved be subtherapeutic, this may only become apparent many hours after the initiation of seemingly optimal therapy. Lidocaine resistance or, more seriously, other diagnoses, such as recurrent myocardial ischemia, might then be entertained. The approach in this situation is to administer small (25 mg) incremental boluses until mild side effects or acceptable plasma concentrations are noted; if a response is seen, the maintenance infusion rate can then be raised. (Raising the maintenance infusion rate in this setting without administering the incremental bolus will result in the eventual attainment of a new higher steady state, but only many hours later.)
4. The common practice of "tapering" lidocaine is based on the misconception that li-

Digitalis	Risk of digitalis intoxication increased with: hypokalemia; hypercalcemia; hypoxemia; hypomagnesemia; acid-base disturbances; hypothyroidism; hypertropic cardiomyopathy; cor pulmonale; acute myocardial infarction; administration to the digitalized patient of: catecholamines, calcium, thyroid hormone, bretylium
Quinidine	Myasthenia gravis (see procainamide)
Disopyramide	Warfarin requirements may rise—monitor prothrombin time
Propranolol	Myasthenia gravis (see procainamide)
Encainide, flecainide	Risk of severe arrhythmia exacerbation in patients with history of sustained ventricular tachycardia and left ventricular dysfunction

docaine is eliminated very rapidly. In fact, when the maintenance dosage is changed, the new steady state is not reached until at least 8 to 10 hours later. It seems more reasonable to stop therapy and observe the effect on rhythm over the subsequent 8 to 10 hours as lidocaine is eliminated.

5. Disease states may require major changes in dosing.

6. Plasma concentrations within or occasionally above the usual therapeutic range have been recorded during lidocaine administration for local anesthesia in many settings. Such concentrations may be clinically important in some drug interactions and may obscure underlying cardiac dysfunction by abolishing the acute onset of ventricular arrhythmias. In addition, accidental intravascular injection of a dose aimed at achieving only local anesthesia has been associated with death due to seizures or cardiac asystole.

Procainamide

Pharmacology. Procainamide is the drug of choice for the acute treatment of lidocaine-resistant ventricular arrhythmias. It is also useful in the therapy of some supraventricular arrhythmias, and it has been used in the treatment of malignant hyperthermia. It can be administered parenterally or orally. Antiarrhythmic effects are usually seen at plasma concentrations above 4 μg/ml. The concentration at which adverse effects occur is not as well defined. In acute studies, some investigators have used dosages that produce concentrations as high as 20 μg/ml, but levels in the range of 8 to 10 μg/ml often produce side effects during chronic therapy. This difference may be due in part to the production of the pharmacologically active metabolite N-acetylprocainamide (acecainide, trademarked NAPA) during chronic treatment. The major side effect during acute procainamide administration is hypotension, often related more to the rate of drug administration than to the dose and possibly refecting myocardial depression and/or a ganglionic blocking property. In addition, QRS and QT widening may occur during acute or chronic administration. If

these changes are pronounced (greater than 25 to 50% prolongation), they are often associated with life-threatening ventricular arrhythmias or hypotension. Side effects during chronic administration include headaches, anorexia, and nausea. In addition, many patients will develop antinuclear antibodies and eventually a lupus erythematosus-type syndrome with chronic administration. The major symptoms are fever, rash, athralgias, arthritis, and pleural and pericardial effusions (which can cause tamponade). This syndrome occurs more often among patients who are phenotypically slow acetylators of procainamide.

Pharmacokinetics. Procainamide is well absorbed following oral administration, but the time taken to achieve peak plasma concentrations is variable (range, 0.5 to 4 hours). Its elimination half-life is 3 to 4 hours in normal patients and is prolonged in patients with decreased renal function. Approximately one-half of a dose is eliminated unchanged by the kidneys, while the remainder (more in rapid acetylators) is metabolized in the liver, primarily to N-acetylprocainamide, prior to elimination by the kidneys.

Suggested Dosage and Administration. In the acute situation, an initial loading dose of 7 to 10 mg/kg should be administered intravenously. This can be accomplished by slow boluses of 100 mg every 5 minutes until the total load is given or, preferably, by a continuous infusion of 20 mg/min for 25 to 50 minutes. In either case, if hypotension occurs, the load should be stopped until blood pressure recovers; in addition, if no antiarrhythmic effect and no adverse effects are seen after a full loading dose (0.6 to 1.0 g) has been given, an additional 5 mg/kg can be administered in the same manner. Maintenance therapy is 20 to 60 μg/kg/min and, as in the case of any drug, steady-state plasma concentrations are not achieved until 4 to 5 elimination half-lives have elapsed, i.e., 12 to 20 hours after maintenance therapy is started or the rate of infusion altered.

While oral therapy is very effective in many patients, doses must be administered every 3 to 4 hours because of the narrow therapeutic window and rapid elimination. A slow release formulation permits dosing every 6 hours; the wax matrix of these tablets often appears in the stool. The adequacy of procainamide absorption should be confirmed by plasma concentration monitoring. The usual starting maintenance dosage is 250 to 500 mg every 3 to 4 hours or 500 mg of slow-release procainamide every 6 hours; if this does not achieve arrhythmia suppression, the dosage can be increased until an antiarrhythmic effect is seen or side effects occur. Monitoring plamsa concentration just before a dose (when arrhythmia is most likely to recur) can be helpful in assessing the adequacy of therapy. If oral therapy is initiated after intravenous therapy, sudden rises in plasma concentration can be avoided by stopping the continuous infusion, waiting 2 to 3 hours, and then starting chronic oral therapy. An oral loading dose is not recommended, since if the clinical situation is urgent enough to require immediate therapy, the intravenous route is preferred. Procainamide can be administered intramuscularly, but this route is rarely if ever indicated.

Precautions and Contraindications. Procainamide and N-acetylprocainamide elimination rates are prolonged in the presence of renal failure. In this setting, intravenous maintenance doses must be reduced. Chronic oral therapy in patients with renal failure requires reduced dosages and less frequent (8 to 12 hours) dosing. In either case, monitoring plasma concentrations of both procainamide and N-acetylprocainamide can be helpful. N-acetylprocainamide has been administered alone to humans: antiarrhythmic effects occurred at concentrations greater than 9 μg/ml, while gastrointestinal side effects occurred above 19 μg/ml. Generalizations on what combination of concentrations is optimal for chronic procainamide therapy are not possible because it is impossible to know how much each agent contributes to antiarrhythmic activity and to toxicity in an individual. It is important to be aware that unexpected antiarrhythmic effects or unexpected side effects during procain-

amide administration may be due to excessive concentrations of N-acetylprocainamide. Plasma concentrations above 20 μg/ml of N-acetylprocainamide in the presence of usual concentrations of procainamide are often toxic, causing gastrointestinal or central nervous system symptoms or hypotension.

The loading dose of procainamide should be reduced in the presence of congestive heart failure. In addition, such patients may be more susceptible to the negative inotropic effects of this and most other antiarrhythmic agents. The effect of liver disease on procainamide requirements is not known. Patients with myasthenia gravis appear to be at increased risk for worsening of neuromuscular blockade during procainamide therapy.

Drug Interactions. The neuromuscular blockade induced by d-tubocurarine may be potentiated by procainamide, but only at high concentrations.

Bretylium

Pharmacology. Bretylium is the only available antiarrhythmic agent which is a quaternary ammonium compound; the other drugs are amines. The unique structure may be responsible for the fact that bretylium is the only currently available agent which can reverse ventricular fibrillation in animal models. It is highly effective in the treatment of refractory ventricular arrhythmias in humans, but adverse effects which are direct extensions of its pharmacological activity frequently complicate its use. Following intravenous administration, bretylium is concentrated in the postganglionic adrenergic neuron, displacing norepinephrine. Further norepinephrine uptake is subsequently blocked. Thus, the major features of bretylium administration include an initial period of hypertension and worsening arrhythmias due to norepinephrine release followed by hypotension which is most pronounced in the upright position due to the subsequent blockade of norepinephrine reuptake. The orthostatic hypotension is accompanied by a suprasensitivity to exogenous catecholamines. The relationship between bretylium's adrenergic effects and its antiarrhythmic and antifibrillatory effects is unclear. Blockade of its uptake into the adrenergic neuron (for example, by tricyclic antidepressant drugs) reverses the adrenergic effects, but appears to leave the antiarrhythmic effects intact. Chronic oral bretylium therapy in combination with tricyclics has been effective but remains investigational, and the use of this agent is confined to parenteral treatment in the acute situation. A number of antifibrillatory agents (clofilium, meobentine) thought to lack the adrenergic blocking properties of bretylium are currently in clinical investigation.

A trial of bretylium therapy is indicated in the presence of life-threatening ventricular arrhythmias which are resistant to lidocaine. Authorities differ on whether such patients should receive a trial of procainamide before bretylium. Because of the prolonged period required to administer adequate doses of procainamide, bretylium may be desirable in life-threatening clinical situations. On the other hand, data from studies in animals indicate that bretylium's effects on cardiac electrophysiology are dependent on myocardial drug uptake which can take sereral hours. Unlike other antiarrhythmics, bretylium does not exert a major negative inotropic effect.

Pharmacokinetics. Bretylium pharmacokinetics are not well understood, and the therapeutic range of plasma concentrations is not defined. This may reflect the fact that the drug concentration in pools which are frequently not in equilibrium with plasma (adrenergic neuron, myocardium) is important for drug action. Renal disease may impair bretylium elimination.

Suggested Dosage and Administration. Bretylium can be administered intravenously or intramuscularly, but the intravenous route is preferred because it can be stopped immediately should adverse effects occur and, in addition, absorption from the intramuscular site is unproven. A loading dose of 5 to 10 mg/kg is administered as a slow infusion over 30 minutes (or more rapidly in urgent situations), followed by a maintenance infusion of 1 to 4 mg/min. An initial period of increased blood pressure and heart rate and worsening arrhythmias may occur in the first 30 minutes, but this is often obscured by other changes in these very ill patients. Orthostatic hypotension is not an indication of excessive doses. It can occur with very small dosages that are not adequate for antiarrhythmic efficacy. If arrhythmias persist, further loading dosages and a higher maintenance dosage should be given. No data are available to define the upper limit on dosage, but responses are generally seen after less than 30 mg/kg. Patients who have required bretylium for control of arrhythmias often require chronic oral antiarrhythmic therapy. This should be instituted under continuous electrocardiogram (ECG) monitoring and delayed if possible until precursor arrhythmias such as frequent VEDs appear so that there is an end point for judging the effectiveness of chronic therapy.

Precautions and Contraindications. Lower maintenance doses are probably required in renal disease but exact recommendations are not possible. Bretylium therapy may actually increase cardiac output in congestive heart failure by reducing afterload. Patients with liver disease have not been studied to detect any differences in bretylium requirements. The use of bretylium should be avoided in clinical situations in which marked reductions in peripheral resistance may be detrimental, such as aortic stenosis or carotid artery disease. Patients with severe pulmonary hypertension should not receive bretylium since pulmonary arterial pressure rises during therapy. In theory, arrhythmias accompanying pheochromocytoma should not be treated with bretylium because of the catecholamine suprasensitivity produced by bretylium. Supine hypotension occurring during bretylium therapy is generally due to peripheral vasodilation and should be treated with volume expansion; a Swan Ganz catheter is often desirable to monitor filling pressure in these patients, but its presence may contribute to ongoing arrhythmias. The use of catecholamines in this setting should be undertaken with caution because of the functional denervation hypersensitivity.

Drug Interactions. Orthostatic hypotension need not be treated, and patients should remain supine while on therapy if necessary. Patients who have received tricyclic antidepressants may be resistant to the adrenergic effects of bretylium, but their antiarrhythmic response is unknown. It is important to note that this effect of the antidepressant drugs may persist for weeks after they have been stopped. Although the digitalized patient may be at an increased risk for arrhythmias during the initial release of catecholamines, this theoretical possibility remains to be documented in humans.

Amiodarone

Pharmacology. This agent has a number of pharmacokinetic, electrophysiologic, and toxicologic attributes which make it unique among antiarrhythmic drugs. It blocks both cardiac sodium and calcium currents, prolongs cardiac repolarization (QT interval), and is a noncompetitive β-blocker. It is a structural analog of thyroid hormone and, although the mechanisms underlying its antiarrhythmic and toxic effects are unknown, some data suggest it interfers with the action of thyroid hormone on the heart. Chronic oral treatment with amiodarone does not usually result in major depression of left ventricular function. It is probably the single most effective agent currently available with demonstrable efficacy in a wide range of arrhythmias (atrial fibrillation, fibrillation/flutter, PSVT, automatic atrial tachycardia, ventricular arrhythmias of all types). However, the potential for serious side effects has blunted enthusiasm for its widespread use in North America. On the other hand, in Europe and South America, it is probably the most commonly used antiarrhythmic agent.

Pharmacokinetics. Amiodarone has an extraordinarily long elimination half-life, estimated to be between 2 weeks and 2 months. A major metabolite, desethylamiodarone, shares many of the parent drug's electrophysiologic properties and accumulates over time; it has been implicated in both arrhythmia suppression and amiodarone toxicity. The time between initiation of therapy and arrhythmia control varies widely but is usually several days to weeks. Because of this lag, it is usual to administer high doses initially, with doses decreasing as efficacy is seen. Also because of the long elimination half-life, the drug does not need to be administered any more often than once daily, and, in fact, missing a dose of amiodarone is less likely to result in arrhythmia recurrence than missing a dose of other antiarrhythmics.

Serious toxicity appears to be more common with chronic dosages above 400 mg/day. An intravenous form, which is still investigational in the United States, is also available; although some data suggest that intravenous amiodarone may acutely control arrhythmias resistant to other therapies such as lidocaine, procainamide, and phenytoin, it can also produce marked hypotension due to depression of left ventricular function. The usual dosage is 300 mg/30 min followed by 0.5 to 1 mg/min. Amiodarone and desethylamiodarone plasma concentrations of 0.5 to 2.0 μg/ml are usual during chronic treatment, and persistently higher levels may be associated with an increased incidence of toxicity.

Precautions and Contraindications. The most serious side effect during amiodarone therapy is pulmonary fibrosis which occurs in 5 to 10% of patients during the first year. If recognized early, this side effect can be reversed by steroid treatment and withdrawal of amiodarone; in some of these patients, amiodarone may even be reinstituted at a later date. In some patients, however, pulmonary fibrosis progresses rapidly to death. The mechanism of this acute lung injury is not known, although inclusion bodies reminiscent of those seen with other forms of lung toxicity, such as that observed after bleomycin, have been observed and have raised the suspicion of free radical-mediated injury. Factors which have been implicated in the development of pulmonary toxicity include high dosages (particularly intravenous dosages through a central catheter), preexisting lung disease (including congestive heart failure), oxygen therapy, and antecedent lung injury from any source. Occasional patients appear to develop acute amiodarone pulmonary toxicity following surgery. Other side effects occurring during amiodarone therapy include abnormal liver function studies (and rare reports of amiodarone-related cirrhosis); corneal microdeposits which are detectable in all patients after 3 months of therapy but only rarely (1 to 2%) cause visual halos and necessitate dose reduction; hypo and hyperthyroidism; peripheral neuropathy which can lead to striking weakness; sinus bradycardia (which may require permanent pacing); photosensitivity; and bluish skin discoloration, particuarly on exposed areas (nose, cheeks). Amiodarone treatment, in contrast to that with other antiarrhythmics, is frequently well tolerated initially and punctuated by chronic organ toxicity later. Because of the drug's long elimination half-life, side effects may persist for weeks or months after the drug is stopped; similarly, it is impossible to judge the efficacy of alternative antiarrhythmic therapy shortly after amiodarone is discontinued. Amiodarone treatment may present problems during the intraoperative period, such as an atropine-resistant bradycardia, myocardial depression, and peripheral vasodilation; invasive monitoring has been recommended for these high-risk patients.

Drug Interactions. Amiodarone interfers with hepatic metabolism and/or renal excretion of a large number of commonly used cardiovascular agents. Coumadin requirements drop dramatically during amiodarone, and bleeding is a real risk unless the dosage is decreased. Similarly, digoxin toxicity due to decreased digoxin clearance can be seen. It is common to use other antiarrhythmics with amiodarone, particularly early in therapy. Plasma concentrations should be monitored since amiodarone is known to decrease the clearance (and therefore to raise plasma concentrations) of quinidine, procainamide, N-acetylprocainamide, and flecainide. No data are yet available on the effects of amiodarone on anesthetic drug pharmacokinetics and efficacy in humans.

Phenytoin (Diphenylhydantoin, Dilantin)

Pharmacology. Phenytoin is a widely used anticonvulsant which can also be effective in the acute parental or chronic oral therapy of ventricular arrhythmias. It is said to be of particular value in the treatment of arrhythmias due to digitalis excess, because it can enhance A-V nodal conduction. However, it has also been effective in the treatment of other ventricular arrhythmias, and its use should be considered in the treatment of lidocaine-resistant arrhythmias or in the oral therapy of chronic ventricular arrhythmias. Combining phenytoin with procainamide or propranolol is occasionally useful in chronic therapy when single-agent therapy fails.

Excessively rapid intravenous administration can result in cardiac conduction abnormalities, such as heart block or asystole and profound hypotension. Other side effects are mainly neurological and are more severe at free plasma concentrations above 2 μg/ml. These are primarily tremor, nystagmus, and dizziness; higher dosages can result in mental slowing and eventually coma. Long-term therapy is regularly accompanied by gingival hypertrophy; lymphadenopathy which resembles lymphoma and macrocytic anemia can also occur. Like many anticonvulsants, phenytoin may be teratogenic.

Pharmacokinetics. There is good evidence that a therapeutic effect is achieved only with plasma concentrations of total (bound and free) drug above 10 μg/ml, while adverse effects often occur above 20 μg/ml. These values are dependent upon protein binding: in normal individuals, phenytoin is approximately 90% bound so the desired therapeutic range of free drug concentrations (i.e., the pharmacologically active fraction) is 1 to 2 μg/ml. Elimination is primarily by hepatic metabolism and subsequent renal excretion; metabolism appears to be saturable over the range of usual phenytoin dosages. Minor dosage changes can therefore result in large increases in plasma free concentrations (see Fig. 1.6) and phenytoin toxicity. Phenytoin has a long elimination half-life (16 to 24 hours), so the institution of maintenance therapy without a loading dose will achieve therapeutic effects only after 3 to 5 days.

Suggested Dosage and Administration. The loading dose of phenytoin for a normal individual is 10 to 15 mg/kg. Intravenous administration is the preferred route for acute therapy, but in order to avoid hypotension, the load must be administered slowly (less than 50 mg/min) under blood pressure and ECG monitoring. Because of incompatibility with most intravenous solutions, the drug should be administered undiluted; otherwise precipitation of phenytoin crystals in the intravenous line can occur. In less urgent situations, the load can be administered in divided oral doses over several hours (e.g., 300 mg every 4 to 6 hours for three to four doses). Phenytoin should not be administered intramuscularly, since the drug may crystallize in tissue and absorption is unpredictable.

Because phenytoin is eliminated so slowly, continuous intravenous maintenance therapy is not usually used. The usual maintenance dosage of phenytoin is variable; while anticonvulsant therapy is often administered on a once daily basis, less fluctuation in plasma concentration might be anticipated with 8 hourly dosing and may be preferable for antiarrhythmic therapy or acute seizure disorders. The usual daily maintenance dosage is 300 to 400 mg/day (5 mg/kg). Because phenytoin elimination does not follow first-order kinetics (see Chapter 1), small increments in dosage may produce large rises in plasma concentration. If usual dosing does not produce therapeutic effects of adequate plasma concentrations at steady state, dosage should be cautiously increased (by 100 mg/day if the clincial condition will permit) and the new steady state then evaluated. Oc-

casional "slow metabolizers" of phenytoin may require only 100 mg/day, while up to 600 to 800 mg/day may be needed to produce adequate plasma concentrations in some patients.

Precautions and Contraindications. Phenytoin requirements are generally reduced in severe liver disease. Binding of phenytoin to plasma albumin is decreased in certain disease states, most notably uremia and hyperbilirubinemia. If total plasma concentration is in the usual therapeutic range, the free concentration may well be elevated and in the toxic range; measurement of unbound drug is thus necessary in these states. However, because clearance and volume of distribution may also change, actual dosages may require little adjustment from the usual wide range required.

Drug Interactions. Hepatic metabolism of phenytoin can be inhibited by a number of agents with resultant decrease in phenytoin requirements and the potential for a fall in plasma concentration if the second agent is stopped. This interaction is known or suspected with barbiturates, carbamazepine, chloramphenicol, disulfiram, isoniazid, and sulphonamides. Phenytoin itself can accelerate hepatic metabolism of a number of other agents, including digitoxin, quinidine, disopyramide, and oral anticoagulants.

Digitalis

Pharmacology. Despite the fact that digitalis glycosides have been used for over two centuries, their mechanism of action is still unclear. The principal clinical uses of digitalis are (a) the treatment of congestive heart failure and (b) the treatment of arrhythmia, for example, to control ventricular rate in atrial fibrillation. Digitalis administration enhances myocardial contractility and automaticity and slows impulse propagation in conducting tissue; in addition to these direct effects, it causes an increase in vagal tone. Digitalis augments calcium's participation in excitation-contraction coupling, providing the basis for current understanding of its positive inotropic effects. The mechanism for this augmentation is uncertain, but digitalis clearly inhibits myocardial Na^+-K^+-ATPase. As a result of this inhibition, intracellular sodium concentration rises, and Na^+-Ca^+ exchange may then result in increased intracellular calcium. Increased intracellular calcium results in both increased inotropic actions as well as arrhythmias. Calcium-dependent delayed afterdepolarizations are demonstrable in preparations treated with digitalis in vitro and are thought to cause many digitalis-related arrhythmias in the intact heart. Because of Na^+-K^+ inhibition, digitalis glycosides also cause a loss of myocardial potassium, and some cardiac effects of severe digitalis overdose may be reversed by potassium administration. Conversely, loss of potassium caused, for example, by concomitant diuretic therapy potentiates digitalis actions. Calcium increases the effects of digitalis in experimental animals, and if calcium is given to digitalized patients, caution is required.

The major clinical effect of the direct and vagomimetic actions on the conduction system is to prolong A-V nodal refractoriness and, thus, to decrease the rate of ventricular response in supraventricular tachyarrhythmias. The effects of digitalis on the sinus node and atria are unpredictable, while ventricular excitability is usually enhanced. Thus, the effects of digitalis administration may be summarized:

1. Direct stimulation of the myocardium leading to increased contractility and a positive inotropic action;
2. Increased risk of arrhythmias, probably due to calcium-dependent afterdepolarizations;
3. Increased vagal activity leading to:
   a. Decreased atrial refractoriness,
   b. Delayed atrioventricular conduction,
   c. Bradycardia.

The toxic effects of digitalis include nausea, high degrees of A-V nodal block, and/or ventricular arrhythmias. The block is occasionally hemodynamically significant requiring temporary pacing, but more often resolves with drug withdrawal alone. Such patients should, however, be monitored because of the risk of serious ventricular arrhythmias. The combination of enhanced atrial automaticity and A-V nodal block produces atrial tachycardia with block; the occurrence of this rhythm is highly suggestive of digitalis intoxication. Ventricular arrhythmias due to digitalis excess are treated with drug withdrawal and lidocaine or phenytoin. Bretylium may be dangerous in this setting and, while the cautious administration of potassium may be beneficial, given in excess, it may also precipitate or augment digitalis-induced A-V nodal block.

It is important to recognize that rhythm disturbances due to digitalis intoxication can occur both when plasma concentrations are excessive or even when trough plasma concentrations are in the therapeutic range, but other complicating factors such as hypokalemia, hypercalcemia, hypothyroidism, acid-base disturbances, hypoxemia, hypomagnesemia, or excess cardiac sensitivity (e.g., some cardiomyopathies) are present. The beneficial effects of digitalis are dose related so there is no true lower limit on the range of therapeutic plasma concentrations.

Pharmacokinetics. A number of forms of digitalis are available, each with its own pharmacokinetic characteristics. The most widely used form is digoxin. Digoxin's bioavailability after oral administration may be only 60% and can vary among manufacturers. It is eliminated primarily by the kidney with a half-life of approximately 36 hours. Following intravenous administration, its onset of action occurs in 20 minutes and its peak effect in 4 hours. Intramuscular use of any digitalis preparation is unreliable, painful, and should be avoided. In the rare situation when an extremely rapid effect is desirable, ouabain or deslanoside can be tried; each has its onset of action within 5 minutes. Otherwise, their pharmacokinetic parameters are less well characterized than digoxin's, and they appear to offer no particular advantage. Digitoxin is a form which is fully bioavailable. It is metabolized by the liver and excreted in the bile (with enterohepatic recirculation); its elmination half-life is 5 to 7 days. The risk of digitalis intoxication increases when the digoxin plasma concentration is greater than 2 ng/ml or the digitoxin plasma concentration is greater than 30 ng/ml.

Indications. The indications for digitalis treatment are congestive heart failure and arrhythmias. Digitalis increases contractility and decreases myocardial oxygen consumption in the acutely failing heart. Its position in the treatment of chronic congestive heart failure has recently become uncertain. Some investigators have reported that withdrawal of digitalis from patients without a history of atrial fibrillation has resulted in no deterioration. However, studies stratified by severity of left ventricular dysfunction demonstrate a clear benefit in patients with advanced heart failure. The administration of digitalis to patients without cardiomegaly may actually increase net myocardial oxygen consumption and, thus, can exacerbate angina. This is particularly true in patients with severe left ventricular hypertrophy due to hypertension, aortic stenosis, or hypertrophic cardiomyopathy in whom subendocardial ischemia or infarction can result. It has also been reported that digitalis may precipitate or exacerbate symptoms of bowel ischemia by decreasing flow to a compromised mesenteric circulation.

Digitalis may be used to slow the rapid ventricular responses associated with atrial fibrillation or flutter. Patients with congestive heart failure appear to respond best. However, in the presence of serious complicating illnesses such as sepsis or thyrotoxicosis, digitalis therapy will not generally slow the ventricular rate to less than 100 beats/min unless high dosages are used. Digitalis therapy should be undertaken with extreme care (if at all) in patients with the Wolff-Parkinson-White syndrome and wide complex superventricular arrhythmias, particularly atrial fibrillation, since acceleration of the ventricular response can occur and ventricular fibrillation has been reported. Because of this small potential risk, some would avoid digitalis entirely in all patients with paroxysmal

supraventricular tachycardia. However, because of its A-V nodal blocking effects, digitalis can be useful in the restoration and maintenance of sinus rhythm in many such patients. Digitalis treatment is occasionally useful for ventricular arrhythmias, especially if congestive heart failure is improved by its use. Some workers have proposed that the parasympathomimetic effects of digitalis may be useful in treating central nervous system and stress-related ventricular arrhythmias.

It is not clear which patients ought to receive prophylactic digitalis preoperatively. Patients with cardiomegaly and overt congestive heart failure and those with a history of atrial tachyarrhythmias will probably benefit from preoperative digitalis. The management of a patient with a history of congestive heart failure without atrial arrhythmia is less clear. If the risks (increased myocardial oxygen consumption, arrhythmias) are thought to outweigh any potential benefit, digitalis should be withheld and the patient carefully monitored and treated if necessary with other modes of drug therapy, such as vasodilators and diuretics.

Suggested Dosage and Administration. Because of their slow elimination rates, loading doses of digitalis glycosides are often used; regardless of loading, steady-state conditions will be achieved four to five half-lives after the institution of maintenance therapy. The total loading dose for digoxin is 10 to 15 μg/kg administered orally in divided doses every 3 to 4 hours. More frequent administration may produce adverse effects. Therapy can then start with an estimated maintenance dose (0.25 mg/day in normal individuals, less in renal failure; see later in this chapter), and adjustments can be made according to clinical response (e.g., ventricular rate), plasma concentrations, and the potential occurrence of side effects. The loading dose for digitoxin is 10 to 15 μg/kg, and the maintenance dosage in patients with normal hepatic function is 0.1 mg/day.

Precautions and Contraindications. Digitalis dosing is profoundly altered by a number of disease states. First, the el-

derly appear to be more sensitive to digitalis toxicity so dosage reduction may be
required. All dosing is on the basis of
lean body weight, and small individuals
should receive less. Hypokalemia, hypercalcemia, hypoxemia, acid-base disturbances, hypomagnesemia, and hypothyroidism all increase the risk of digitalis
intoxication and should be corrected, if
possible, prior to the administration of
any form of digitalis

Digoxin's elimination is markedly
slowed in the presence of renal insufficiency. Elaborate nomograms exist for
adjusting dosage, but the principles are
that digoxin clearance generally falls in
parallel with decreases in creatinine
clearance and that monitoring plasma
concentrations may help avoid digoxin
intoxication. In 24 hours, the anephric
patient eliminates 14% of a daily dose of
digoxin (in contrast to the 36% eliminated by normals). Thus, an anephric patient should receive the same dose less
frequently (e.g., 0.25 mg every 3 to 4
days) or, more usually, 0.125 mg every
second day. Patients undergoing hemodialysis require the same dosage reductions, since digoxin is not appreciably
dialyzed.

Digitoxin's elimination is not affected
by renal disease, and this has been used
as an argument in favor of its use. However, should toxicity occur, it is likely to
be more prologed. Digitoxin elimination
is impaired in the presence of hepatic
disease and dosage reduction is required.
Congestive heart failure probably does
not alter elimination of either digoxin or
digitoxin, although gastrointestinal absorption of digoxin may be impaired in
the presence of severe right-sided heart
failure and bowel edema. Patients with
hypertrophic cardiomyopathies or cor
pulmonale appear to be especially sensi
tive to digitalis intoxication. It is uncertain whether digitalis in the setting of
acute myocardial infarction predisposes
to increased arrhythmias; its use should
be undertaken only when a clear indication (e.g., atrial fibrillation with a rapid
ventricular response) is present. The
commonly cited risk of provoking ventricular fibrillation by cardioverting a

digitalized patient has probably been exaggerated: the possiblity of this outcome
is largely confined to those with digitalis
toxicity.

Drug Interactions. The administration of
thyroid hormone, calcium, or catecholamines to a digitalized patient may be
harmful, and the catecholamine release
induced by bretylium may in theory exacerbate digitalis intoxication. Arrhythmias have been reported in digitalized
patients who have been given succinylcholine, possibly due either to a direct effect or to the hyperkalemia which can be
induced by succinylcholine. Administration of quinidine, verapamil, or amiodarone to a digitalized patient causes a rise
in digitalis plasma levels (digoxin or digitoxin) and may precipitate toxicity (see
Chapter 4). In some patients, digoxin is
metabolized by gut flora, so that alteration of flora by antibiotic therapy can result in increased plasma digoxin and
toxicity.

Quinidine

Pharmacology. Quinidine is the d-isomer of the antimalarial drug quinine and
has been used in the treatment of atrial
fibrillation since the turn of the century.
While elective DC countershock is probably the current treatment of choice for
conversion of paroxysmal atrial fibrillation to sinus rhythm, quinidine is often
used to prevent recurrence. It is also
effective in suppressing ventricular arrhythmias. In addition to its direct antiarrhythmic actions, quindine has vagolytic properties which can result in
increased A-V nodal conduction, particularly in patients not receiving digitalis.

The most common adverse effects are
gastrointestinal (diarrhea, nausea, anorexia), and these may prevent chronic
therapy in up to one-half of the patients.
QRS and/or QT prolongation, hypotension, and increasing ventricular arrhythmias, including torsade de pointes (a distinct type of ventricular tachycardia seen
when QT intervals are markedly prolonged, e.g., > 600 milliseconds) and
ventricular fibrillation, may occur with
excessive plasma concentrations; this

cardiotoxic symptom complex is occasionally seen after only a few doses and when quinidine plasma concentrations are low. Serious quinidine-associated arrhythmias occur in 2 to 3% of patients, regardless of the underlying heart disease or the arrhythmia being treated; hypokalemia is a very frequent exacerbating factor. Treatment of torsades de pointes depends on recognition, withdrawal of any offending agent, correction of serum K^+ or Mg^{++} abnormalities, and maneuvers to increase heart rate (pacing, isoproterenol); conventional antiarrhythmias are less effective (lidocaine) or contraindicated (procainamide). Other side effects include dose-related psychosis and cinchonism (tinnitus, vertigo). The idiosyncratic syndromes of quinidine-related hepatitis and fever and quinidine-induced thrombocytopenia are immunologically mediated and recur promptly on rechallenge. Patients who have had such reactions should not receive quinidine or quinine (contained in tonic water).

Pharmacokinetics. Quinidine is well absorbed with peak plasma concentrations occurring 2 to 4 hours after a dose. Quinidine undergoes hepatic metabolism, and some of its metabolites are active and may be responsible for some of the efficacy or toxicity observed during treatment. Approximately 35% of the administered dose is cleared by the kidneys. The mean elimination half-life is approximately 6 hours, but can vary widely in normal individuals (range, 4 to 19 hours). The range of therapeutic plasma concentrations depends upon the analytical method used. Using the double-extraction method to exclude inactive metabolites, an antiarrhythmic effect generally occurs above 1.5 to 2 $\mu g/ml$, and adverse effects above 5 to 8 $\mu g/ml$.

Quindine sulfate tablets have been the most widely studied. Other salts (gluconate, polygalacturonase) are available, and some believe that they are associated with fewer gastrointestinal side effects. They have variable amounts of quinidine and differ from the sulfate in their rates of absorption, sometimes allowing less frequent dosing. However, comparative studies are not available, and lesser toxicity may be due to the poorer bioavailability of the other salts that some studies have found.

Suggested Dosage and Administration. Parenteral administration of quinidine is associated with hypotension and is rarely indicated. Many authorities recommend an initial "screening" dose of 100 to 200 mg orally to detect patients at risk from the cardiotoxic side effects. However, because most patients develop these symptoms only after multiple doses, quinidine should be started in the hospital, preferably under monitored conditons for 2 to 3 days. Patients with atrial flutter or fibrillation should receive digitalis prior to quinidine to prevent acceleration of their ventricular rate. For either atrial or ventricular arrhythmias, therapy should start at 200 to 300 mg every 6 hours and the response observed. If the response is inadequate once steady state is achieved (1 to 2 days), if the QRS and QT complexes are not markedly prolonged (QT < 500 milliseconds), and if plasma concentrations are less than 2 $\mu g/ml$, the dosage can be cautiously increased. Monitoring (estimated) peak plasma concentration is frequently recommended but of little practical value except in confirming a clinical suspicion of toxicity. Monitoring trough levels (prior to the next dose) is the preferred method to assist in determining adequacy of dosage. The final dosage is highly variable (200 to 600 mg every 4 to 6 hours). Plasma concentrations in the range of 2 to 5 $\mu g/ml$ are usually clincially effective, while toxicity is frequently seen above 5 $\mu g/ml$.

Precautions and Contraindications. Both clearance and the intitial volume of distribution are reduced in the elderly, resulting in a lower dose requirement. In the postoperative or postmyocardial infarction period, the plasma binding of quinidine increases, resulting in a fall in the free fraction, probably due to a rise in α_1-acid glycoprotein levels (see Chapter 1). This should be taken into account in the interpretation of total quinidine levels in the postoperative period. Quinidine, like procainamide, can potentiate neuromuscular blockade in patients suffering from myasthenia gravis. Congestive heart failure, liver disease, and renal disease are thought to require no particular dosage adjustment. Quinidine should be avoided in patients who have preexisiting QT prolongation.

Drug Interactions. The administration of quinidine to the digitalized patient (a common occurrence) decreases digitalis (digoxin and digitoxin) clearance, increases digitalis concentrations, and can produce digitalis intoxication. Quinidine requirements can be dramatically increased by drugs which induce hepatic mixed-function oxidase, such as phenytoin, rifampin, and phenobarbital. Like many other antiarrhythmics, quinidine can potentiate the neuromuscular blockade induced by d-tubocurarine. Recently, quinidine has been found to be a potent inhibitor of one specific hepatic cytochrome ($P450_{db1}$). Thus, for drugs whose clearance is entirely dependent on metabolism by $P450_{db1}$, doses of quinidine as low as 50 mg may increase plasma concentrations and action of such concomitantly administered drugs. Debrisoquin and flecainide are theoretical examples.

Disopyramide

Pharmacology. Disopyramide has electrophysiologic characteristics similar to those of quinidine and is generally used to treat ventricular arrhythmias. Like quinidine, it has also been used for atrial arrhythmias. Cardiodepression and anticholinergic side effects (urinary retention, constipation, dry mouth) occur frequently and have limited the drug's widespread use. Like quinidine, disopyramide has also been associated with acceleration of the ventricular rate in atrial fibrillation, excessive QT prolongation, ventricular arrhythmias, and sudden death.

Pharmacokinetics. Disopyramide is well absorbed after oral administration, and peak levels occur in 2 to 3 hours. It undergoes hepatic metabolism and subsequent renal elimination with a half-life of 4 to 10 hours in normal individuals. Therapeutic concentrations are not as well established as with older agents, but some reports have indicated the range to

be 2 to 7 μg/ml. Plasma protein binding is 30 to 50% but varies over the therapeutic range, so the concentration of free drug may in the future be a more helpful guide to treatment.

Suggested Dosage and Administration. In the absence of widespread availability of plasma concentration monitoring, therapy is empiric. Loading doses, particularly intravenous boluses, are associated with an excessively high incidence of side effects and are not recommended. Treatment usually starts with 100 mg orally every 6 to 8 hours. The dosage can be increased every 1 to 2 days if no antiarrhythmic effect is seen and side effects are absent. Therapy with more than 800 mg/day should only be attempted under monitored conditions.

Precautions and Contraindications. Dosage should be reduced and/or dosing intervals lengthened in the presence of renal disease or hepatic disease. While a reduction in dosage in the presence of heart failure is recommended, disopyramide should probably be avoided altogether in this setting. Diseases in which the anticholinergic effects would be detrimental (prostatism, glaucoma) are contraindications to disopyramide therapy.

Drug Interactions. Warfarin requirements may rise during disopyramide therapy.

Propranolol and Other β-Adrenergic Blocking Agents

Propranolol and other β-adrenergic blocking agents are fully discussed in Chapter 15, and this section is confined to their use in the treatment of arrhythmias.

Pharmacology. Propranolol is highly effective in the treatment of supraventricular arrhythmias and catecholamine-mediated arrhythmias (e.g., VEDs in pheochromocytoma). It also has been shown to suppress chronic ventricular arrhythmias of any etiolgy. In this setting, some patients require plasma concentrations associated with β-blockade (40 to 100 ng/ml), while an additional subset respond only to much higher dosages and concentrations, suggesting that a non-β-blocking property of propranolol may be important for this antiarrhythmic activity. In addition, occasional patients exhibit arrhythmia suppression at lower dosages and recurrence at higher dosages which is also consistent with a dual mechanism of action. Propranolol reduces sodium conductance in vitro at concentrations which may be achieved by high doses in humans. Chronic therapy with propranolol and some other β-blocking agents (atenolol, timolol, metopolol, alprenolol) has been associated with a decreased risk of sudden death following myocardial infarction.

Suggested Dosage and Administration. Propranolol can be administered intravenously in small doses (1 mg every few minutes) to achieve a rapid antiarrhythmic action (for example, in the treatment of paroxysmal supraventricular tachycardia). Chronic oral therapy (for any indication) should start at low dosages (20 mg 6 hourly) and gradually increase until a satisfactory effect is seen. Oral dosages up to 320 mg/day usually control supraventricular arrhythmias, but up to 640 mg/day may be required for chronic ventricular arrhythmias. Antiarrhythmic therapy on an 8- to 12-hour basis is feasible, but patients should be observed carefully for recurrence of arrhythmia just before the next dose is required. Antiarrhythmic dosing recommendations for other β-blockers have in general not been determined, but "usual" dosages are frequently used. Acebutolol has been shown to suppress ventricular ectopics at a dosage of 200 to 600 mg 3 times daily.

Precautions and Contraindications. Lower dosages of propranolol are required in severe liver disease, but renal disease is unlikely to require major dosing schedule adjustments. β-Blockers should be avoided in congestive heart failure, although they can occasionally be used along with digitalis in asymmetric septal hypertrophy and in hypertensive heart disease. Myasthenics may be at risk from increased neuromuscular blockade.

β-Blockers should be avoided in those individuals in whom withdrawal of β-receptor-mediated sympathetic support would be detrimental (asthma, congestive heart failure, sinus node dysfunction). The use of β-blocking agents alone in situations of catecholamine excess (phenochromocytoma, clonidine withdrawal, epinephrine administration) may cause severe hypertension due to unopposed α-mediated vasoconstriction. Patients with pheochromocytoma who are undergoing preoperative medical treatment should receive an α-adrenergic blocking agent such as phenoxybenzamine or phentolamine before being given β-blockers to control any arrhythmias. β-Blockers will block catecholamine-mediated symptoms of hypoglycemia and should be used with caution in insulin-treated diabetics. The major side effects of propranolol are otherwise limited to fatigue and depression, presumably reflecting the drug's accumulation in the central nervous system. Other β-blockers may offer theoretical advantages such as cardioselectivity, less penetration into the central nervous system, or intrinsic sympathomimetic activity. However, the antiarrhythmic activity of these agents has not yet been studied as extensively as that of propranolol.

Drug Interactions. Propranolol-mediated cardiodepression can be accentuated by the use of other potential cardiodepressant agents, especially disopyramide. Interactions during clonidine withdrawal, epinephrine administration, and hypoglycemia (induced by insulin or oral hypoglycemic agents) have all been mentioned above. Concomitant use of parenteral β-blockers and calcium channel antagonists such as verapamil should be avoided (see later in this chapter).

ESMOLOL

Pharmacology. Esmolol is a cardioselective β-blocker which may be particularly useful in acute care situations, since it has a very short elimination half-life. Its pharmacologic effects appear confined to those of β-blockade with minimal intrinsic sympathomimetic activity or sodium channel blocking effect. It is metabolized by red cell esterases, and its major metabolite is a much less potent β-blocker than is the parent drug. Methanol is another metabolite, but methanol intoxication does not appear to be a clinically important problem during esmolol treatment. The major advantage of esmolol therapy is that it has a very short elimination half-life (9 minutes), and its pharmacologic effects disappear very rapidly when esmolol is discontinued. Thus, in the acute care situation, esmolol offers the advantage that, should side effects due to β-blockade develop with parenteral therapy, the drug can be stopped and adverse effects rapidly reversed. Esmolol has been shown to be both safe and effective for the acute management of supraventricular tachycardias and to control ventricular rate in atrial fibrillation or flutter. It has also been used to control heart rate and thus treat myocardial ischemia both in the coronary care unit and during the perioperative period. It appears to be a useful agent in the management of postoperative hypertension. The mechanism of its hypotensive effect is unclear; parenteral administration of other β-blockers, such as propranolol, often results in increased peripheral vascular resistance and no change in blood pressure. Hypotension, in fact, is the major dose-limiting side effect during esmolol treatment.

Suggested Dosage and Administration. The usual dosage is 500 μg/kg/min given over 5 minutes followed by a constant infusion of 100 to 300 μg/kg/min.

Precautions and Contraindications. Like all β-blockers, esmolol should be used with caution in patients who may be at risk for adverse effects (as outlined above).

Drug Interactions. Data from animal studies suggest that cardiodepression by esmolol may be enhanced in the presence of halothane or enflurane, although studies in patients are not yet available. Because it is metabolized by red cell esterases, its duration of action is not prolonged in patients with atypical plasma esterase whose metabolism of succinylcholine is impaired.

SOTALOL

Pharmacology. Sotalol is a nonselective β-blocker which is particlarly useful in antiarrhythmic therapy because it also prolongs cardiac repolarization. The mechanism underlying this action is unclear, but block of repolarizing potassium currents in cardiac tissue is probably re-

sponsible. Both the β-blocking l-isomer as well as the weakly β-blocking d-isomer prolong action potential in a variety of in vitro and in vivo tests systems and exert antiarrhythmic actions. Sotalol is effective in a wide range of rhythm disturbances including PSVT, arrhythmias related to the presence of an accessory pathway, and ventricular arrhythmias. It can also be used, like other β-blockers, to treat angina or hypertension.

Suggested Dosage and Administration. β-Blocking effects of the drug become apparent at dosages as low as 80 to 160 mg every 12 h, while higher dosages (160 to 480 mg every 12 h) are generally required to suppress ventricular arrhythmias. The drug has also been used intravenously at a dose of 1 to 2 mg/kg over 15 to 30 minutes. Its elimination half-life is fairly long (10 to 28 hours), and dosage reduction is generally required in renal failure.

Precautions and Contraindications. Therapy with racemic sotalol, the form which is currently available, carries with it the risks associated with β-blockade which are outlined above. Sotalol also slows sinus rate to an extent greater than that seen with other β-blocking drugs. In addition, it prolongs the QT interval and has been associated with quinidine-like induction of torsades de pointes, particularly in the presence of hypokalemia. Thus patients with underlying conduction system disturbances, particularly abnormalities of sinus node function, as well as those with prolonged QT intervals should not receive sotalol. Because the d-isomer exerts electrophysiologic effects similar to the l-isomer but is only a weak β-blocker, it is currently being evaluated as a potential alternative therapy for patients in whom β-blockade is contraindicated but in whom sotalol might be a useful antiarrhythmic.

Verapamil

Pharmacology. Entry of calcium into myocardial cells following depolarization by rapid influx of sodium has become recognized as a critical event in the cardiac cycle. Agents designed to block the slow calcium current have been valuable in the treatment of supraventricular arrhythmias and of angina. Calcium channel blockers prolong A-V nodal refractoriness, thereby terminating PSVT and slowing ventricular rate in atrial fibrillation or flutter. Verapamil has been most widely used in antiarrhythmic therapy, although diltiazem appears to have similar antiarrhythmic effects. The dihydropyridines such as nifedipine have less activity at the A-V node and more on coronary smooth muscle, making them more useful for the treatment of angina. Ventricular arrhythmias are usually unaffected by verapamil, although a small group of patients with otherwise normal hearts and VEDs or ventricular tachycardia may respond.

Suggested Dosage and Administration. Verapamil undergoes extensive (and stereoselective) first-pass hepatic metabolism. As a consequence, usual oral doses (40 to 120 mg 3 to 4 times daily) are much higher than the intravenous doses necessary for the acute treatment of supraventricular arrhythmias (1 mg/min up to a total dose of 5 to 15 mg). Paroxysmal supraventricular tachycardia will usually convert to sinus rhythm with verapamil, while the ventricular response rate in atrial flutter or fibrillation is decreased. Recent reports indicate that verapamil treatment of multifocal atrial tachycardia can not only reduce ventricular rate but also convert the rhythm to sinus.

Precautions and Contraindications. The widespread use of verapamil in PSVT has been accompanied by its misuse in patients with wide complex sustained arrhythmias of all types. As discussed previously, use of verapamil in misdiagnosed ventricular tachycardia often results in catastrophic hemodynamic collapse and/or ventricular fibrillation. Verapamil may shorten accessory A-V pathway refractoriness and increase ventricular rate during atrial fibrillation in patients with Wolff-Parkinson-White syndrome. Side effects are uncommon with oral therapy (dizziness, flushing, nausea), but parenteral administration, especially in patients with heart failure, can cause marked hypotension due to peripheral vasodilation and depression of cardiac output, especially in patients receiving other vasodilators (nitrates, quin-

idine). Patients with preexisting abnormalities of the sinus or A-V nodes and patients receiving digitalis or propranolol should receive parenteral verapamil only under careful monitoring, because high grades of heart block (up to asystole) can occur. If verapamil is given to patients at risk for side effects, very low initial doses should be used. Parenteral calcium may be useful in reversing adverse effects (particularly hypotension), and a small number of reports have suggested that calcium pretreatment may help avoid hypotension while still permitting antiarrhythmic actions. Calcium antagonists are further discussed in Chapter 18.

Lidocaine Analogs: Mexiletine and Tocainide

Mexiletine and tocainide are lidocaine analogs whose long elimination half-lives (10 to 15 hours) allow chronic oral therapy with dosing only 2 or 3 times per day. Side effects (tremor, ataxia, nausea) are common with the use of either agent, and idiosyncratic hematologic abnormalities (including agranulocytosis in 0.1%) are a particular problem with tocainide. The latter is reversible with discontinuation of the drug, although fatalities due to overwhelming sepsis have occurred. These agents are indicated for the chronic oral treatment of ventricular arrhythmias. Lidocaine-sensitive arrhythmias respond better to mexiletine or tocainide than those which are lidocaine resistant. Therapeutic plasma concentrations are 0.5 to 2.0 $\mu g/ml$ (mexiletine) and 3 to 11 $\mu g/ml$ (tocainide). Dosages (300 to 1200 mg/day for mexiletine and 800 to 2400 mg/day for tocainide) should be adjusted to the minimum required to eliminate transient side effects and maintain an antiarrhythmic action. Both are almost completely absorbed and, while administration of a dose with food delays absorption, the total amount of drug absorbed is unaltered. Thus, transient side effects associated with rapid absorption can often be avoided by giving doses with food. Both drugs have been used parenterally, but they do not appear to offer any advantage over lidocaine. Administration of lidocaine to a patient already receiving chronic mexiletine or tocainide therapy frequently results in side effects (tremor, nausea, etc.); if the use of lidocaine is anticipated in such a patient (e.g., for endoscopy), the oral analogue should be withheld for 1 to 2 doses. Aprindine is another antiarrhythmic with some lidocaine-like properties; although it is still available in some countries in Europe, its use has become severely limited because of potentially fatal agranulocytosis in approximately 1 of 500 patients.

Encainide and Flecainide

Pharmacology. These drugs are newly developed sodium channel blockers with unusual potency and electrocardiographic effects. With an increased understanding of the molecular mechanisms of antiarrhythmic drug action, it has become useful to subclassify sodium channel blocking drugs. Drugs can be classified either by their effects of *(a) action potential duration* (lengthen, shorten, no change) or on the basis of their *(b) kinetics of interaction with the sodium channel* (very fast, intermediate, slow).

The kinetics of interaction with sodium channels and, in particular, the kinetics of recovery from drug-induced sodium channel block appear to be important determinants of drug effects at normal heart rates versus those at fast heart rates (or with premature beats). Drugs are thought to bind to sodium channels with each depolarization and to unbind during diastole. Thus, drugs with rapid recovery kinetics which unbind quickly (e.g., lidocaine) produce virtually no sodium channel block at slow rates, while block accumulates at faster ones. In contrast, drugs with slower recovery kinetics, such as flecainide, do not unbind significantly during diastole even at normal heart rates, so sodium channel block accumulates. Interestingly, classifying drugs by these recovery kinetics or by drug effects on action potential duration yields similar patterns despite the fact that changes in action potential duration are almost certainly dependent on factors other than depression of cardiac sodium currents. Quinidine and similar agents (disopyramide, procainamide) prolong action potential duration (QT interval on the surface ECG) and have intermediate kinetics of interaction with sodium channels; lidocaine and similar drugs (mexiletine, tocainide) shorten action potential duration and QT and have rapid interaction kinetics with cardiac sodium channels. Encainide and flecainide do not fall readily into either of the above categories. The drugs are very potent sodium channel blockers which exert relatively little effect on action potential duration; they have very slow kinetics of interaction with cardiac sodium channels.

In contrast to quinidine-like (often termed "class Ia") or lidocaine-like drugs ("class Ib"), encainide and flecainide (class Ic") typically prolong PR and QRS up to 50%. These agents are particularly effective in suppressing isolated VEDs and nonsustained episodes of ventricular tachycardia, especially in patients with near-normal left ventricular function. In patients with severe left ventricular dysfunction and sustained ventricular tachyarrhythmias, the drugs are less predictably effective and, in up to 20% of this group, an increase in frequency of sustained ventricular tachycardia episodes or difficulty cardioverting sustained ventricular tachycardia is seen. This form of arrhythmia aggravation, unlike quinidine-induced torsades de pointes, is not accompanied by marked QT prolongation. This arrhythmia-promoting property may also account for the increased mortality attributable to encainide or flecainide therapy in patients with VEDs and a history of myocardial infarction. (see page 467.) Difficulty with visual accommodation and, occasionally, a metallic taste are common side effects at higher dosages.

Other drugs with similar activity [recainam, indecainide, ethmozine (also called moricizine)] are currently under investigation. Propafenone is another agent with class Ic properties which has been available for some time in Germany. In addition to their efficacy in ventricular arrhythmias, the drugs have also been useful in the management of a variety of supraventricular tachyarrhythmias, including PSVT, and of automatic atrial tachycardia and for the maintenance of sinus rhythm in patients with atrial fibrillation or flutter.

Pharmacokinetics. Flecainide undergoes hepatic biotransformation to largely inactive metabolites which are, along with the parent drug, excreted by the kidneys. Its elimination half-life is sufficiently long (18 to 24 hours) that twice daily dosing is feasible in most patients.

In most patients, encainide undergoes extensive first-pass hepatic metabolism to the potent active metabolities O-desmethyl encainide (ODE) and 3-methoxy-O-desmethyl encainide (MODE). Encainide itself is eliminated with a half-life of approximately 2 hours, while the metabolites accumulate with time and appear to have much longer elimination half-lives (6 to 18 hours). In 7% of the Caucasian and black populations, the specific cytochrome P450 responsible for encainide biotransformation is absent on a genetic basis. In the subset of patients, first-pass hepatic metabolism is largely absent, encainide clearance is strikingly reduced, encainide plasma concentrations are increased, and encainide elimination half-life is prolonged (7 to 13 hours). In extensive metabolizers, ODE and MODE almost certainly account for arrhythmia suppression, while in the poor metabolizer group, encainide itself accumulates to plasma concentrations which suppress arrhythmias; the dosages required for arrhythmia suppression are, interestingly, no different between the two groups. Encainide, ODE, and MODE all undergo hepatic conjugation and renal excretion.

Precautions and Contraindications. The incidence of arrhythmia aggravation by class Ic drugs appears to be dose dependent, concentration dependent, and substrate dependent. That is, patients with normal left ventricular function may tolerate high dosages and plasma concentration of these agents without adverse effects, while lower dosages and concentrations in patients with severe left ventricular dysfunction and a history of sustained ventricular tachyarrhythmias are associated with a higher risk of developing arrhythmia aggravation. The risk during flecainide therapy appears to be greatest with dosages above 400 mg/day and plasma concentrations above 1000 ng/ml. Guidelines for encainide therapy are not as clearly defined, probably because of the complexities of monitoring plasma concentrations of parent drug and metabolites in these patients. Encainide dosages above 200 mg/day are thought to be associated with an increased risk of arrhythmia exacerbation.

Because of their potent effect on cardiac conduction, these agents should be used with caution in patients with known conduction system disturbances, since profound bradyarrhythmias (sinus bradycardia, A-V block) have been reported.

Flecainide appears to be a particularly potent depressor of left ventricular function, while encainide is better tolerated by these patients. Moreover, flecainide clearance is reduced in congestive heart failure, leading to higher concentrations and presumably an increased risk of left ventricular dysfunction. The dosage of both agents should be reduced in patients with advanced renal disease. Dosage adjustments are not thought to be required for either drug in hepatic disease. A parenteral form of flecainide is under investigation; because of encainide's complex pharmacokinetic profile, an intravenous form is not currently under investigation.

Drug Interactions. Since these are relatively new agents, little information is available on drug interactions, particularly those which may be important in anesthetic practice. Cimetidine, an inhibitor of hepatic drug oxidation, increases plasma encainide, ODE, and MODE. Mechanisms other than just inhibition of metabolism may be involved. Quinidine also inhibits encainide biotransformation (see p. 484), but the clinical consequences of this genetically determined drug interaction have not been fully evaluated. Neither agent exerts a significant effect on plasma digoxin concentrations.

BIBLIOGRAPHY

Antiarrhythmic Drug Pharmacology: General

Bertrand CA, Steiner NV, Jameson AG, Lopez M: Disturbances of cardiac rhythm during anesthesia and surgery. *JAMA* 216:1615–1617, 1971.

Clarkson CW, Hondeghem LM: Evidence for a specific receptor site for lidocaine, quinidine, and bupivacaine associated with cardiac sodium channels in guinea pig ventricular myocardium. *Circ Res* 56:496–506, 1985.

Clarkson CW, Hondeghem LM: Mechanism for bupivacaine depression of cardiac conduction: fast block of sodium channels during the action potential with slow recovery from block during diastole. *Anesthesiology* 62:396–405, 1985.

Drugs for cardiac arrhythmias. *Med Lett* 28:111–116, 1986.

Johnston RR, Eger E, Wilson CA: Comparative interaction of epinephrine with enflurane, isoflurane, and halothane in man. *Anesth Analg* 55:709–712, 1976.

Katz RL, Bigger JT Jr: Cardiac arrhythmias during anesthesia and operation. *Anesthesiology* 33:193, 1970.

Kendig JJ: Clinical implications of the modulated receptor hypothesis: local anesthetics and the heart (editorial). *Anesthesiology* 62:382–384, 1985.

Morganroth J, Anderson JL, Gentzkow GD: Classification by type of ventricular arrhythmia predicts frequency of adverse cardiac events from flecainide. *J Am Coll Cardiol* 8:607–615, 1986.

Roden DM, Thompson KA, Hoffman BF, Woosley RL: Clinical features and basic mechanisms of quinidine-induced arrhythmias. *J Am Coll Cardiol* 8:73A–78A, 1986.

Stewart RB, Bardy GH, Greene HL: Wide complex tachycardia: misdiagnosis and outcome after emergent therapy. *Ann Intern Med* 104:766–771, 1986.

Woosley RL, Echt DS, Roden DM: The treatment of ventricular arrhythmias in the failing heart. Pharmacologic and clinical considerations. *Ration Drug Ther* 19:1–7, 1985.

Woosley RL, Roden DM: Pharmacologic aspects of arrhythmia aggravation by antiarrhythmic drugs. *Am J Cardiol* 59:19E–25E, 1987.

Woosley RL, Shand DG: Pharmacokinetics of antiarrhythmic drugs. *Am J Cardiol* 41:986–995, 1978.

Zipes DP, Troup PJ: New antiarrhythmic agents: amiodarone, aprindine, disopyramide, ethmozin, mexiletine, tocainide, verapamil. *Am J Cardiol* 41:1005–1024, 1978.

Specific Antiarrhythmic Drugs

Lidocaine

Collingsworth KA, Sumner MK, Harrison, DC: The clinical pharmacology of lidocaine as an antiarrhythmic drug. *Circulation* 50:1217–1230, 1974.

Thompson PD, Melmon KL, Richards JA, Cohn K, Steinbrunn W, Cudihee R, Rowland M: Lidocane pharmacokinetics in advanced heart failure, liver disease, and renal failure in man. *Ann Intern Med.* 78:499, 1973.

Procainamide

Karlsson E: Clinical pharmacokinetics of procainamide. *Clin Pharmacokinet* 3:97, 1978.

Roden DM, Reele SG, Higgins SB, Smith R, Oates JA, Woosley RL: Antiarrhythmic efficacy, pharmacokinetics, and safety of N-acetylprocainamide in man: comparison of procainamide. *Am J Cardio* 46:463–468, 1980.

Bretylium

Koch-Weser J: Drug therapy: bretylium. *N Engl J Med* 300:473–477, 1979.

Amiodarone

Mason JW: Amiodarone. *N Engl J Med* 316:455–466, 1987.

Zipes DP, Prystowsky EN, Heger JJ: Amiodarone: electrophysiologic actions, pharmacokinetics, and clinical effects. *J Am Coll Cardiol* 3:1059–1071, 1984.

Phenytoin

Bigger JT, Steiner C, Burris JO: Relationship between the plasma level of diphenylhdantoin sodium and its cardiac antiarrhythmic effects. *Circulation* 38:363–374, 1968.

Stone N, Klein MD, Lown B: Diphenylhydantoin in the prevention of recurring ventricular tachycardia. *Circulation* 43:420–427, 1971.

Digitalis

Antman EM, Smith TW: Digitalis toxicity. *Mod Concepts Cardiovasc Dis* 55:26–30, 1986.

Aronson JK: Clinical pharmacokinetcs of digoxin 1980. *Clin Pharmacokinet* 5:137–149, 1980.

Byington R, Goldstein S: Association of digitalis therapy with mortality in survivors of acute myocardial infarction: observations in the beta-blocker heart attack trial. *J Am Coll Cardiol* 6:976–982, 1985.

Hager WD, Fenster P, Mayersohn M, Perrier D, Graves P, Marcus F, Goldman S: Digoxin-quinidine interaction: pharmacokinetic evaluation. *N Engl J Med 300:*1238–1241, 1979.

Lindenbaum J, Rund DG, Butler VP Jr, Tse-Eng D, Saha JR: Inactivation of digoxin by the gut flora: reversal by antibiotic therapy, *N Engl J Med* 305:789–794, 1981.

Lown B: Cardioversion and the digitalized patient. *J Am Coll Cardiol* 5:889–890, 1985.

Mulrow CD, Feussner JR, Velez R: Reevaluation of digitalis efficacy. *Ann Intern Med* 101:113–117, 1984.

Disopyramide

Koch-West J: Disopyramide. *N Engl J Med* 300:957–962, 1979.

Morady F, Scheinman MM, Desia J: Disopyramide. *Ann Intern Med* 96:337–343, 1982.

Propranolol and Other β-Blockers

Nies, AS, Shand DG: Clinical pharmacology of propranolol. *Circulation* 52:6–15, 1975.

Sleight P: Beta-adrenergic blockade after myocardial infarction. *N Engl J Med* 304:837–838, 1981.

Sonnenblick EH: Esmolol—an ultrashort-acting intravenous beta blocker. *Am J Cardiol* 56 (suppl):1F-62F, 1985.

Turi ZG, Braunwald E: The use of β-blockers after myocardial infarction.*JAMA* 249:2512–2516, 1983.

Woosley RL, Kornhauser D, Smith R, Reele S, Higgins SB, Nies AS, Shand DG; Oates JA: Suppression of chronic ventricular arrhythmias with propranolol. *Circulation* 60:819–827, 1979.

Verapamil

Gulamhusein S, Ko P, Carruthers SG, Klein GJ: Acceleration of the ventricular response during atrial fibrillation in the Wolff-Parkinson-White syndrome after verapamil. *Circulation* 65:348, 1982.

Haft JI, Habbab MA: Treatment of atrial arrhythmias: effectiveness of verapamil when preceded by calcium infusion. *Arch Intern Med* 146:1085–1089, 1986.

Levine JH, Michael JR, Guarnieri T: Treatment of multifocal atrial tachycardia with verapamil. *N Engl J Med* 312:21–44, 1985.

Mauritson DR, Winniford MD, Walker WS, Rude RE, Cary JR, Hillis LD: Oral verapamil for paroxysmal supraventricular tachycardia. *Ann Intern Med*.96:409–412, 1982.

Shenasa M, Fromer M, Faugere G, Nadeau R, Leblanc RA, Lambert C, Sadr-ameli MA: Efficacy and safety of intravenous and oral diltiazem for Wolff-Parkinson-White syndrome. *Am J Cardiol* 59:301–306, 1987.

Talano JV, Tommaso C: Slow channel calcium antagonists in the treatment of supraventricular tachycardia. *Prog Cardiovasc Dis* 25:141–156, 1982.

Waxman HL, Myerbug RJ, Appel R, Sung RJ: Verapamil for control of ventricular rate in paroxysmal supraventricular tachycardia and atrial fibrillation or flutter. *Ann Intern Med* 94:1–6, 1981.

Mexiletine and Tocainide

Campbell RWF: Mexiletine. *N Engl J Med* 316:29–34, 1987.

Roden DM: **Editorial.** Tocainide and mexiletine: orally effective lidocaine analogs. *Arch Intern Med* 145:417–418, 1985.

Roden DM, Woosley RL: Tocainide. *N Engl J Med* 315:41–45, 1986.

Encainide and Flecainide

Roden DM, Wood AJJ, Wilkinson GR, Woosley RL: Disposition kinetics of encainide and metabolites. *Am J Cardiol* 58:4C–9C, 1986.

Roden DM, Woosley RL: Flecainide. *N Engl J Med* 315:36–41, 1986.

Woosley RL, Wood, AJJ, Roden DM: Encainide. *N Engl J Med* 318:1107–1115, 1988.

The CAST Investigators: Preliminary Report: Effect of encainide and flecainide on mortality in a randomized trial of arrythmia suppression after myocardial infarction. *N Engl J Med* 321:406–412, 1989.

17

Diuretics

ROBERT A. BRANCH

Diuretic drugs are one of the most widely used group of drugs in clinical practice and represent a powerful tool in the clinical pharmaceutical armamentarium. There are now a large number of drugs that can induce a diuresis. This, by definition, is "An increase in sodium loss from the kidney." The diuretics can be grouped and classified on the basis of their site of action in the nephron:

1. Proximal renal tubule—**osmotic diuretics**—carbonic anhydrase inhibitors
2. Ascending limb of loop of Henle—**loop diuretics**
3. Distal tubule—**thiazides**
4. Distal tuble—**potassium sparing diuretics**

RENAL PHYSIOLOGY

Urine is formed from the blood by a process of filtration followed by selective tubular reabsorption. The basic unit for urine production is the nephron (Fig. 17.1). The kidney has three major functions; these are: (a) homeostatic regulation of the internal environment of water, sodium, potassium, calcium, magnesium, and phosphate, and maintenance of acid-base balance; (b) excretion of the end metabolic products particularly of protein metabolism including urea, creatinine, uric acid, guanidino metabolites, and others; (c) endocrine function in relation to vitamin D metabolism, parathormone metabolism, and erythropoietin and renin release.

GLOMERULAR FILTRATION

The glomerulus of each nephron filters the blood. It is a passive process and allows blood constituents having a molecular weight of less than 68,000 to pass through into the tubule, but retains cellular elements and large molecular weight substances, such as proteins. The determinants of glomerular filtration are total renal blood flow, the balance of afferent and efferent glomerular arteriolar tone, pore size of the endothelium basement membrane, and probably most importantly clinically, the total number of functioning glomeruli.

RENAL TUBULAR EPITHELIUM TRANSPORT MECHANISMS

Following glomerular filtration, the filtrate enters the renal tubule, where both tubular reabsorption and secretion of inorganic and organic compounds take place. There has recently been an improved understanding of the mechanisms involved in renal tubular transport. Figure 17.2 is a simplified schematic illustration that illustrates the differential localization of transport proteins between the luminal membrane and the basolateral membrane of epithelial cells with special reference to sodium. Sodium transport occurs at two levels across tubular epithelium: (a) movement of sodium across the luminal membrane from tubular fluid into the renal tubular cell; and (b) extrusion of sodium from the cell into the peritubular fluid or interstitial fluid space. The fundamental energy supply that drives transport in tubular cells is provided by the hydrolysis of adenosine triphosphate (ATP). This provides energy to the enzyme Na^+,K^+-ATPase, a single protein, located on the basolateral membrane in contact with peritubular fluid. The protein has now been purified, and the structure of its catalytic site has been characterized. It is often referred to as the "sodium pump," since it provides energy for the active extrusion of sodium. Under experimental conditions, Na^+,K^+-ATPase can be inhibited by high concentrations of the cardiac glycosides, which thus prevent active reabsorption of sodium. This does not occur at therapeutic doses.

In contrast to a single transport process on the basolateral membrane for the extrusion of sodium, the luminal membrane has a number of separate transport mechanisms regulated by proteins. The specificity of these proteins for transporting substances varies, and each has a preferential location within the nephron. Three major routes of sodium transporter proteins have been defined. These are responsible for: (a) facilitated diffusion along a favorable electrochemical gradient; (b) cotransport with either an anion, such as chloride or phosphate, or a non-

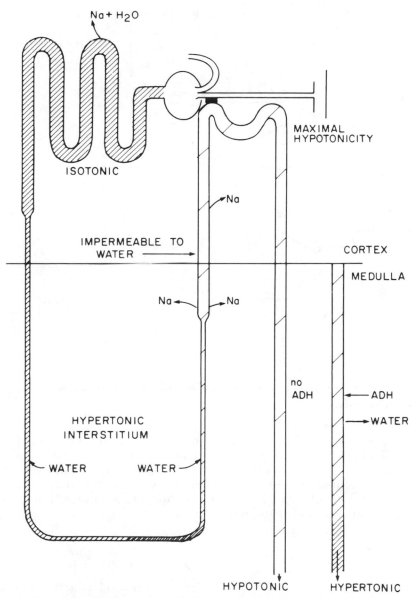

Figure 17.1.   Schematic diagram of nephron to indicate the relative function of individual components of the nephron with respect to sodium and water homeostasis.   Intensity of shading represents osmolarity.

electrolyte, such as glucose or amino acids; such transport proteins have been called synporters and are predominant in the proximal convoluted tubule and ascending limb of the loop of Henle; and (c) exchange of sodium for a cation, such as hydrogen ion or potassium. These transport proteins have been called antiport-

ers and are predominant in the distal tubule and collecting duct.

PROXIMAL CONVOLUTED TUBULE

Under normal circumstances, over 99% of the water entering the tubule from the glomerulus has been reabsorbed before the ureter is reached. Although reabsorp-

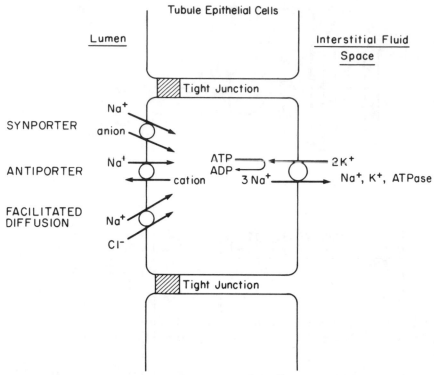

Figure 17.2.   Schematic diagram to indicate sodium transport mechanisms across renal tubular epithelial cells.

tion of water takes place in the proximal, distal, and collecting tubules, over 70% of total water reabsorption takes place in the proximal convoluted tubule. About seven-eighths of sodium chloride is reabsorbed in the proximal tubules, and only one-eighth in the loop of Henle and distal tubules.

The proximal convoluted tubule is also the site of numerous active transport processes; these include pumps for reabsorbing glucose, amino acids, low molecular weight proteins, phosphate and sodium, and for excreting anions, bases and neutral drugs such as ouabain into the filtrate. In this part of the tubule, movement of osmotically active molecules is accompanied by a free flow of water so that the filtrate remains isoosmotic with respect to plasma.

One specific pump of relevance to diuretics in this part of the tubule is the bicarbonate-conserving, acid-secreting mechanism controlled by the enzyme carbonic anhydrase (Fig. 17.3). In excess

of 90% of filtered bicarbonate (HCO_3^-) is reabsorbed in the proximal tubule via an exchange for hydrogen (H^+) ion produced by the dissociation of carbonic acid aided by the intracellular action of the enzyme carbonic anhydrase:

$$\text{Carbonic} \atop \text{Anhydrase}$$
$$H_2CO_3 \rightleftarrows H^+ + HCO_3^-$$

This is followed by active transport of the H^+ ion into the nephron lumen. When the hydrogen ion reaches the lumen, it combines with HCO_3^- to form carbonic acid (H_2CO_3), which dissociates to water (H_2O) and carbon dioxide (CO_2). The CO_2 is membrane soluble, passes through the tubular cell to the blood stream, and is excreted by the lungs. Thus, the net effect is excretion of an acid load and reabsorption of HCO_3^-. At the time H^+ ion is being actively secreted, electrical balance has to be maintained, and this is achieved by the passive reabsorption of sodium; thus, sodium ions enter the tu-

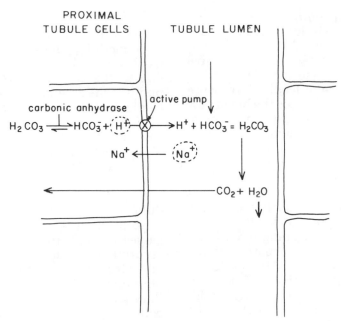

PROXIMAL
TUBULE CELLS   TUBULE LUMEN

carbonic anhydrase   active pump

$$H_2CO_3 \rightleftharpoons HCO_3^- + H^+ \quad -\!\!\otimes\!\!\rightarrow \quad H^+ + HCO_3^- = H_2CO_3$$

$$Na^+ \leftarrow \quad Na^+$$

$$\leftarrow \quad CO_2 + H_2O$$

Figure 17.3.   Schematic diagram of the bicarbonate-conserving, acid-secreting mechanism in the proximal tubule that is regulated by carbonic anhydrase.

bular cells from the filtrate in exchange for hydrogen ions. Because the reabsorption of sodium ions in exchange for hydrogen ions can proceed only so long as there is an adequate supply of the enzyme carbonic anhydrase, alterations in the activity of carbonic anhydrase will influence the passive reabsorption of sodium.

LOOP OF HENLE

The function of this section of the nephron is to generate hypertonic interstitial fluid within the renal medulla which subsequently will facilitate water reabsorption from the collecting tubule as it passes through the same area. The thin descending limb is permeable to water but impermeable to sodium. Once around the loop, the ascending limb of the loop of Henle undergoes a sudden anatomical change, with the external nephron diameter widening into the so-called "thick component" of the ascending limb of the loop of Henle, part of which is in the outer medulla, and part of which is in the cortex (Fig. 17.1). This change in structure is associated with a change in function. The two principal changes

are that an active chloride pump reabsorbs chloride, with sodium and calcium following passively, and secondly, this part of the nephron is impermeable to water. Thus, the extracellular fluid becomes hypertonic, and the filtrate in the lumen hypotonic with respect to plasma. This pump, via a counter-current-multiplying effect is responsible for generating the hypertonic medullary interstitium required for maximal free water reabsorption (urine concentration) and also for generating a hypotonic filtrate required for maximal free water clearance (urine dilution).

DISTAL CONVOLUTED TUBULE

The distal convoluted tubule is the area of fine control of filtrate, and its initial anatomical starting point is at the macula densa, which is situated where the distal convoluted tubule contacts its glomerulus, an ideal anatomical location for placing regulatory sensing and control mechanisms to achieve precise modulation (Fig. 17.1). Sensing mechanisms at the macula densa assess the delivery of sodium chloride to the early part of the distal tubule and influence distal tubular function through the renin, angiotensin, and aldosterone axis. It can even "sense" situations of proximal tubule failure. When inappropriate and excessive amounts of electrolytes are delivered to it, a tubuloglomerular feedback response is activated which reduces the blood flow to that individual nephron in order to prevent massive electrolyte loss in situations such as acute tubular necrosis or acute drug-induced toxicity.

Sodium reabsorption in the distal tubule, which can account for 5 to 10% of the filtered sodium, probably takes place by an active transport mechanism which, in contrast to the ascending limb, is independent of calcium transport. As in the ascending limb, the distal tubule is impermeable to water so that sodium reabsorption results in further dilution of filtrate, but because this part of the nephron is in the cortex, medullary interstitial tonicity is unaffected. Thus, the distal tubule sodium pump does influence maximal free water clearance (ability to produce a dilute urine), but does not influence maximal urine concentrating ability.

The distal part of the distal tubule and the proximal part of the collecting tubule are the major sites which regulate urinary potassium excretion. Up to this point, the potassium concentration in the filtrate is approximately that of plasma. Potassium excretion is regulated predominantly through an aldosterone-controlled sodium-potassium exchange pump. Aldosterone causes sodium reabsorption and potassium loss at this site. Because the aldosterone-controlled loss of potassium occurs in exchange for sodium, the urinary excretion of potassium is determined by both the rate of delivery of sodium to this site and the activity of the aldosterone system. Thus, in hyperaldosteronism whether of primary or secondary etiology, excessive loss of urinary potassium only occurs when there is appreciable concomitant sodium loss. Even when the rate of potassium-sodium exchange is high, the extent of sodium reabsorption is small, accounting for less than 0.5% of the filtered load.

COLLECTING TUBULES

The collecting tubules pass through the renal medulla where the interstitial fluid has been rendered markedly hypertonic due to the counter-current multiplying pump of the ascending limb of the loop of Henle (previously discussed). The collecting tubules are responsible for urine concentration and the final modification of the electrolyte content (Na^+ and K^+) of the filtrate. Prior to the collecting duct, the filtrate in the distal tubule is hypotonic, while interstitial fluid in the medulla is hypertonic, creating a marked concentration gradient as the filtrate passes through the collecting duct. Reabsorption of water in the collecting tubules is under the control of antidiuretic hormone (ADH) from the posterior pituitary gland. In the absence of ADH, the collecting duct remains impermeable to water, and dilute urine is passed (increased free water clearance). In the presence of ADH, the membrane is permeable, and water is reabsorbed across the concentration gradient, creating concentrated urine (negative free water clearance). In addition, it has recently been suggested that local production of the prostaglandin, PGE_2 (see Chapter 24), in the collecting tubule may modulate water reabsorption for any given level of ADH activity. This may explain the potential for nonsteroidal antiinflammatory drugs to be associated with impaired free water clearance, which can result in water intoxication with a dilutional hyponatremia.

INDIVIDUAL DIURETICS

Osmotic Diuretics

Mode of Action. Small molecular weight substances, if they are filtered at the glomerulus and not reabsorbed in the tubule, will exert an osmotic force to retain water within the nephron and, thus, will increase the rate of urine production. If the amount of osmotically active substance is substantial, then there will be a greater rate of flow through the nephron lumen, resulting in reduced efficiency of sodium reabsorption and a true diuresis (i.e., sodium loss). Clinically, the most important osmotic diuretics are found in disease states such as uncontrolled diabetes, uremia, and hypercalcemia, which can all be associated with marked sodium loss and dehydration. Examples of osmotic diuretics used therapeutically include **mannitol** and **urea**. In addition to initiating a sodium diuresis, mannitol increases renal blood flow and reduces the rate of secretion of renin. It also washes out the hypertonic medullary interstitial gradient and, hence, reduces the kidney's ability to produce concentrated urine. Delivery of increased amounts of sodium to the distal tubule can be associated with high urinary potassium loss if there is high aldosterone activity.

Pharmacokinetics. Mannitol is unreliably absorbed via the oral route and therefore has to be administered intravenously. It is initially contained within the intravascular space and then slowly distributed to expand the extracellular fluid volume. Mannitol is not metabolized but is excreted unchanged in urine.

Therapeutic Use. Mannitol is administered by anesthesiologists for rapid reduction of intracranial pressure during neurosurgical procedures. It is also frequently used in the management of shocked patients to maintain renal function and prevent acute tubular necrosis.

Toxicity. Mannitol has the potential to increase extracellular fluid volume which may compromise cardiac function in patients in heart failure. It should be remembered that, when this drug is used in neurological emergencies, it causes a sodium diuresis, and this sodium deficit must be replaced. It may occasionally cause hypersensitivity reactions.

Carbonic Anhydrase Inhibitors

Mode of Action. Acetazolamide (Diamox) is a potent inhibitor of the renal enzyme, carbonic anhydrase. Normally, sodium is reabsorbed in exchange for hydrogen ions which are excreted (see above) in the proximal and distal tubules. Inhibition of carbonic anhydrase reduces the

supply of hydrogen ions, and so sodium and bicarbonate ions remain within the renal tubule. Thus, acetazolamide administration results in the production of an alkaline urine with a high sodium bicarbonate content. The increase in sodium excretion causes a diuresis. Although acetazolamide acts in the proximal tubule where the major portion of sodium reabsorption occurs, it influences a mechanism which only accounts for a small proportion of the total amount of filtered sodium that is reabsorbed. Therefore, acetazolamide causes only a relatively modest diuresis. The alkaline diuresis results in a metabolic acidosis and a lowered plasma bicarbonate, which reduces the amount of sodium bicarbonate in the glomerular filtrate. This may be a factor in explaining the rapid tachyphylaxis that occurs with repeated acetazolamide administration, even though the urine remains persistently alkaline.

Pharmacokinetics. Acetazolamide is well absorbed with peak plasma concentrations occurring within 2 hours of administration. It is a weak acid and is actively transported into renal tubular fluid. Its elimination is essentially complete within 24 hours, and it does not undergo any appreciable metabolism.

Therapeutic Use. Acetazolamide can be used to initiate an alkaline diuresis in the management of salicylate overdose. Otherwise its therapeutic uses are for nonrenal objectives, namely, the management of glaucoma, familial periodic paralysis, acute mountain sickness, and petit mal epilepsy.

Toxicity. Toxicity is rare. Large doses may cause paresthesia and drowsiness. Drug rashes are rare. Teratogenicity has been reported in animals. Drug-induced osteomalacia has been reported when given concurrently with phenytoin.

Loop Diuretics

The loop diuretics comprise a group of structurally dissimilar drugs which appear to have a common mechanism of action.

Furosemide is the most widely used member of this group. In addition, ethacrynic acid, bumetanide, and mercurial diuretics act at this site. Furosemide, an anthranilic acid derivative, has been shown to inhibit active chloride reabsorption in the thick portion of the ascending limb of the loop of Henle (Fig. 17.3). The extent of the response is determined by the amount of furosemide presented to this section of the tubule in the filtrate. As the ascending limb accounts for approximately 25% of sodium chloride reabsorption in the total nephron, inhibition of reabsorption results in a marked diuresis. Following the initiation of diuresis, homeostatic mechanisms (increased aldosterone activity and probably increased proximal tubule sodium reabsorption) tend to retain sodium; thus, repeated dosage will result in an attenuation of the response. However, the initial diuresis is so marked that even moderate reduction in response still leaves a clinically useful diuretic effect. Although the active transport process that is inhibited is chloride reabsorption, anions such as calcium and sodium are also reabsorbed with chloride to maintain electrical neutrality. Thus, inhibition of chloride reabsorption will cause an increased urinary rate of excretion of sodium and calcium.

Loss of sodium chloride reabsorption results in a reduced ability to form a hypertonic medullary interstitium and, therefore, a hypotonic distal tubule filtrate osmolality. As a consequence, both maximal urine-concentrating and diluting ability are reduced (Table 17.1). A further consequence of loss of chloride reabsorption is an immediate stimulus to the macula densa to release renin and thereby activate the renin, angiotensin, aldosterone axis. This response is mediated via prostaglandins as is the ability of furosemide to increase renal blood flow and cause a redistribution of renal blood flow such that outer cortical blood flow is unchanged, while inner corticomedullary flow is increased. The increases in renin and blood flow can be inhibited by inhibiting prostaglandin biosynthesis with cyclooxygenase inhibitors such as indomethacin (see Chapter 24).

As with any diuretic, sodium delivery to the distal tubule can potentiate potassium loss in the presence of high aldosterone activity. As the diuresis is so potent and continues even in the presence of substantial secondary hyperaldosteronism, substantial potassium deficits can occur.

Pharmacokinetics. Furosemide may be administered intravenously, orally, or intramuscularly. Following oral administration, 50 to 60% of the dose rapidly reaches the systemic circulation to achieve peak levels 0.5 to 1.5 hours after administration. Furosemide is approximately 90% bound to plasma proteins. Its volume of distribution (0.1 L/kg) is low in comparison to many other drugs and approximates extracellular fluid volume. Probenecid, an inhibitor of anion transport, reduces the volume of distribution so that it is possible that part of distribution occurs as an active rather than a passive diffusion process. Furosemide is eliminated either unchanged in urine, in which case it has been actively secreted by the anion pump, or is eliminated by alternative mechanisms. These include metabolism to glucuronide and active secretion into the gastrointestinal tract. Total clearance in normal subjects is 2

Table 17.1.
Comparison of Common Orally Administered Diuretics

Diuretic	Sodium diuresis	Impaired urine concentrating ability	Impaired urine diluting ability	Potassium excretion
Loop diuretics	+++	++	++	++
Thiazides	++	−	+	++
Potassium-sparing diuretics	+	−	−	−

ml/min/kg, and the elimination half-life is approximately 60 minutes. Both renal and nonrenal routes of elimination are impaired in association with decreased renal function and in neonates, but neither is influenced by liver disease.

Therapeutic Use. Furosemide is the diuretic of choice in acute life-threatening situations of fluid overload, such as congestive cardiac failure; furosemide may be able to reduce pulmonary wedge pressure even before a diuresis has occurred. Similar observations of acute changes in capacitance vessels have been made in the dog in response to furosemide. These only occur when the kidneys are intact and can be abolished by prior treatment with indomethacin, suggesting that these acute changes might be due to renal release of a circulating vasodilator prostaglandin.

Furosemide is also the diuretic of choice in excessive fluid overload, in patients with fluid retention resistant to milder diuretics, and in patients with chronic renal insufficiency who require diuretic therapy. Even though it is an effective hypotensive agent in the management of hypertension, it has no advantage over thiazide diuretics, while potential disadvantages of excessive furosemide therapy include prerenal uremia and hypokalemia. It may be used in nonedematous conditions to reduce intracerebral pressure and to reduce serum calcium levels in malignant hypercalcemia provided rehydration and sodium replacement are also performed. It can also be used to induce water loss in water intoxication; in this instance, urinary sodium losses should be replaced, so that there is a net increase in free water clearance and no change in total-body sodium content.

Toxicity. The major toxicity is due to excessive therapy, which causes dehydration and hypokalemia. Hyperuricemia secondary to diuresis may precipitate an acute attack of gout in a patient with preexisting gouty diathesis, but does not cause clinical complications in subjects who do not have the primary metabolic abnormality. Drug rashes and idiosyncratic reactions are rare, although interstitial nephritis has been reported. The one major dose-related toxicity is the development of VIII nerve damage when plasma levels exceed 100 μg/ml. This is thought to be due to electrolyte changes in the endolymph. These levels can be avoided even when using large-dose intravenous therapy if furosemide is only administered slowly (i.e., no faster than 4 mg/min). There is some evidence of synergy between aminoglycosides and furosemide in the production of VIII nerve toxicity. Eighth nerve damage has been observed more frequently with ethacrynic acid, where it has been suggested that the accumulation of an ototoxic metabolite may occur if the patient has renal failure.

ETHACRYNIC ACID

Ethacrynic acid, an unsaturated ketone derivative of aryloxyacetic acid, is structurally dissimilar from furosemide but has almost identical pharmacological properties.

Following intravenous administration, it is highly bound to plasma proteins and distributed in a space approximating extracellular volume. It is eliminated by active secretion into the renal tubule and, as with furosemide, it is this component that contributes to the pharmacological response. In addition to a cysteine adduct, other minor metabolites are found in urine, and up to one-third is excreted in bile.

It has been suggested that the peak response to ethacrynic acid is lower than furosemide and that the risk of ototoxicity, when large doses are given to patients with impaired renal function, is greater. However, it is more likely that these two drugs are equivalent in pharmacological action and risk of toxicity.

BUMETANIDE

Bumetanide is a melanidamide derivative, structurally similar to furosemide but with a 40 times greater potency. This characteristic does not confer any advantage or disadvantage in comparison to furosemide, providing equivalent doses are administered. Pharmacokinetically, bumetanide and furosemide are handled similarly, with the exception that bumetanide is completely absorbed following oral administration, and its rate of elimination is less influenced by impaired renal function.

Thiazides

Mode of Action. Thiazides were first synthesized during structure-activity studies on compounds which inhibited carbonic anhydrase. Their essential difference from carbonic anhydrase inhibitors is that they induce a sodium chloride rather than a sodium bicarbonate diuresis.

There are now a large number of thiazides which, although they have different potencies on a molar basis, have identically shaped dose-response curves, with each compound achieving the same maximal rate of diuresis. Their toxic effects and handling by the body are similar, and the only distinguishing features (apart from cost) are minor differences in their rates of elimination.

The site of action of the thiazide diuretics is in the distal convoluted tubule (Fig. 17.4). This portion of the nephron accounts for less than 5% of total sodium reabsorption, so that even under optimal conditions, the diuresis achieved by this group of drugs can never be as intense as with loop diuretics. In sodium-depleted situations, or following successful initiation of diuretic therapy, homeostatic mechanisms tend to conserve sodium and can markedly reduce the diuretic response. Thus, if thiazides are given to the point of inducing severe sodium depletion, the body adapts by reducing their efficacy. This acts as a safety factor and contrasts with the persistent diuretic response associated with loop diuretics.

The thiazides inhibit an active pump for sodium reabsorption but, in contrast to the loop diuretics, they decrease renal excretion of calcium and hypercalcemia may result. As thiazides act on the distal tubule, urine-concentrating mechanisms are not impaired, but maximal urine dilution is modestly reduced (Table 17.1). As with the loop diuretics, thiazides increase the rate of delivery of sodium to the lower nephron and, in the presence of high aldosterone activity, large quantities of potassium may be lost. Thiazides also reduce renal uric acid clearance and cause hyperuricemia.

Pharmacokinetics. The thiazides are rapidly absorbed from the gastrointestinal tract to reach peak levels between 0.5 and 1.5 hours after oral administration. The principal difference between the numerous thiazides available is in their rate of elimination, with chlorthiazide having a half-life of about 6 hours and bendrofluazide 12 hours at each extreme. These drugs are distributed within the extracellular fluid space and are eliminated predominantly by active anion secretion into the proximal tubule of the nephron.

Therapeutic Uses. The major use of thiazide diuretics is in the management of edematous states associated with congestive cardiac failure, cirrhosis, and the nephrotic syndrome, where they provide a mild but sustained diuresis. They are also extensively used in the management of hypertension, where they can reduce blood pressure when given as single drug therapy with or without sodium depletion. Low-sodium diets will potentiate the hypotensive action, and also increase urinary potassium loss. The combination of thiazide and a low-sodium diet acts synergistically with many of the other drugs available for reducing blood pressure. A rarer use of thiazides concerns their curious effect in reducing water loss in patients with nephrogenic diabetes insipidus. It is probable that sodium depletion associated with thiazides is the major factor in helping such patients' polyervia. In patients with recurrent urinary calculi, hypercalciuria can be reduced with thiazide therapy.

Toxicity. The most common side effect is due to excessive therapy causing dehydration and hypokalemia. Thiazides cause hyperuricemia; this only requires treatment if it precipitates symptomatic gout. Thiazides decrease carbohydrate tolerance, particularly in patients who have developed hypokalemia which alters insulin tolerance. Diabetes may be precipitated in a prediabetic subject, while insulin requirements may be in-

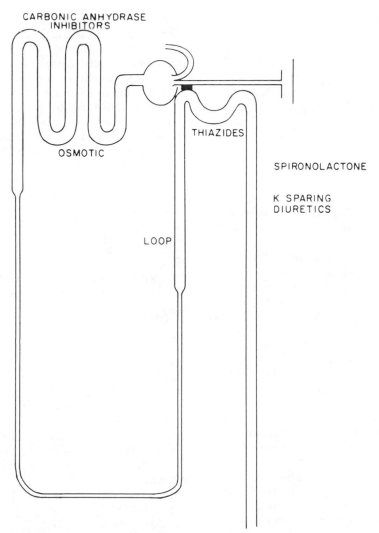

Figure 17.4.   Schematic diagram of nephron to indicate the site of action of different diuretics.

creased in the diabetic patient. However, they probably do not cause diabetes in a normal subject. Hypersensitivity reactions are rare, but occur more frequently than with loop diuretics. Purpura, dermatitis with photosensitivity, antibody-induced thrombocytopenia, bone marrow depression, and necrotizing vasculitis have all been reported.

Potassium-sparing Diuretics

This group of drugs consists of two subgroups: (a) aldosterone antagonists, e.g., spironolactone, and (b) those that act in-

dependently of aldosterone, i.e., amiloride or triamterine. Because the site of action of these drugs is in the lower part of the distal tubule and in the collecting duct (Fig. 17.4), the extent to which they can inhibit sodium reabsorption is limited. They do, however, augment the diuretic response to loop or thiazide diuretics when given concurrently. They have the further advantage that, as they reduce the exchange of sodium for potassium, they prevent the excessive loss of potassium that occurs with thiazide and loop diuretics. They do not influence renal handling of water (Table 17.1) and slightly increase urinary calcium excretion.

SPIRONOLACTONE

Aldosterone causes sodium reabsorption and potassium loss in the distal renal tubule. Spironolactone competes with aldosterone for specific receptors in the renal tubule; thus, in the absence of aldosterone, spironolactone has no effect. It is a complex molecule in which a steroid nucleus has been modified to allow gastrointestinal absorption. Following absorption, spironolactone is metabolized almost immediately ($t_{1/2}$ = 5 minutes) to a number of metabolites, the predominant one being canrenoate sodium. This active metabolite has a half-life of about 15 hours in normal subjects, which can be prolonged 2-fold in liver disease.

The major therapeutic uses are as (a) a single diuretic in the management of patients with ascites due to cirrhosis who have marked secondary hyperaldosteronism and (b) a concurrent treatment with other diuretics to reduce the risk of hypokalemia in other situations of excess sodium retention.

Disadvantages of spironolactone (apart from being expensive with respect to alternatives) include an appreciable incidence of nausea with higher doses, the risk of inducing hyperkalemia if renal function is impaired, and the development of gynecomastia in men (a reflection of its steroid structure).

AMILORIDE

Amiloride is a potassium-sparing diuretic acting on the distal tubule and collecting duct which can conserve potassium and increase sodium loss even in the absence of hyperaldosteronism. Recently, it has been suggested that it can bind specifically to kallikrein in the collecting duct and that this protein is involved in the sodium-potassium exchange pump.

Amiloride is an organic base which is partially absorbed after oral administration (15 to 25%) and excreted almost entirely unchanged in urine. Its peak activity occurs within 6 hours of administration and is over within 24 hours.

Amiloride is almost always given in combination with either a loop diuretic or thiazide, where it acts synergistically in terms of diuresis but opposes potassium loss. It should be appreciated that, in patients with normal renal function, increasing the dose of combination diuretics increases the sodium loss, but rapidly attenuates the potassium-conserving properties, so that with high sodium losses, hypokalemia can occur. Conversely, patients with impaired renal function may develop hyperkalemia with this combination, and the use of potassium-sparing diuretics in renal failure is usually contraindicated.

RATIONAL USE OF DIURETICS IN EDEMATOUS STATES

Diuretics are administered to edematous patients with the therapeutic objective of decreasing the extracellular fluid volume by reducing the total-body sodium content. Under normal conditions, water is distributed throughout the body. Potassium is predominantly an intracellular ion, while sodium is predominantly extracellular. As sodium is the major osmotically active cation in the extracellular fluid, the extracellular fluid volume is directly proportional to the total amount of sodium in the body. It should also be recognized that there is no simple relationship between plasma sodium concentration and total-body sodium. The former parameter simply reflects the ratio of sodium to water and is, in fact, a better indicator of water homeostasis than sodium homeostasis. Thus, diuretics, by decreasing total-body sodium, decrease interstitial fluid volume and reduce edema.

Under physiological conditions, decreases in extracellular fluid volume activate hormonal reflexes including the renin, angiotensin, aldosterone axis to conserve sodium by enhancing tubular reabsorption. Conversely, increases in extracellular fluid volume stimulate the release of *atrial natriuretic factor* (ANF) to result in enhanced urinary sodium excretion. Since the seminal observation in 1981 that an extract of rat atria could induce a natriuresis, there has been a dramatic increase in our knowledge of this hormone. The active hormone in humans is a 28-amino acid peptide, originally formed from a 151-amino acid peptide precursor. Within 3 years of identification, this protein was purified and sequenced, its RNA and complementary DNA clones identified, and many factors of its role in sodium homeostasis elucidated.

The precursor of ANF is synthesized predominantly in the atria. Its release is stimulated by increased stretch and contraction within the atria, indicating that blood volume is a critical determinant to release. Once released, it is the most potent natriuretic factor yet known; for example, it can achieve well over twice the maximal diuretic response of furosemide in renal failure models, implying an action on proximal and distal segments of the nephron. In addition, it is a potent renal vasodilator and, in pharmacological doses, will reduce blood pressure.

Its major disadvantage from a therapeutic perspective is that it has to be administered intravenously and has a short duration of action. However, it is anticipated that structural analogs will be available for therapeutic use in the future. It should also be noted that, despite its desirable properties and its elevation in clinical situations associated with edema, such as congestive cardiac failure and cirrhosis, these conditions are characterized by sodium retention rather than sodium loss. Thus, activation of endogenous release of ANF has been ineffective in correcting the initial abnormality, and it remains to be shown that exogenous administration of ANF will have a major therapeutic role.

Diuretics are extensively used in clinical practice. Three important considerations should be kept in mind when considering the use of diuretics in patients with edema:

1. Therapy is only palliative and does not influence the underlying cause for the edema.
2. Apart from acute pulmonary edema, a dramatic response is rarely required and can be dangerous; thus, the maxim is—"the mildest diuresis consistent with a sustained response." This approach reduces the major adverse effect of the diuretics, namely, overtreatment causing dehydration and prerenal uremia.
3. Whenever a diuretic is being administered, specific consideration must be given to potassium homeostasis.

SODIUM DIURESIS

Acute pulmonary edema is the one therapeutic indication when a rapid reduction in extracellular fluid volume is required. This is most rapidly achieved with intravenous administration of furosemide or another loop diuretic. There is evidence that pulmonary wedge pressure falls even before a diuresis occurs, and this response has been attributed to the ability of furosemide to release vasodilator prostaglandins from the kidney. Thus, furosemide provides an immediate acute reduction in pulmonary pressure which is subsequently sustained by the diuresis. Once pulmonary edema is under control, the rate of diuresis needs to be reduced by dosage modification to prevent overtreatment.

In situations of sodium retention due to cirrhosis, nephrotic syndrome, cor pulmonale, or chronic congestive cardiac failure, a more gradual diuresis is indicated. This is particularly important in cirrhotic patients with ascites and a predisposition to portasystemic encephalopathy. Sudden diuretic induced hypokalemia can rapidly put such patients into coma. Furthermore, ascitic fluid only exchanges slowly with the rest of extracellular fluid so that it is possible in the presence of marked ascites to reduce circulating blood volume to such an extent that prerenal failure is produced if diuresis is too rapid. In such patients, a reasonable therapeutic objective is to try and achieve a urinary sodium loss of approximately 100 mEq/day. At the same time, dietary intake of sodium should be reduced to 20 to 40 mEq/day so that a net loss of 60 to 80 mEq results.

If the dose-response relationship of thiazides and loop diuretics is compared (Fig. 17.5), it can be seen that low doses of thiazides result in a modest diuresis,

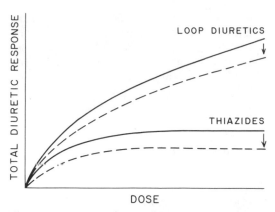

Figure 17.5. Schematic comparison of dose to total diuretic response relationships between loop diuretics and thiazides. ——, response to initial dose; – – –, reduced response to the same doses with increased attempts by the body to conserve sodium.

which to a limited extent increases with increasing doses. However, a ceiling effect is achieved such that doses above this level fail to result in further diuretic response. Following repeated therapy, the body responds to induced sodium depletion by attempting to conserve more sodium, and thus, the ceiling response becomes reduced. The variability in this ceiling response between subjects is due in part to differences in glomerular filtration rate and in part to avid sodium retention even before administering the diuretic. In contrast to thiazides, loop diuretics have a steeper dose-response curve such that a response can be achieved in almost anyone even in the presence of impaired renal function, and although increasing attempts at sodium conservation reduce the response, it remains significant. However, very high doses of furosemide may be required.

These observations imply firstly, that for the majority of subjects a low dose of thiazide will be adequate; secondly, that there is little advantage in trying high doses of thiazides, and thirdly, that in the patient who becomes resistant to thiazides, an adequate diuresis can still be achieved by giving appropriate doses of a loop diuretic.

POTASSIUM DEPLETION

As has already been indicated, urinary potassium elimination is determined by a sodium-for-potassium exchange mechanism in the distal tubule and collecting duct. This active transport system is dependent on sodium delivery and aldosterone activity. Many edematous conditions are associated with secondary hyperaldosteronism, particularly cirrhosis with ascites. Furthermore, successful diuretic therapy will potentiate a secondary hyperaldosteronism in an attempt to conserve sodium. In the presence of high aldosterone activity, urinary potassium loss will reflect sodium delivery. The administration of both thiazides and loop diuretics increases such a delivery and therefore results in hyperkaluria and the potential to induce hypokalemia. This is of particular consequence in cirrhotic patients and patients with heart disease receiving digoxin.

It is mandatory to consider potassium in any patient on a diuretic. One simple guide to assess whether specific action is required is to measure the urinary Na/K ratio. A Na/K ratio of less than one is a fairly good indicator of hyperaldosteronism. Furthermore, if a therapeutic objective of a urinary excretion of 100 mEq of sodium per day is being achieved, then it is apparent that more than 100 mEq of potassium is being excreted. As the normal dietary intake of potassium varies between 60 and 80 mEq, a cumulative deficit will inevitably result unless active steps are taken to prevent hypokalemia (Fig. 17.6).

Alternative therapies are:

1. Potassium supplements which if taken can provide adequate homeostasis; however, noncompliance by patients is high because of their unpleasant taste;
2. Coadministration of potassium-sparing diuretics either as separate tablets or in combination tablets.

The major hazard of giving either of these two forms of therapy is that dangerous hyperkalemia can develop in patients with impaired renal function. Active consideration of potassium as an

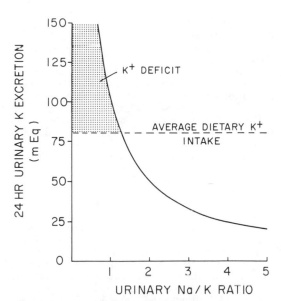

Figure 17.6. The relationship between urinary Na/K ratio and 24-hour urinary potassium excretion assuming a diuresis of 100 mEq of sodium is being excreted in urine per day.

independent factor can prevent either low or high levels of potassium.

BIBLIOGRAPHY

Alison MEM, Kennedy AC: Diuretics in chronic renal disease: a study of high dosage frusemide. *Clin Sci* 41:171–187, 1971.

Aranda JV, Perez J, Sitar DS, Collinge J, Portuguez-Malavasi A, Duffy B, Dupont C: Pharmacokinetic disposition and protein binding of furosemide in newborn infants. *J Pediatr* 93:507–511, 1978.

Barclay JE, Lee HA: Clinical and pharmacokinetic studies on bumetanide in chronic renal failure. *Postgrad Med J* 51:43–46, 1975.

Björnberg A, Gisslén H: Thiazides: a cause of necrotising vasculitis. *Lancet* 2:982–983, 1965.

Burg M, Good D: Sodium chloride coupled transport in mammalian nephrons. *Annu Rev Physiol* 45:533–547, 1983.

Burg MB, Green N: Function of the thick ascending limb of Henle's loop. *Am J Physiol* 224:659–668, 1973.

de Bold A: Atrial natriuretic factor. A hormone produced by the heart. *Science* 230:767–770, 1985.

Dollery CT: Diabetogenic effect of long-term diuretic therapy. In Lant AF, Wilson GM (eds): *Modern Diuretic Therapy in the Treatment of Cardiovascular and Renal Disease*. Amsterdam, Excerpta Medica, 1973, pp 320–330.

Espiner EA, Tucci JR, Jagger PI, Pauk GL, Lauler DP: The effect of acute diuretic induced extracellular volume depletion on aldosterone secretion in normal man. *Clin Sci* 33:125–134, 1967.

Flezzani P, McIntryre RW, Xuan YT, Su YF, Leslie JB, Watkins WD: Atrial natriuretic peptide during cardiac surgery: a comparison of valvular heart disease and ischemic heart disease. *Anesthesiology* 65:A511, 1986.

Hedner J, Towle A, Saltzman L, Mueller RA, Pettersson A, Norfleet EA, Watson CB, Hedner T: Atrial natriuretic factor (ANF) in plasma of patients undergoing cardiopulmonary bypass surgery. *Anesthesiology* 65:A509, 1986.

Horky K, Gutowska J, Garcia R, Thibault G, Genest J, Cantin M: Effect of different anesthetics on immunoreactive atrial natriuretic factor concentrations in rat plasma. *Biochem Biophys Res Commun* 129:651–657, 1985.

Jacobsen HR, Kokko JP: Diuretics: sites and mechanisms of action. *Annu Rev Pharmcol* 16:201–214, 1976.

Karim A: Spironolactone: disposition, metabolism, pharmacodynamics, and bioavailability. *Drug Metab Rev* 8:151–188, 1978.

Kim KE, Onesti G, Moyer JH, Swartz C: Ethacrynic acid and furosemide, diuretic and hemodynamic effects and clinical uses. *Am J Cardiol* 27:407–415, 1971.

Liddle GW: Specific and nonspecific inhibition of mineralocorticoid activity. *Metabolism* 10:1021–1030, 1961.

Liddle GW: Aldosterone antagonists and triamterene. *Ann NY Acad Sci* 139:466–470, 1966.

Lyons H, Pinn VW, Cartell S, Cohen JJ, Harrington JT: Allergic interstitial nephritis causing reversible renal failure in four patients with idiopathic nephrotic syndrome. *N Engl J Med* 288:124–128, 1973.

Maren TH: Carbonic anydrase: chemistry, physiology, and inhibition. *Physiol Rev* 47:595–781, 1967.

Muth RG: Diuretics in chronic renal insufficiency. In Lant AF, Wilson GM (eds): *Modern Diuretics Therapy in the Treatment of Cardiovascular and Renal Disease*. Amsterdam, Excerpta Medica, 1973, pp 294–305.

Needleman P: Atriopeptins as cardiac hormones. *Hypertension* 7:469–482, 1985.

Needleman P, Greenwalk JE: Atriopeptin: a cardiac hormone intimately involved in fluid, electrolyte, and blood-pressure homeostasis. *N Engl J Med* 314:828–834, 1986.

Pentikainen PJ, Pentilla A, Neuvonen PJ, Gothoni G: Fate of [¹⁴C]bumetanide in man. *Br J Clin Pharmacol* 4:39–44, 1977.

Prazma J, Thomas WG, Fischer ND; Preslar MJ: Ototoxicity of ethacrynic acid. *Arch Otolar* 95:448–456, 1972.

Ramsey L, Shelton J, Harrison J, Tidd M; Asbury N: Spironolactone and potassium canrenoate in normal man. *Clin Pharmacol Ther* 20:167–177, 1971.

Rane A, Villeneuve JP, Stone WJ, Nies AS, Wilkinson GR, Branch RA: Plasma binding and disposition of furosemide in the nephrotic syndrome and in uremia. *Clin Pharmacol Ther* 24:199–207, 1978.

Rodeheffer RJ, Tanaka I, Imada T, Hollister AS, Robertson D, Inagami T: Atrial pressure and secretion of atrial natriuretic factor into the human central circulation. *J Am Coll Cardiol* 8:18–26, 1986.

Rupp W: Pharmacokinetics and pharmacodynamics of Lasix. *Scott Med J* 19:5–13, 1974.

Sadee W, Schroder R, Leitner E, Dagcioglu M: Multidose kinetics of spironolactone and canrenoate-potassium in cardiac and hepatic failure. *Eur J Clin Pharmacol* 7:195–200, 1974.

Schwab TR, Edwards BS, Heublein DM, Burnett JC Jr: Role of atrial natriuretic peptide in volume-expansion natriuresis. *Am J Physiol* 251:R310–R313, 1986.

Sherlock S: Diuretics in hepatic disease. In Lant AF, Wilson GM (eds): *Modern Diuretic Therapy in the Treatment of Cardiovascular and Renal Disease.* Amsterdam, Excerpta Medica, 1973, pp 270–280.

Sherlock S, Walker JG, Seneviratue B, Scott A: The complications of diuretic therapy in patients with cirrhosis. *Ann NY Acad Sci* 139:497–505, 1966.

Suki WN, Eknoyan G; Martinez-Maldonado M: Tubular sites and mechanisms of diuretic action. *Ann Rev Pharmacol* 13:91–106, 1973.

Suki WN, Yium JJ, Von Minden J, Saller-Hebert C, Eknoyan G, Martinez-Maldonado M: Acute treatment of hypercalcemia with furosemide. *N Engl J Med* 283:836–840, 1970.

Sulton RAL, Dinks JH: Renal handling of calcium. *Fed Proc* 37:2112–2119, 1978.

Thibault G, Garcia R, Gutkowska J, Genest J, Cantin M: Atrial natriuretic factor: a newly discovered hormone with significant clinical implications. *Drugs* 31:369–375, 1986.

Wales JK, Krees SV, Grant AM, Viktora JK, Wolff FW: Structure-activity relationships of benzothiadizine compounds as hyperglycemic agents. *J Pharmacol Exp Ther* 164:421–432, 1968.

Walker WG: Indications and contraindications for diuretic therapy. *Ann NY Acad Sci* 139:481–496, 1966.

Walker WG, Sapir DG, Turin M, Cheng JT: Potassium homeostasis with diuretic therapy. In Lant AF, Wilson GM (eds): *Modern Diuretic Therapy in the Treatment of Cardiovascular and Renal Disease.* Amsterdam, Excerpta Medica, 1973, pp 331–342.

Weiner IM: Transport of weak acids and bases. In Orloff J, Berliner RW (eds): *Renal Physiology. Handbook of Physiology.* Washington DC, American Physiological Society, 1973, sect 8, pp 521–554.

Wigand ME, Heidland A: Ototoxic side effects of high doses of furosemide in patients with uremia. *Postgrad Med J* 47:54–56, 1971.

Wood M, Bullington J, Hammon JW, Imada T, Inagami T: Control of circulatory volume and sodium excretion during cardiac surgery by atrial natriuretic factor. *Anesthesiology* 67:A18, 1987.

Calcium Antagonists

R. G. McALLISTER, JR.

Drugs which are "calcium antagonists" or calcium-blocking agents act selectively on specialized membrane channels to inhibit movement of calcium into cardiac and smooth muscle cells. In contrast to skeletal muscle, which contains adequate endogenous stores of calcium ion, both cardiac muscle and vascular smooth muscle require extracellular calcium for contractile function. Since the calcium antagonists compounds can reduce transmembrane calcium flux in these tissues, they have been found useful in the management of conditions in which pathologic vasoconstriction occurs, such as hypertension, Raynaud's disease, Prinzmetal's angina, and migraine syndromes. Similarly, calcium antagonists can decrease cardiac contractility, thereby reducing myocardial oxygen demand and providing a basis for therapeutic use in angina pectoris. In hypertrophic cardiomyopathy, in which a hypercontractile state leads to ventricular diastolic dysfunction, calcium antagonists may improve cardiac function by reducing contractility parameters to normal levels.

MECHANISM OF ACTION

The entrance of calcium into cells occurs through discrete passageways or gates which may be open or closed. Some of them are opened by stimulation of nearby adrenergic receptors (receptor-operated channel; Fig. 18.1), while others are opened by depolarization of the cellular membrane (voltage-dependent channel; Fig. 18.1). The receptor-operated gate on the intracellular surface is opened by cyclic AMP which allows the inward movement of calcium and is closed by cyclic GMP. These calcium passageways are sometimes referred to as "slow channels" in contrast to the so-called "fast channels" which conduct sodium ion (see Chapter 16). The fast sodium channels can be selectively blocked by lidocaine, procainamide, and tetrodotoxin, while the slow channels are blocked by nifedipine, verapamil, diltiazem, and certain other calcium antagonists.

At rest, the electrical potential inside the myocardial cell is negative (Fig. 18.2).

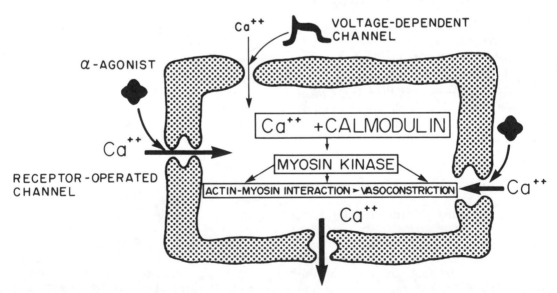

Figure 18.1. Mechanisms of calcium entry into cells. Calcium enters cells by a receptor-operated channel or a voltage-dependent channel to bind to calmodulin. (With permission from Ferlinz J: Nifedipine in myocardial ischemia, systemic hypertension, and other cardiovascular disorders. *Ann Intern Med* 105:714–729, 1986.)

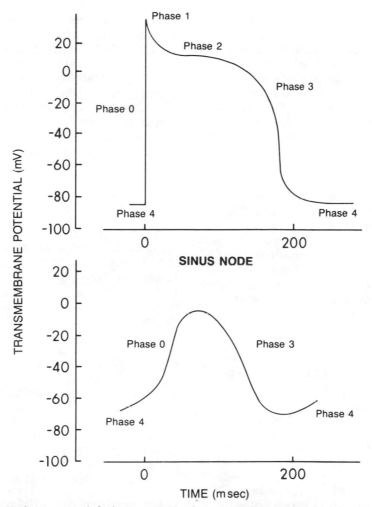

Figure 18.2.   Action potentials from ventricular myocardium (Purkinje cell) and the sinus node, contrasting the "fast" channel mediated by sodium flux in the ventricular myocardium with the "slow" calcium channel activity seen in the sinus node.   Note the rapid depolarization during phase 0 in the myocardium *(top)* and the slower depolarization of phase 0 in the sinus node pacemaker tissue *(bottom)*. Phase 4 is relatively stable in myocardial tissue, whereas slow spontaneous depolarization (characteristic of pacemaker tissue) occurs with the automatic rise of phase 4 in calcium flux-dependent nodal cells.

Excitation produces a brief depolarization due to inward sodium current (phase 0); positively charged calcium ions then begin to move through the cell prolonging the action potential (through phases 1 and 2). Thus, the fast sodium channels are important for the rapid upstroke of the action potential (phase 0), while phase 2 of the cardiac action potential is thought to be due to inward calcium movement. Most myocardial tissues de-

pend upon the fast sodium current in the initiation of activation, but areas with pacemaker activity [such as specialized pacemaker cells in the sinoatrial node, atrioventricular (A-V) node, and ischemic myocardial tissue] depolarize only as a result of the slow inward flux of calcium ion.

The calcium channel blockers are heterogeneous. They can be thought of electrophysiologically as selectively inhibiting the inward flux of calcium through slow calcium channels. Some act exclusively on the slow channel, either by physically obstructing or by interfering with the function of the gating machinery. Others such as verapamil inhibit the fast (sodium) channel as well as the slow channel. Verapamil also appears to bind to postsynaptic α-adrenergic receptors in some situations. Furthermore, the available calcium antagonists appear to have differing affinities for their various target tissues in vivo, thus making their effects appear relatively tissue selective. Verapamil, for example, acts on the A-V node at doses and plasma concentrations below those generally required for depressant effects on myocardial function; nifedipine has pronounced effects on arterial smooth muscle at doses lower than those required for direct cardiac effects. Therefore, although their in vitro properties and mechanisms of action are similar, there are important *clinical* differences in their pharmacologic activity and clinical application.

THE ROLE OF CALCIUM ION

Calcium is essential to the contractile function of vascular and myocardial smooth muscle cells and plays an important role in coupling depolarization of the surface membrane of myocardial and vascular smooth muscle cells to muscle contraction, i.e., excitation-contraction coupling. Extracellular calcium ion concentrations are about 10,000-fold higher than those within resting smooth muscle cells, and, in general, minor alterations in serum calcium concentrations do not significantly affect the availability of intracellular calcium ion for smooth muscle function. A rise in intracellular calcium sets in motion a chain of events leading to contraction.

Two stimuli are primarily responsible for the opening of membrane channels which are relatively selective for inward calcium ion movement: (*a*) activation of adrenergic receptors coupled to calcium channels; and/or (*b*) increases in the resting membrane potential (partial or full depolarization). Therefore, the vaso-

constrictor effects of the α-adrenergic agonist norepinephrine can be attenuated by prior administration of a calcium antagonist, whose action at calcium channel sites distal to the α-adrenergic receptor may mimic those of a true adrenoceptor blocker; similarly, the cardiostimulant actions of the β-adrenergic agonist isoproterenol can be opposed by pretreatment with a calcium antagonist agent.

Role of Calcium in Smooth Muscle Contraction

In vascular smooth muscle cells, the opening of calcium channels is the first step in the cascade of contraction. The inward flux of calcium ions produces release of additional calcium from intracellular storage sites. This newly released calcium binds to the regulatory protein calmodulin, a ubiquitous 16,500-dalton protein. The calcium-calmodulin complex then binds to myosin light-chain kinase, which phosphorylates myosin. The myosin-actin interaction then occurs, resulting in muscle contraction. Calcium antagonists inhibit the initial inward ion movement, thereby affecting the subsequent contractile process.

Role of Calcium in Cardiac Excitation

The electrical potential inside the resting myocardial cell is negative (Fig. 18.2). Excitation produces a brief depolarization due to inward sodium current (phase 0); positively charged calcium ions then begin to move into the cell prolonging the action potential (through phases 1 and 2) as described previously. With depolarization, the myoplasmic calcium concentration rises, and calcium binds to the cardiac regulatory protein troponin, releasing the inhibitory effect of troponin on the interaction between the contractile proteins, actin and myosin, and muscle contraction therefore results.

Thus, the calcium ion plays an important role in both cardiac and smooth vascular muscle contraction and on cardiac pacemaker tissues. This knowledge allows the prediction of the pharmacological effects of the calcium blocking agents:

1. Decrease in myocardial contractility;
2. Decrease in heart rate;
3. Decrease in rate of conduction through the A-V node;
4. Vasodilation and reduction in blood pressure.

CLASSIFICATION OF CALCIUM ANTAGONISTS

Calcium antagonists differ in their relative potency for peripheral vascular and myocardial tissue; for example, verapamil exerts a relatively greater effect on the myocardium than nifedipine, while nifedipine exerts a relatively greater effect on the vasculature than verapamil. The calcium antagonists have been classified into four types based on their relative specificity for cardiac or peripheral activity.

TYPE I, AGENTS WITH IN VIVO MYOCARDIAL, ELECTROPHYSIOLOGIC, AND VASCULAR EFFECTS

These agents, typified by verapamil and diltiazem, have predominant electrophysiologic effects and produce prolonged A-V nodal conduction and refractoriness with little effect on the ventricular or atrial refractory period. They are moderately potent peripheral and coronary vasodilators.

TYPE II, AGENTS WITH PREDOMINANT IN VIVO VASCULAR EFFECTS— DIHYDROPYRIDINES

These agents do not exhibit cardiac electrophysiologic effects in vivo at usual dosage levels but are potent peripheral vasodilators. Examples in this group include nifedipine, nicardipine, and nitrendipine. The dihydropyridines produce profound peripheral vasodilation so that increases in heart rate and contractility commonly result from the reflex increase in sympathetic stimulation.

TYPE III, AGENTS WITH HIGHLY SELECTIVE VASCULAR EFFECTS— PIPERAZINES

These agents are highly selective for calcium channels in vascular smooth muscle with no corresponding calcium-blocking actions in the heart. Cinnarizine and flunarizine are examples of type III calcium antagonists.

TYPE IV, AGENTS WITH A COMPLEX PHARMACOLOGIC PROFILE

These calcium antagonists have complex effects and may have a selective action for vascular tissues or have effects on both cardiac and smooth muscle with associated fast sodium channel blockade. Examples of this group include bepridil, lidoflazine, and perhexilene.

INDIVIDUAL CALCIUM ANTAGONISTS

Three drugs—verapamil, nifedipine, and diltiazem—can be viewed as prototypes for derivative compounds, which appear to have properties generally similar to those of the parent drug. Verapamil, the first calcium-channel blocker introduced into clinical practice, is a papaverine derivative; nifedipine is the progenitor of a variety of dihydropyridine analogs; and diltiazem is a benzothiazepine. While each has similar properties in vitro, the clinical effects of each drug reflect striking differences in affinity for various target tissues; therefore, the clinical indications and applications for each compound have different emphases. Table 18.1 compares and contrasts the hemodynamic effects of some of the important calcium antagonists.

Verapamil

Verapamil (Fig. 18.3) was the first of the calcium antagonists to become available for clinical use. It has dose-related effects on the sinus and A-V nodes, vascular and cardiac smooth muscle, the gastrointestinal tract, and the uterus—evidence of broad interference with transmembrane calcium flux.

PHARMACOKINETICS

The drug is available for both intravenous and oral use. It is eliminated exclusively by hepatic metabolism. Although well absorbed after oral administration, verapamil is subject to extensive first-pass hepatic extraction, resulting in an oral bioavailability of only 10 to 20%.

Table 18.1.
Comparison of the Hemodynamic Effects of the Calcium Antagonists

	Nifedipine	Nicardipine	Verapamil	Diltiazem
Vasodilation	+++	+++	++	+
Negative inotropic effect	0	0	++	+
Negative chronotropic effect	0	0	+++	+++
Positive chronotropic effect*	+	+	0	0
Negative dromotropic effect (A-V conduction)	0	0	+++	+++
Cardiac output increase*	+	+	0	0

*Due to reflex stimulation.

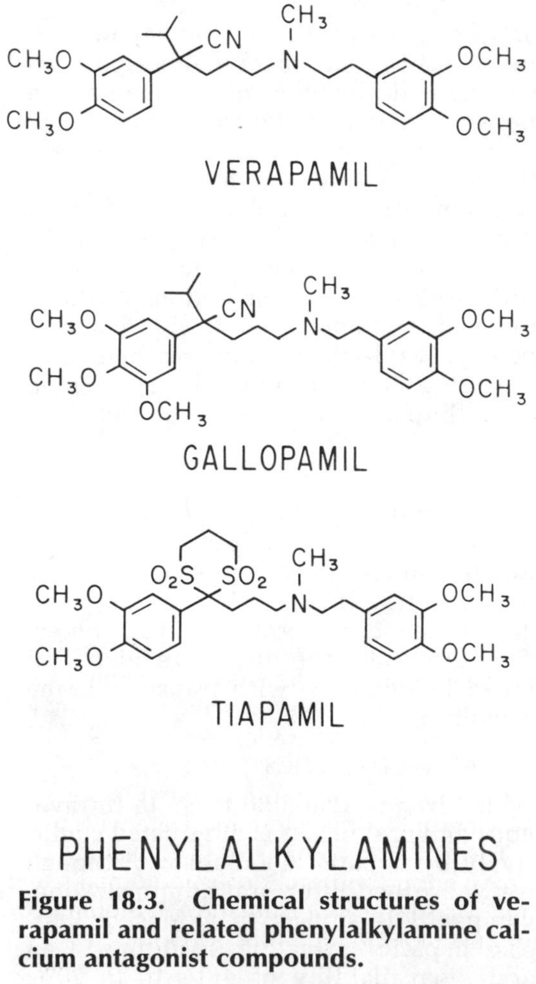

VERAPAMIL

GALLOPAMIL

TIAPAMIL

PHENYLALKYLAMINES

Figure 18.3. Chemical structures of verapamil and related phenylalkylamine calcium antagonist compounds.

Oral doses of the drug are, therefore, severalfold greater than those required by the intravenous route. The observation that the liver is the only site of drug clearance implies that the elimination of verapamil will be substantially prolonged in the presence of significant hepatic dysfunction; this has been confirmed in several studies. In patients with cirrhosis, oral verapamil doses must be reduced to levels near those used intravenously. The pharmacokinetic parameters for verapamil are shown in Table 18.2.

Verapamil clearance has been shown to be reduced during chronic oral administration; this is possibly due to the drugs' vasodilator effects, which may redistribute blood flow away from the liver and, thereby, decrease drug delivery to its site of elimination. In addition, the decrease in clearance may also be related to saturation of specific uptake and metabolizing enzyme systems. Regardless of mechanism, the reduction in clearance of verapamil permits a decrease in the required frequency of dosing during chronic drug administration.

Verapamil is administered as a racemic compound, but the L-isomer is the active moiety. After oral dosing, the liver appears to remove the L-isomer from the circulation more avidly than the relatively less active D-isomer; thus, the proportion of total plasma verapamil concentration accounted for by the inactive D-form is higher after oral drug administration than after intravenous administration (Fig. 18.4). For this reason, meas-

Table 18.2.
Pharmacokinetics of Calcium Antagonists

Drug	Route	Elimination half-life (hr)	Clearance (ml/min)	F* (%)	Protein binding (%)
Verapamil	i.v.	4.8 ± 2.4†	828 ± 345		
	p.o.	4.8 ± 3.8	980 ± 350	20 ± 12	> 90
Nifedipine	i.v.	1.8 ± 0.3	759 ± 110		
Capsule	p.o.	3.4 ± 10.4	600 ± 110	45 ± 9	> 90
Tablet	p.o.	10.4 ± 2.4‡	553 ± 121		
Diltiazem	i.v.	4.4 ± 1.3	828 ± 152		80
	p.o.	3.7 ± 0.6		38 ± 11	

Most of the data are from McAllister RG, Hamann SR, Blouin RA: Pharmacokinetics of calcium entry blockers. *Am J Cardiol* 55:30B–40B, 1985.
*F (%), bioavailability.
†Mean ± SE.
‡The apparent elimination half-life of nifedipine tablets is increased because of the prolonged absorption from the slow-release formulation.

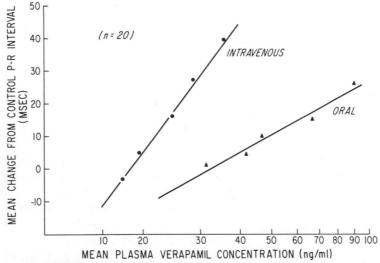

Figure 18.4.   Contrasting effects of verapamil following oral and intravenous administration. Plasma verapamil concentrations plotted against mean change in electrocardiographic PR interval from control predrug values, after 10 mg intravenous and 80 mg orally in 20 normal subjects. Note that the same *total* verapamil concentrations produce less PR prolongation after oral therapy than after intravenous therapy, reflecting the rapid metabolism of the active L-isomer following oral administration, so that more of the total verapamil concentration consists of the D-isomer following oral administration. (Data with permission from McAllister RG, Kirsten EB: The pharmacology of verapamil. IV. Pharmacokinetics and drug effects after single intravenous and oral doses in normal subjects. *Clin Pharmacol Ther* 31:418–426, 1982; and McAllister RG, Hamann SR, Blouin RA: Pharmacokinetics of calcium entry blockers. *Am J Cardiol* 55:30B–40B, 1985.)

urements of verapamil plasma levels which do not discriminate between the two isomers show less impressive correlations between blood levels and effect after oral than after intravenous administration.

Verapamil is widely distributed throughout the body, reaching relatively high concentrations in the liver, kidney, lung, and heart. The drug is highly bound to plasma proteins (>90%), and the binding is independent of plasma drug concentrations over the therapeutic concentration range. Verapamil is bound to both albumin and to α_1-acid glycoprotein and may be displaced from its binding sites by its major metabolite, norverapamil, as well as several weak bases, including propranolol, diazepam, lidocaine, and disopyramide. However, no clinically significant interactions deriving from bind-

ing site displacement of verapamil have been demonstrated.

After an inital intravenous dose, plasma verapamil levels are linearly related to both electrophysiologic (i.e., suppression of A-V nodal function) and the negative inotropic (i.e., depression of left ventricular dp/dt) effects. The electrophysiologic effects on the A-V node occur at lower plasma concentrations than those producing depression of left ventricular dp/dt (Fig. 18.5), reflecting a differential affinity for target tissues. Therefore, the antiarrhythmic effects of the drug can usually be achieved at doses and plasma levels associated with minimal negative inotropic activity. However, following an initial oral dose, a similar correlation between verapamil plasma concentrations and cardiac effects can be found, but the dose-response relation-

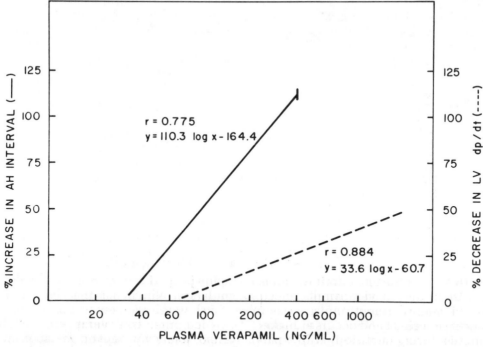

Figure 18.5. Effects of verapamil on cardiac conduction and contractility. Lower concentrations of verapamil are required to prolong cardiac conduction (increase the interval from atrium to bundle of His, i.e., the AH interval) (———) than are required to produce the negative inotropic effects (decrease in left ventricular dp/dt) (– – –). Thus, virtually complete A-V block can be achieved at drug levels associated with only modest negative inotropic activity. (With permission from McAllister RG: Clinical pharmacology of slow channel blocking agents. *Prog Cardiovasc Dis* 25:83–102, 1982.)

ship for orally administered drug is shifted to the right by a factor of 3- to 4-fold. This probably reflects stereoselective isomeric extraction and accumulation of the relatively less active D-isomer after oral drug dosing and first-pass hepatic metabolism, as discussed previously.

During chronic oral verapamil treatment, the correlation between plasma drug levels and clinical pharmacologic effects is poor, with up to a 10-fold variation in the verapamil concentration required to produce a fixed reduction in blood pressure in hypertensive patients. Nonetheless, the oral dose of verapamil generally associated with "therapeutic" effects ranges from about 160 to 480 mg/day.

SUGGESTED DOSAGE AND ADMINISTRATION

The usual initial oral dose of verapamil is 240 mg per day, either as one dose of the sustained release preparation, or as three divided doses (80 mg) of the regular preparation. Intravenous doses are smaller because of the extensive first-pass hepatic metabolism; 5 to 10 mg (75 to 150 μ/kg) should be given over 2 minutes. This can be repeated 30 minutes later.

PRECAUTIONS AND CONTRAINDICATIONS

The side effects of verapamil are extensions of its pharmacologic effect. Myocardial depression and hypotension may occur, but are unusual in the absence of significant preexisting ventricular dysfunction. Advanced A-V nodal block is more commonly seen, especially following intravenous drug administration. Constipation, due to verapamil's effects on gastrointestinal smooth muscle, is an important side effect and occurs at higher drug doses during chronic therapy, particularly in elderly patients.

Overdoses of verapamil of several grams have been reported; treatment with volume expansion, intravenous administration of calcium salts, and temporary pacemakers has been successful in supporting the patients until drug lev-

els decline; on a few occasions, supplemental insulin has been required for management of elevated blood glucose concentrations.

Nifedipine

Nifedipine acts in vivo almost exclusively as an arterial vasodilator, reflecting its strong affinity for vascular tissue. Its effects are dose related, both after acute administration and during long-term therapy. The structure of nifedipine and other selected dihydropyridine derivatives is shown in Figure 18.6. Nifedipine is unstable when exposed to light and poorly soluble; it is, therefore, not available for clinical use as an intravenous formulation.

PHARMACOKINETICS

In the United States, nifedipine is available as 10- and 20-mg capsules, filled with a gelatinous substance containing the drug. After oral dosing, nifedipine is rapidly absorbed, with peak levels generally occurring between 30 and 60 minutes after administration; in about 25% of subjects, however, drug absorption may be substantially delayed.

Although the drug has been widely used sublingually, it appears that sublingual doses are poorly absorbed through the buccal mucosa and that the effects of such doses are actually due to the drug being swallowed and then absorbed; thus, drug effects may be slightly hastened by having the patient bite the capsule and promptly swallow the contents, thereby delaying any lag in absorption due to the need for capsule dissolution (Fig. 18.7). Outside the United States, nifedipine is also available as a tablet formulation, which has the characteristics of a slow-release preparation.

Nifedipine, like verapamil, is eliminated solely by hepatic metabolism, although first-pass extraction is less, about 45 to 55%. The metabolites are inactive. The pharmacokinetic properties of nifedipine are shown in Table 18.2. The drug is strongly bound (92 to 98%) to plasma proteins, primarily albumin, although it also binds to α_1-acid glycoprotein and β-

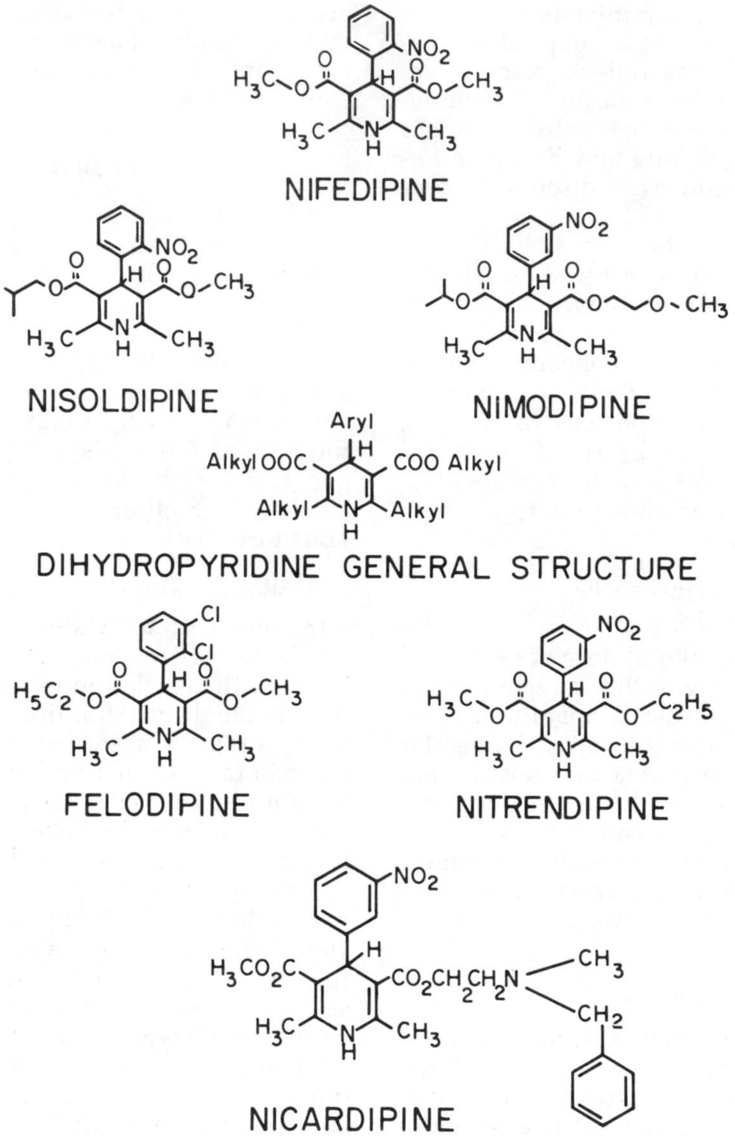

Figure 18.6. Chemical structure of nifedipine and related dihydropyridine calcium antagonists.

globulin. There is no evidence that the clearance of nifedipine is altered during chronic oral dosing.

The net clinical effect of nifedipine is the result of its direct and indirect effects. Because of its powerful direct vasodilatory effects, nifedipine activates baroreceptor reflexes which, in turn, alter the overall cardiovascular effects of the drug. Clinical doses reduce coronary and peripheral vascular resistance and lower blood pressure. Baroreceptor activation and increased sympathetic drive are then manifest in a reflex increase in heart rate, myocardial contractility, and cardiac output during therapy. Circulating norepinephrine and plasma renin levels also rise. Because of the sympathetic activation, nifedipine cannot be used in the treatment of arrhythmias. Its powerful vascular effect has made it the treatment of choice in coronary artery spasm in patients who can tolerate the drug.

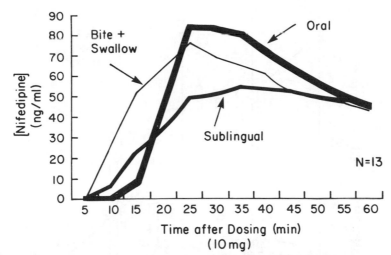

Figure 18.7. Comparison of routes of administration of nifedipine.   Plasma nifedipine concentrations in 13 healthy subjects given single doses of 20 mg of nifedipine. Subjects swallowed the capsule whole (oral), bit through the capsule and swallowed the contents (bite and swallow), or bit through the capsule and held the contents in their mouths for 5 minutes (sublingual). (Data with permission from McAllister RG: Kinetics and dynamics of nifedipine after oral and sublingual doses. *Am J Med* 81 (Suppl 6A):2–5, 1986.)

Both the fall in blood pressure and the reflex increase in heart rate are related to dose and to drug concentration in plasma (Figs. 18.8 and 18.9). Limited information suggests that this relationship is maintained during chronic drug administration, although tolerance to the reflex tachycardia occurs rather rapidly.

SUGGESTED DOSAGE AND
ADMINISTRATION

The usual starting oral dose is 10 mg given 3 times daily, but up to 30-mg doses 4 times daily may sometimes be given. To acutely lower blood pressure, a single capsule of 10 mg can be bitten and swallowed for rapid control of the blood pressure.

PRECAUTIONS AND
CONTRAINDICATIONS

Side effects are related to nifedipine's pharmacologic activity as a powerful vasodilator; vascular headaches and flushing are the most common, and both may resolve if drug dosage is reduced. At higher doses, during chronic therapy, pedal edema may occur resulting from third-space fluid sequestration, not cardiac failure or sodium retention. Hypo-

tension may occur, but is uncommon in the absence of intravascular volume depletion. In patients with migraine syndromes, headaches may be precipitated by the initial dose of nifedipine. Gastrointestinal side effects are uncommon during nifedipine therapy, and the drug has no effect on gastric emptying time.

Diltiazem

Diltiazem is a benzothiazepine derivative (Fig. 18.10), which appears to have more balanced effects on the myocardium and vasculature than nifedipine. It has less negative inotropic effect but about the same intensity of action on the sinoatrial and atrioventricular nodes as verapamil (see Table 18.1).

PHARMACOKINETICS

Diltiazem is well absorbed after oral dosing, with a systemic bioavailability of about 40%.

The pharmacokinetic parameters for diltiazem are shown in Table 18.2. This drug is extensively metabolized to inactive products in the liver, with the major route of metabolism being by deacetylation. With chronic administration, non-

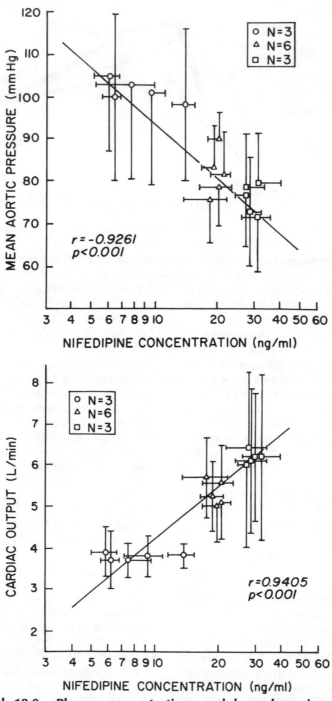

Figures 18.8 and 18.9. Plasma concentrations and hemodynamic effects of nifedi-pine. Relationship between mean plasma nifedipine concentration and mean arterial (aortic) pressure (Fig 18.8) and cardiac output (Fig 18.9), during nifedipine infusion in dogs. These figures demonstrate the hypotensive effect of nifedipine, accompanied by the reflex increase in cardiac output which occurs as arterial pressure falls. (Data with permission from Hamann SR, McAllister RG: Plasma concentrations and hemodynamic effects of ni-fedipine. *J Cardiovasc Pharmacol* 5:920–927, 1983.)

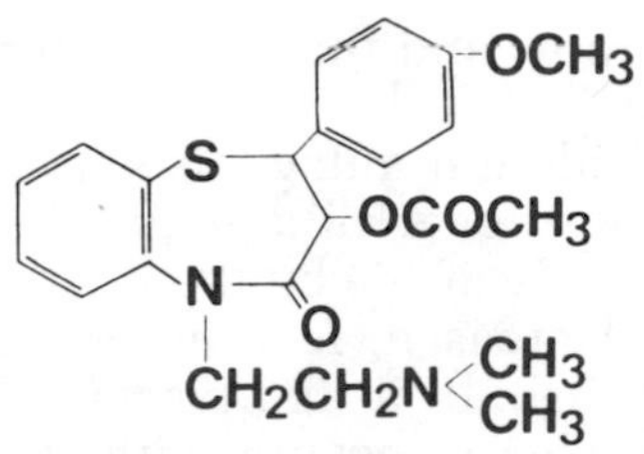

Figure 18.10. Chemical structure of diltiazem.

linear kinetics may be seen, with accumulation of both the drug and its major metabolite, deacetyldiltiazem. At modest doses, however, this is not a constant observation among patients. It is thus important to recognize that the dose of diltiazem and the plasma levels produced must be carefully titrated on the basis of clinical response. In addition, diltiazem may be subject to enterohepatic recirculation, as two distinct plasma level peaks may be seen after oral administration.

Diltiazem is about 80% bound in plasma, with plasma protein binding being independent of drug concentration. Drug binding is not altered by therapeutic concentrations of other cardioactive drugs.

SUGGESTED DOSAGE AND ADMINISTRATION

Diltiazem is usually given 3 times daily in a dose range of 180 to 480 mg/day, similar to that for verapamil.

PRECAUTIONS AND CONTRAINDICATIONS

Side effects of diltiazem, like the other calcium-entry blockers, can be predicted from a knowledge of its pharmacologic effects. Vasodilation may result in headache and flushing, and occasionally in hypotension. Pedal edema may occur, as is seen with both nifedipine and verapamil, presumably resulting from precapillary sphincter dilation and capillary leakage. The effects of diltiazem on the sinoatrial and A-V nodes may result in sinus node depression or prolongation of A-V conduction time. Although side effects following diltiazem are generally regarded as less frequent than those for

nifedipine and verapamil, the low incidence of adverse reactions may result from the general clinical practice of using rather low doses of diltiazem. At equivalent therapeutic doses, the incidence of side effects with all three drugs is relatively low, and those side effects which occur are rapidly reversible on discontinuation of the drug.

A few cases of overdosage with diltiazem have been reported, each presenting with hypotension and A-V block. Management should include volume expansion, use of atropine or temporary pacemaker insertion if required, administration of calcium gluconate and isoproterenol for cardiac support as needed, and other general supportive measures.

Nicardipine

Nicardipine is a second generation dihydropyridine calcium antagonist with peripheral vasodilatory actions similar to those of nifedipine. The chemical structure is given in Figure 18.6. It is a potent coronary and peripheral arterial vasodilator. The reduction in systemic vascular resistance leads to reflex sympathetic stimulation accompanied by an increase in heart rate, myocardial contractility, and cardiac index. In contrast to nifedipine, intracoronary administration of nicardipine does not appear to produce negative inotropic effects. Nicardipine can be prepared for both oral and intravenous use, in contrast to nifedipine. It is well absorbed following oral administration and undergoes extensive presystemic metabolism so that bioavailability is low. Peak plasma concentrations are achieved between 20 minutes and 2 hours after oral administration. Nicardipine is metabolized to inactive metabolites by the liver. Plasma protein binding of nicardipine is about 90%, and the volume of distribution is about 0.6 L/kg. The elimination half-life has been reported to range from about 44 to 107 minutes with a clearance value of 0.4 to 0.9 L/kg/hour. Nicardipine is excreted mainly through the bile and feces and, thus, elimination is not impaired in renal failure. Nicardipine should, however, be used cautiously in patients with liver disease.

Side effects are related to the vasodilatory properties of nicardipine: flushing; headache; and peripheral edema. Other effects include increased anginal symptoms, palpitations, myocardial infarction, and exercise-induced hypotension.

Important uses for nicardipine include angina and hypertension. Nifedipine is not available for parenteral administration and thus nicardipine, either as an intravenous bolus or intravenous infusion, may be a useful drug in the management of acute hypertension when a calcium antagonist is selected.

Perhexiline

Perhexiline is rapidly and completely absorbed following oral administration. Plasma levels peak in 1 hour and are still detectable after 6 hours. The drug is 90% protein bound.

The usual starting dose of perhexiline is 100 mg twice daily, and doses as high as 200 mg twice daily are commonly given. Perhexiline appears to be associated with more side effects than the other calcium channel blockers discussed previously. Mild elevations of serum glutamic-oxaloacetic transaminase (SGOT), serum glutamic-pyruvic transaminase (SGPT), alkaline phosphatase, and lactate dehydrogenase (LDH) sometimes occur. These elevations reverse after discontinuation of the drug. In addition, a mild diuretic effect, weight loss, and reduced creatinine clearance have been described. The nature of this effect is uncertain. In patients who are poor metabolizers of debrisoquine (see Chapter 2), metabolism of perhexiline is also impaired, and in these patients, a proximal sensorimotor neuropathy has been seen. Regression after discontinuation of perhexiline therapy occurs slowly.

DRUG INTERACTIONS

The calcium antagonists have found broad application in patients with many types of cardiovascular disorders. These patients are likely to require multiple drug therapy, and thus drug interactions are likely.

When calcium antagonists are administered together with digoxin, the excretion of the glycoside by the renal tubules may be decreased, leading to increased levels of digoxin in the plasma. This interaction clearly occurs with verapamil and has been inconsistently observed with nifedipine and diltiazem. In some clinical studies, the rise in digoxin plasma concentration when verapamil was added was thought to be responsible for glycoside toxicity. However, it should be recognized that arrhythmias from digitalis preparations are related to calcium-dependent afterdepolarizations, which are, of course, suppressed by the calcium antagonist drugs. Therefore, although the pharmacokinetic aspects of the interaction between verapamil and digoxin are well demonstrated, the clinical consequences are not at all clear, and the need to decrease glycoside doses when verapamil is added is not well established.

Because of the intrinsic negative inotropic and electrophysiologic effects of interference with transmembrane calcium ion flux, the interaction of calcium antagonists and *β-adrenoceptor blocking agents* can produce profound depression of cardiac conduction and contractile function. In the presence of normal ventricular function, such adverse consequences may not be clinically significant. When even modest impairment of cardiac contractility is present, however, dose-related depression of ventricular function can be seen when verapamil and a *β*-blocker are administered together (Fig. 18.11). Since *β*-blocking drugs decrease liver blood flow, the clearance of a simultaneously administered calcium antagonist may be decreased, and accumulation of the calcium antagonists may occur with possible resultant toxicity. Less information is available about diltiazem given together with *β*-blockers, but prudence would dicate avoidance of this combination. Since nifedipine's myocardial depressant effects tend to be masked by its pronounced arterial vasodilating properties, *β*-blockers in modest doses have

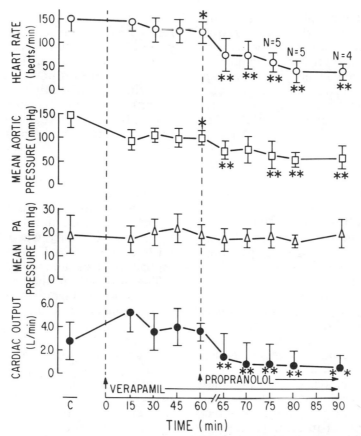

Figure 18.11.   Drug interaction between verapamil and propranolol.   Both drugs were given in doses which produce therapeutic plasma concentrations. The combination resulted in significant (**) decreases in heart rate, aortic pressure, and cardiac output. (Data with permission from Hamann SR, Kaltenborn KE, Vose M, Tan G, McAllister RG: Cardiovascular and pharmacokinetic consequences of combined administration of verapamil and propranolol in dogs. *Am J Cardiol* 56:147–156, 1985.)

been used effectively to blunt the reflex tachycardia which may result from the vascular effects of nifedipine. Thus, this may be a *beneficial* drug interaction, based upon the rational use of the various component drugs. In the presence of impaired ventricular function, however, the potential for electrophysiologic and hemodynamic toxicity may be evident, even with nifedipine.

The H_2 receptor blocking agent, *cimetidine*, might be expected to alter the hepatic elimination of verapamil, nifedipine, and diltiazem, because of its pronounced effects on both liver blood flow and drug-metabolizing enzyme systems (see Chapter 23). Results of clinical trials, however, have shown either variable results or pharmacokinetic alterations of no real clinical importance. Ranitidine and famotidine have less or no effect on hepatic drug-metabolizing ability, and interactions are rare with these two compounds.

CALCIUM ANTAGONISTS AND ANESTHESIA

VOLATILE ANESTHETICS

Calcium entry blocking drugs have multiple cardiovascular effects: vasodilation and negative inotropic, negative chronotropic, and negative dromotropic (conduction velocity) effects. The volatile anesthetics have been shown to interfere with calcium ion movement across cell membranes, and their hemodynamic effects are well recognized. Halothane, enflurane, and isoflurane depress conduction at the sinoatrial node and have negative inotropic and vasodilatory effects. Thus, the calcium channel blocking drugs and inhalational anesthetics possess similar cardiovascular properties, and it is not surprising that interactions have been demonstrated between the inhalational anesthetics and calcium blocking drugs. It is thought that the cardiovascular effects of isoflurane more closely resemble the dihydropyridines (nifedipine and nicardipine), while those of halothane and enflurane are more similar to verapamil and diltiazem.

In the laboratory, increasing infusion rates of verapamil during enflurane, isoflurane, and halothane anesthesia have been shown to produce dose-dependent reductions in arterial blood pressure, heart rate, cardiac index, and an increase in the electrocardiographic PR interval. The cardiovascular depressant effects were more marked in animals anesthetized with enflurane than halothane or isoflurane. Other workers have shown that verapamil infusions (3.0 and 6.0 μg/kg/min preceded by 200-μ/kg bolus) during low concentrations of halothane [approximately 1.0 minimum alveolar concentration (MAC)] produce minimal effects but produce significant cardiovascular depression during anesthesia with high concentrations of halothane (2.0 MAC) (Fig. 18.12). The effects of verapamil during enflurane and isoflurane administration appear to be qualitatively similar (Fig. 18.12), but overall verapamil is better tolerated during isoflurane and halothane anesthesia than during comparable concentrations of enflurane anesthesia. Dogs given nifedipine during halothane anesthesia develop exaggerated hypotension, because higher concentrations of halothane attenuate the reflex compensatory increase in heart rate normally elicited by nifedipine. Similarly, when dogs are given the dihydropyridine vasodilator nicardipine in the presence of isoflurane anesthesia, high

concentrations of isoflurane prevent the reflex increase in heart rate and cardiac output that normally accompany nicardipine administration (Fig. 18.13). Thus, laboratory studies have generally shown that the administration of low doses of calcium channel blockers during low concentrations of inhalational anesthesia produces minimal hemodynamic interaction. However, in experiments with open-chest animal preparations, marked depression of ventricular function has resulted from the interaction of diltiazem and verapamil with halothane and isoflurane; in closed-chest animals, electrophysiologic toxicity was more common, with depressed A-V nodal conduction and sinus arrest and/or bradycardia.

The interaction that occurs between the calcium antagonists and the volatile anesthetics is not solely pharmacodynamic in nature. The volatile anesthetics have been shown to inhibit drug metabolism and to reduce hepatic blood flow, resulting in reduced elimination of calcium antagonists during inhalational anesthesia. This may lead to higher plasma concentrations and thus increased pharmacological effect.

Many patients now present for anesthesia and surgery who have been chronically treated with calcium channel blocking agents, often in combination with β-adrenergic blocking drugs. In addition, the calcium channel blocking agents may be useful when given intravenously during anesthesia to treat supraventricular tachyarrhythmias and to control coronary vascular spasm. The administration of verapamil (150 μg/kg over 10 minutes) to patients with normal left ventricular function undergoing coronary artery bypass surgery produces small reductions in blood pressure even in the presence of chronic low-dose β-adrenergic blocker therapy. However, caution should be exercised in the administration of verapamil to patients with left ventricular dysfunction, since myocardial depression and a fall in cardiac output may occur. Chronic administration of calcium channel and β-adrenergic blockers to patients undergoing coronary artery bypass grafting does not appear to adversely affect cardiac conduction in

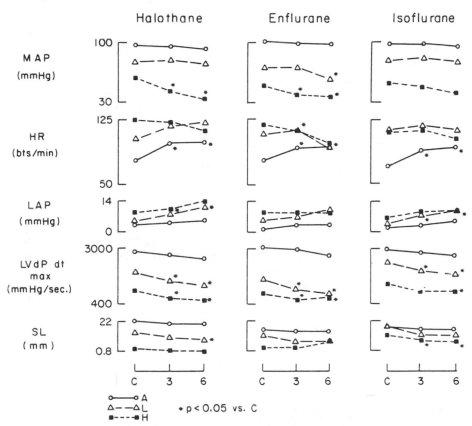

Figure 18.12.   Comparison of the effects of verapamil infusion during halothane, enflurane, and isoflurane anesthesia in dogs.   Measurements were made without verapamil (C, control) and during verapamil infusions of 3.0 μg/kg/min and 6.0 μg/kg/min. The dogs were studied awake (O), during low dose, i.e., approximately 1.0 MAC (Δ), and during high dose, i.e., 2.0 MAC (■) halothane, enflurane, and isoflurane anesthesia. *MAP*, mean aortic pressure; *HR*, heart rate; *LAP*, left atrial pressure; *LV dp/dt max*, maximum rate of rise of left ventricular pressure; *SL*, myocardial segment length shortening. (With permission from Rogers K, Hysing ES, Merin RG, Taylor A, Hartley C, Chelly JE: Cardiovascular effects of and interaction between calcium blocking drugs and anesthetics in chronically instrumented dogs. II. Verapamil, enflurane, and isoflurane. *Anesthesiology* 64:568–575, 1986.)

the perioperative period and, although these patients have a decreased heart rate and an increase in PR interval, they do not develop complete heart block. In addition, it has been shown that patients treated with a combination of β-blockers and nifedipine tolerate high-dose fentanyl anesthesia for coronary artery surgery without adverse effect.

Thus, clinical experience with these drugs during the perioperative period suggests that they are beneficial, and if potential problems are recognized and the anesthetic regimen titrated to clinical effect, patients can be safely anesthetized while continuing to receive this group of drugs. In patients with good ventricular function, therapeutic doses of the calcium antagonists and clinical concentrations of volatile anesthetics are well tolerated, and these drugs should be continued until the time of surgery. In patients with poor left ventricular function or hypovolemia, low doses of volatile anesthetics should be administered (or even avoided), and invasive monitoring may be required. Varying degrees of hypotension, bradycardia, and heart block may occur during surgery and anesthesia. Attention to the maintenance of

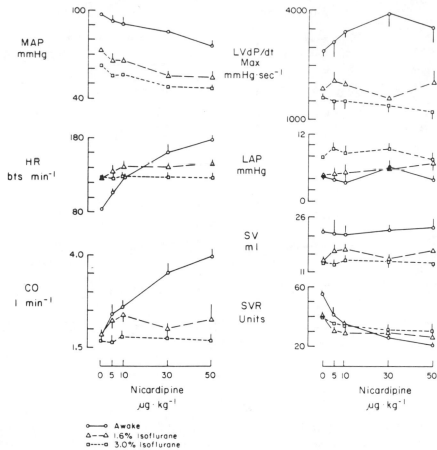

Figure 18.13. Hemodynamic interaction between nicardipine and isoflurane. Maximum changes produced by nicardipine (5, 10, 30, and 50 μg/kg) on mean arterial pressure *(MAP)*, heart rate *(HR)*, cardiac output *(CO)*, left ventricular dp/dt *(LV dp/dt)*, left atrial pressure *(LAP)*, stroke volume *(SV)*, and systemic vascular resistance *(SVR)* in awake dogs (O) and during 1.6 (Δ) and 3.0% (□) end-tidal isoflurane anesthesia. Note the isoflurane-induced inhibition of the reflex tachycardia and increase in cardiac output normally elicited by nicardipine. (With permission from Hysing ES, Chelly JE, Doursout MF, Hartley C, Merin RG: Cardiovascular effects of and interaction between calcium blocking drugs and anesthesia in chronically instrumented dogs. III. Nicardipine and isoflurane. *Anesthesiology* 65:385–391, 1986.)

intravascular volume is important; adverse effects may be managed by the administration of large doses of calcium, β-agonists, or appropriate inotrope.

NEUROMUSCULAR BLOCKING DRUGS

The calcium channel blocking drugs have been shown to potentiate the effects of the depolarizing and nondepolarizing neuromuscular blocking drugs in the laboratory. Clinical reports suggest that verapamil might potentiate neuromuscular

blockade in humans and that caution should be exercised. Limited data suggest that the calcium antagonists may also interact with some local anesthetics; verapamil exerts effects on the fast sodium channel and has itself been shown to possess local anesthetic activity.

OTHER EFFECTS

Verapamil decreases the MAC for halothane in dogs, and thus anesthetic requirements are reduced. Adjustment in anesthetic dosage may therefore be necessary in patients receiving verapamil.

Verapamil has been suggested as a useful agent in the treatment of malignant hyperpyrexia, since it inhibits intracellular calcium flux. However, it is interesting that the administration of dantrolene to swine pretreated with verapamil induces hyperkalemia and cardiovascular collapse. The mechanism is unknown.

THERAPEUTIC USES OF CALCIUM ANTAGONISTS

ARRHYTHMIAS

Both verapamil and diltiazem prolong the effective and functional refractory periods of A-V nodal tissue, resulting in a slowing of ventricular rate response in the presence of atrial fibrillation and other supraventricular tachyarrhythmias. Verapamil, available for clinical use as an intravenous formulation, has become widely used in the acute management of supraventricular tachycardias with excessively rapid ventricular rates. In those arrhythmias where reentry circuits in the A-V node are responsible for continuation of the arrhythmias [paroxysmal supraventricular tachycardia (PSVT)], verapamil is rapidly effective; in over 90% of patients, conversion to sinus rhythm results within 5 minutes of administration of 5 or 10 mg of the drug, and the efficacy appears to be dependent upon achieving, even briefly, "therapeutic" verapamil concentrations of about 100 ng/ml. In patients with atrial fibrillation or flutter, acutely administered verapamil reduces the ventricular rate in a dose-dependent fashion, but conversion to sinus rhythm is uncommon (Fig. 18.14).

Chronic oral dosing with either verapamil or diltiazem is useful in controlling ventricular rates in patients with chronic atrial fibrillation. The doses required vary widely among patients and must be gradually increased until the desired clinical result is obtained. Verapamil is occasionally combined with quinidine in the management of atrial tachyarrhythmias. However, since both drugs

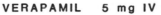

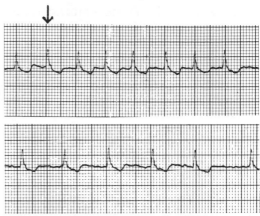

Figure 18.14. Use of verapamil in atrial fibrillation. Result of administration of 5 mg of verapamil intravenously, in a patient with atrial fibrillation; the predrug ventricular rate of 150/min rapidly falls to less than 100/min following verapamil administration. (McAllister RG: Unpublished observation.)

may produce hypotension (presumably through α-adrenoceptor-mediated effects), the combination of quinidine and verapamil may result in dramatic orthostatic decreases in arterial pressure, especially in hypertensive patients. This is infrequent but requires careful clinical monitoring when the two agents are given together.

The calcium antagonists are not generally effective in the management of ventricular arrhythmias. One exception appears to be exercise-related ventricular tachycardia, which can be suppressed by both intravenous and oral verapamil. The mechanism for this response is obscure. In ventricular arrhythmias produced by myocardial ischemia, the calcium antagonists may be useful by reducing the ischemic stimulus, but not by direct antiarrhythmic effects.

Nifedipine is not effective as an antiarrhythmic agent, because doses producing direct myocardial effects are associated with profound vasodilation, hypotension, and reflex sympathetic stimulation.

ISCHEMIC HEART DISEASE

It is useful to divide ischemic heart disease syndromes into (a) chronic stable angina, resulting from fixed atherosclerotic obstructions within the coronary vasculature, and (b) Prinzmetal's, or variant, angina, produced by intermittent coronary arterial vasospasm. In truth, the syndromes often overlap, and vasospasm is more common in patients with preexisting atheromatous lesions. Nonetheless, the division is useful clinically and conceptually.

All of the calcium antagonists are remarkably effective in preventing coronary vasospasm, and the group, collectively, is first-choice therapy for Prinzmetal's angina.

Patients with chronic stable angina develop symptoms when myocardial oxygen demands exceed the ability of the compromised coronary circulation to provide oxygen to the distal tissues. In the absence of alteration of the diseased vessels, as with revascularization surgery or angioplasty procedures, the traditional therapeutic approach involves pharmacologic attempts to decrease myocardial oxygen demand and to prevent deleterious increases. The nitrates decrease venous return and decrease preload; the β-blockers decrease heart rate and ventricular contractility. Both are effective, alone and in combination, and have emerged as important therapy in patients with angina, although each has unwanted effects, such as reflex tachycardia with nitrates and an increase in left ventricular end diastolic volume with β-blockers. In contrast, the calcium antagonists not only decrease myocardial oxygen demand but also may improve coronary flow, thereby increasing oxygen supply. They have, therefore, assumed an important position in the pharmacologic management of angina pectoris.

Both verapamil and diltiazem decrease heart rate (though effects on the sinoatrial node); they decrease afterload (through peripheral vasodilation); they decrease ventricular contractility (by altering calcium channel flux); and they have no major effects on preload. Thus,

these agents are often effective as the sole agents (or, together with nitrates, if required) in the management of patients with angina. Nifedipine is less effective, since its peripheral vasodilating effects may induce a reflex tachycardia, which in itself may precipitate anginal symptoms. However, in combination with a β-blocker to prevent tachycardia, nifedipine may be remarkably effective.

HYPERTENSION

The calcium antagonists have emerged as important new agents in the treatment of hypertension. In patients with severe hypertension in whom rapid reduction of arterial pressure is clinically indicated, nifedipine is promptly effective when given either orally or by biting a capsule and swallowing the contents; sublingual administration, as shown in Figure 18.8, may result in lower plasma concentrations and less intense effects. Either 10 or 20 mg are generally sufficient to produce significant reductions in blood pressure within 15 to 30 minutes. Clinically significant hypotension is uncommon with this drug (in the absence of diuretic-induced hypovolemia), giving it an additional advantage over other antihypertensive agents in the acute management of hypertension. Nicardipine administered intravenously is also effective in the acute management of hypertension and may supersede the use of nifedipine in this situation.

In the chronic management of hypertension, nifedipine in capsule formulations is less attractive, as it must generally be given at least thrice daily, and a β-blocker is often required to blunt the reflex tachycardia. Following the use of slow-release nifedipine, little, if any, tachycardia results, and the sustained effects permit twice daily dosing.

Verapamil has been the most widely studied calcium antagonist in patients with hypertension. It reduces elevated peripheral vascular resistance, the constant hallmark of established essential hypertension, while its effects on the sinoatrial node prevent significant increases in heart rate. During chronic administration, it may have a mild natriuretic effect, and sodium retention does not occur; therefore, a diuretic is not commonly required, and verapamil may be effective as monotherapy (Fig. 18.15). An additional advantage is that it has no important effects on serum lipids. The doses required range from 160 to 480 mg daily. Since the drug's clearance falls and the half-life increases during chronic dosing, administration twice daily is usually sufficient. Sustained-release formulations possibly permitting once daily treatment are now available.

Diltiazem is also effective in patients with essential hypertension. In modest doses (up to 360 mg daily), it appears to be about as effective as thiazide diuretics. At higher doses, it should be equal in efficacy to verapamil, and it may be better tolerated in patients who develop constipation with verapamil.

The calcium antagonists act primarily as vasodilators in hypertensive patients, and previously established left ventricular hypertrophy may regress during chronic treatment. This has not occurred with previously available vasodilators. Since ventricular hypertrophy may, in itself, be an important risk factor for the development of arrhythmias and death in hypertensive patients, pharmacologic treatment, which not only lowers elevated arterial pressure but also permits regression of ventricular abnormalities, is particularly desirable. The combination of vasodilation and regression of ventricular hypertrophy has made the calcium antagonists especially attractive in the treatment of hypertensive patients.

HYPERTROPHIC CARDIOMYOPATHY

The functional hallmark of hypertrophic cardiomyopathy is an abnormality in ventricular compliance, i.e., failure of the ventricle to relax adequately during diastole. This results in elevation of ventricular filling pressures and may lead to pulmonary congestion, with patients developing symptoms of cardiac failure in the presence of normal or supranormal systolic ventricular function. This hypercontractile state responds well to calcium antagonists, and the elevated filling pressures frequently fall to normal levels, restoring normal diastolic function and improving ventricular functional parameters.

In contrast to patients with ischemic heart disease, in whom systolic function is commonly compromised and calcium antagonists may have undesirable nega-

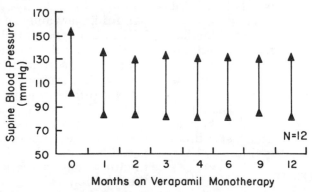

Figure 18.15. Use of verapamil in hypertension. Results of verapamil monotherapy in 12 hypertensive patients studied over 1 year, at doses ranging from 160 to 480 mg/day. The data reflect changes in blood pressure for the group. No evidence of tachyphylaxis was seen, and all patients remained under good control during the study period. (With permission from McAllister RG, Frazier PE, Schloemer GL: Long-term antihypertensive therapy with verapamil: efficacy and electrocardiographic changes. *Clin Res* 33:873A, 1985.)

tive inotropic effects, patients with hypertrophic cardiomyopathy who have diastolic dysfunction benefit from the negative inotropic actions of these drugs. Verapamil is the most widely studied and can be therapeutically useful in patients whose symptoms are refractory to treatment with β-blockers. The dose of verapamil varies widely in these patients and must be adjusted on an individual basis; the range is, however, similar to that found for other applications of this drug, i.e., 160 to 480 mg daily. Nifedipine can also be effective, but its vascular effects may produce poorly tolerated hypotension in such patients, and the reflex sympathetic stimulation resulting from the fall in arterial pressure may worsen the hypercontractile ventricular activity. The therapeutic role of diltiazem in hypertrophic cardiomyopathy is less well defined.

As might be expected, side effects with any of the calcium antagonists are more common in cardiomyopathic patients than in subjects with more stable cardiac function. A particular risk appears to occur when verapamil is combined with quinidine to manage atrial arrhythmias in patients with the obstructive variant of hypertrophic cardiomyopathy; the hypotension which may result is potentially lethal.

The long-term results of treatment with calcium antagonists in hypertrophic cardiomyopathy are not known. Whether regression of the hypertrophy will occur and whether the incidence and complications of arrhythmias in these patients are reduced have not yet been defined. However, the calcium antagonists represent a rational approach to the pharmacologic management of the major functional disorder in this condition.

PERIOPERATIVE PERIOD

Perioperative uses of the calcium antagonists include the treatment of intraoperative arrhythmias, myocardial ischemia, systemic hypertension and pulmonary hypertension, to provide myocardial protection during cardiac surgery and to produce deliberate hypotensive anesthesia. The calcium antago-

nists have also been used to treat postoperative hypertension.

OTHER CLINICAL APPLICATIONS

Recent studies have shown that the calcium antagonists are particularly useful in the prophylaxis of migraine syndromes. Such patients appear to have inappropriate vasoconstriction in extracranial vessels in a unihemispheric distribution, leading to the "aura" of migraine; subsequent vasodilation results in the headache. The calcium antagonists can prevent the initial vasoconstrictive episode, and comparative studies have shown that they are at least as effective as β-blockers in prophylaxis. A new dihydropyridine derivative, nimodipine, has a strong affinity for cerebral vasculature, with relatively little effect on peripheral vessels; it is effective in preventing migraine headaches and has little other clinical effect. In addition, clinical studies have also shown that nimodipine substantially reduces mortality from subarachnoid hemorrhage, presumably by preventing local vasoconstriction in bleeding areas and extension of ischemic cerebral damage.

Raynaud's phenomenon is a condition where severe peripheral vasospasm occurs, either spontaneously or, more commonly, in response to cold and emotional stimuli. It typically presents as cold, painful fingers and can be incapacitating. Nifedipine appears to be the most effective of the calcium antagonists in preventing these attacks, and it is now the drug of first choice.

Myocardial preservation during acute myocardial ischemia and/or infarction would seem a logical application of these drugs, as they produce coronary arterial vasodilation, reduced myocardial contractility, and decreased afterload, and they inhibit calcium overload in ischemic myocardial cells. In a variety of animal models, administration of calcium antagonists can reduce the area of myocardium at risk for infarction. However, studies in patients have not shown similar results, and these drugs are not indicated for such use at this time. Nifedipine and other calcium antagonists are, however, being widely studied as cardioplegic agents during hypothermic cardiac arrest, primarily because they can prevent calcium overload on rewarming.

Patients with asthma have inappropriate constriction of bronchial smooth muscle in response to various stimuli. Although calcium antagonists are effective in preventing such bronchoconstriction in in vitro experiments, results with oral or inhaled administration of these drugs have not shown significant therapeutic benefit at this time.

The calcium antagonist drugs can prevent calcium-dependent aspects of platelet aggregation, but no important clinical application for this property has yet been identified. In selected animal models, they appear to retard the development of lipid-laden plaques; as such, they may have important antiatherosclerotic activity. Finally, verapamil has been combined with adriamycin to prevent or ameliorate the cardiomyopathy which is a limiting factor in the administration of this important oncolytic drug.

FUTURE DIRECTIONS

The development of the calcium antagonist compounds provided vital tools for exploration of calcium-dependent systems, especially in relation to smooth muscle function. As our understanding of the role of calcium in normal physiology expands, our ability to use these compounds wisely and well will grow. New calcium antagonists with greater vascular selectivity are likely to become available. Minor molecular modifications of the dihydropyridine nucleus have resulted in a calcium agonist compound, whose effects are the reverse of those seen with nifedipine; further studies in this area may result in the development of clinically useful vasopressor and cardiotonic drugs.

BIBLIOGRAPHY

General

Allen JC: The current status of the mechanism of the calcium channel antagonists. *Prog Cardiovasc Dis* 25:133–139, 1982.

Awan NA, DeMaria AN, Mason DT: Therapeutic importance of calcium antagonists in coronary artery disease and congestive heart failure: an overview. *Drugs* 23:235–241, 1982.

Braunwald E: Mechanism of action of calcium-channel-blocking agents. *N Engl J Med* 307:1618–1627, 1982.

Cheung JY, Bonventre JV, Malis CD, Leaf A: Calcium and ischemic injury. *N Engl J Med* 314:1670–1676, 1986.

Echizen H, Eichelbaum M: Clinical pharmacokinetics of verapamil, nifedipine, and diltiazem. *Clin Pharmacokinet* 11:425–449, 1986.

Fleckenstein A: Calcium antagonism in heart and vascular smooth muscle. *Med Res Rev* 5:395–425, 1985.

Freedman DD, Waters DD: "Second generation" dihydropyridine calcium antagonists. *Drugs* 34:578–598, 1987.

Jenkins LC, Scoates PJ: Anaesthetic implications of calcium channel blockers. *Can Anaesth Soc J* 32:436–447, 1985.

Kates RE: Calcium antagonists: pharmacokinetic properties. *Drugs* 25:113–124, 1983.

McAllister RG, Hamann SR, Blouin RA: Pharmacokinetics of calcium-entry blockers. *Am J Cardiol* 55:30B–40B, 1985.

McCleskey EW, Fox AP, Feldman D, Tsien RW: Different types of calcium channels, *J Exp Biol* 124:177–190, 1986.

Motulsky HJ, Snavely MD, Hughes RJ, Insel PA: Interactions of verapamil and other calcium channel blockers with alpha$_1$ and alpha$_2$ adrenergic receptors. *Circ Res* 82:226–231, 1983.

Rasmussen H: The calcium messenger system (first of two parts). *N Engl J Med* 314:1094–1101, 1986.

Rasmussen H: The calcium messenger system (second of two parts). *N Engl J Med* 314:1164–1170, 1986.

Reves JG, Kissin I, Lell WA, Tosone S: Calcium entry blockers: uses and implications for anesthesiologists. *Anesthesiology* 57:504–518, 1982.

Singh BN: The mechanism of action of calcium antagonists relative to their clinical applications. *Br J Clin Pharmacol* 21:109S–121S, 1986.

Walsh MP: Calmodulin and its roles in skeletal muscle function. *Can Anaesth Soc J* 30:390–398, 1983.

Verapamil

Bonow RO, Rosing DR, Bacharach SL, Green MV, Kent KM, Lipson LC, Maron BJ, Leon MB, Epstein SE: Effects of verapamil on left ventricular systolic function and diastolic filling in patients with hypertrophic cardiomyopathy. *Circulation* 64:787–796, 1981.

Buhler FR, Hulthen UL, Kiowski W, Muller FB, Bolli P: The place of the calcium antagonist verapamil in antihypertensive therapy. *J Cardiovasc Pharmacol* 4:S350–S357, 1982.

Eichelbaum M, Somogyi A, Von Unruh GE, Dengler HJ: Simultaneous determination of the intravenous and oral pharmacokinetic parameters of D,L-verapamil using stable isotope-labelled verapamil. *Eur J Clin Pharmacol* 19:133–137, 1981.

Hamann SR, Blouin RA, McAllister RG Jr: Clinical pharmacokinetics of verapamil. *Clin Pharmacokinet* 9:26–41, 1984.

McAllister RG, Kirsten EB: The pharmacology of verapamil. IV. Pharmacokinetics and drug effects after single intravenous and oral doses in normal subjects. *Clin Pharmacol Ther* 31:418–426, 1982.

Shand DG, Hammill SC, Aanonsen L, Pritchett EL: Reduced verapamil clearance during long-term administration. *Clin Pharmacol Ther* 30:701–705, 1981.

Somogyi A, Albrecht M, Kliems G, Schafter K, Eichelbaum M: Pharmacokinetics, bioavailability, and ECG response of verapamil in patients with liver cirrhosis. *Br J Clin Pharmacol* 12:51–60, 1981.

Wit AL, Cranefield PF: Effects of verapamil on the sinoatrial and atrioventricular nodes. *Circ Res* 35:415–425, 1974.

Nifedipine

Banzet O, Colin JN, Thibonnier M, Singlas E, Alexandre JM, Corvol P: Pharmacokinetic studies of nifedipine tablet. Correlation with antihypertensive effects. *Hypertension* 5 (Suppl 2):29–33, 1983.

Ferlinz J: Nifedipine in myocardial ischemia, systemic hypertension, and other cardiovascular disorders. *Ann Intern Med* 105:714–729, 1986.

Foster TS, Hamann SR, Richards VR, Bryant PJ, Graves DA, McAllister RG Jr: Nifedipine kinetics and bioavailability after single intravenous and oral doses in normal subjects. *J Clin Pharmacol* 25:161–170, 1983.

Raemsch KD, Sommer J: Pharmacokinetics and metabolism of nifedipine. *Hypertension* 5 (Suppl 2):18–24, 1983.

Sorkin EM, Clissold SP, Brogden RN: Nifedipine. A review of the pharmacodynamic and pharmacokinetic properties, and therapeutic efficacy, in ischaemic heart disease, hypertension, and related cardiovascular disorders. *Drugs* 30:182–275, 1985.

Diltiazem

Chaffman M, Brogden RN: Diltiazem: a review of its pharmacological properties and therapeutic efficacy. *Drugs* 29:387–454, 1985.

Hermann PH, Rodger SD, Remones G, Thenot JP, London DR, Morselli PL: Pharmacokinetics of diltiazem after intravenous and oral administration. *Eur J Clin Pharmacol* 24:349–352, 1983.

Smith MS, Verghese CP, Shand DG, Pritchett EL: Pharmacokinetic and pharmacodynamic effects of diltiazem. *Am J Cardiol* 51:1369–1374, 1983.

Nicardipine

Sorkin EM, Clissold SP: Nicardipine. *Drugs* 33:296–345, 1987.

Drug Interactions

Babich M, Hamann SR, McAllister RG, Reddy CP, Piascik MT: Effects of verapamil on the arrhythmogenic action of acetylstrophanthidin. *Pharmacology* 29:224–232, 1984.

Belz GG, Doering W, Munkes R, Matthews J: Interaction between digoxin and calcium antagonists and antiarrhythmic drugs. *Clin Pharmacol Ther* 33:410–417, 1983.

Dargie HJ, Lynch PG, Krikler DM, Harris L, Krikler S: Nifedipine and propranolol: a beneficial drug interaction. *Am J Med* 71:676–682, 1981.

Hamann SR, Kaltenborn KE, Vore M, Tan TG, McAllister RG: Cardiovascular and pharmacokinetic consequences of combined administration of verapamil and propranolol in dogs. *Am J Cardiol* 56:147–156, 1985.

Joshi PI, Dalal JJ, Ruttley MS, Sheridan EJ, Henderson AH: Nifedipine and left ventricular function in beta-blocked patients. *Br Heart J* 45:457–459, 1981.

Klein HO, Kaplinsky E: Verapamil and digoxin: their respective effects on atrial fibrillation and their interaction. *Am J Cardiol* 50:894–902, 1982.

Packer M, Meller J, Medina N, Yushak M, Smith H, Holt J, Guerrero J, Todd GD, McAllister RG, Gorlin R: Hemodynamic consequences of combined beta-adrenergic and slow calcium channel blockade in man. *Circulation* 65:660–668, 1982.

Calcium Antagonists and Anesthesia

Adam LP, Henderson EG: Augmentation of succinylcholine-induced neuromuscular blockade by calcium channel antagonists. *Neurosci Lett* 70:148–153, 1986.

Chelly JE, Hysing ES, Abernethy DR, Doursout MF, Hartley CJ, Guerret M, Merin RG: Role of isoflurane on hemodynamic properties and disposition of nicardipine. *J Pharmacol Exp Ther* 241:899–906, 1987.

Chelly JE, Hysing ES, Abernethy DR, Doursout MF, Merin RG: Effects of inhalational anesthetics on verapamil pharmacokinetics in the dog. *Anesthesiology* 65:266–271, 1986.

Chelly JE, Hysing ES, Hill DC, Abernethy DR, Dewati A, Doursout MF, Merin RG: Cardiovascular effects of and interaction between calcium blocking drugs and anesthetics in chronically instrumented dogs. V. Role of pharmacokinetics and the autonomic nervous system in the interactions between verapamil and inhalational anesthetics. *Anesthesiology* 67:320–325, 1987.

Chelly JE, Rogers K, Hysing ES, Taylor A, Hartley C, Merin RG: Cardiovascular effects of and interaction between calcium blocking drugs and anesthetics in chronically instrumented dogs. I. Verapamil and halothane. *Anesthesiology* 64:560–567, 1986.

Durant NN, Nguyen N, Katz RL: Potentiation of neuromuscular blockade by verapamil. *Anesthesiology* 60:298–303, 1984.

Gorven AM, Cooper GM, Prys-Roberts C: Haemodynamic disturbances during anaesthesia in a patient receiving calcium channel blockers. *Br J Anaesth* 58:357–360, 1986.

Henling CE, Slogoff S, Kodali SV, Arlund C: Heart block after coronary artery bypass—effect of chronic administration of calcium-entry blockers and β-blockers. *Anesth Analg* 63:515–520, 1984.

Hysing ES, Chelly JE, Doursout MF, Hartley C, Merin RG: Cardiovascular effects of and interaction between calcium blocking drugs and anesthetics in chronically instrumented dogs. III. Nicardipine and isoflurane. *Anesthesiology* 65:385–391, 1986.

Jones RM, Cashman JN, Casson WR, Broadbent MP: Verapamil potentiation of neuromuscular blockade: failure of reversal with neostigmine but prompt reversal with edrophonium. Anesth Analg 64:1021–1025, 1985.

Kapur PA, Bloor BC, Flacke WE, Olewine SK: Comparison of cardiovascular responses to verapamil during enflurane, isoflurane, or halothane anesthesia in the dog. Anesthesiology 61:156–160, 1984.

Kapur PA, Campos JH, Buchea OC: Plasma diltiazem levels, cardiovascular function, and coronary hemodynamics during enflurane anesthesia in the dog. Anesth Analg 65:918–924, 1986.

Kapur PA, Campos JH, Tippit SE: Influence of diltiazem on cardiovascular function and coronary hemodynamics during isoflurane anesthesia in the dog: correlation with plasma diltiazem levels. Anesth Analg 65:81–87, 1986.

Kapur PA, Norel EJ, Dajee H, Cohen G, Flacke W: Hemodynamic effects of verapamil administration after large doses of fentanyl in man. Can Anaesth Soc J 33:138–144, 1986.

Kates RA, Kaplan JA: Cardiovascular responses to verapamil during coronary artery bypass graft surgery. Anesth Analg 62:821–826, 1983.

Kates RA, Kaplan JA, Guyton RA, Dorsey L, Hug CC, Hatcher CR: Hemodynamic interactions of verapamil and isoflurane. Anesthesiology 59:132–138, 1983.

Kates RA, Zaggy AP, Norfleet EA, Heath KR: Comparative cardiovascular effects of verapamil, nifedipine, and diltiazem during halothane anesthesia in swine. Anesthesiology 61:10–18, 1984.

Kraynack BJ, Lawson NW, Gintautas J, Tjay HT: Effects of verapamil on indirect muscle twitch responses. Anesth Analg 62:827–830, 1983.

Lawson NW, Kraynack BJ, Gintautas J: Neuromuscular and electrocardiographic responses to verapamil in dogs. Anesth Analg 62:50–54, 1983.

Marshall AG, Kissin I, Reves JG, Bradley EL Jr, Blackstone EH: Interaction between negative inotropic effects of halothane and nifedipine in the isolated rat heart. J Cardiovasc Pharmacol 5:592–597, 1983.

Maze M, Mason DM, Kates RE: Verapamil decreases MAC for halothane in dogs. Anesthesiology 59:327–329, 1983.

Merin RG: Calcium channel blocking drugs and anesthetics: is the drug interaction beneficial or detrimental? Anesthesiology 66:111–113, 1987.

Priebe HJ, Skarvan K: Cardiovascular and electrophysiologic interactions between diltiazem and isoflurane in the dog. Anesthesiology 66:114–121, 1987.

Reilly CS, Wood AJJ, Koshakji RP, Wood M: The effect of halothane on drug disposition: contribution of changes in intrinsic drug metabolizing capacity and hepatic blood flow. Anesthesiology 66:70–76, 1985.

Reves JG: The relative hemodynamic effects of Ca++ entry blockers. Anesthesiology 61:3–5, 1984.

Rogers K, Hysing ES, Merin RG, Taylor A, Hartley C, Chelly JE: Cardiovascular effects of and interaction between calcium blocking drugs and anesthetics in chronically instrumented dogs. II. Verapamil, enflurane, and isoflurane. Anesthesiology 64:568–575, 1986.

Saltzman LS, Kates RA, Corke BC, Norfleet EA, Heath KR: Hyperkalemia and cardiovascular collapse after verapamil and dantrolene administration in swine. Anesth Analg 63:473–478, 1984.

Schulte-Sasse U, Hess W, Markschies-Hornung A, Tarnow J: Combined effects of halothane anesthesia and verapamil on systemic hemodynamics and left ventricular myocardial contractility in patients with ischemic heart disease. Anesth Analg 63:791–798, 1984.

Schulte-Sasse U,Tarnow J: Effects of short-term infusion of nifedipine or verapamil on systemic hemodynamics and left ventricular myocardial contractility in patients prior to coronary artery bypass surgery. Anesthesiology 67:492–497, 1987.

Sullivan KB, Kapur PA: The effect of β-adrenergic blockade on the cardiovascular response to diltiazem or verapamil in dogs. Anesth Analg 65:1099–1106, 1986.

Tosone SR, Reves JG, Kissin I, Smith LR, Fournier SE: Hemodynamic responses to nifedipine in dogs anesthetized with halothane. Anesth Analg 62:903–908, 1983.

Therapeutic Uses

Bala Subramanian V, Bowles MJ, Khurmi NS, Davies AB, Raftery EB: Rationale for the choice of calcium antagonists in chronic stable angina. An objective double-blind placebo-controlled comparison of nifedipine and verapamil. Am J Cardiol 50:1173–1179, 1982.

Erne P, Bolli P, Bertel O, Lennart U, Hulthen L, Kiowski W, Muller F, Buhler FR: Factors influencing the hypotensive effects of calcium antagonists. Hypertension 5 (Suppl 2):97–102, 1983.

Frishman W, Charlap S, Kimmel B, Saltzberg S, Stroh J, Weinberg P, Monuszko E, Weizner J, Dorsa F, Pollack S, Strom J: Twice-daily oral verapamil in essential hypertension. Arch Intern Med 146:561–565, 1986.

Frishman WH, Charlap S, Michelson EL: Calcium channel blockers in systemic hypertension. Am J Cardiol 58:157–160, 1986.

Gunther S, Green L, Muller JE, Mudge GH, Grossman W: Prevention by nifedipine of abnormal coronary vasoconstriction in patients with coronary artery disease. Circulation 63:849–855, 1981.

Hossack KF, Pool PE, Steele P, Crawford MH, Demaria AN, Cohen LS, Ports TA: Efficacy of diltiazem in angina of effort: a multicenter trial. Am J Cardiol 49:567–572, 1982.

Inouye IK, Massie BM, Benowitz N, Simpson P, Loge D: Antihypertensive therapy with diltiazem and comparison with hydrochlorothiazide. Am J Cardiol 53:1588–1592, 1984.

Johnson GJ, Leis LA, Francis GS: Disparate effects of calcium channel blockers, nifedipine and verapamil, on alpha₂-adrenergic receptors and thromboxane A₂-induced aggregation of human platelets. Circulation 73:847–854, 1986.

Kaltenbach M, Hopf R, Kober G, Bussmann WD, Keller M, Petersen Y: Treatment of hypertrophic obstructive cardiomyopathy with verapamil. *Br Heart J* 42:35–42, 1979.

Klein HO, Kaplinsky E: Digitalis and verapamil in atrial fibrillation and flutter. *Drugs* 31:185–197, 1986.

Littler WA: Use of nifedipine as monotherapy in the management of hypertension. *Am J Med* (Suppl 4A):36–40, 1985.

Meyer JS: Calcium channel blockers in the prophylactic treatment of vascular headache. *Ann Intern Med* 102:395–397, 1985.

Ochs HR, Anda L, Eichelbaum M, Greenblatt DJ: Diltiazem, verapamil, and quinidine in patients with chronic atrial fibrillation. *J Clin Pharmacol* 25:204–209, 1985.

Rogan AM, Hamilton TC, Young RC, Klecker RW, Ozols RF: Reversal of adriamycin resistance by verapamil in human ovarian cancer. *Science* 224:994–995, 1984.

Rosing DR, Condit JR, Maron BJ, Kent KM, Leon MB, Bonow RO, Lipson LC, Epstein SE: Verapamil therapy. A new approach to the pharmacologic treatment of hypertrophic cardiomyopathy. III. Effects of long-term administration. *Am J Cardiol* 48:545–553, 1981.

Rozanski JJ, Zaman L, Castellanos A: Electrophysiologic effects of diltiazem hydrochloride on supraventricular tachycardia. *Am J Cardiol* 49:621–628, 1982.

Singh BN, Nademanee K, Baky SH: Calcium antagonists. Clinical use in the treatment of arrhythmias. *Drugs* 25:125–153, 1983.

Spicer RL, Rocchini AP, Crowley DC, Vasiliades J, Rosenthal A: Hemodynamic effects of verapamil in children and adolescents with hypertrophic cardiomyopathy. *Circulation* 67:413–420, 1983.

Sung RJ, Elser B, McAllister RG: Intravenous verapamil for termination of re-entrant supraventricular tachycardias. Intracardiac studies correlated with plasma verapamil concentrations. *Ann Intern Med* 93:682–689, 1980.

Theroux P, Taeymans Y, Waters DD: Calcium antagonists. Clinical use in the treatment of angina. *Drugs* 25:178–195, 1983.

Waters DD, Theroux P, Szlachcic J, Dauwe F: Provocative testing with ergonovine to assess the efficacy of treatment with nifedipine, diltiazem, and verapamil in variant angina. *Am J Cardiol* 48:123–130, 1981.

Weinstein DB, Heider JG: Antiatherogenic properties of calcium antagonists. *Am J Cardiol* 59:163B–172B, 1987.

Woelfel A, Foster JR, McAllister RG, Simpson RJ, Gettes LS: Efficacy of verapamil in exercise induced ventricular tachycardia. *Am J Cardiol* 56:292–297, 1985.

GENERAL THERAPEUTICS

19

Drugs and the Respiratory System

MARGARET WOOD

PHYSIOLOGICAL CONTROL OF BRONCHOMOTOR TONE

The trachea, bronchi, lungs, and pulmonary vessels are innervated by cholinergic and adrenergic fibers of the autonomic nervous system. In humans, bronchial smooth muscle has a rich parasympathetic nerve supply via the vagus, stimulation of which causes smooth muscle contraction (evident clinically as bronchoconstriction) and an increase in respiratory tract secretions. In addition, bronchial smooth muscle also contains β-adrenergic receptors, stimulation of which causes bronchial smooth muscle relaxation and bronchodilation. The β-receptors have been divided by Lands (1967) into β_1- and β_2-subgroups (see Chapter 13), and β_2-receptors predominate in the smooth muscle of the bronchus and bronchiole. The activity of the β-receptor is thought to be mediated through the production of cyclic adenosine monophosphate (cAMP) (see Chapter 3). β-Receptor agonists (either endogenous circulating catecholamines or exogenously administered drug) bind to the receptor and stimulate adenylate cyclase, which is closely linked to the receptor (Fig 19.1); stimulation of adenylate cyclase results in the formation of cAMP

from ATP. cAMP which is formed is then released into the cytoplasm and acts to alter cellular function. Thus, cAMP is thought of as the "second messenger" while the neurotransmitter (norepinephrine or epinephrine, for example) is the "first messenger." An increasing concentration of cAMP in bronchial smooth muscle is associated with bronchodilation, while decreasing concentrations of cAMP lead to bronchoconstriction. cAMP is then broken down to the inactive 5'-adenosine monophosphate (5-AMP) by the enzyme, phosphodiesterase. Thus, increases in intracellular concentrations of cAMP may be due to either:

1. Stimulation of the enzyme adenylate cyclase which causes the conversion of ATP to cAMP; or
2. Inhibition of the enzyme phosphodiesterase, thus preventing the breakdown of cAMP to 5-AMP.

Figure 19.1 illustrates diagramatically the role of the adrenergic system in the control of bronchodilation. Sympathomimetic β_2-agonists stimulate the β_2-adrenergic receptor causing an increase in intracellular cAMP concentrations which initiates a series of events resulting in bronchodilation, while methylxanthines such as theophylline inhibit the break-

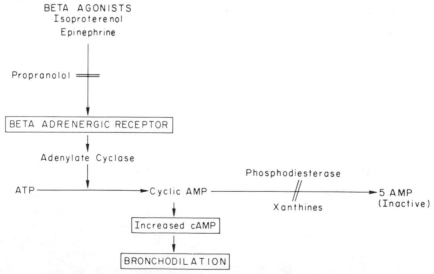

Figure 19.1. Role of the β-adrenergic system in the production of bronchodilation. ATP, adenosine triphosphate; cyclic AMP, cyclic adenosine 3', 5'-monophosphate.

down of cAMP by phosphodiesterase. Prostaglandins E_1 and E_2 increase cAMP concentrations, while corticosteroids act at least in part by stimulating the β-adrenergic receptor, but their main role is to reduce inflammation. Prostaglandin $F_{2\alpha}$ decreases cAMP concentrations, resulting in bronchoconstriction. Decreased concentrations of cAMP lead to bronchoconstriction.

Cyclic guanosine monophosphate (cGMP) is another second messenger which appears to be under the control of the parasympathetic nervous system. cGMP causes contraction of bronchial smooth muscle, resulting in bronchoconstriction. Stimulation of cholinergic receptors by vagal stimulation or cholinergic drugs such as carbachol or methacholine increases cGMP concentrations. Thus, bronchomotor tone is probably regulated in part by a balance between intracellular cAMP and cGMP concentrations.

Allergic responses mediated by the immunoglobulin, IgE, play an important role in the production of an asthmatic attack, and serum levels of IgE are often elevated in the patient with allergic asthma. When an individual is "sensitized" by exposure to an antigen (such as pollen), antibodies are produced in the IgE class of the serum immunoglobulins. Mast cells and basophils contain a surface receptor which has a high affinity for IgE and, therefore, binds IgE. Subsequent reexposure to the antigen causes the activation of the target tissue mast cell, which has previously been sensitized by IgE antibody and initiates a series of complex biochemical events culminating in the degranulation of the mast cell and release of many chemical mediators, such as histamine, slow-reacting substance of anaphylaxis (SRS-A) (see Chapter 24), and eosinophil chemotatic factor of anaphylaxis (ECF-A). Platelet-activating factor (PAF) is another mediator that is now thought to be important in the production of bronchial constriction, and a number of PAF antagonists have been developed that might be useful in the management of asthmatic patients. The release of chemical mediators results in

bronchial smooth muscle constriction. The maintenance of intracellular cAMP concentrations is probably required for stability of the mast cell granules, and agents which act to increase these levels tend to inhibit anaphylaxis; release of chemical mediators from the mast cell is inhibited by cAMP and, thus, β-agonists and methylxanthines inhibit mediator release. Cholinergic stimulation increases mediator release; this may be due to increased cGMP concentrations. Figure 19.2 depicts the sequence of events which are thought to cause the release of chemical mediators of bronchospasm, while Table 19.1 lists the receptors situated in respiratory smooth muscle and summarizes the effects resulting from receptor stimulation. It is now recognized that the airway narrowing associated with asthma is due not only to constriction of airway smooth muscle but also to inflammation, and therefore the therapeutic management of asthma dictates the use of (a) bronchodilators and (b) antiinflammatory drugs, such as corticosteroids and cromolyn.

β-RECEPTOR AGONISTS

Sympathomimetic bronchodilators are effective because β-adrenergic receptor stimulation leads to an increase in intracellular cAMP concentrations, which then triggers a sequence of intracellular events leading to bronchodilation. They also inhibit the release of chemical mediators which cause bronchospasm and stabilize mast cells.

The endogenous adrenergic agonists epinephrine and norepinephrine are both potent β-receptor stimulants. However, their hemodynamic effects are different due to epinephrine's greater potency at the β_2-receptor and norepinephrine's greater potency at the α-receptor (see Chapter 13). In order to minimize the unwanted α-effects of both epinephrine and norepinephrine, β-receptor stimulating drugs with little α-effect, such as isoproterenol, were developed. The pharmacological differences between the β-receptor agonists are due to differences in their potency at β_1- and β_2-receptors

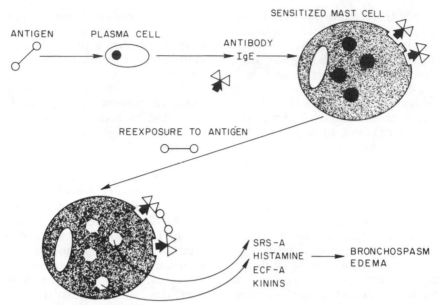

Figure 19.2.   Chemical mediators of bronchospasm.   Sensitization of the mast cell by the binding to the cell membrane of the immunoglobulin E (IgE) occurs on first exposure to the antigen. Subsequent reexposure to the same antigen causes mast cell degranulation and release of chemical mediators following interaction of antigen and bound IgE. Increased cAMP and cromolyn sodium prevent the release of chemical mediators.

and also in their resistance to degradation by the enzyme catechol-O-methyltransferase (COMT). Because this enzyme is present in high concentrations in the liver, little of an absorbed dose of substrates for COMT can enter the systemic circulation following oral administration.

NONSELECTIVE AGONISTS

Isoproterenol is a relatively nonselective β_1- and β_2-receptor stimulant. Its

Table 19.1.
Smooth Muscle Receptors of the Respiratory Tract

Receptor type	Effect
Adrenergic	
α_1 and α_2	Contraction, bronchoconstriction
β_2	Relaxation, bronchodilation
Cholinergic	Contraction, bronchoconstriction
Histamine	
H_1	Contraction, bronchoconstriction
H_2	Relaxation, bronchodilation

pharmacological actions can be predicted from a knowledge of the location of β_1- and β_2-receptors and the effects of their stimulation (Table 14.2, page 411). Stimulation of cardiac β_1-receptors causes positive chronotropic and inotropic effects. The rise in heart rate and cardiac output is further reflexly increased by the fall in peripheral resistance produced by the β_2-induced relaxation of vascular smooth muscle. This is particularly seen in skeletal muscle beds resulting in increased venous return. In addition to vascular smooth muscle, smooth muscle relaxation also occurs in the bronchi, gastrointestinal tract, and uterus.

The ability to cause bronchial dilation and reverse airway obstruction gave isoproterenol an important therapeutic role in asthma in the past. However, selective β_2-agonists have now replaced isoproterenol because they produce less β_1-induced cardiac effects at a given degree of bronchodilation. There is therefore no indication today for the administration of nonselective β-agonists. The use of isoproterenol was associated with fatal cardiac arrhythmias in the 1960s. Isoproterenol aerosols may have been used excessively by asthmatics whose attacks were unresponsive at a time when they were also hypoxic, perhaps resulting in fatal cardiac arrhythmias.

Isoproterenol is metabolized by COMT, and therefore very little enters the systemic circulation following an oral dose. However, it is highly effective in producing bronchial dilation when given by inhalation.

SELECTIVE AGONISTS

The high incidence of undesirable side effects associated with the use of isoproterenol for the treatment of bronchospasm has led to the development of a series of compounds that are more potent agonists at β_2-receptors than at β_1-receptors. Therefore, at doses of these drugs which produce equivalent bronchial dilation, less cardiac effects are produced than with isoproterenol. It is important to remember, however, that these drugs do still have β_1-effects at high concentrations, so that increasing the dosage leads to tachycardia, arrhythmias, and increased myocardial oxygen consumption. Also there may be an additive effect on cardiac toxicity when these drugs are combined with theophylline. Examples of such selective β-agonists include metaproterenol (orciprenaline), terbutaline, isoetharine, albuterol (salbutamol), fenoterol, and rimiterol.

Biotransformation of sympathomimetic agents has an important influence on duration of action and route of administration. The term catecholamine has been applied to sympathomimetic amines that have hydroxyl substitutions in the 3 and 4 positions of the benzene ring (see Chapter 13). Catechol-O-methyltransferase (COMT) methylates the 3-hydroxy group causing a reduction in pharmacological activity. The enzyme monoamine oxidase (MAO) metabolizes catecholamines by the process of oxidative deamination. Thus, the duration of action of catecholamines is limited primarily by rapid removal from their site of action (reuptake) and to some extent by metabolism by COMT and MAO. They are not effective

when given orally due to presystemic metabolism; oral isoproterenol, for example, is inactivated by being sulfated in the intestine and broken down in the liver and, thus, must be given by the intravenous or inhalational route. Ephedrine has a longer duration of action and good oral absorption since it is resistant to metabolism by COMT and MAO. Terbutaline, albuterol, and fenoterol do not possess the catechol nucleus and, therefore, are not metabolized by COMT (Figure 19.3). This means that they can reach effective levels when given orally. However, rimiterol does possess the catechol nucleus, is metabolized by COMT, and is ineffective when administered orally.

Prolonged use of β-receptor agonists can result in tachyphylaxis, i.e., desensitization or tolerance. This takes 1 to 2 weeks to occur and is due to a decrease in β-receptor density (number) or affinity ("down regulation," see page 68). Restoration of normal responsiveness takes about 2 weeks to occur following discontinuation of therapy.

Thus, the noncatechol β_2-agonists have increased β_2 selectivity, increased duration of action, and greater oral bioavailability. Inhalation of β-agonist drugs, however, offers the advantage of maximum bronchodilation at lower doses accompanied by lower systemic concentrations and, consequently, fewer adverse effects. The onset of action when β-agonists are given by the inhalational route is almost as rapid as that seen with intravenous administration, and it may be the only route available to the anesthesiologist. The metered inhalers can be administered via a T-connector placed between the anesthesia circuit and the endotracheal tube, or a solution can be made up in normal saline and given via a nebulizer placed in the inspiratory limb of the anesthesia circuit. The dose of a metered inhaler should be reduced when given by endotracheal tube, since it is likely that a larger proportion of the dose will be received by the lung. Administration of respiratory solutions by nebulizers appears to be less efficient than the correct administration of metered-dose inhalers, and recommended nebulizer solution

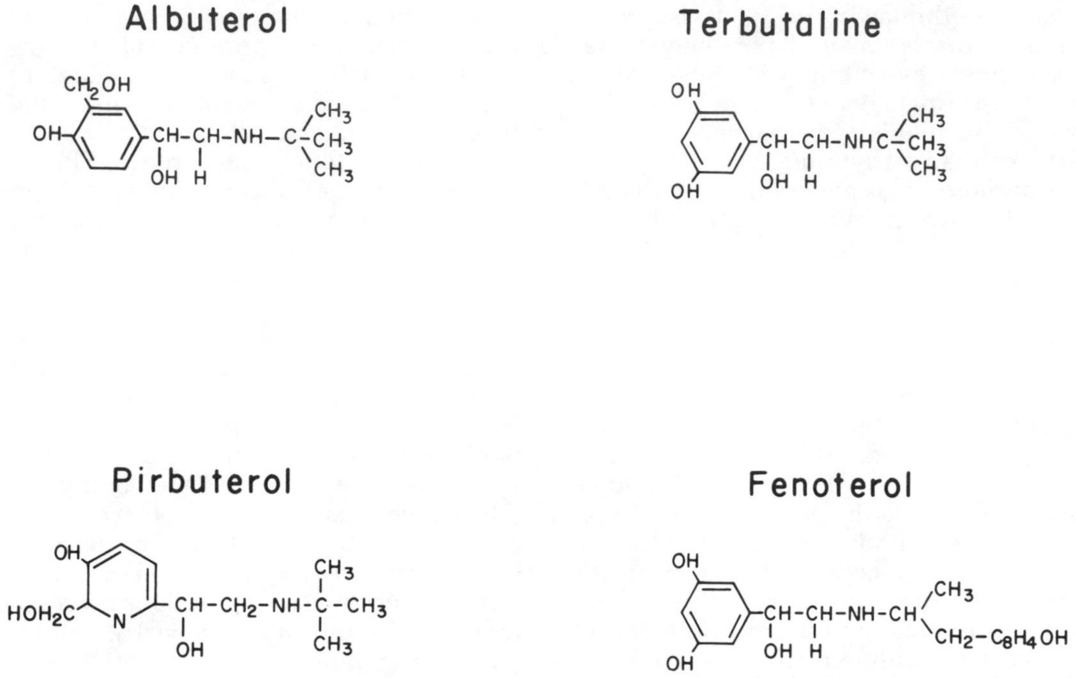

Albuterol

Terbutaline

Pirbuterol

Fenoterol

Figure 19.3.   Structural formulae of some important selective β_2-agonists.

doses are 3 to 10 times the dose for metered-dose inhalers.

Figure 19.3 gives the structural formula of some important selective β_2-agonists.

INDIVIDUAL β-AGONIST DRUGS

The general pharmacology of the sympathomimetic amines, and epinephrine and isoproterenol in particular, is discussed in more detail in Chapter 13, and only the use of sympathomimetic amines in respiratory disease will be discussed here.

Epinephrine

Epinephrine possesses both α- and β-effects. β-Stimulation results in bronchodilation, while α-effects, by producing vasoconstriction of bronchial mucosal vasculature, may reduce congestion and edema, especially if given by the inhalational route. Epinephrine is metabolized by catechol-O-methyl transferase (COMT) and by monoamine oxidase

(MAO) and, thus, cannot be given by the oral route. Epinephrine can be given subcutaneously as 0.2 to 0.5 ml of a 1:1000 solution to adults (it may need to be repeated after 15 to 20 minutes), while the pediatric dose is 0.01 ml/kg of body weight every 4 hours as required. Tolerance often develops, and the patient may become refractory to therapy. For inhalational therapy, the use of epinephrine has largely been superseded by selective β_2-adrenergic agonists. **Racemic epinephrine** is a synthetic preparation; it is a racemic mixture of d- and l-epinephrine (50:50), whereas the natural compound exists only in the l-form. α-Agonist effects make racemic epinephrine a useful drug in the treatment of bronchial mucosal congestion, and it has been successfully used in the treatment of croup and epiglottitis. Racemic epinephrine, 0.25 to 0.7 ml of 2.25% solution (4.5 to 15.75 mg), is diluted in 2.0 to 5.0 ml of normal saline and administered by a hand-held nebulizer or intermittent positive pressure breathing (IPPB); the therapy may be repeated every 3 to 4 hours.

Isoproterenol

Isoproterenol has β_1- and β_2-effects and is a potent bronchodilator. It is ineffective when given orally. It may be given by the inhalational route either as a 1:100 or 1:200 solution. Isoproterenol, 0.25 to 0.5 ml of 1:200 solution (1.25 to 2.5 mg), is diluted with 2.0 to 5.0 ml of normal saline and delivered by a hand-held nebulizer or IPPB. It can be repeated every 2 hours if necessary. Metered-dose inhalers are available for patient use. They require the use of 1 or 2 inhalations ("puffs"), to be repeated every 4 to 6 hours if required. The dose of isoproterenol per puff varies among the different commercial preparations, but is in the region of 0.075 to 0.125 mg per puff. The patient should be instructed not to use more than two puffs at a time of an aerosol containing up to 0.1 mg of isoproterenol per puff; if this dose does not relieve bronchospasm, the patient should see a physician and may require alternate therapy. Adverse effects of isoproterenol include tachycardia, arrhythmias, and increased myocardial oxygen consumption. Selective β_2-adrenergic stimulants should be used in preference to isoproterenol to avoid unwanted cardiac stimulation. The dosage and duration of action of isoproterenol are given in Table 19.2.

Metaproterenol (Orciprenaline)

Metaproterenol is a noncatechol relatively selective β_2-agonist which is effective when given orally and has a longer duration of action than isoproterenol when administered by the inhalational route. It is available in metered-dose inhalers and as tablets for oral use. When administered by the inhalational route, it has a rapid onset of action and a duration of effect of 1 to 4 hours. Oral administration has a slower onset of action and a duration of effect of 1 to 5 hours. Side effects are predictable and include tachy-

Table 19.2
Comparison of Selective β_2-Adrenergic Bronchodilators

Drug	Dose (mg)	Onset of effect (min)	Peak of effect (min)	Duration of effect (hr)
Isoproterenol (inhaled)	0.1–0.3	2–5	5–30	1–3
Ephedrine (oral)	15–50	~60	120–180	3–5
Isoetharine (inhaled)	0.5	5	15–60	1–3
Metaproterenol (inhaled)	1.0–1.5	2–10	60	1–4
Metaproterenol (oral)	10–20	~30	120–150	1–5
Terbutaline (subcutaneous)	0.25–0.5	5–15	30–60	3–4
Terbutaline (oral)	5	30	120–180	4–8
Terbutaline (inhaled)	0.4	5–10	60	4–6
Albuterol (inhaled)	0.1–0.4	5–10	30–60	3–6
Albuterol (oral)	2–4	30	60–120	3–4
Pirbuterol (inhaled)	0.4	5–10	30–60	4–6

cardia, hypertension, tremor, palpitations, nausea, and vomiting. Side effects occur in about 4 to 8% of patients when the drug is given by aerosol and in about 17% of patients when administered orally. The dosage of metaproterenol is given in Table 19.2.

Terbutaline

Terbutaline is a relatively selective β_2-agonist that is effective in the treatment of asthma. It is not a catechol and, thus, is not metabolized by COMT. It is available for oral and subcutaneous administration. The duration of action is long (4 to 8 hours) following oral administration. When administered subcutaneously, it has a rapid onset and a duration of action of 3 to 4 hours. It appears to lose β_2 selectivity when administered by the subcutaneous route, and cardiovascular side effects should be anticipated. Side effects include those commonly associated with sympathomimetic drugs but, in addition, muscle tremor is a notable adverse effect. Terbutaline, in common with other selective β_2-agonists, has been shown to cause hypokalemia which results from β_2-receptor stimulation which drives potassium into the cells (see page 412). Tachyphylaxis may occur with chronic administration. The dosage of terbutaline is given in Table 19.2. Terbutaline has also been given by intravenous infusion using a loading dose of 250 to 500 μg and a maintenance infusion of 1.5 to 5.0 μg per minute. Terbutaline has also been administered by nebulizer as a solution, when 2 to 10 mg are recommended. It should be diluted in 2 ml of normal saline and given up to a maximum of every 6 hours.

Isoetharine

Isoetharine is a selective β_2-agonist available for the treatment of reversible obstructive airway disease as a solution for nebulization (Bronkosol) and a metered-dose inhaler (Bronkometer). Isoetharine may be administered as 0.25 to 1.0 ml of a 1% solution (2.5 to 10 mg) diluted with 2.0 to 5.0 ml of normal saline delivered by a hand-held nebulizer or IPPB.

The treatment may be repeated every 3 to 4 hours.

Albuterol (Salbutamol)

Albuterol is a selective β_2-agonist that has been administered by oral, inhalational, and intravenous routes. When administered by the inhalational route, it has a rapid onset of action and reduces airway resistance for 4 to 6 hours. Side effects are similar to other selective β_2-agonists and include β_1-induced cardiac effects and β_2-induced hypokalemia. Albuterol causes tremor as frequently as terbutaline.

Albuterol is available as a "Ventolin" metered-dose aerosol for inhalation, as a solution for inhalation, and as tablets and syrup for oral use. Albuterol solution for inhalation is prepared as a 0.5% solution; the usual starting dose is 2.5 mg, and 0.5 ml of 0.5% solution (i.e., 2.5 mg of albuterol) is diluted to 3.0 ml with normal saline solution and then given by nebulization. This mode of administration may be particularly useful during anesthesia. It may be given every 6 hours. Although albuterol is not available in the United States for parenteral use, it can be administered both subcutaneously and intravenously: 8.0 μg/kg subcutaneously and intravenously as a loading dose of 250 μg followed by a maintenance infusion of 5 to 20 μg/min. The dosage of albuterol for oral and inhalational use is given in Table 19.2.

Ritodrine

Ritodrine is another selective β_2-adrenergic agonist that, although used in obstructive airway disease, was actually developed for use as a uterine relaxant in obstetric practice to delay or prevent premature delivery. Ritodrine is available in a solution of 10 mg/ml for parenteral administration and 10-mg oral tablets. A solution of ritodrine (0.3 mg/ml) is administered intravenously at a rate of 0.1 mg per minute and titrated to clinical effect when used to inhibit premature labor. Although ritodrine is primarily used to inhibit uterine contractions, its respiratory effects are similar to other selective

β_2-agonists (see Chapter 12). The maximum recommended infusion rate is 0.35 mg per minute. Side effects are similar to those for other selective β_2-agonist drugs.

Pirbuterol

Pirbuterol is a selective β_2-agonist which has been shown to produce bronchodilatory effects and is used in the management of reversible obstructive airway disease. It is structurally similar to albuterol. Pirbuterol can be given either orally or via an aerosol. It is available in the United States as an aerosol, 200 μg per inhalation, with the recommendation that the adult dose is 1 to 2 inhalations (0.2 or 0.4 mg) every 4 to 6 hours. When given by inhalational aerosol, it has a rapid onset of action, with a maximum effect at 30 to 60 minutes and a duration of action of 4 to 6 hours (Table 19.2). Side effects include tremor, tachycardia, and palpitations. Pirbuterol has a plasma half-life of about 2 to 3 hours.

Rimiterol

Rimiterol is another selection β_2-agonist that is effective in reversible airway obstruction. Side effects are similar to other sympathomimetic drugs.

Table 19.2 compares the dosages and duration of action of selective β_2-adrenergic bronchodilators with isoproterenol and ephedrine.

METHYLXANTHINES

Theophylline, caffeine, and theobromine are three closely related methylated xanthines that are found in plants widely distributed throughout the world. Tea, coffee, cocoa, and cola-flavored beverages contain caffeine and other xanthine-related alkaloids. The solubility of the xanthines is low but is increased by formation of compounds with a wide range of salts; for example, aminophylline is the ethylenediamine salt of theophylline. The structural formulae of xanthine, caffeine, theophylline, and theobromine are given in Figure 19.4.

MECHANISM OF ACTION

Theophylline administration is known to inhibit the enzyme phosphodiesterase, leading to increased levels of cAMP and resulting in physiological responses such as bronchodilation (Fig 19.1). However, this effect is produced only at high concentrations, and it is unlikely that inhibition of phosphodiesterase is the major factor in causing bronchodilation. Selective inhibition of an isoenzyme, phosphodiesterase F-III (relatively specific for cAMP degradation), has, however, been proposed as a possible mode of action. Other mechanisms, such as theophylline-mediated catecholamine release, alterations in intracellular calcium, adenosine receptor antagonism, and

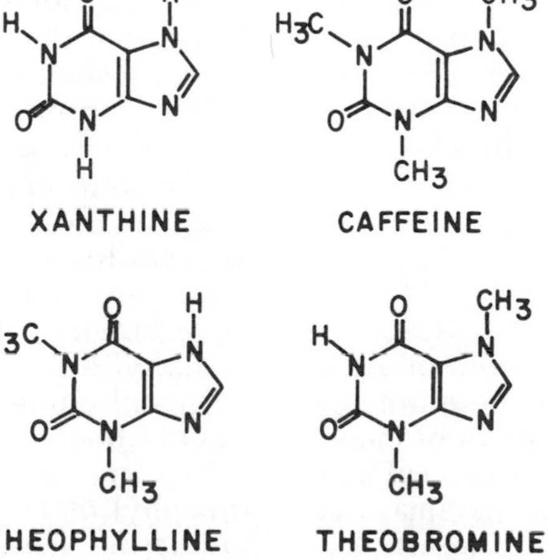

Figure 19.4. Structural formulae of xanthine and three important methylated derivatives.

prostaglandin antagonism may all contribute to the clinical effects of the methylxanthines. In addition, theophylline has been shown to interact synergistically with other agents that increase cAMP through the stimulation of adenylate cyclase.

CENTRAL NERVOUS SYSTEM

Theophylline and caffeine are potent central nervous system stimulants. Persons ingesting caffeine or caffeine-containing beverages report less drowsiness, less fatigue, and clearer intellectual thinking. Methylxanthines also stimulate the medullary respiratory center, increasing the sensitivity of the medullary center to the stimulatory effects of carbon dioxide. Other central nervous system effects of theophylline include nervousness, anxiety, insomnia, and nausea and vomiting.

The xanthines cause a marked increase in cerebrovascular resistance, resulting in a decrease in cerebral blood flow. This effect may be responsible for the alleviation of hypertensive headaches by caffeine.

CARDIOVASCULAR SYSTEM

In humans, aminophylline produces a modest chronotropic effect at therapeutic plasma concentrations, accompanied by an increase in stroke volume and cardiac output. There is a decrease in peripheral vascular resistance, resulting in lowered right and left ventricular end-diastolic filling pressures. Thus, at one time, aminophylline was used in the management of congestive cardiac failure. Cardiac arrhythmias are associated with theophylline toxicity at high serum concentrations. Theophylline also has a diuretic effect.

RESPIRATORY SYSTEM

The xanthines relax smooth muscle, including that of the bronchi; aminophylline administration results in bronchodilation and has been shown to be of benefit in the treatment of asthma and bronchospasm in humans. The effect of aminophylline on the medullary respiratory center and the carbon dioxide-ventilatory response curve has been described earlier in this section; aminophylline is widely used in pediatric practice to treat neonatal apnea.

OTHER EFFECTS

Caffeine has been shown to increase the capacity for muscular work. Theophylline stimulates the neuromuscular junction, and it is interesting that, in patients with myasthenia gravis, theophylline causes an improvement in symptoms. Antagonism of pancuronium-induced neuromuscular block by high concentrations of theophylline has been reported. It has been suggested that aminophylline might facilitate neuromuscular transmission by raising cAMP concentrations at the neuromuscular junction via phosphodiesterase inhibition (see Chapter 10).

PHARMACOKINETICS

Theophylline is eliminated from the body by biotransformation in the liver and urinary excretion of its metabolites, 1,3-dimethyl uric acid, 1-methyl uric acid, and 3-methylxanthine. Seven to 13% is excreted unchanged in the urine. One of its metabolites, 3-methylxanthine, is pharmacologically active but less potent than theophylline. Since theophylline is metabolized in the liver, hepatic disease or cardiac disease accompanied by chronic passive hepatic venous congestion will increase the plasma half-life of the drug (see Chapter 1), and the dose should be reduced accordingly.

Plasma protein binding is in the range of 53 to 65% while the apparent volume of distribution at steady state is about 0.5 L/kg in the adult. Premature neonates and adults with hepatic cirrhosis have reduced protein binding and also tend to have larger volumes of distribution for theophylline.

Theophylline has a mean plasma half-life of about 4.5 hours in adults and 3.6 hours in children. The elimination of theophylline is markedly decreased in premature neonates, but increases during childhood, and it is not until the late teens that the rapid clearance of childhood approaches adult values. Factors affecting theophylline clearance include age, weight, cigarette smoking, drugs (phenobarbital, allopurinol), and cardiorespiratory or hepatic disease. The plasma clearance for theophylline in the adult has been reported as varying from 0.05 to 0.07 L/kg/hour.

Cimetidine administration decreases theophylline metabolism resulting in increased plasma theophylline concentrations. Ranitidine administration does not appear to cause this effect (see Chapter 23).

SUGGESTED DOSAGE AND ADMINISTRATION

The determination of plasma theophylline concentrations is extremely useful in adjusting dosage and preventing side effects. The therapeutic range of plasma theophylline is from 10 to 20 mg/L. Serious adverse effects are rare at plasma theophylline concentrations below 20 mg/L, while clinical effect is not usually significant at levels below 10 mg/L. The most frequent side effects include gastrointestinal (anorexia, nausea, vomiting, abdominal discomfort) and nervous (headache, nervousness, anxiety, agitation) system symptoms. At plasma theophylline levels between 20 and 40 mg/L, sinus tachycardia and atrial or ventricular arrhythmias may occur, while at levels above 40 mg/L, seizures or cardiorespiratory arrest may ensue. Signs of toxicity are evident in 75% of patients at plasma theophylline concentrations above 25 mg/L. The measurement of plasma theophylline concentrations is the only reliable method of assessing risk of toxicity and should be routinely undertaken.

Theophylline base is quite insoluble in aqueous solution, and the only intravenous preparation available is aminophylline, which contains about 80% theophylline by weight. Aminophylline may be administered by the oral, rectal, or intravenous route, but the intravenous route is the most reliable and rapid in the acute emergency situation.

Intravenous dosage schedules for aminophylline have been developed to rapidly achieve and maintain therapeutic theophylline concentrations in most patients. For rapid clinical effect, a loading dose is essential. A loading dose of 6 mg/kg of aminophylline is administered to adults intravenously over 20 minutes, followed by a maintenance infusion of 0.9 mg/kg/hour which will produce theophylline concentrations around 10 mg/L (Table 19.3). If the patient does not develop symptoms of toxicity but has not attained relief of symptoms, another loading dose of 3 mg/kg should be ad-

Table 19.3.
Intravenous Dose Schedule for Aminophylline

Subjects	Load (mg/kg over 20 min)	Maintenance (mg/kg each hr)	Plasma theophylline* (mg/L)
Children			
Low dose	6	1.10	10 (5–15)†
High dose	9‡	1.65	15 (10–20)
Adults			
Low dose	6	0.90	10 (5–15)
High dose	9‡	1.35	15 (10–20)

With permission from Piafsky KM, Ogilvie R: Dosage of theophylline in bronchial asthma. *N Engl J Med* 292:1218–1222, 1975.
*Predicted plasma theophylline concentrations are given as mean values.
†Numbers in parentheses, range.
‡This is an accumulated loading dose. If the patient has previously received a 6-mg/kg load, only the difference or 3 mg/kg should be administered for dose schedule.

ministered over 20 minutes, and the maintenance infusion dose increased to 1.35 mg/kg/hour, which should raise the plasma theophylline concentration into the range of 15 to 20 mg/L. In children, the loading dose is the same, but because there is increased elimination of theophylline in this age group, the maintenance dose is increased (Table 19.3).

The disposition of theophylline is altered in patients with congestive cardiac failure and severe liver disease; the plasma half-life increases as clearance decreases, but the apparent volume of distribution is unchanged. Because the apparent volume of distribution of theophylline is relatively unaffected by factors that affect clearance, the loading dose is essentially unaltered in patients with severe congestive cardiac failure and severe liver disease. However, to prevent toxicity, the rate of maintenance dose infusion must be reduced by one-third of the usual dose in the presence of congestive cardiac failure and reduced by half the usual dose in patients with severe hepatic disease. It is important to monitor therapy by measurement of plasma theophylline concentrations. If the patient has previously received oral theophylline therapy, the usual loading dose may produce toxicity, and the recommended loading dose should be reduced.

Oral theophylline is useful in the chronic treatment of mild to moderate asthma, and dose recommendations are given in Table 19.4.

TOXICITY, PRECAUTIONS, AND CONTRAINDICATIONS

Aminophylline toxicity is largely due to overdose with resultant high plasma concentrations. Aminophylline should be administered via a peripheral vein and not via a central venous catheter, since exposure of the heart to a high bolus drug concentration may result from inadequate distribution. As previously described, aminophylline is optimally effective when serum theophylline concentrations range from 10 to 20 mg/L. The main adverse effects observed with chronic therapy are gastrointestinal, such as anorexia, nausea, vomiting, and abdominal discomfort. In this situation, the plasma theophylline concentration is usually over 20 mg/L. Serious toxicity (seizures, arrhythmias, coma, cardiorespiratory arrest) is usually associated with intravenous therapy and can be prevented by careful administration in conjunction with the monitoring of serum theophylline levels. Treatment of theophylline intoxication includes cessation of the drug and supportive therapy. Anticonvulsant therapy with intravenous diazepam may be required while cardiac arrhythmias may be treated with lidocaine or a cardioselective β-adrenergic blocking agent. (Propranolol may worsen airway obstruction.) The altered dosage

Table 19.4.
Oral Dose Schedule for Aminophylline

Subjects	Oral dose (mg/kg/6 hr)		Plasma Theophylline* (mg/L)	
	Aminophylline	Theophylline	Maximum	Minimum
Children				
Initial	5	4.0	7 (3–12)	2 (1–6)†
Optimal	8	6.4	12 (9–25)	4 (2–10)
Adults				
Initial	3	2.4	7 (4–12)	3 (1–4)
Optimal	6	4.8	14 (10–24)	6 (3–16)

With permission from Piafsky KM, Ogilvie R: Dosage of theophylline in bronchial asthma. *N Engl J Med* 292:1218–1222, 1975.
*Predicted plasma theophylline concentrations are given as mean values.
†Numbers in parentheses, range.

schedules due to age and disease outlined in the previous sections should be followed to prevent the development of toxic plasma theophylline concentrations.

Perioperative administration of aminophylline has been reported to result in arrhythmias during halothane anesthesia, and there is evidence to suggest that levels of theophylline that are safe in the awake patient may be arrhythmogenic when followed by halothane anesthesia in dogs. Isoflurane may be safer than halothane in this situation.

CROMOLYN SODIUM

Cromolyn sodium has no direct bronchodilator, antihistaminic, or antiinflammatory actions but rather inhibits the release of chemical mediators of bronchospasm from the sensitized mast cell (Fig. 19.2). Consequently, it can only be used prophylactically and is of no use in the management of the acute asthmatic attack. It is most effective in young patients with extrinsic allergic asthma and in the prevention of exercise-induced asthma when it should be taken about half an hour before exercise.

Cromolyn sodium is supplied as a dry powder in capsules and is inhaled by the patient using a "Spinhaler." The capsule is punctured by depressing a sleeve on the Spinhaler, and the powder is inhaled with the aid of a propeller inside the device. The usual dose is 20 mg, inhaled 4 times a day. Because airway obstruction may reduce the amount inhaled, the use of a sympathomimetic bronchodilator aerosol prior to cromolyn therapy may allow better access to the bronchi. When administered by a Spinhaler, only about 75% of the dose of cromolyn is delivered, and of that, only 10% reaches the peripheral airways. The remainder is swallowed. No biotransformation is known to occur.

CORTICOSTEROIDS

Although corticosteroids have been used to treat asthma for many years, their exact mode of action is still far from clear. They can effectively reverse bronchospasm due to asthma that is unresponsive to other bronchodilators, and thus they are an important mode of therapy. Steroids probably have multiple actions in reversing asthmatic obstruction; these include reduction of inflammatory mucosal swelling and edema, bronchial smooth muscle relaxation, and direct effects on bronchial vasculature resulting in vasoconstriction and reduced capillary permeability. Steroids appear to have only a small effect on the acute reaction to mast cell mediators and more effectively inhibit the delayed, late inflammatory phase of the response. They may also be useful in restoring the responsiveness of asthmatic patients to sympathomimetic bronchodilators. Unfortunately, with oral therapy the well-recognized side effects of long-term steroid therapy are frequently encountered; details of corticosteroid pharmacology are further described in Chapter 20.

Corticosteroids can be administered orally or preferably by inhaled aerosol for the management of chronic asthma, but should be administered intravenously for the treatment of status asthmaticus. A dose of 3 to 4 mg/kg of hydrocortisone hemisuccinate, intravenously, will achieve plasma concentrations around 100 to 150 μg/100 ml, a level considered to be within the therapeutic range.

Beclomethasone dipropionate is a synthetic steroid which is administered using a metered-dose inhaler. It provides an effective means of delivering steroid to the bronchi with minimal systemic absorption, so that systemic steroid side effects are not a problem at usual doses. Side effects of note include oropharyngeal *Candida* infection and hoarseness at higher doses. Inhaled steroid preparations have been shown to be a major advance in the management of the asthmatic patient, since side effects are relatively uncommon and they have allowed many previously steroid-dependent asthmatic patients to reduce or stop regular oral steroid therapy. However, they still may require increased dosage for exacerbation of disease or surgery.

The usual daily dose of beclomethasone is 0.4 mg (two puffs 4 times daily) and is approximately equivalent in efficacy to 7.5 mg of prednisone orally in treating asthma.

Other steroids that have also been administered by the inhalational route include **triamcinolone, flunisolide,** and **budesonide.**

IPRATROPIUM

Anticholinergic drugs cause bronchodilation by antagonizing the action of acetylcholine at the cholinergic receptor (Table 19.1) and by decreasing mediator release through inhibition of cGMP, as outlined earlier in the chapter. Ipratropium is a derivative of atropine that is used to treat asthma and chronic obstructive airway disease. It is probably most effective in the treatment of chronic obstructive airway disease. The clinical pharmacology of ipratropium bromide is described in detail in Chapter 6, page 120.

BIBLIOGRAPHY

Physiology

Aarons RD, Nies AS, Gerber JG, Molinoff PB: Decreased beta adrenergic receptor density on human lymphocytes after chronic treatment with agonists. *J Pharmacol Exp Ther* 224:1–6, 1983.

Chung KF, Barnes PJ: PAR antagonists. Their potential therapeutic role in asthma. *Drugs* 35:93–103, 1988.

Editorial: Autonomic abnormalities in asthma. *Lancet* 1:1224–1225, 1982.

Goetzl EJ: Asthma: new mediators and old problems. *N Engl J Med* 311:252–253, 1984.

Hardy CC, Robinson C, Tattersfield AE, Holgate ST: The bronchoconstrictor effect of inhaled prostaglandin D_2 in normal and asthmatic men. *N Engl J Med* 311:209–213, 1984.

Holgate ST, Baldwin CJ, Tattersfield AE: β-Adrenergic agonist resistance in normal human airways. *Lancet* 2:375–377, 1977.

β-Receptor Agonists

Brogden RN, Speight TM, Avery GS: Terbutaline. *Drugs* 6:324–332, 1973.

Heel RC, Brogden RN, Speight TM, Avery GS: Fenoterol: a review of its pharmacological properties and therapeutic efficacy in asthma. *Drugs* 15:3–32, 1978.

Manders WT, Vatner SF, Braunwald E: Cardioselective beta adrenergic stimulation with prenalterol in the conscious dog. *J Pharmacol Exp Ther* 215:266–270, 1980.

Pinder RM, Brogden RN, Speight TM, Avery GS: Rimiterol: a review of its pharmacological properties and therapeutic efficacy in asthma. *Drugs* 14:81–104, 1977.

Richards DM, Brogden RN: Pirbuterol. A preliminary review of its pharmacological properties and therapeutic efficacy in reversible bronchospastic disease. *Drugs* 30:6–21, 1985.

Thiagarajah S, Grynsztejn M, Lear E, Azar I: Ventricular arrhythmias after terbutaline administration to patients anesthetized with halothane. *Anesth Analg* 65:417–418, 1986.

Wolfe JD, Yamato M, Biedermann AA, Chu TJ: Comparison of the acute cardiopulmonary effects of oral albuterol, metaproterenol, and terbutaline in asthmatics. *JAMA* 253:2068–2072, 1985.

Methylxanthines

Aitken ML, Martin TR: Life-threatening theophylline toxicity is not predictable by serum levels. *Chest* 91:10–14, 1987.

Berger JM, Stirt JA, Sullivan SF: Enflurane, halothane, and aminophylline—uptake and pharmacokinetics. *Anesth Analg* 62:733–737, 1983.

Cochrane GM: Slow release theophyllines and chronic bronchitis. *Br Med J* 289:1643–1644, 1984.

Haley TJ: Metabolism and pharmacokinetics of theophylline in human neonates, children, and adults. *Drug Metab Rev* 14:295–335, 1983.

Hendeles L, Iafrate RP, Weinberger M: A clinical and pharmacokinetic basis for the selection and use of slow release theophylline products. *Clin Pharmacokinet* 9:95–135, 1984.

Hendeles L, Weinberger M, Johnson G: Monitoring serum theophylline levels. *Clin Pharmacokinet* 3:294–312, 1978.

Hirshman CA, Krieger W, Littlejohn G, Lee R, Julien R: Ketamine-aminophylline-induced decrease in seizure threshold. *Anesthesiology* 56:464–467, 1982.

Jonkman JHG, Upton RA: Pharmacokinetic drug interactions with theophylline. *Clin Pharmacokinet* 9:309–334, 1984.

Lesko LJ, Tabor KJ, Johnson BF: Theophylline serum protein binding in obstructive airways disease. *Clin Pharmacol Ther* 29:776–781, 1981.

Ogilvie RI: Clinical pharmacokinetics of theophylline. *Clin Pharmacokinet* 3:267–293, 1978.

Piafsky KM, Ogilvie RI: Dosage of theophylline in bronchial asthma. *N Engl J Med* 292:1218–1222, 1975.

Prokocimer PG, Nicholls E, Gaba DM, Maze M: Epinephrine arrhythmogenicity is enhanced by acute, but not chronic, aminophylline administration during halothane anesthesia in dogs. *Anesthesiology* 65:13–18, 1986.

Stirt JA, Berger JM, Ricker SM, Sullivan SF: Aminophylline pharmacokinetics and cardiorespiratory effects during halothane anesthesia in experimental animals. *Anesth Analg* 59:186–191, 1980.

Stirt JA, Berger JM, Ricker SM, Sullivan SF: Arrhythmogenic effects of aminophylline during halothane anesthesia in experimental animals. *Anesth Analg* 59:410–416, 1980.

Stirt JA, Berger JM, Roe SD, Eicker SM, Sullivan SF: Halothane-induced cardiac arrhythmias following administration of aminophylline in experimental animals. *Anesth Analg* 60:517–520, 1981.

Stirt JA, Berger JM, Roe SD, Ricker SM, Sullivan SF: Safety of enflurane following administration of aminophylline in experimental animals. *Anesth Analg* 60:871–873, 1981.

Stirt JA, Berger JM, Roe SD, Ricker SM, Sullivan SF: Cardiovascular effects of ketamine following administration of aminophylline in dogs. *Anesth Analg* 61:685–688, 1982.

Stirt JA, Berger JM, Sullivan SF: Lack of arrhythmogenicity of isoflurane following administration of aminophylline in dogs. *Anesth Analg* 62:568–571, 1983.

Stirt JA, Sullivan SF: Aminophylline: review article. *Anesth Analg* 60:587–602, 1981.

Tattersfield AE: Airway pharmacology. *Br J Anaesth* 51:681–691, 1979.

Tserng KY, King KC, Takieddine FN: Theophylline metabolism in premature infants. *Clin Pharmacol Ther* 29:594–600, 1981.

Cromolyn

Brogden RN, Speight TM, Avery GS: Sodium cromoglycate (cromolyn sodium). *Drugs* 7:164–282, 1974.

Gonzalez JP, Brogden RN: Nedocromil sodium. A preliminary review of its pharmacodynamic and pharmacokinetic properties, and therapeutic efficacy in the treatment of reversible obstructive airways disease. *Drugs* 34:560–577, 1987.

Corticosteroids

Brogden RN, Pinder RM, Sawyer PR, Speight TM, Avery GS: Beclomethasone dipropionate inhaler. *Drugs* 10:166–210, 1975.

Editorial: Steroids for bronchitic exacerbations? *Lancet* 1:84, 1981.

Smith MJ: The place of high-dose inhaled corticosteroids in asthma therapy. *Drugs* 33:423–429, 1987.

General

Banner AS, Sunderrajan EV, Agarwal MK, Addington WW: Arrhythmogenic effects of orally administered bronchodilators. *Arch Intern Med* 139:434–437, 1979.

Barnes PJ: A logical and pharmacological approach to asthma therapy. *N Engl J Med* in press, 1989.

Cole P: Drug-induced lung disease. *Drugs* 13:422–444, 1977.

Editorial: Beclomethasone dipropionate aerosol in asthma. *Lancet* 2:1239–1240, 1972.

Greenberger PA, Patterson R: Management of asthma during pregnancy. *N Engl J Med* 312:897–902, 1985.

Kingston HGG, Hirshman CA: Perioperative management of the patient with asthma. *Anesth Analg* 63:844–855, 1984.

Mawhinney H, Spector SL: Optimum management of asthma in pregnancy. *Drugs* 32:178–187, 1986.

Morr-Strathmann U, Morr H: Influence of inhalational anaesthetics on bronchomotor tone—animal experiments on vago-vagal reflex bronchoconstriction. *Acta Anaesth Scand Suppl* 71:39–42, 1979.

Newhouse MT, Dolovich MB: Control of asthma by aerosols. *N Engl J Med* 315:870–874, 1986.

Rodentsein D, DeCoster A, Gazzaniga A: Pharmacokinetics of oral acetylcysteine: absorption, binding, and metabolism in patients with respiratory disorders. *Clin Pharmacokinet* 3:247–254, 1978.

Webb-Johnson DC, Andrews JL: Bronchodilator therapy (first of two parts). *N Engl J Med* 297:476–482, 1977.

Webb-Johnson DC, Andrews JL: Bronchodilator therapy (second of two parts). *N Engl J Med* 297:758–763, 1977

20

Drugs and the Endocrine System

JOHN FEELY

This chapter is primarily concerned with the pharmacology of agents used to treat hypo- or hyper- function of the endocrine organs. Drug therapy of endocrine disorders during the perioperative period is emphasized.

Hormones, in general, react with two types of receptors. Steroid hormones (sex, adrenocorticoid) and thyroid hormones penetrate the cell and form a complex with intracellular proteins such as those in the cell nucleus which are the intracellular receptors. The other class of receptors is located within the plasma membrane at the cell surface. These membrane receptors are large glycoproteins which bind with a high affinity for polypeptide and adrenergic hormones. The hormone receptor complex may then activate, through guanine nucleotides, cyclic AMP which then, in turn, acts as a second messenger of hormone action within the cell (see Chapter 3).

DIABETES MELLITUS

The objectives of the management of the diabetic patient are physiological control of metabolism and the prevention of diabetic complications. Central to good diabetic control is diet which, in combination with insulin (insulin-dependent, type I diabetics) or with oral hypoglycemic agents (insulin-independent, or type II, usually maturity onset diabetics), forms the basis of all therapy. The effectiveness of diabetic control can be monitored by blood glucose measurements (fasting and postprandial) in addition to urine tests. It is important to know the threshold at which glycosuria occurs in an individual patient if urinalysis is to be used as a guide in therapy. The renal threshold is higher in the elderly long-standing diabetic and in those with renal disease.

Rapid measurement of blood glucose using impregnated strips and pinprick blood samples allows many patients to make appropriate adjustments to insulin therapy and is also useful to the anesthesiologist during the perioperative period. The level of glycosylated hemoglobins provides an index of the degree of hyper-

glycemia present during the previous weeks and, thus, a retrospective index of diabetic control. A glycosylated hemoglobin fraction of less than 8% indicates acceptable control, while greater than 10% indicates poor control.

Insulin

The introduction of insulin in 1922 by Banting and Best revolutionized the treatment of diabetes. In humans, the daily insulin output by the pancreatic β-cell is 30 to 40 units (comprised of a basal output of 1 unit per hour with surges or increases in response to food) which represents about a quarter of the total pancreatic insulin content. Insulin is a polypeptide hormone with two peptide chains A and B of 21 and 30 amino acids, respectively, joined by two disulfide bridges. Secreted as proinsulin, the more active insulin portion is cleaved in the liver. Some patients require more than 40 units/day of insulin to control their diabetes, suggesting that in such patients a reduction in the number or function of receptor sites for insulin on the surface of target cells or, less commonly the development of insulin antibodies, has occurred. Bovine insulin has three and the porcine has one amino acid different from human insulin. Recent improvements in fractionation techniques have greatly increased the purity of insulin preparations, reducing contaminating proteins to less than 2%. Highly purified insulin such as monocomponent insulin (>99% pure) is particularly useful in patients with insulin allergy or lipodystrophy (either hypertrophy or atrophy of subcutaneous tissues at the site of injection).

Human insulin (i.e., insulin identical in chemical structure to human pancreatic insulin) can be produced either by enzymatic modification of porcine insulin or by recombinant DNA technology. It is less antigenic than other insulins and is frequently used today. In clinical use, the therapeutic efficacy of human insulin is very similar to that of porcine insulin. Although patients whose diabetes is well controlled with purified porcine insulin do not necessarily require to be changed to human insulin, human insulin is now the insulin of "first choice" for newly diagnosed diabetics requiring insulin.

EFFECTS OF INSULIN

1. *Reduction in blood glucose* due to increased glucose uptake and metabolism in the periphery and reduced hepatic output of glucose.
2. *Reduction in gluconeogenesis.*
3. *Promotion of the formation of protein from amino acids.*
4. *Promotion of glycogen synthesis.*

Insulin deficiency allows the blood glucose to rise above the renal threshold, and the resultant glycosuria produces an osmotic diuresis with dehydration and sodium and potassium depletion. Insulin deficiency encourages the use of fat as an alternate energy source. The production of ketones causes acidosis and contributes to diabetic coma.

USE OF INSULIN

In addition to its use in insulin-dependent diabetics (type I, who usually have circulating antibodies to islet cells), insulin is necessary for the mild diabetic during periods of stress. The release of insulin antagonists (cortisol, growth hormone, catecholamines) during surgery may be sufficient to lead to a marked deterioration in glucose homeostasis in the previously well-controlled subject. Fre-

quent injections of rapid acting insulin are required for good physiological control. Intermediate or long-acting insulins (produced by changing the pH of insulin and forming larger crystals or by the addition of zinc or protamine to retard absorption) will, although practically more attractive, rarely control the postprandial peak in glucose. Table 20.1 describes the commonly used insulins. Combinations of short and longer acting insulin given once or twice daily may provide good control. It must be stressed that the time course of activity varies considerably from patient to patient and, in general, the duration of action is prolonged as dosage is increased. Only insulins with rapid action should be used to control diabetes during stress. Their prompt onset of action and short duration of effect allow rapid control of hyperglycemia without the risk of prolonged hypoglycemia. In nearly all Western countries the 100-U/ml strength for insulin is now in use.

Oral Hypoglycemic Agents

Oral hypoglycemic drugs are of two kinds, sulfonamide derivatives (sulfonylureas) and guanidine derivatives (biguanides). The mechanism of action of the two major groups (sulfonylureas and biguanides) is different. Sulfonylureas initially stimulate insulin release by the

Table 20.1.
Approximate Time Course (Hours) of Activity of Commonly Used Insulin Preparations after Subcutaneous or Intramuscular Administration

Insulin preparations	Onset	Peak effect	Duration
Rapid action			
Regular (soluble)			
Neutral	0.25	2–5	5–8
Intermediate action			
Semilente (zinc suspension)	1–2	3–8	10–20
Isophane (NPH)			
Lente—Insulin zinc suspension	2–3	6–14	18–28
Prolonged action			
Ultralente—extended insulin			
zinc suspension			
PZI—protamine zinc insulin	4–5	12–24	24–36
suspension			

pancreatic β-cells and, thus, some endogenous insulin secretion is required for their efficacy. Later, however, glucose continues to fall without any change in insulin levels. This further fall in glucose may result from an improved sensitivity to insulin. Biguanides increase the peripheral uptake of glucose and, thus, also require endogenous or exogenous insulin for activity. Additional suggested mechanisms for the biguanides include decreased glucose absorption and anorexia. Biguanides also inhibit lactate catabolism and may, particularly in patients with renal insufficiency (common in diabetics), give rise to lactic acidosis.

Sulfonylureas

In general, the sulfonylureas are well absorbed from the gastrointestinal tract. The most important difference among this group of drugs lies in their duration of action, relative potency, and elimination half-life (Table 20.2). Their high degree of plasma protein binding to albumin (Table 20.2) makes them susceptible to displacement by other drugs and results in a small volume of distribution (0.1 to 0.3 L/kg). Displacement interactions are not usually seen with second generation sulfonylureas, such as glibenclamide. Because of extensive hepatic metabolism, the hypoglycemic action of some of these drugs may be enhanced in patients with liver disease. The metabolism of tolbutamide exhibits wide interindividual variability in metabolism. This wide interindividual variability led to the suggestion that the ability to metabolize tolbutamide might be bimodally distributed in the population similar to that seen with debrisoquine (see Chapter 2). However, more detailed studies have

Table 20.2.
Oral Hypoglycemic Agents

Dosage range (per day)	Relative potency	Plasma half-life (hr) (effect)	Route of elimination	Comments
Sulfonylureas				
Tolbutamide, 0.5–2.0 g	1	4–10 (6–10)*	Hepatic	Marked interindividual differences in clearance
Acetohexamide, 0.5–1.5 g	2.5	3–11 (10–16)	Hepatic	Forms active metabolite
Chlorpropamide, 100–500 mg	6	24–42 (20–60)	Mainly renal, some hepatic	Avoid in elderly, takes 1 to 2 weeks to reach steady state
Tolazamide, 100–1000 mg	5	12–24	Hepatic	Active metabolite
Glyburide (Glibenclamide), 5–15 mg	150	10–16 (10–15)	Hepatic	Some biliary excretion
Glipizide, 2.5–30 mg	100	3–7 (12–24)	Hepatic	May cause hypoglycemia
Biguanides				
Metformin, 0.5–2.0 g		1–2 (5–6)	Renal excretion of unchanged drug	Avoid in renal and cardiac disease

*,numbers in parentheses, effect in hours.

demonstrated a wide interindividual scatter but no suggestion of bimodality. Similarly the elimination of these drugs may be subject to changes due to hepatic enzyme induction or inhibition by other agents (Table 20.3). A considerable (20%) fraction of chlorpropamide is excreted unchanged in the urine and, therefore, the half-life is prolonged in patients with renal disease. Because of the long plasma and biological half-life of chlorpropamide, it may take some weeks after starting therapy (four drug half-lives) to approximate steady state and similarly many days for its effects to wear off when therapy is stopped. Thus, when hypoglycemia occurs, careful monitoring of blood sugar and dextrose administration for a prolonged period after cessation of therapy is required. The newer sulfonylureas (second generation) such as glibenclamide and glipizide are somewhat more potent than chlorpropamide with a shorter half-life. However, like chlorpropamide they are usually effective when given once daily, whereas tolbuta-mide requires twice daily administration.

Side effects consist of gastrointestinal upsets, skin rashes, muscle weakness, and unpleasant taste. Cholestatic jaundice and blood disorders are rare. Alcohol intolerance, characterized by facial flush, lightheadedness, and breathlessness (resembling the disulfiram-antabuse reaction), is occasionally seen with chlorpropamide and is usually avoided by the use of a second generation sulfonylurea. Inappropriate antidiuretic hormone activity leading to hyponatremia and water intoxication has also been reported following sulfonylurea administration.

DIABETIC COMA

Our inability to mimic true physiological blood sugar control (except with an "artificial pancreas" in which blood glucose is continuously monitored and the rate of insulin infusion is calculated and then administered via a pump and to a lesser extent with continuous subcuta-

Table 20.3.
Clinically Important Endocrine Drug Interactions

Endocrine drug	Mechanism	Interaction with and consequence
Sulfonylureas	Displaced from binding sites	Aspirin, phenylbutazone, sulfonamide—enhanced hypoglycemic effect
	Inhibition of metabolism	Chloramphenicol, dicoumarol, anticoagulants—enhanced hypoglycemia effect
Insulin	Antagonism	Corticosteroids, oral contraceptives, thiazide, and loop diuretics
	Pharmacodynamic	β-Blockers—mask signs and may prolong hypoglycemia
Thyroxine	Decreased absorption	Cholestyramine
Corticosteroids (hydrocortisone, dexamethasone, prednisolone)	Increased metabolism	Phenytoin, phenobarbital rifampin—decreased efficacy of steroids
Oral contraceptives	Increased metabolism, decreased absorption	Rifampin, anticonvulsants Ampicillin—pregnancy
Diethylstilbestrol	Decreased plasma cholinesterase	Succinylcholine—prolongs paralysis

neous insulin infusions) becomes most obvious in the perioperative setting when marked fluctuations in both glucose intake and elevated counterregulatory and stress hormone levels make patients susceptible both to hypo- and hyperglycemia. Excessive insulin intake in the face of reduced demands and reduced carbohydrate intake (e.g., fasting) may result in *hypoglycemia*. The onset is usually sudden. The clinical diagnosis is confirmed by biochemical evidence of hypoglycemia—a bedside dextrostix with a blood sugar (taken simultaneously for subsequent accurate quantitation of hypoglycemia). Treatment with parenteral glucose usually quickly restores the patient to consciousness.

Hyperglycemic coma may be precipitated by surgery or infection and is insidious in onset.

During the last decade, the approach to the management of diabetic ketoacidosis has changed considerably. For a review of studies comparing the conventional to the new low-dose methods, the reader is referred to Kitabichi *et al.* (1979). The older method employed a high (>50 U) insulin dosage initially, usually intravenously, followed by similar doses. Available evidence now suggests that a low loading dose (10 U) followed by regular low dose (5 to 10 U/hour or 0.1 U/kg/hour intravenously) gives a more reliable and practical method of treatment. Thus, diabetic ketoacidosis is now often treated with relatively small dose of continuous intravenous infusions of insulin, and furthermore is less likely to be associated with the common complications of high-dose therapy, hypoglycemia, and hypokalemia. The initial response in terms of fall in blood sugar may not be as marked with the low-dose approach; however, the use of the intravenous route appears to reduce the number of patients who are initially slow to respond. As the half-life of intravenous insulin is in the region of 3 to 5 minutes, a continuous infusion of insulin is also both rational and effective. One factor that contributes greatly to increasing the efficacy and, thus, facilitating the use of the low-dose technique is adequate hydration. Fluid deficits of up

to 6 L are common. The importance of prompt fluid and electrolyte (sodium and potassium) replacement cannot be overemphasized. Isotonic saline is the fluid of choice, and 1 L may be given in the first hour followed by another 1 L over the subsequent 2 hours. If the patient is hyperosmolar or serum sodium exceeds 155 mEq/L, then hypotonic (1/2 normal saline or even 5% dextrose) solutions are preferred in order to avoid cerebral edema. Care should be exercised, and the central venous pressure (CVP) should be monitored in patients with renal or cardiovascular impairment to avoid overhydration. Rehydration alone will commonly lead to a reduction in blood sugar. The intracellular influx of potassium accompanied by volume expansion will result in a prompt and potentially lethal fall in serum potassium. Potassium supplements may wrongly be omitted because the initial serum potassium may be raised despite a marked intracellular deficit. Potassium should be given from the outset (provided it is not elevated above 5.5 mEq/L) or when the potassium falls to within the normal range. Alkali therapy has long been used to correct the metabolic acidosis. Recent evidence, however, suggests that rapid correction of acidosis with bicarbonate may initially raise PCO_2 which will exaggerate the intracellular acidosis in the central nervous system before the bicarbonate enters the brain. Alkali therapy also aggravates hypokalemia and may reduce the oxygen-carrying capacity of blood. Many clinicians, therefore, restrict its use to patients with a pH < 7.1. Antibiotics are not routinely indicated. Phosphate replacement therapy has also been recommended. Following correction of diabetic ketosis, patients may conveniently be managed by an insulin sliding scale (discussed later in this chapter), while their dosage requirements are being determined.

Nonketotic coma in the absence of ketonuria or ketonemia occurs in some patients, particularly the elderly, and those with renal disease. Such patients are severely dehydrated and, therefore, develop hyperosmolar coma (plasma osmolality >350 mOsm/L) with a very high blood glucose.

MANAGEMENT OF THE DIABETIC UNDERGOING SURGERY

A confusing variety of regimens exist for the management of the diabetic patient during the perioperative period. It has been traditional in the past to maintain moderate hyperglycemia during surgery to minimize the occurrence of hypoglycemia, since hypoglycemia is difficult to recognize during anesthesia. However, perioperative hyperglycemia may lead to the development of diabetic ketoacidosis and hyperosmolar, hyperglycemic nonketotic coma. The cumulative consequences of starvation, stress hormone release, and surgical trauma in a patient who is already deficient in one of the major adaptive metabolic hormones are not always easy to predict. It is not surprising that regimens advocated for the maangement of the diabetic in the perioperative period vary widely, ranging from omission of all antidiabetic therapy to combined insulin/glucose infusions with frequent monitoring of blood sugar.

For elective surgery, diabetics should be admitted prior to surgery to allow stable control of their disease. Ideally physiological control should be achieved avoiding postprandial hyperglycemia (> 160 mg/100 ml) or a tendency to fasting hypoglycemia (<60 mg/100ml). It is also important that secondary conditions such as dehydration and infection are adequately managed prior to surgery.

Insulin-independent Diabetics

Minor surgery in well-controlled subjects receiving oral hypoglycemic agents who will be able to recommence eating on the day of surgery often requires only careful monitoring of the blood glucose pre- and postoperatively. A change from a long-acting sulfonylurea to a short-acting one may be preferable. For major surgery in well-controlled subjects, the morning dose of oral hypoglycemic should be omitted. Although many of these patients can undergo major surgery without any changes in treatment, there are situations when diabetic control with insulin may be required, such as intercurrent surgical infection, prolonged surgery, and inability to resume a normal regimen in the immediate postoperative period. All poorly controlled patients should first be stabilized on insulin.

Insulin-dependent Diabetics

Suggested protocols for the management of insulin-dependent diabetics during surgery are of three types:

1. Preoperative insulin is omitted and insulin is given intra- and/or postoperatively depending on blood glucose concentrations;
2. A partial dose of long-acting insulin is given in the preoperative period;
3. Intravenous regular insulin is given to titrate the blood glucose, either as a bolus or continuous intravenous infusion.

Many anesthesiologists prefer not to use arbitrary insulin programs but rather maintain the blood glucose level within a tight range of perhaps 100 to 200 mg/dl by administering single intravenous injections of regular insulin (5 to 7 U) titrated to frequent blood glucose estimations.

Continuous glucose-insulin-potassium infusion for the management of insulin-dependent diabetic patients, proposed by Alberti in 1979, has been adopted by many anesthesiologists for major surgery. Patients ideally should be stabilized in the hospital before surgery. This commonly requires twice daily insulin. Patients on long-acting insulins undergoing *major* surgery where normal oral feeding will not be possible should be changed to rapid acting insulin prior to surgery to ensure adequate control and avoid hypoglycemia. Where possible, surgery should be scheduled for early in the day, i.e., the morning. Under the Alberti regimen, patients receive a continuous infusion consisting of 500 ml of 10% dextrose (with 10 mEq of potassium chloride) to which 10 units of regular insulin have been added at a rate of 100 ml/hour, delivering 2 U insulin, 2 mEq of KCl, and 10 g of glucose hourly. The morning dose of insulin is omitted, no breakfast is given, blood glucose and potassium are checked, and the infusion is started 30 minutes before surgery and continued until the first postoperative meal. Thereafter, postoperative diabetic control is attained with thrice daily short-acting insulin. The blood glucose is frequently checked intraoperatively (every 15 minutes) using reagent strips and/or a reflectance meter, and appropriate adjustments of the infusion rate are made. Blood glucose estimations are also frequently carried out to confirm the adequacy of therapy.

Postoperatively, glucose and potassium levels should be checked every 4 and 8 hours, respectively. Once the patient resumes normal feeding, the normal daily insulin dose is given as rapid acting insulin with one-third of the daily dose being given 3 times a day for 2 to 3 days, after which the patient can usually be changed over to his or her normal regimen.

It is important to recognize that no studies have shown that long-term outcome is changed with the glucose-insulin intravenous infusion approach as compared to more traditional insulin regimens (e.g., 50 to 75% of the usual morning dose of insulin accompanied by 25 g of glucose intravenously), although control of plasma glucose and other metabolic indices, e.g., lactate, nonesterified fatty acids, is better at 4 hours after the operation in patients receiving the glucose-insulin-potassium infusion. Some workers using intravenous infusion insulin regimens have reported problems with hypoglycemia, and frequent blood glucose estimations should be carried out.

Many other regimens have been successfully used, e.g., giving insulin, subcutaneously, immediately before and after operation (depending on the blood glucose) with an infusion of 5% dextrose before and during surgery; for example, the following protocol may be used:

1. Nothing by mouth after midnight;
2. At 6:00 AM on the day of surgery an intravenous infusion of 5% dextrose is commenced at a rate of 100 ml/hour/70 kg after obtaining a blood sample for estimation of blood glucose;
3. After the intravenous infusion has been commenced, one-third to one-half of the patient's daily morning dose of insulin is given subcutaneously;
4. The intravenous infusion is continued up to and during surgery to prevent the development of hypoglycemia.

Postoperatively, patients can be managed by a sliding scale of insulin dosage depending on urinalysis and blood glucose estimations (Table 20.4). This sliding scale may also be used in poorly controlled diabetics and, in addition, during certain situations such as emergency surgery, myocardial infarction, and infection. It should be noted that patients with sepsis or receiving steroids have a higher insulin requirement. Irrespective of which regimen is used, close monitoring of blood glucose will prevent a major deviation from the desired range (90 to 180 mg/100 ml).

Table 20.4.
An Example of a Sliding Scale of Insulin Dosage

Urinary glucose* (%)	Soluble insulin dosage (IU s.c.)	Blood glucose (mg/100 ml)	Soluble insulin dosage (IU s.c.)
Negative	4	<60	Omit
½	8	60—90	4–6
1	12	90–180	8–10
1½	16	180–300	12–16
2 or >	20	>300	20

*Empty bladder and take urine sample 30 minutes later. Add 8 units of insulin for ketonuria.

ADRENAL HORMONES

Adrenal Cortex and Adrenal Steroids

The adrenal cortex produces the hormones hydrocortisone (cortisol) and aldosterone. Few hormones or drugs have produced such dramatic beneficial and adverse effects as the adrenal steroids. In the late 1940s, synthetic steroids were shown to produce a dramatic symptomatic response in patients with rheumatoid arthritis. Since that time, the list of indications has become legion. In addition to replacement therapy, steroids are used to suppress inflammation (in collagen disorders) and as immunosuppressants in autoimmune, neoplastic, and allergic disorders. These properties are associated with the glucocorticoid action of cortisol and not with mineralocorticoid (aldosterone) or adrenal adrogen activity. Numerous steroids have been synthesized over the years with varying glucocorticoid and mineralocorticoid activity (Table 20.5).

The secretion of cortisol is controlled by the pituitary secretion of adrenocorticotrophin (ACTH). This, in turn, is regulated by the hypothalamic corticotrophin releasing hormone which is influenced by negative feedback from circulating cortisol, higher centers, stress, and a di-

urnal rhythm. Cortisol may also feedback directly on the pituitary. Exogenous corticosteroids initially suppress the normal diurnal rhythm (highest cortisol in the morning and lowest at midnight) before suppressing the stress-associated rise in ACTH. In general, cortisol is a catabolic hormone, and when given in pharmacological doses (greater than the daily production of 25 mg), the side effects are an extension of its physiological effects.

Cortisol increases gluconeogenesis in part by binding to a cellular cytoplasmic receptor, promoting the transcription of messenger RNA for certain enzymes. It reduces peripheral glucose utilization, and glycosuria may occur; latent diabetes may become overt. Negative nitrogen balance is produced by a reduced conversion of amino acids to protein with increased catabolism. Growth retardation in children, osteoporosis, skin atrophy, and increased capillary fragility result. This may lead to bruising, striae, delayed wound, and possibly delayed peptic ulcer healing. The change in fat distribution, to the trunk face and shoulders, coupled with the wasting of peripheral muscles gives the characteristic appearance of glucocorticoid excess. The mineralocorticoid action of cortisol will cause sodium retention and contribute to the development of hypertension. Depression or eu-

Table No. 20.5.
Pharmacology of Commonly Used Steroids

Drug	Approximate potency		Equivalent dosage for antiinflammatory (glucocorticoid) effect (mg)	Biological half-life of effects (hr)	Daily dose producting supression of hypothalamic-pituitary-adrenal axis (mg)
	Glucocorticoid	Mineralocorticoid			
Cortisol (hydrocortisone)	1	1	20	8–12	20–30
Cortisone	0.8	0.8	25	8–12	25–35
Prednisolone (prednisone)	4	0.8	5	12–36	7.5–10
Triamcinolone	5	0	4	12–36	6–10
Dexamethasone (Betamethasone)	25	0	0.8	36–54	1–1.5
Aldosterone	0.1	400			
Fludrocortisone	10	300			

phoria may also cocur in patients receiving pharmacological doses of corticosteroids. However, more important in terms of the considerable mortality associated with the use of these drugs, is the suppression of the inflammatory response and of the hypothalamic-pituitary-adrenal axis. Cortisol also appears to be essential for maintaining a normal circulation in response to shock. The increased permeability of capillary endothelium leading to exudation of inflammatory cells and the in vivo chemotaxis of these cells to the site of inflammation is inhibited by corticosteroids. Thymus dependent (T)-lymphocytes, which subserve the function of cell-mediated immunity, but not antibody-producing lymphocytes, are suppressed by cortisol. This is of potential advantage in suppressing the rejection of transplanted organs. On the other hand, impairment of cellular immunity predisposes to infections caused by intracellular organisms such as viruses, fungi (*Monilia, Histoplasma, Cryptococcus*), and protozoa (*Pneumocystis carinii* and toxoplasmosis). Dormant tuberculosis may also be activated.

Suppression of the hypothalamic-pituitary-adrenal axis and adrenal cortical atrophy may occur when the dose of exogenous steroid exceeds physiological levels. This is more likely with chronic therapy and where dosage does not mimic the circadian rhythm. Alternate day therapy produces less suppression of the axis. Suppression of the axis may persist for up to 1 year following a course of steroids. The period of suppression may be considerably less after a short course of high-dose steroids. To determine the degree of suppression, the adrenal response to ACTH or, better, the response of the entire axis to hypoglycemia should be tested. Where this is inappropriate or doubt exists, it is safer to give steroids during the period of stress. As there is often difficulty in defining the "end" of the stress situation, a gradual withdrawal over 5 to 7 days is more appropriate than an abrupt cessation of therapy. In this way, one may more easily separate a deterioration of the patient's condition from

steroid withdrawal. Steroid cover is, therefore, required for patients on maintenance therapy (whose axis has lost the ability to respond with increased endogenous output) and in those who have received a course of steroids in pharmacological doses in the previous year and have not been shown to have a normal axis. Cover is given during intercurrent illness or stress such as infection or trauma.

ANESTHESIA AND ADRENAL CORTICOSTEROIDS

The first postoperative death due to adrenocortical suppression following steroid therapy was reported in 1952. Suppression of the hypothalamic-pituitary-adrenal axis following cessation of steroid therapy may occur for as long as 9 months in some individuals, so that stress, including anesthesia and surgery, fails to elicit a normal increase in adrenocortical output. Perioperative steroid supplementation is therefore required for patients who have received oral corticosteroid therapy during the year prior to surgery and do not have the ability to respond to stress with a rise in plasma cortisol. However, the administration of steroid cover in patients who do have an intact hypothalamic-pituitary-adrenal axis is undesirable since perioperative steroid treatment itself has side effects such as increased susceptibility to infection, delayed wound healing, hypertension, venous thrombosis, and electrolyte imbalance. Unfortuantely, it is not possible to recognize on clinical grounds which patients receiving long-term steroid therapy have adrenocortical insufficiency and therefore require perioperative steroid supplementation. Ideally, the use of the insulin hypoglycemia test to assess the integrity of the hypothalamic-pituitary-adrenal axis would allow the withholding of unnecessary steroids where the test is positive, since the patient has been shown to respond to stress with increased endogenous output.

Since in most patients the adrenal "stress" responsiveness returns to normal very rapidly after cessation of steroid therapy, many anesthesiologists now accept that routine steroid supplement is unnecessary more than 2 months following cessation of therapy. For patients currently receiving corticosteroid therapy, cover is probably required.

A suitable regimen for steroid supplementation in the perioperative period is:

Preoperatively: hydrocortisone, 100 mg intramuscularly 1 hour before surgery, usually with premedication.

Intraoperatively: hydrocortisone, 100 mg intravenously at induction of anesthesia, and repeated if required during prolonged surgery.

Postoperatively: hydrocortisone, 100 mg intramuscularly every 6 hours for 72 hours. Provided the patient can take medication orally, this can be followed by return to maintenance therapy.

For minor surgery and dental extractions, hydrocortisone, 100 mg orally approximately 2 hours before and 4 hours following surgery, should provide adequate cover. For emergency surgery or where a patient has not been controlled preoperatively, the dosage regimen above should be doubled and, in addition, a saline and glucose infusion should be given with central venous pressure monitoring.

A number of drugs—mitolane (o,p'-DDD), metyrapone, aminoglutamide, and the antifungal ketoconozole—inhibit steroid production and are sometimes used in inoperable adrenal carcinoma or in Cushing's syndrome preoperatively to reduce steroid levels.

PHARMACOKINETICS OF SYNTHETIC STEROIDS

Synthetic steroids are rapidly absorbed, although the extent of absorption of prednisolone shows wide intersubject variation. They are metabolized in the liver and the metabolites are then excreted renally. The plasma half-life (e.g., cortisol, 90 minutes; prednisolone, 2 to 3.5 hours, and prednisone, 3.5 to 4.0 hours) does not, however, reflect the biological half-life of effect (Table 20.5). Cortisone and prednisone are converted in the liver to their active metabolites, cortisol and prednisolone. Only in severe liver disease does the conversion of cortisone and prednisone to their active metabolites appear to be impaired. Liver disease prolongs prednisolone half-life, while hepatic enzyme-inducing agents reduce the half-life of both cortisol and prednisolone. In the blood, these drugs are approximately 95% bound (to transcortin, a high-affinity, low-capacity globulin, and to albumin), leaving 5% free for pharmacological effect. In patients with liver disease and/or the nephrotic syndrome, the concentration of these binding proteins may be reduced, resulting in higher free concentrations. In patients with these disorders, the side effects of steroids are more severe at "normal dosages"; therefore, dosage may require to be reduced.

Prednisolone exhibits dose-dependent kinetics (see Chapter 1), possibly due to nonlinear binding of the drug to plasma proteins. Increased prednisolone dosage will increase both the volume of distribution and clearance due to the increase in free fraction. The metabolism of prednisolone also appears to be age dependent with a reduced half-life in children.

SUBSTITUTION THERAPY WITH STEROIDS

Cortisol given in divided doses (e.g., 20 mg AM, 10 mg PM) is the preferred agent in chronic adrenal insufficiency because of its mineralocorticoid activity. Most patients will require additional therapy with a mineralocorticoid such as fludrocortisone (0.1 to 0.2 mg/day) to maintain normotension and electrolyte homeostasis. Patients should be advised to double the cortisol dosage during stress or infection and seek parenteral therapy if this is not feasible because of vomiting.

Acute adrenal insufficiency (Addisonian crisis) requires prompt treatment to correct the marked dehydration, hypotension, hyponatremia, and hypoglycemia. Hydrocortisone (100 mg), hemisuccinate, or hydrocortisone sodium phosphate intravenously should be followed by another 100 mg in a liter of normal saline over 2 hours with a further 100 mg every 8 hours. In the transition from intravenous to oral therapy, intramuscular dosage, 25 mg every 6 hours, may be employed. Fluid replacement will be determined by the degree of dehydration, central venous pressure, and response to therapy.

PHARMACOLOGICAL USES OF STEROIDS

As outlined earlier, the lowest therapeutically effective dose for the shortest time should be used to avoid the pharmacological sequellae of iatrogenic Cushing's syndrome. Unfortunately, many inflammatory disorders require higher doses initially (e.g., prednisolone, 60 mg/day). If the maintenance dose can be kept at or below prednisolone, 7.5 mg, or hydrocortisone, 30 mg, daily, few problems will be encountered. In emergency situations such as shock, cardiogenic shock, or status asthmaticus, very high doses of steroids (2 to 3 g of hydrocortisone/day) have been used, but there is no good evidence to justify the use of high-dose steroids in shock. High-dose dexamethasone is also used to reduce cerebral edema.

Adrenal Medulla

The adrenal medulla produces the catecholamines epinephrine and norepinephrine. The pharmacology of these hormones is fully discussed in Chapter 13.

DRUG THERAPY OF PHEOCHROMOCYTOMA

Since the first operative removal of a pheochromocytoma by Charles Mayo in 1927, the mortality associated with surgery has fallen considerably. Nevertheless, a high standard of care is essential throughout the perioperative period. This usually pathologically benign adenoma of sympathetic chromaffin cells arises within the adrenals in 90% of patients. The right adrenal is more commonly involved than the left, but the condition is occasionally bilateral (hyperplasia or adenoma) or multiple, particularly in children. Only 2% are located outside the abdomen, usually in the thorax or neck. Those which arise outside the adrenals usually originate on the sympathetic chain near the kidney or bladder or in the organ of Zuckerkandl.

The cardinal clinical features of the condition are due to excess catecholamine secretion and include hypertension, paroxysmal attacks of palpitations, sweating, anxiety, headache, and abdominal pain.

As soon as biochemical evidence for a diagnosis of pheochromocytoma has been obtained, pharmacological control of the excess catecholamine secretion should be begun to allow time for safe tumor localization by imaging and surgical and anesthetic planning. Emergency surgery to remove a pheochromocytoma from an unprepared patient is extremely dangerous.

Preoperative α-adrenergic blockade is essential, as this not only controls blood pressure, but allows expansion of the intravascular volume to overcome the marked volume depletion present in many patients. Phenoxybenzamine (beginning with 20 mg/day, and increasing by 10 mg/day to a dose just below that producing orthostatic hypotension) is the preferred agent because of its long elimination half-life (>24 hours; Chapter 14). Immediately before and during surgery, phentolamine infusion is preferable to the use of phenoxybenzamine as it has a shorter duration of effect which is of advantage in avoiding hypotension following removal of the tumor. Furthermore, a marked rise in blood pressure following cessation of the infusion may suggest another tumor, whereas the long-acting preparation would mask its presence. Phenoxybenzamine and phentolamine are α-adrenergic blocking agents (see Chapter 14) and therefore block not only postsynaptic α_1-receptors, but also presynaptic α_2-receptors. Thus, both these drugs block the negative feedback effect of presynaptic α_2-stimulation that limits catecholamine release leading to an increase in norepinephrine release and tachycardia. Prazosin (a selective α_1-blocking agent) has been advocated in the treatment of hypertension from pheochromocytoma. However, treatment failures have been reported. Although labetalol (α- and β-blocking agent) has also been used successfully in the management of pheochromocytoma, it is important to recognize that its β-blocking effects predominate and that the α-effects are much less than those produced by prazosin or phentolamine. For that reason, despite the introduction of new vasodilators, phenoxybenzamine remains the first-line agent for the management of hypertension in pheochromocytoma.

Tachycardia and arrhythmias are treated by the use of a β-adrenergic blocking agent. β-Blockers, by allowing unopposed α-adrenergic vasoconstriction, can aggravate hypertension when administered alone and should only be used following adequate α-blockade. α-Methylpara-tyrosine, by blocking tyrosine hydroxylase and thereby inhibiting the rate-limiting step that converts tyrosine to dopa, may decrease catecholamine synthesis by up to 30%. Although it is particularly useful in the management of inoperable tumors, it is now widely used in the preoperative preparation of patients to reduce catecholamine concentration.

It is wise in the anesthetic management to avoid drugs that have been implicated in causing a pressor response or tachycardia. Morphine, by causing histamine release, might provoke catecholamine secretion. Most anesthesiologists omit atropine from the premedication as excessive tachycardia may result. The need for adequate rehydration (using pulmonary capillary wedge pressure as a guide) is stressed, and the safety of sodium thiopental is well established. Many different inhalational anesthetic agents have been used over the years. Neuromuscular blocking agents that stimulate histamine release should be avoided, and therefore vecuronium is the muscle relaxant of choice. Succinylcholine should be avoided as the involuntary fasciculations can provoke catecholamine release from the tumor. Opioids such a fentanyl and alfentanil have been successfully employed. Increased doses of phentolamine may be required to control hypertensive responses during endotracheal intubation and tumor manipulation. Sodium nitroprusside has also been used successfully to control large intraoperative swings in blood pressure. Hypotensive episodes may be treated by phenyleph-

rine or dopamine and by the infusion of large quantities of fluid. Propranolol and lidocaine are used to treat intraoperative tachyarrhythmias and ventricular ectopic beats.

Postoperatively hypotension, tachycardia, and a decreasing urinary output may indicate inadequate fluid replacement, pump failure due to myocardial infarction, or possible hemorrhage. Blood transfusion will almost invariably correct hypotension due to hypovolemia, and it should be emphasized that considerable volume replacement may be required.

THYROID HORMONES

Almost all circulating thyroxine and triiodothyronine (T_3) are protein bound to thyroxine binding globulin. Although the serum concentration of thyroxine is about 30 times that of T_3, the latter is less firmly bound. The unbound fraction penetrates cells and is available for metabolism; thus, the half-life of the more highly bound thyroxine is 7 days compared to 1 day for T_3. The majority of thyroxine undergoes deiodination to either active T_3 or biologically inactive reverse T_3 in peripheral tissues. Stress, steroids, surgery, propylthiouracil, and propranolol all favor the conversion to reverse T_3. Only a small fraction of thyroxine is metabolized or conjugated. T_3 interacts with a receptor on the nuclear chromatin and mitochondria. Nuclear transcription, mitochondrial activation, and stimulation of the Na^+-K^+-ATPase pump are the postulated mechanisms whereby basal metabolic rate, protein synthesis, and degradation of fats are stimulated. There is, however, a latent period of hours to days, depending on the tissue studied, between administration of T_3 and manifestation of the response. This is even more prolonged with thyroxine which must first undergo conversion to T_3. Thyroxine, however, appears to be more important than T_3 in the negative feedback on pituitary thyrotrophin (TSH).

Thyroid hormones are used as replacement therapy and to suppress thyroid function in patients with goiter and thyroid tumors. The efficacy of thyroxine in the management of obesity has never been established.

HYPOTHYROIDISM

Replacement therapy in primary auto-immune, postradioiodine, or postsurgery hypothyroidism must be given cautiously to the elderly and those with heart disease. A starting dose of 25 μg of thyroxine increasing each month is commonly given while in younger subjects one can commence with 50 μg and increase more rapidly. The average replacement dose is 150 μg (0.15 mg) and can be given once daily. In addition to measuring free hormone concentrations, the plasma level of TSH gives an indication of adequacy of dosage.

HYPERTHYROIDISM

The choice of treatment for the hyperthyroid patient remains controversial. Antithyroid drugs are effective and relatively free of side effects, but relapse of hyperthyroidism follows their withdrawal in approximately 50% of patients. The initial fears that the use of radioactive iodine would be associated with an increased risk of thyroid carcinoma or leukemia have proved unfounded. However, given time, the majority of radioiodine-treated patients become hypothyroid. Partial thyroidectomy therefore enjoys a place in the management of hyperthyroidism.

Antithyroid Drugs

Antithyroid drugs (propylthiouracil, carbimazole, methimazole) are commonly employed to treat hyperthyroidism. They inhibit thyroid hormone synthesis primarily by interfering with the iodination of the tyrosol residues of thyroglobulin. They also prevent coupling of iodotyrosines to form thyroxine and T_3. Propylthiouracil (PTU), which is the more commonly employed drug in the U.S., also reduces the conversion of thyroxine (T_4) to the biologically more active and important thyroid hormone triiodothyronine (T_3) in peripheral tissues. As these drugs inhibit synthesis of new hormone and do not affect the stored hormone, it is some days before an effect of these drugs is seen, limiting their usefulness in thyroid crisis. On average, it takes 1 to 2 months of therapy before biochemical euthyroidism is achieved.

Apart from rashes, the major uncommon (approximately 1 in 500) side effects are agranulocytosis and aplastic anemia. These are usually reversible on withdrawal of therapy and rarely anticipated by routine blood counts. All patients on these drugs should be instructed to report all infections, particularly pharyngitis, to their physician. Hepatitis is also a rare side effect of PTU. A mild papular or occasionally purpuric rash is the most common side effect in up to one-fifth of patients. Although it may subside spontaneously, physicians usually change preparations as cross-sensitivity is rare. Arthralgia, hair loss, and drug fever are uncommon. The plasma half-life of PTU is in the region of 1 to 2 hours and for carbimazole, 4 to 8 hours. Carbimazole is rapidly converted to methimazole in the body which contributes significantly if not totally to the antithyroid activity. Metabolites are excreted renally.

Thyroidectomy: Perioperative Drug Therapy

Thyroidectomy for hyperthyroidism should always be elective. The traditional and safest method is to initially render the patient euthyroid with antithyroid drugs followed by 7 to 10 days preoperative treatment with iodide (potassium or Lugols) to reduce gland vascularity. An alternative approach is to prepare the patient with propranolol, a β-blocker which reduces many of the symptoms (palpitations, nervousness, sweating, and tremor) and some of the clinical (heart rate, weight loss) manifestations of thyrotoxicosis. The use of propranolol (usually without iodide) reduces, to about a week, the time required to prepare patients for surgery. Propranolol levels, however, vary considerably from patient to patient, and dosage in excess of 160 mg/day is frequently required in the younger and more severely thyrotoxic patient to achieve an adequate degree of β-blockade. Thyroid storm occurs in 3% of patients prepared with propranolol alone and is commonly attributable to omission of the crucial postoperative dosage. This is important because of propranolol's short half-life and increased clearance in hyperthyroidism. Dosage is continued for 7 to 10 days postoperatively because of the long half-life (approximately 1 week) of circulating thyroxine. Sympatholytic drugs such as reserpine and guanethidine are outmoded. The addition of iodide to the propranolol regime for 7 to 10 days preoperatively will temporarily reduce thyroid hormone secretion and thyroid hormones to the normal range in many patients before surgery and is to be recommended if surgery is required in a patient who is incidentally found to be thyrotoxic preoperatively.

Adequate attention should be given to preoperative sedation. There is little evidence that omission of anticholinergics is necessary. Thiopental is the most widely used agent for induction, and there is a theoretical suggestion that agents which "sensitize" the heart to catecholamine should be avoided. However, halothane and enflurane have been widely used without ill effect. Cardiac monitoring is important, particularly for patients prepared with propranolol. All patients must be followed closely for the first 24 hours following surgery, especially to detect thyroid crisis (pyrexia, tachycardia, sweating, and confusion). This should be treated promptly with propranolol (0.1 mg/kg given slowly, intravenously) and propylthiouracil (1 g orally or via nasogastric tube) followed by 200 mg every 6 hours. Some 2 to 3 hours after PTU, potassium iodide should be given orally or intravenously to prevent further release of thyroid hormone. Corticosteroids (300 mg intravenously) are usually given. If propranolol, which in the absence of cardiac failure may be continued (240 mg/day), has been unsuccessful in relieving anxiety and agitation, diazepam or chlorpromazine is used. A high caloric intake and

parenteral feeding, particularly carbohydrates and fluids to correct dehydration due to vomiting and sweating, are indicated. Oxygen therapy and cooling blankets (but not salicylates which displace bound thyroxine) may also be used.

Drug Metabolism and Sensitivity in Thyroid Disease

Because of the marked effects of thyroid hormones on many metabolic functions, it is not unexpected that hyperthyroidism and hypothyroidism might influence drug clearance. In general, the clearance of drugs that are metabolized by the mixed-function oxidase system (see Chapter 1), such an antipyrine, tolbutamide, carbimazole, and propranolol, is increased in hyperthyroidism, and the half-life of antipyrine and carbimazole is prolonged in hypothyroidism. Serum digoxin levels are reduced in hyperthyroidism and increased in hypothyroidism in part due to disease-induced changes in the renal clearance and volume of distribution of digoxin. It has also been suggested that hyperthyroid patients are particularly insensitive to the effects of digoxin. The anticoagulant effect of warfarin is enhanced in hyperthyroidism, probably due to an increased catabolism of clotting factors. The clincial suggestion that hypothyroid patients are very sensitive to the effects of sedative remains to be evaluated.

Endocrine drug interactions are described in Table 20.3.

BIBLIOGRAPHY

Diabetes Mellitus

Alberti KGMM, Thomas DJB: The management of diabetes during surgery. Br J Anaesth 51:693–710, 1979.

Bowen DJ, Daykin AP, Nancekievill ML, Norman J: Insulin-dependent diabetic patients during surgery and labour. Anaesthesia 39:407–411, 1984.

Bressler R: Control of the blood glucose in diabetes mellitus: is it valuable? Is it feasible? Drugs 17:461–470, 1979.

Brogden RN, Heel RC: Human insulin. A review of its biological activity, pharmacokinetics, and therapeutic use. Drugs 34:350–371, 1987.

Christiansen CL, Schurizek BA, Malling B, Knudsen L, Alberti KGMM, Hermanson K: Insulin treatment of the insulin-dependent diabetic patient undergoing minor surgery. *Anaesthesia* 43:533–537, 1988.

Dunnet JM, Holman RR, Turner RC, Sear JW: Diabetes mellitus and anaesthesia. *Anaesthesia* 43:538–542, 1988.

Elliott MJ, Gill GV, Home PD, Noy GA, Holden MP, Alberti KGMM: A comparison of two regimens for the management of diabetes during open-heart surgery. *Anesthesiology* 60:364–368, 1984.

Ferner RE, Caplin S: The relationship between the pharmacokinetics and pharmacodynamic effects of oral hypoglycaemic drugs. *Clin Pharmacokinet* 12:379–401, 1987.

Foster DW, McGarry JD: The metabolic derangements and treatment of diabetic ketoacidosis. *N Engl J Med* 309:159–169, 1983.

Hall GM: Diabetes and anesthesia—a promise unfulfilled? *Anaesthesia* 39:627–628, 1984.

Hall GM, Desborough JP: Diabetes and anaesthesia—slow progress? *Anaesthesia* 43:531–532, 1988.

Jackson JE, Bressler R: Clinical pharmacology of sulphonylurea hypoglycemic agents: part 1. *Drugs* 22:211–245, 1981.

Jackson JE, Bressler R: Clinical pharmacology of sulphonylurea hypoglycemic agents: part 2. *Drugs* 22:295–320, 1981.

Kitabchi AE, Young R, Sachs H, Morris L: Diabetic ketoacidosis—reappraisal of therapeutic approach. *Annu Rev Med* 30:339–357, 1979.

Kraegen EW, Chisholm DJ: Pharmacokinetics of insulin. Implications for continuous subcutaneous insulin infusion therapy. *Clin Pharmacokine* 10:303–314, 1985.

MacPherson JN, Feely J: Insulins. *Br Med J* 286:1502–1505, 1983.

O'Connor P, Feely J: Clinical pharmacokinetics and endocrine disorders. Therapeutic implications. *Clin Pharmacokinet* 13:345–364, 1987.

Palumbo PJ: Blood glucose control during surgery. *Anesthesiology* 55:94–95, 1981.

Sutherland HW, Pearson DWM, Powrie JK: Management of the pregnant diabetic patient. *Drugs* 36:239–248, 1988.

Thomas DJB, Hinds CJ, Rees GM: The management of insulin dependent diabetes during cardiopulmonary bypass and general surgery. *Anaesthesia* 38:1047–1052, 1983.

Thomas DJB, Platt HS, Alberti KGMM: Insulin-dependent diabetes during the postoperative period. *Anaesthesia* 39:629–637, 1984.

Walts LF, Miller J, Davidson MB, Brown J: Perioperative management of diabetes mellitus. *Anesthesiology* 55:104–109. 1981.

Ward GM: The insulin receptor concept and its relations to the treatment of diabetes. *Drugs* 33:156–170, 1987.

Watson BG, Elliott MJ, Pay DA, Williamson M: Diabetes mellitus and open heart surgery. *Anaesthesia* 41:250–257, 1986.

Woodruff RE, Lewis SB, McLeskey CH, Graney WF: Avoidance of surgical hyperglycemia in diabetic patients. *JAMA* 244:166–168, 1980.

Adrenal Hormones

Cubeddu LX, Zarate NA, Rosales CB, Zschaeck DW: Prazosin and propranolol in preoperative management of pheochromocytoma. *Clin Pharmacol Ther* 32:156–160, 1982.

Desmonts JM, Marty J: Anaesthetic management of patients with phaeochromocytoma. *Br J Anaesth* 56:781–789, 1984.

Gilsanz FJ, Luengo C, Conejero P, Peral P, Avello F: Cardiomyopathy and phaeochromocytoma. *Anaesthesia* 38:888–891, 1983.

Hull CJ: Phaeochromocytoma. *Br J Anaesth* 58:1453–1468, 1986.

Juiz W, Meikle AW: Alterations of glucocorticoid actions by other drugs and disease states. *Drugs* 18:113–121, 1979.

Kohlet H, Binder C: Adrenocortical function and clinical course during and after surgery in unsupplemented glucocorticoid-treated patients. *Br J Anaesth* 45:1043–1048, 1973.

Kehlet H, Engquist A, Griebe J: Plasma volume during surgery in unsupplemented glucocorticoid-treated patients. *Br J Anaesth* 46:452–454, 1974.

Pickup ME: Clinical pharmacokinetics of prednisone and prednisolone. *Clin Pharmacokinet* 4:111–128, 1979.

Plumpton FS, Besser GM, Cole PV: Corticosteroid treatment and surgery. 1. An investigation of the indications for steroid cover. *Anaesthesia* 24:3–11, 1969.

Plumpton VS, Besser GM, Cole PV: Corticosteroid treatment and surgery. 2. The management of steroid cover. *Anaesthesia* 24:12–18, 1969.

Pooler HE: A planned approach to the surgical patient with iatrogenic adrenocortical insufficiency. *Br J Anaesth* 40:539–542, 1968.

Pullerits J, Ein S, Balfe JW: Anaesthesia for phaeochromocytoma. *Can J Anaesth* 35:526–534, 1988.

Swartz SL, Dluhy RG: Corticosteroids: clinical pharmacology and therapeutic use. *Drugs* 16:238–255, 1978.

Symreng T, Karlberg BE, Kagedal B, Schildt B: Physiological cortisol substitution of long-term steroid-treated patients undergoing major surgery. *Br J Anaesth* 53:949–953, 1981.

Udelsman R, Ramp J, Gallucci WT, Gordon A, Lipford E, Norton JA, Loriaux DL, Chrousos GP: Adaptation during surgical stress. A reevaluation of the role of glucocorticoids. *J Clin Invest* 77:1377–1381, 1986.

Weatherill D, Spence AA: Anaesthesia and disorders of the adrenal cortex. *Br J Anaesth* 56:741–749, 1984.

Thyroid Hormones

Cooper DS: Antithyroid drugs. *N Engl J Med* 311:1353–1362, 1984.

Feely J, Peden N: Use of β-adrenoceptor blocking drugs in hyperthyroidism. *Drugs* 27:425–446, 1984.

Hamilton WFD, Forrest AL, Gunn A, Peden NR, Feely J: Beta-adrenoceptor blockade and anaesthesia for thyroidectomy. *Anaesthesia* 39:335–342, 1984.

Murkin JM: Anesthesia and hypothyroidism: a review of thyroxine physiology, pharmacology, and aesthetic implications. *Anesth Analg* 61:371–383, 1982.

Stehling LC: Anesthetic management of the patient with hyperthyroidism. *Anesthesiology* 41:585–595, 1974.

Strube PJ: Thyroid storm during beta blockade. *Anaesthesia* 39:343–346, 1984.

General

Marble A, Selenkow HA, Rose LJ, Dluhy RG, Williams GH, Feely J: Endocrine diseases. In *Drug Treatment*, ed 3. New York, Adis Press, 1989.

21

Drugs and the Central Nervous System

RICHARD C. SHELTON
MICHAEL H. EBERT

A knowledge of the pharmacology of the drugs affecting the central nervous system is important for the anesthesiologist, since it is common to encounter patients who are receiving one or more of these agents preoperatively. In addition, the anesthetic management of patients receiving electroconvulsive therapy presents a special problem.

CLASSIFICATION OF PSYCHOTROPIC DRUGS

The underlying mechanisms of depression and anxiety are incompletely understood, and psychotropic drugs only provide symptomatic treatment. The classifcation of drugs used in the treatment of psychiatric disorders is based on the symptoms they are used to relieve, rather than mechanism of action.

ANTIPSYCHOTIC DRUGS

Introduction of the antipsychotic drugs in the early 1950s exerted a profound influence on the understanding and treatment of major psychiatric illnesses. While efficacy has been demonstrated in a wide range of disorders, the effects on psychosis (i.e., reversal of hallucinations and delusions) per se should be considered the most significant. In psychiatry, the use of antipsychotics is largely limited to the treatment of schizophrenic, manic, and "organic" psychoses, and occasionally for acute, severe behavioral disturbances that are unresponsive to more conservative measures.

The important chemical classes of neuroleptic or antipsychotic drugs are as follows:

1. Phenothiazines, e.g., chlorpromazine (considered the prototype of the phenothiazine class, the structural formula is shown in Fig. 21.1);
2. Butyrophenones, e.g., haloperidol (droperidol, a butyrophenone used commonly in anesthesia but not as an antipsychotic agent is discussed in Chapter 8);
3. Thioxanthenes.

Drugs from the dibenzoxapine class (loxapine) and an indole derivative (mol-

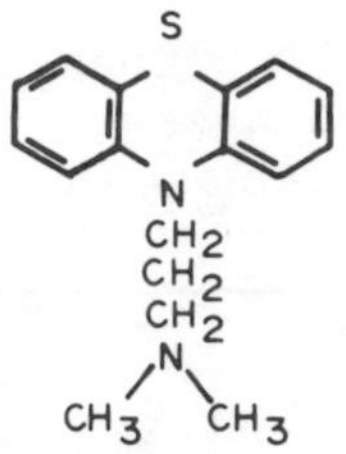

CHLORPROMAZINE

Figure 21.1. Chemical structure of chlorpromazine.

indone) are also used in the United States. The dibenzodiazepines (clozapine) hold considerable research and therapeutic promise. The rauwolfia alkaloids (e.g., reserpine) are largely of theoretical and historical interest. Table 21.1 summarizes the pharmacological properties of the important antipsychotics.

Mechanism of Action of Antipsychotics

Antipsychotics, like the antidepressants discussed in the next section and other drugs active in the central nervous system, are lipophilic amines that bind to many receptor sites on neuronal membranes. These binding sites include pre- and postsynaptic receptors and reuptake sites for the endogenous "biogenic amines," such as dopamine, norepinephrine, acetylcholine, histamine, and serotonin. The relative affinity for such binding sites determines the degree to which certain desired pharmacological actions and unwanted side effects occur (see Chapter 3). The affinity for specific receptors varies widely between compounds, and this is reflected in their relative therapeutic and adverse effects, as shown in Table 21.2.

DOPAMINE RECEPTOR

The therapeutic effects of the antipsychotics are most closely related to their receptor binding action on dopamine receptors. The desired reversal of hallucinations and delusions is directly related to the relative degree of blockade of central dopamine receptors that inhibit adenylate cyclase (dopamine$_2$ receptors). Thus, blockade of dopaminergic receptors is responsible for many of the side effects of the compounds.

Dopamine receptors are distributed in five main areas in the central nervous system:

1. The retina;
2. The tuberoinfundibular area;
3. The mesocortical area;
4. The mesolimbic area;
5. The nigrostriatal area.

The primary antipsychotic effects are thought to occur in the mesolimbic and mesocortical dopamine systems, resulting in a reduction in hallucinations, delusions, and agitation. The significance of dopaminergic blockade in the retina is unclear. Actions on the tuberoinfundibular (hypothalamic) dopamine neurons produce the characteristic endocrine effects, such as inhibition of growth hormone, stimulation of prolactin release, and other actions which cause gynecomastia, galactorrhea, amenorrhea, and reduction of sexual drive.

Some of the most characteristic side effects of antipsychotics are produced by their actions on the nigrostriatal system. Loss of dopamine neurons in the nigrostriatum is pathognomonic of Parkinson's disease. Blockade of these neurons by antidopaminergic drugs can produce a Parkinsonian-like state (including tremor, bradykinesia, etc.) as well as other motor effects to be discussed later.

HISTAMINE RECEPTOR

Antipsychotics have varying degrees of affinity for histamine receptors, but are all potent antihistamine agents. The blockade of central histamine$_1$ receptors (along with the dopamine blocking effects discussed above) produces sedation without depressing vital centers or producing unconsciousness.

α_1-ADRENERGIC RECEPTOR

α_1-Adrenergic blockade produced by the antipsychotic drugs is responsible for a reduction in peripheral vascular resistance and a decreased pressor response to postural changes. This results in orthostatic hypotension and is a greater problem in the drugs that have a relatively low potency in binding to dopamine$_2$ receptors. This can cause fainting (a particular problem in the elderly) and can be a special problem in the anesthetized patient through lowering of blood pressure, failure of vascular response to volume loss, and heat loss from peripheral vasodilation.

CHOLINERGIC RECEPTOR

Antipsychotics also bind to the muscarinic cholinergic receptor which causes the common problems of dry mouth, blurred vision, constipation, tachycardia, and retrograde ejaculation. These difficulties are often compounded by the concomitant administration of other anticholinergic agents (such as benztropin, trihexphenidyl) used to counteract the motor side effects discussed below. Additive effects with other anticholinergic agents such as atropine can be very important in anesthesia.

Clinical Pharmacology

CENTRAL NERVOUS SYSTEM

Antipsychotics produce so-called "neuroleptic" effects centrally (related to the dopamine blocking properties of the drugs), yielding changes in affect (emotional quieting, indifference), cognition (psychomotor slowing), and motor performance (reductions in spontaneous motor activity). The electroencephalogram (EEG) is slowed with increases in both θ-activity and voltage. The action on the brainstem reticular formation differs from the sedative agents that simply reduce activity; it has been hypothesized that antipsychotics increase the activity of this system, which selectively reduces the inflow of stimuli to the cortex. Further, the compounds (especially chlorpromazine and other phenothiazines) have significant antiemetic effects that are likely mediated through actions on the medullary chemoreceptor trigger zone.

By most criteria of improvement, the antipsychotics have been clearly established to be more effective than sedatives, antianxiety agents, psychotherapy, custodial care, and placebo in treating schizophrenia. This is predominantly through reduction in (and subsequent prevention of) "positive" symptoms of schizophrenia, including hallucinations, delusions, agitation, etc. The drugs usually have little effect on the important "negative" symptoms such as apathy, loss of energy, flat affect, social isolation, and vocational impairment and, therefore, cannot be considered truly "antischizophrenic." While results are more dramatic in acute than chronic schizophrenia, sustained reductions of symptoms, preventing relapse and rehospitalization, do occur. Doses of 400 to 600 mg of chlorpromazine or its equivalent are usually required for the control of acute psychosis (with a somewhat lower dose in the elderly). There is growing evidence that maintenance therapy with antipsychotics can be achieved with chronic use of lower doses, or even the elimination of the drugs with targeted intervention as dictated by symptoms.

Acute manic episodes often respond well to antipsychotic drug therapy. Lithium carbonate is considered a more specific and safe treatment of mania; its antimanic effects are, however, usually delayed by 10 days or more. Control of the florid symptoms of agitation, combativeness, and psychosis is usually achieved acutely with antipsychotics. Further, there is a role for antipsychotic medications in the treatment of the agitation and psychosis sometimes seen in severe depression, particularly in the elderly. The use of these drugs should not be considered the primary treatment and should be discontinued as soon as possible because of the risk of tardive dyskinesia (see below).

Antipsychotic drugs are often prescribed for psychosis, agitation, and insomnia associated with "organic mental disorders" (e.g., dementias), as well as other severe behavioral disturbances. Such treatment should occur only after other means have been exhausted and should be for the shortest duration possible. In general, the use of these drugs to treat anxiety or insomnia alone should be discouraged because of the unfavorable

risk/benefit ratio, largely engendered again by the tardive dyskinesia problem.

Finally, the antipsychotics are directly useful to the anesthesiologist as part of neuroleptanalgesia and neuroleptanesthesia, discussed in Chapter 8. In addition, neuroleptics have been used to treat postoperative nausea and vomiting.

Pharmacokinetics

All of the antipsychotic drugs are cyclic compounds that are strongly lipophilic. They are, therefore, readily absorbed when administered orally or intramuscularly, highly protein bound, and rapidly cross the blood-brain barrier. Peak plasma levels of, for example, chlorpromazine occur 2 to 3 hours after oral administration, with wide (greater than 10-fold) intersubject variability. The half-life of elimination tends to be long (20 to 30 hours), and for this reason the compounds can be administered on a once-per-day basis. Elimination of chlorpromazine from plasma includes a rapid ($t_{1/2}=$ 2 hours) and prolonged ($t_{1/2}=30$ hours) phase, while metabolites are excreted in urine for 2 to 6 weeks after chronic administration. The drugs are degraded via microsomal oxidative metabolism in the liver, followed by the formation of water-soluble glucoronides. Impairment of liver function or competition with other drugs (such as steroids) can, therefore, significantly prolong metabolism and elimination; this will produce accumulation of active drug, either parent compound or metabolite. Alternatively, induction of liver enzymes, such as seen in smoking (with exposure to polycyclic hydrocarbons), yields lower plasma levels. Since the metabolites are hydrophilic and excreted via the kidney, their elimination can be slowed by renal impairment. Fortunately, most of the metabolic products are biologically inactive.

Adverse Effects of Antipsychotic Drugs

Many of the adverse effects of the antipsychotic drugs are either directly or inversely related to the clinical potency of the compounds (expressed in mg dose per day in Table 21.1).

CENTRAL NERVOUS SYSTEM

Sedation is a commonly occurring side effect and often resolves to some degree with continued treatment. This effect is due to histamine-1 receptor blockade and is inversely related to potency (i.e., is more common in drugs like chlorpromazine and thioridazine). Depressive symptoms (often part of the drug-induced motor symptoms, including akinesia), confusional episodes (especially in impending delirium from other causes, dementia, or overdosage), and rarely worsening of psychotic symptoms can also occur. The latter may be related to agitation secondary to severe motor side effects that occur somewhat more commonly in the high-potency drugs. All antipsychotics can lower the seizure threshold and, therefore, should always be used with care in persons with a history of epilepsy.

Motor Side Effects. Acute effects are caused by actions in the nigrostriatal (extrapyramidal) system, usually within the first few weeks of treatment. These include (a) actue dystonia: severe, painful, spasmatic contractions of muscles, particularly the extraocular, sternocleidomastoid, and trapezius muscles. These reactions generally occur within the first 24 to 36 hours of initial administration or increase in dose. (b) Drug-induced Parkinsonism: rigidity, tremor, bradykinesia, drooling, mask-like facies, etc., occurring days to weeks after initiating treatment. (c) Akathisia: motor restlessness accompanied by subjective muscular discomfort and often a desire to move or pace. These side effects are responsive to anticholinergic medications such as benztropin, although akathisia tends to remit incompletely with anticholinergics. Akathisia may be more responsive to low-dose β-blockers (e.g., propranolol, 20 to 40 mg/day). The extrapyramidal side effects are directly related to the potency of the drugs in blocking the dopamine$_2$ receptors in the nigrostriatal

tract and are, therefore, directly related to clinical potency.

Tardive Dyskinesia. Tardive dyskinesia is a relatively late-appearing side effect of antipsychotic medication, presenting months to years after initiating treatment. The syndrome includes persistent abnormal buccofaciolingual movements, multiple tics, and/or choreoathetotic movements, and can involve any or all muscle groups. Total dose and duration of treatment are relative risk factors, but older age, female sex, affective illness, and history of brain injury are considered to put an individual at greater risk overall. Withdrawal dyskinesias can be seen after abrupt discontinuation or reduction of dose; these generally disappear within 3 months. Persistent dyskinesias occur in about 20% of all patients who receive antipsychotics chronically. The syndrome may be unmasked by withdrawing the medications, and symptoms are often worsened by anticholinergics. For some patients the syndrome is irreversible, although there is recent evidence showing that even those movements present for a long period of time may gradually remit. Treatments have generally been disappointing in the past. Currently, limiting the total exposure to antipsychotic drugs and symptomatic use of benzodiazepines may be helpful. In addition, syndromes involving chronic, recurring spasms of muscles ("tardive dystonia") may respond to anticholinergic agents in some patients. All of the antipsychotic drugs are linked to the development of tardive dyskinesia, although clozapine (a drug not yet available in the United States) is thought by some to not produce the syndrome with great frequencyl

CARDIOVASCULAR SIDE EFFECTS

Orthostatic hypotension due to α_1-adrenergic blockade is the most common cardiovascular problem associated with antipsychotic treatment. This effect is generally manifested as dizziness or syncope on standing. The resultant peripheral vasodilation can antagonize the pressor effects of certain sympathomimetics and can also produce signifcant heat loss.

Table 21.1.
Pharmacological Properties of Neuroleptic Drugs

	Therpeutically equivalent oral dose (mg)	Sedation	Adrenergic blockade	Extrapyramidal reactions
Phenothiazines				
Aliphatic compounds				
Chlorpromazine hydrochloride (Thorazine)	100	High	Moderate to high	Moderate
Triflupromazine hydrochloride (Vesprin)	25	High	Moderate to high	Moderate
Piperidine compounds				
Thioridazine hydrochloride (Mellaril)	100	High	Moderate (peripheral effects high)	Low
Mesoridazine besylate (Serentil)	50	High	High	Low
Piperacetazine (Quide)	10	Moderate	Low	Moderate
Piperazine compounds				
Trifluoperazine hydrochloride (Stelazine)	5	Moderate	Low	High
Acetophenazine maleate (Tindal)	20	Moderate	Low	Moderate
Butaperazine maleate (Repoise)	10	Moderate	Low	High
Carphenazine maleate (Proketazine)	25	Moderate	Low	High
Fluphenazine (Permitil, Prolixin)	2	Low to moderate	Low	High
Perphenazine (Trilafon)	8	Low to moderate	Low	High
Prochlorperazine (Compazine)	15	Moderate	Low	High
Thioxanthene compounds				
Chlorprothixene (Taractan)	100	High	High	Low to moderate
Thiothixene (Navane)	5	Low	Low	High
Butyrophenone compounds				
Haloperidol (Haldol)	2	Low	Low	High
Indole compounds				
Molindone (Moban)	15–20*	Moderate	Moderate	High
Dibenzoxazepine compounds				
Loxapine succinate (Loxitane)	(10–25)*	High	Low to moderate	High

*Tentative equivalency.

This effect is inversely related to clinical antipsychotic potency. All antipsychotic agents, particularly the low-potency phenothiazines, have quinidine-like effects and produce electrocardiogram (ECG) changes such as an increase in PR, QRS, and QT intervals. Though not as potent as the tricyclic antidepressants in this regard, they can aggravate any preexisting heart block. Alternatively, the anticholinergic side effects produce a positive chronotropic action with resultant tachycardia, an effect inversely related to potency. Sudden death due to arrythmia has been associated with antipsychotic treatment, most commonly reported with high doses of phenothiazines.

AUTONOMIC NERVOUS SYSTEM SIDE EFFECTS

In addition to orthostatic hypotension (mediated by α_1-adrenergic blockade) and tachycardia (via blockade of muscarinic cholinergic receptors) mentioned earlier, other autonomic side effects are related primarily to cholinergic blockade: dry mouth; blurred vision; urinary hesitancy and retention (especially in face of prostatic disease); constipation; and retrograde ejaculation. As with all anticholinergic side effects in this class of drugs, this is inversely related to potency. There are also impairments of the temperature regulation through peripheral vasodilation and direct effects on hypothalamic thermoregulation via blockade of dopamine neurons. This produces a relative "poikilothermia" and can cause problems in temperature regulation in surgery.

ENDOCRINE EFFECTS

Side effects due to actions on the endocrine system include amenorrhea, gynecomastia, galactorrhea, weight gain, and inhibition of sexual drive.

HEPATIC TOXICITY

Cholestatic jaundice was a common occurrence in the early history of antipsychotic use and associated with the use of chlorpromazine. The incidence of hepatotoxicity has declined significantly in recent years. The primary manifestations include anorexia, malaise, fever, jaundice, and elevations of alkaline phosphatase, bilirubin, and (less commonly) serum glutamic-oxaloacetic transaminase (SGOT).

HEMATOLOGIC TOXICITY

Blood dyscrasias develop as hypersensitivity reactions to certain antipsychotic drugs. Mild and transient leucocytosis, eosinophilia, or leukopenia have been reported. Much more rarely, agranulocytosis may occur and represents a medical emergency. Almost all cases develop within the first 3 months of treatment. These reactions may be seen more commonly with the aliphatic phenothiazines (Table 21.1).

SKIN REACTIONS

A maculopapular erythematous rash can develop with any of the compounds; such reactions disappear with discontinuation of the offending agent. Symptomatic relief can be given with antihistaminic compounds. More severe allergic (anaphylactic) reactions or exfoliative dermatitis can occur, but these are rare. Increased sensitivity to sunlight with resultant sunburn is commonly seen and can be prevented by the use of sun-blocking agents, especially those containing **para-aminobutyric** acid or its congener padimate-O. An irreversible, dark purple pigment that develops on sunlight exposure has been reported with high doses of aliphatic phenothiazines (Table 21.1).

OPHTHALMIC SIDE EFFECTS

Epithelial keratopathy, conjunctival melanosis, and opacities of the lens or cornea are sometimes seen. In addition, the more serious pigmented retinopathy has been reported, especially with thioridazine, and for that reason the dose of this compound should at all times be kept below 800 mg per day.

TERATOGENICITY

All neuroleptics cross the placenta and have been identified in amniotic fluid and fetal plasma. Aliphatic phenothiazines (Table 21.1) have been implicated as teratogens, but all antipsychotics should be considered to have adverse potential. Use in pregnancy should, therefore, only be undertaken when absolutely required and after informing the patient of the attendant risk.

NEUROLEPTIC MALIGNANT SYNDROME (NMS)

NMS is a relatively uncommon but very important side effect of neuroleptics. The cardinal features of this idiosyncratic reaction include fever, muscular rigidity, altered consciousness, leukocytosis, elevated serum creatinine phosphokinase, and autonomic dysfunction (tachypnea, tachycardia, diaphoresis, blood pressure changes, tremor, etc.). Death occurs in approximately 20% of all cases. The reaction usually occurs early in the course of neuroleptic treatment, though it can happen at any point. Risk factors include high ambient temperature, malnutrition, dehydration, and physical exertion (as when restraints are used). NMS shares many features with malignant hyperthermia (see Chapter 10), and common mechanisms have been postulated but not established. Treatment of NMS includes discontinuing the antipsychotic, fluid and electrolyte resuscitation, and cooling blankets to reduce fever. Further, Dantrolene (0.8 to 2.5 mg/kg intramuscularly or orally every 6 hours; see Chapter 10) or bromocriptine (2 to 20 mg intravenously or orally every 8 hours) has been used with some success in controlling symptoms until resolution of the syndrome. Rechallenge with antipsychotics after resolution often results in reemergence of symptoms and should therefore be undertaken with great care and only when absolutely necessary.

ANTIDEPRESSANT DRUGS

At about the same time that the antipsychotic medications were introduced into general use, two classes of antidepressants emerged: (a) the tricyclic antidepressants and (b) the monoamine oxidase inhibitors. The tricyclics are by far the most widely used antidepressants today. The tricyclic compounds have two benzene rings joined by a central seven member ring. Some newer antidepressant compounds that are neither tricyclics nor monoamine oxidase inhibitors have entered into clinical use in the United States (e.g., trazodone, amoxipine, maprotiline, and fluoxetine; see Table 21.2).

Tricyclic Antidepressants

The tricyclic antidepressant, imipramine, was developed by modification of the phenothiazine nucleus. Since the first report of the drug's efficacy in 1956, imipramine and amitriptyline have become the most widely used drugs to treat depression. Table 21.2 lists some of the important antidepressant drugs available in the United States, while Figure 21.2 gives the structural formulae of imipramine, amitriptyline, protriptyline, and doxepin. Amitriptyline results from replacement of the ring nitrogen of imipramine with a carbon atom.

CENTRAL NERVOUS SYSTEM

The "amine hypothesis" of depression developed from the observation that drugs that augmented catecholamine and indoleamine neurotransmission at central nervous system synapses usually had antidepressant effects, whereas drugs that diminished neurotransmission at the same synaptic regions were therapeutic in mania. This led to the hypothesis that an alteration in neural activity in central catecholamine and/or indoleamine pathways plays an etiologic role in major depression and bipolar affective disorder, and that pharmacological correction of these processes results in effective treatment. The understanding of the complexity of brain neurotransmitter systems has rendered such a simple explanation unlikely, but the pharmacological effects of tricyclics are nonetheless consistent with many aspects of this hypothesis. Tricyclic antidepressants facilitate noradrenergic and serotonergic neurotransmission by inhibiting reuptake of the released neurotransmitter into the presynaptic nerve ending, a major mechanism of deactivation of the neurotransmitter in the synaptic cleft.

Table 21.2.
Antidepressant Drugs

	Initial dose (mg)	Daily dose (mg)	Central action	Dose schedule	Anti-cholinergic	Sedation	Hypo-tension
Tricyclics							
Imipramine (Tofranil)	15–50	75–300	Norepinephrine, serotonin	q.d.	4+	2+	3+
Desipramine (Norpramine)	15–50	75–300	Norepinephrine	q.d.	2+	1+	2+
Amitriptyline (Elavil)	15–50	75–300	Serotonin (norepinephrine)	q.d.	4+	3–4+	4+
Nortriptyline (Aventyl)	15–50	50–100	Norepinephrine, serotonin	q.d.	2+	1+	2+
Protryptyline (Vivactil)	5–10	20–60	Norepinephrine	t.i.d.	2+	0–1+	2+
Trimipramine	15–50	75–200+	Serotonin (norepinephrine)	q.d.	1–2+	3+	2+
Doxepin (Sinequan)	25–50	75–300	Serotonin	q.d.	2+	1+	2+
Nonpolycyclics							
Maprotiline (Ludiomil)	25–75	75–300	Norepinephrine	q.d.	1–2+	2+	1–2+
Bicyclics							
Fluoxetine (Prozac)	10–20	20–80	Serotonin	q.d.–t.i.d.	0	0–1+	0
Noncyclics							
Amoxapine (Asendin)	100–150	150–300+	Norepinephrine, dopamine	q.d.	1+	1+	1+
Trazodone (Desyrel)	50–150	150–300	Serotonin	b.i.d.	0–1+	3–4+	1+
Bupropion (Wellbutrin)	200	300–450		t.i.d.	0	0	0
Monoamine oxidase inhibitors							
Phenelzine (Nardil)	15–30	45–90	MAO inhibition	b.i.d.	0–1+	2–3+	3+
Tranylcypromine (Parnate)	10–20	10–30+	MAO inhibition	t.i.d.	0–1+	2+	3+
Isocarboxazid (Marplan)	10–20	20–30	MAO inhibition	t.i.d.	0–1+	2+	3+

They also have delayed effects on adrenergic receptor sensitivity at pre- and post-synaptic sites. The clinical response to tricyclics usually occurs after a delay of several weeks. Some investigators have hypothesized that clinical response is most closely correlated with changes in noradrenergic receptor sensitivity.

Tertiary amines (amitriptyline, imipramine, doxepin, trimipramine) are more potent serotonin reuptake inhibitors than the secondary amines (desipramine, pro- triptyline, nortriptyline), which are more potent norepinephrine reuptake inhibitors. In addition, the tertiary agents are generally more sedating than the secondary amines. Whether these biochemical differences reflect clinically significant response patterns in patients has not been determined.

Tricyclic antidepressants cause sedation in normal subjects, and no improvement in mood state occurs. In fact, dysphoric effects are often reported in

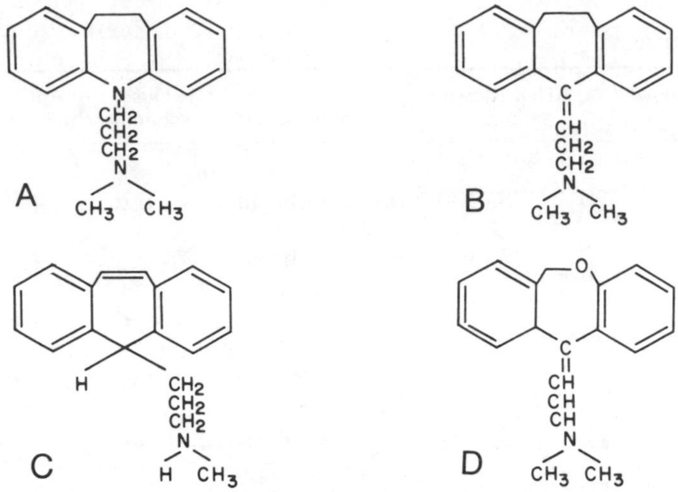

Figure 21.2.   Chemical structure of imipramine (*A*), amitriptyline (*B*), protriptyline (*C*), and doxepin (*D*).

addition to transient deterioration of psychomotor performance. In contrast, if the tricyclic antidepressants are given to depressed patients, they produce an elevation of mood and improvement of psychomotor and cognitive function.

AUTONOMIC NERVOUS SYSTEM

Anticholinergic effects are prominent with all the tricyclics; antihistamine (H_1-receptor) effects are most marked with doxepin.

CARDIOVASCULAR SYSTEM

Mild postural hypotension may occur in approximately 20% of patients, and this is a serious concern in the elderly and patients with cardiovascular disease. The tricyclics occasionally have effects on cardiac rhythm. The most common effects are atrial tachycardia (due to anticholinergic actions) and decreases in cardiac conduction (a quinidine-like effect on cardiac excitability).

PHARMACOKINETICS

Metabolism occurs via sequential oxidative demethylation, *N*-oxidation of the side chain, hydroxylation, and glucuronidation. As the methyl group is metabolically removed from imipramine and amitriptyline, the pharmacologically active secondary amines desmethylimipramine (desipramine) and nortriptyline are formed. Thus, patients treated with the tertiary agents imipramine or amitriptyline will have substantial levels of active secondary metabolite present.

Pharmacokinetic studies have demonstrated a wide interindividual variation in steady-state concentrations. Genetic differences, age, race, and volume of distribution account for much of this difference. Monitoring of plasma levels may be used therapeutically, but is not firmly established. One agent (nortriptyline) has a relatively clear decrement in efficacy at plasma levels exceeding 150 mg/ml, while for most other tricyclics a linear relationship between plasma concentration and therapeutic response has been suggested, but not proven.

INDICATIONS

The chief indication for tricyclic antidepressants is the treatment of major depression (endogenous depression). Patients with major depression exhibit a good response to the tricyclic antidepressants, while patients suffering from reactive or neurotic depression are less responsive. These drugs are relatively contraindicated in schizophrenia, where psychotic symptoms are likely to deteriorate.

Adverse Effects of Tricyclic Antidepressants

Autonomic. Adverse effects include those characteristics of anticholinergic action and have been reported in 15% of patients. Nausea, vomiting, constipation, achalasia, hiatal hernia, adynamic ileus, blurred vision and, rarely, exacerbation of narrow angle glaucoma have all been reported. Tricyclic treatment frequently results in increased bladder sphincter tone, and urinary retention may develop, especially in the elderly.

Central Nervous System Effects. Confusional states may result from the central anticholinergic effects of the tricyclic antidepressants. These reactions have been estimated to be as high as 35% in older patients; a less severe forgetfulness has been observed in younger patients. Patients on other anticholinergic agents (e.g., neuroleptics, antiparkinsonian drugs) are more susceptible to these reactions.

Tremor may frequently occur, and lowering of the seizure threshold has been described occasionally.

Cardiovascular and Cardiac Effects. Brief increases in blood pressure have been observed following routine treatment with tricyclic drugs in geriatric patients. However, orthostatic hypotension is much more common.

Cardiac arrhythmias have been reported, possibly due to prolongation of repolarization. Congestive heart failure may also be precipitated or worsened, probably due to a negative inotropic effect on the myocardium.

Other effects. These include agranulocytosis and hepatotoxicity.

Poisoning. Overdose is extremely serious, especially in children. Overdose symptoms include respiratory depression, agitation, delirium, neuromuscular irritability, seizures, apnea, coma, and cardiac arrhythmias with conduction disturbances. Supraventricular tachycardia with intraventricular block should suggest tricyclic overdose. Patients with exceptionally high plasma concentrations show QRS intervals of greater than 0.10 second. High plasma concentrations are associated with cardiac arrest, grand mal seizures, and death. Intensive cardiorespiratory support is required. The use of antiarrhythmic drugs with effects on cardiac conduction (quinidine, procainamide) should be avoided. Lidocaine, propranolol, and diphenylhydantoin have been safety used. Oral administration of activated charcoal may reduce absorption of tricyclics. Electrical pacemaking or cardioversion has been occasionally necessary. Physostigmine (1 to 4 mg intravenously) may assist in diagnosis and treatment of anticholinergic toxicity, but may increase the risk of grand mal seizures, and itself produces bradycardia and hypotension and is not recommended.

Anesthesia and the Tricyclic Antidepressants. Severe arrhythmias including ventricular ectopic beats have been reported in patients undergoing oral surgery anesthetized with halothane while receiving tricyclic antidepressants. Intraoperative cardiac monitoring is important in this situation.

Monoamine Oxidase Inhibitors

Tricyclic antidepressants are generally considered the drugs of first choice for the treatment of severe depression, and monoamine oxidase inhibitors are used when tricyclic antidepressants fail to achieve a satisfactory result. There has been a renewal of interest in the monoamine oxidase inhibitors in psychiatry, so that the anesthesiologist may see them in use more frequently. Their use became controversial due to interactions between monoamine oxidase inhibitors and many drugs and certain foods, but they are now used for special indications (atypical depression) and as a second choice in depression not responding well to tricyclics. Currently available monoamine oxidase inhibitors for psychiatric use include isocarboxazid, phenelzine, and tranylcypromine. Of the monoamine oxidase inhibitors, phenelzine and tranylcypromine are the most widely used and investigated, and their chemical structures are given in Figure 21.3.

Monomaine oxidase inhibitors inhibit

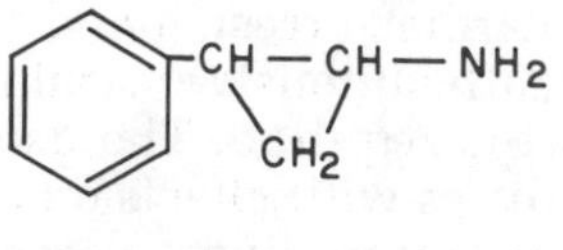

TRANYLCYPROMINE

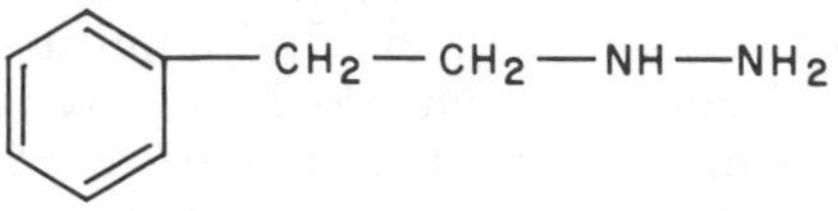

PHENELZINE

Figure 21.3. Chemical structure of tranylcypromine and phenelzine.

monoamine oxidase, an enzyme present in the central nervous system, adrenergic nerve endings, the liver, and the gastrointestinal tracts. This enzyme is involved in the metabolic degradation of epinephrine, norepinephrine, dopamine, and 5-hydroxytryptamine (see Chapter 13). Monoamine oxidase inhibitors bind to monoamine oxidase to form stable complexes which inactivate the enzyme, resulting in increases in the intraneuronal stores of epinephrine, norepinephrine, dopamine, and 5-hydroxytryptamine in the brain, heart, and intestine. Monoamine oxidase is only one of several oxidase enzymes. Since monoamine oxidase inhibitors are not specific for monoamine oxidase, they may interfere with the metabolic degradation of a wide variety of drugs. The antidepressant activity of the monoamine oxidase inhibitors is thought to be due to their augmenting effect on central noradrenergic and serotonergic neurotransmission. Signs of central stimulation are more commonly associated with the monoamine oxidase inhibitors than with the tricyclics. Inhibition of monomaine oxidase is usually achieved within a few days of therapy, although the antidepressant effect develops more slowly over as long as 4 to 6 weeks. In addition, the termination of drug effect is dependent upon enzyme regeneration, which may take as long as 2 weeks.

ADVERSE EFFECTS

Monoamine oxidase inhibitors are more stimulating and less sedating than the tricyclic antidepressants. Monoamine oxidase inhibitors have less anticholinergic side effects than tricyclic antidepressants, and so are less likely to cause urinary hesitancy and retention, constipation, and other autonomic effects. Toxic overdose may occur causing agitation, hallucinations, hyperpyrexia, and convulsions. Hepatotoxicity has occurred with iproniazid, but is rare with the currently available agents. Orthostatic hypotension is a common side effect, particularly in elderly patients.

DRUG INTERACTIONS

The most notorious adverse effect associated with monoamine oxidase inhibitors is a hypertensive crisis caused by an interaction with certain food stuffs containing tyramine. The mechanism is not completely understood, but normally, ingested tyramine is inactivated by monoamine oxidase in the gastrointestinal tract and liver. When this inactivation is prevented by monoamine oxidase inhibitors, severe headaches and a hypertensive crisis can result. Intravenous phentolamine, a short-acting α-adrenergic blocking agent, is recommended to treat the crisis. The foods most commonly implicated are aged cheeses, (blue, Liederkrantz, New York cheddar), pickled herring, chicken liver, Chianti wines, beef liver, broad beans, and avocado pears.

Monoamine oxidase inhibitors also interfere with the metabolism of other drugs. The actions of some sympathomimetic amines are potentiated (see Chapter 13), while the concurrent administration of levodopa and a monoamine oxidase inhibitor may also produce hypertension. In addition, the effects of the barbiturates, alcohol, and opiate analgesics are prolonged and intensified, and adverse effects with meperidine have been reported (see below). Antiparkinsonian agents and tricyclic antidepressants are also potentiated. Hypertension and excitability have followed the use of monoamine oxidase inhibitors with guanethidine, methyldopa, and reserpine. Interactions may also occur between two monoamine oxidase inhibitors, the effects of each being accentuated.

Anesthesia and the Monoamine Oxidase Inhibitors

When some vasopressors are used in the presence of monoamine oxidase inhibitor therapy, a hypertensive crisis may result (see Chapter 13), and their use should be avoided if possible during anesthesia and surgery. The concurrent administration of anesthetic agents, particularly narcotics, is often of concern to anesthetists. There are two types of interactions: an "excitatory" form in which hypertension, hyperpyrexia, and convulsions have been reported; and a "depressive" form in which depression of the central nervous system (including respiratory depression) occurs. Hyperthermia and muscular rigidity have been observed in cats premedicated with monoamine oxidase inhibitors and anesthetized with halothane. A minimum of 2 weeks of abstinence from monoamine oxidase inhibitors should be allowed if the decision is made to discontinue monoamine oxidase inhibitor therapy prior to anesthesia for elective surgery.

Nontricyclic Antidepressants

In the early 1970s, the so-called "second generation" antidepressants were introduced into the United States. These drugs have different chemical structures than the tricyclics but the same mechanism of action: reuptake blockade of norepinephrine or serotonin. These drugs include trazodone, maprotiline, amoxipine and, most recently, fluoxetine. As can be seen in Table 21.2, these drugs have a somewhat improved side effect profile than the tricyclics, though relative efficacy has been questioned. Special problems have been associated with these drugs. The use of trazodone has been connected with increased sexual arousal, including priapism in males, as well as cardiac arrythmias. Maprotiline can induce seizures, especially when the dosage is rapidly escalated or when the total daily dose exceeds 225 mg. Amoxapine is chemically related to the antipsychotic loxipine, and it has attendant dopamine, receptor blocking properties, which can produce extrapyramidal ef-

fects and (at least theoretically) tardive dyskinesia. Fluoxetine has been recently introduced in the United States and has been reported to be of benefit in obsessive-compulsive disorder as well as depression. This drug can cause nausea (and more rarely vomiting), overstimulation, insomnia, headache, and a paradoxical increase in anxiety.

Finally, Bupropion is a new antidepressant with an unknown direct mechanism of action. It has limited side effects except for seizures seen most commonly with rapid dose titration or the use of doses greater than 450 mg per day. This drug should be avoided in persons with active CNS disease, a history of seizures or head trauma, eating disorders, or in persons taking other drugs that lower seizure threshold.

DRUG TREATMENT OF ANXIETY AND INSOMNIA

This group of agents is the most widely prescribed in American medicine. In most cases, they are prescribed for symptoms of anxiety or insomnia associated with a variety of syndromes. The number of agents that have been used for the treatment of anxiety traces the search for a satisfactory compound, that is, a drug useful for anxiety yet without excessive sedation or abuse liability. These agents do not share a common mechanism of action; even the pathophysiology of anxiety itself is poorly understood. Drugs used in the treatment of anxiety include those from the following groups:

1. Benzodiazepines
2. Buspirone
3. Antihistamines
4. Chloral derivatives
5. Propanediols
6. Barbiturates
7. Other sedative-hypnotics

Table 21.3 lists some drugs commonly used in the treatment of anxiety and insomnia and their daily dosage.

Benzodiazepines

The benzodiazepines available in the United States for the treatment of anxiety

are listed in Table 21.3. Chlordiazepoxide and diazepam are considered prototypes for the benzodiazepine class of
drugs. The benzodiazepines are widely
used by anesthesiologists and are further
discussed in Chapter 8; the structure of
the benzodiazepine nucleus and diazepam are both given in Figure 8.10, while
the chemical structure of chlordiazepoxide is depicted in Figure 21.4.

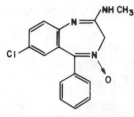

CHLORDIAZEPOXIDE

Figure 21.4. Chemical structure of chlordiazepoxide.

CENTRAL NERVOUS SYSTEM

Central nervous system effects of the
benzodiazepines include:

1. Antianxiety
2. Sedation
3. Anticonvulsant

4. Amnesia
5. Muscle relaxation

With all the benzodiazepines, overse-
dation is the major adverse effect. Ataxia,
slurred speech, and impaired psychomo-

Table 21.3.
Drug Treatment of Anxiety

Drug	Trade name	Daily dosage for anxiety (mg)	Hypnotic dose (mg)
Benzodiazepines			
Alprazolam	Xanax	0.5–2	
Chlorazepate	Tranxene	5–20	
Chlordiazepoxide	Librium	25–100	
Diazepam	Valium	5–25	
Flurazepam	Dalmane		15–30
Halazepam	Paxipam	60–160	
Lorazepam	Ativan	2–8	
Oxazepam	Serax	30–90	
Prazepam	Centrax	5–25	
Temazepam	Restoril		30–60
Triazolam	Halcion		0.25–0.5
Buspirone	Buspar	20–60	
Chloral derivatives			
Chloral hydrate	Noctec		500–1000
Antihistamines			
Diphenhydramine	Benedryl	25–150	50
Hydroxyzine	Atarax, Vistaril	25–150	
Promethazine	Phenergan	50–200	
Propanediols*			
Meprobamate	Miltown, Equanil	400–1200	
Tybamate	Tybatran, Solacren	500–1500	
Piperidinediones*			
Glutethimide	Doriden		500
Methyprylon	Noludar		300
Acetylinols*			
Ethclorvynol	Placidyl		750

*These drugs have a high potential for abuse and addiction and are not recommended for use.

tor function are less frequent; paradoxical excitement (unexpected increase in activation or anxiety) and occasional hostile and aggressive behavior have been noted. The tolerance which develops to benzodiazepines has particular significance for the treatment of anxiety. Benzodiazepine tolerance develops more slowly than with meprobamate, but still probably occurs after approximately 6 weeks of constant treatment, though some antianxiety effect persists. Physical dependence generally requires a substantial increase in dosage above normal therapeutic levels; however, withdrawal reactions have been observed in variable dosage ranges, though these are usually mild.

OTHER EFFECTS

Cardiovascular effects are minimal, and the drugs are used with relative safety in patients with cardiovascular illness.

PHARMACOKINETICS

Knowledge of pharmacokinetic differences allows clinicians to provide short-term relief from episodes of anxiety utilizing short-acting agents (oxazepam, lorazepam), while longer acting agents are employed when more persistent pharmacological effects are required. In addition, since accumulation of active metabolites can be a problem for the elderly, drugs with multiple active metabolites should be avoided in this group, and doses should be kept *low*.

The metabolic pathways for the biotransformation of the benzodiazepines are depicted in Figure 21.5. These pathways are important in the differentiation between long-acting agents (for example, diazepam and chlordiazepoxide) and the shorter acting drugs (for example, lorazepam and oxazepam) which require only conjugation for excretion.

Benzodiazepines are well absorbed from the gastrointestinal tract, with peak

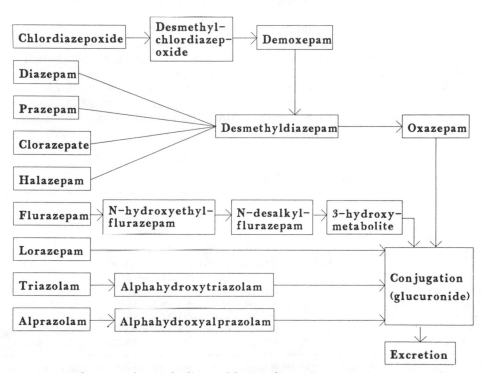

Figure 21.5. Pathways of metabolism of benzodiazepines. Lorazepam and oxazepam are directly glucuronidated, while active metabolites are formed from some of the other compounds.

blood concentrations being achieved in approximately 1 hour. Intramuscular absorption of diazepam and chlordiazepoxide is slower and more irregular than the oral route, though lorazepam is well absorbed intramuscularly and can be effectively delivered via this route.

Diazepam undergoes demethylation by hepatic enzymes to yield the pharmacologically active metabolite, N-desmethyldiazepam. The elimination half-life of diazepam ranges from 20 to 60 hours (Table 21.4). although redistribution to peripheral compartments limits its acute effects. Plasma protein binding of diazepam is high (Table 21.4), and pharmacological effects are increased when albumin concentrations are low. The elimination of diazepam is delayed in the elderly and in patients with liver disease. The half-life of desmethyldiazepam (48 to 96 hours) is longer than that of diazepam.

Oxazepam and lorazepam undergo glucuronidation (Fig. 21.5) followed by urinary excretion of the inactive glucuronide metabolite. Oxazepam is the hydroxylated metabolite of desmethyldiazepam and has an elimination half-life of 5 to 15 hours, volume of distribution of 0.6 to 2.0 L/kg, and a clearance of 0.9 to 2.0 ml/min/kg. Its metabolism is largely independent of age and liver disease, but renal disease is associated with

a prolonged half-life and increased volume of distribution.

Lorazepam has a slightly longer duration of action than oxazepam with an elimination half-life of 8 to 25 hours, volume of distribution of 1.0 to 1.3 L/kg, and a clearance of 0.7 to 1.2 ml/min/kg. Both oxazepam and lorazepam are highly bound in plasma; the free fraction of lorazepam (8 to 12%) is greater than that of oxazepam (2 to 4%).

BUSPIRONE

Buspirone is an azaspirodecandedione that has been shown in clinical trials to have antianxiety efficacy similar to benzodiazepines, particularly diazepam and alprazolam. Studies in animals and humans suggest that this drug does not have the abuse potential of benzodiazepines. Buspirone does not develop cross-tolerance with benzodiazepines. Its mechanism of action is unclear at present, but it does not appear to exert its action on γ-aminobutyric acid (GABA) receptors or benzodiazepine binding sites.

ANTIHISTAMINES

Antihistamines are occasionally used to treat anxiety, particularly with individuals at risk to become dependent on other agents (e.g., benzodiazepines). Hydroxyzine is the most satisfactory of these agents. Its bronchodilatory, anti-

Table 21.4.
Pharmacokinetic Parameters of Antiepileptic Drugs

Drug	Protein binding (%)	V_d (L/kg)	Half-life (hr)	Clearance (L/kg/hr)	Therapeutic plasma concentration (μg/ml)	Toxic concentration (μg/ml)
Phenytoin	87–93	0.51–0.81	15–20*	0.008–0.055	8–20	>20
Phenobarbital	45	0.6–1.01	50–160	0.003–0.013	10–25	>40–45
Primidone	<20	0.06	4–12	0.013–0.041	5–10	<10–15
Carbamazepine	70–80	0.8–1.8	20–55†	0.025–0.096‡	4–12	> 8–10
Ethosuximide	Negligible	0.6–0.7	40–60	0.012–0.016	40–120	>100
Valproic acid	87–94	0.14–0.20	11–20	0.006–0.027	50–100	>100–150
Diazepam	90–97	1.6–2.3	20–60	0.013–0.046	600–1200 ng/ml	>800 ng/ml
Clonazepam	85	2.0–4.8	19–60		20–70 ng/ml	>60 ng/ml

Most of the data are from Morselli PL, Franco-Morselli R: Clinical pharmacokinetics of antiepileptic drugs in adults. *Pharmacol Ther* 10:65–101, 1980.
*Half-life is dependent on plasma concentration (see Chapter 1).
†Following single oral dose in normal volunteers (see text).
‡Following repeated doses in patients.

emetic, antiarrhythmic, and anxiolytic properties have also made it a popular part of a preanesthetic medication regimen. No tolerance develops to hydroxyzine, nor does cross-tolerance develop to other anxiolytics. Doxepin, a tricyclic antidepressant, may owe its anxiety-relieving effects to its potent antihistaminic profile.

CHLORAL DERIVATIVES

Chloral hydrate is a short-acting hypnotic which is relatively safe for short-term use in treating insomnia, particularly difficulty in falling asleep. It is rapidly effective and has a mean half-life of 8 hours. Tolerance to the hypnotic action develops within 5 weeks. It has physical and psychological dependence potential and is not a satisfactory long-term treatment for insomnia.

BARBITURATES

Barbiturates have historical importance as both anxiolytic and hypnotic agents, but have been replaced by the benzodiazepines. The barbiturates are considered further in Chapter 8. The barbiturates generally should not be used for the treatment of anxiety or sleep problems.

PROPANEDIOLS

In 1951, a structural analogy of mephenesin, meprobamate, was introduced with prolonged muscle-relaxant and sedative actions. Within 10 years, the drug was widely used for the treatment of anxiety. The pharmacological profile of meprobamate is similar to the barbiturates, although meprobamate has no specific action on the reticular activating system. Peak effects occur within 3 hours of administration; meprobamate has a half-life of approximately 19 hours. Metabolism is primarily by the hepatic microsomal enzyme system and, as with the barbiturates, enzyme induction occurs. Adverse effects of propanediols include ataxia and drowsiness, allergic reactions, dermatological effects, and the exacerbation of acute intermittent porphyria. Death may result from respiratory depression at high doses. The use of as little as 2 g/day of meprobamate has been associated with tolerance, physical dependence, and a withdrawal syndrome of delirium and convulsions. These drugs are not in wide use, though the anesthesiologist may come across a patient being treated with a drug of this class. The propanediols have no current place in clinical practice.

LITHIUM

Lithium was discovered by Cade to be an effective agent for the treatment of bipolar disorder (manic-depressive illness) in 1949. Concerns about the safety of treatment with lithium salts prevented their widespread use in the United States until the early 1970s, though they had been widely used in Europe before then. Lithium is the treatment of choice for acute manic states and the maintenance therapy of bipolar disorder. Because initial response to lithium may be delayed 10 to 14 days in acute mania, the short-term use of antipsychotics, benzodiazepines, or sedative agents may be required for management of uncontrolled behavior. In the long-term management of patients with bipolar affective disorder, lithium has a prophylactic effect on both manic and depressive episodes. Lithium has also been used for the treatment of other episodic behavioral disorders (such as intermittent violence) and as an adjunctive agent to the standard antidepressants in treatment-resistant depression.

PHARMACOLOGY

The mechanism of action of lithium in treating bipolar affective disorder is unknown. The actions of lithium ion on the release of dopamine and norepinephrine, on the distribution of ions (sodium, potassium, calcium) across cellular membranes, and on neuronal adenylate cyclase systems have been postulated to be significant in its psychotropic effects. Lithium ion is rapidly and nearly completely absorbed from the gastrointestinal tract with peak plasma levels occurring 2 to 4 hours after oral administration. The apparent volume of distribution is 0.7 to 0.9 L/kg, and there is essentially no protein binding. Lithium is excreted almost entirely by the kidney and, therefore, renal impairment can cause significant accumulation and toxicity. The elimination half-life is about 22 hours. Lithium is treated by the body somewhat like sodium; i.e., it is retained when sodium intake is low and excreted along with sodium when intake is high. Therefore, salt restriction or thiazide diuretics may decrease renal clearance of lithium and precipitate toxicity. Alternatively, increases of salt intake, as well as osmotic diuretics, aminophylline, and acetazolamide will increase renal excretion of lithium.

SUGGESTED DOSAGE AND ADMINISTRATION

Lithium toxicity is closely related to serum lithium levels, and there is a very narrow therapeutic range. Because of the low therapeutic index of lithium, dosage is begun at a low level and titrated upward with careful monitoring of blood levels. Levels of 0.8 to 1.2 mEq/L are usually required for management of acute manic states, but maintenance therapy can generally be achieved at lower levels (i.e., 0.4 to 0.8 mEq/L). This corresponds to a maintenance dose in adults of 900 to 1500 mg/day, usually administered 3 or 4 times per day. Slow-release preparations are available and can be given on a twice per pay schedule. Plasma lithium levels should be checked frequently (i.e., every 2 to 3 days) in the acute titrating phase and much less often during maintenance. Weekly blood levels should be checked until stabilization is assured, then again every 2 to 3 months. Toxicity is more commonly seen at blood levels above 1.5 mEq/L and this should be avoided.

ADVERSE REACTIONS

Gastrointestinal side effects including nausea, vomiting, and diarrhea are common with lithium carbonate and occasionally respond to substitution of the citrate salt of lithium. Cardiac arrhythmias, hypotension, peripheral edema, lowered seizure threshold, as well as a fine tremor that tends to worsen as plasma levels of lithium increase are known to occur. Teratogenic effects have been reported. Lithium produces polydipsia and polyuria, possibly via an antagonistic effect on antidiuretic hormone. Renal impairment associated with chronic treatment with lithium has been reported and, therefore, renal function should be periodically assessed. This is generally done by following serum creatinine levels, though some investigators have advocated creatinine clearance determinations, especially in older patients.

Enlargement of the thyroid and less commonly clinical hypothyroidism can occur in patients treated with lithium. There is some evidence to indicate that certain bipolar patients have preexisting thyroid disease and that lithium may "unmask" or aggravate the condition.

Toxicity generally occurs at plasma concentrations above 1.5 to 2.0 mEq/L, although some signs (such as confusion, tremor, or sedation) may be seen at lower serum levels in certain patients (e.g., the elderly). Ataxia, dysarthria, aphasia, confusion, sedation, choreoathetoid movements, vomiting, diarrhea, and coarse tremor are common toxic symptoms. This can progress on to include focal neurological signs, hyperreflexia, seizures, coma, and death as very high levels are achieved.

ANESTHETIC CONSIDERATIONS

It has been reported that lithium may potentiate the actions of both depolarizing and nondepolarizing muscle relaxants (see Chapter 10) and, therefore, lithium should be discontinued prior to major surgical procedures if possible. Concomitant treatment with lithium and electroconvulsant therapy has been associated with increased frequency of adverse neuropsychological reactions and, therefore, the lithium should be stopped before electroconvulsive therapy is initiated.

ANTIEPILEPTIC DRUGS

Nearly 100 years ago, John Hughlings Jackson postulated that seizures resulted from "occasional, sudden, excessive, rapid, and local discharges of the gray matter." Anticonvulsant drugs are agents that inhibit the original abnormal discharge (spike) or its propagation through brain tissue. **Primary** or **idiopathic** epilepsy, where no cause for the seizure can be identified, is generally more easily controlled by drugs than **secondary** or **symptomatic** seizures that are due to demonstrable brain disease such as trauma, tremor, infection, or congenital abnormalities. Seizures are classified by their clinical manifestations; Table 21.5 reviews the classification of seizure types. Drug therapy is generally dependent on the type of seizure.

PHARMACOLOGY

Many fundamental pharmacological actions of the anticonvulsants leading to inhibition of neuronal membrane activation are known to occur. The specific mechanisms by which the drugs exert their effects are generally unknown. The benzodiazepines (diazepam, clonazepam,

etc.) exert their primary pharmacological effect by their augmentation of the inhibitory neurotransmitter gamma aminobutyric acid (GABA) Several other anticonvulsants, including phenytoin, phenobarbital, ethosuximide, and valproic acid, produce at least transient increases in GABA levels. Another possible mechanism of anticonvulsant effects may be the hyperpolarization of neuronal membranes by alterations in gradients of sodium, potassium, and less commonly calcium ions. This is true of phenytoin, phenobarbital, and valproic acid. The mechanisms will be discussed more fully under the specific drugs listed below.

Table 21.4 summarizes important pharmacokinetic parameters of the anticonvulsants. As can be seen, several of the drugs have a high degree of protein binding; anything that alters the availability of binding sites can increase the free fraction (and therefore the bioactivity) of the compounds. Factors that decrease protein binding (such as competition with other drugs or protein depletion through starvation) can cause unexpected toxicity if only total concentrations are considered.

Elimination of the antiepileptic drugs involves hepatic oxidative metabolism. Here again, changes in the activity of the liver oxidative enzymes can cause variability in plasma levels of the compounds. Liver disease or competition with other drugs can cause a relative reduction in metabolism and raise blood levels; induction of the enzymes will lower the available drug concentrations. Several of the anticonvulsants, including primidone, carbamazepine, diazepam, and valproic acid, have active metabolites that can significantly prolong their biological half-lives. Finally, a substantial proportion of phenobarbital, primidone, and ethosuximdie is excreted unchanged in the urine. Renal impairment can, therefore, result in accumulation of drug.

Table 21.5.
Classification of Seizures and Corresponding Pharmacological Agents

Seizure type	Effective anticonvulsants
Partial seizures	Carbamazepine
Simple partial seizures	Phenytoin
Complex partial seizures	Phenobarbital
Partial seizures with secondary generalization	Primidone Clonazepam
Generalized seizures	
Absence seizures	Ethosuximide
Atypical absence seizures	Valproic acid Clonazepam
Myoclonic seizures	Valproic acid Clonazepam
Clonic seizures	Phenytoin
Tonic seizures	Phenobarbital
Tonic-clonic seizures	Carbamazepine
Atonic seizures	Primidone Clonazepam

Adapted from the Commission on Classification and Terminology of the International League against Epilepsy, 1981.

Management of Antiepileptic Therapy

GENERAL CONSIDERATIONS

Knowledge of the pharmacokinetics of antiepileptic drugs is important in determining dosage and schedule of administration. Monitoring of drug concentrations in plasma or serum under steady-state conditions has become routine practice in order to maximize therapeutic benefits while minimizing adverse effects. Such concentrations are usually estimates of total drug in plasma, and plasma protein binding, discussed in the previous section, must be taken into consideration.

In general, choice of drug therapy is dependent upon the type of seizure manifestation. Table 21.5 matches drug choice with seizure subtype. Therapy is usually started with a single anticonvulsant; the dose is increased in accordance with the drug's pharmacokinetic properties and measured plasma concentrations. If control remains poor, a second drug can be added to the regimen, or the first can be slowly withdrawn while the second drug is substituted. Table 21.5 lists primary and secondary choices for antiepileptic therapy. Usually one or more primary drugs, alone or in combination, will be used prior to utilizing a secondary compound. Certain seizures such as myoclonus and epilepsy in young children are difficult to treat effectively, and drugs like valproic acid, primidone, and clonazepam are often employed.

ANESTHETIC CONSIDERATIONS

Anesthesia and surgery in epileptic patients or chronic anticonvulsant therapy requires careful planning so that the plasma concentrations of these agents are maintained within the therapeutic range during the perioperative period. Severe renal and hepatic disease may alter the plasma drug concentrations. The anesthesiologist should be aware of the possible occurrence of adverse drug interactions. Postoperatively, reduced protein binding of phenytoin has been reported, possibly due to altered albumin and α_1-acid glycoprotein concentrations and significantly increased free fatty acid levels. Alterations in acid-base balance may influence drug binding and distribution (see barbiturates, Chapter 8).

INDIVIDUAL ANTIEPILEPTIC DRUGS

Hydantoins—Phenytoin

Available as an effective anticonvulsant since the late 1930s, phenytoin (diphenylhydantoin) remains a mainstay of epilepsy treatment. It is considered a primary drug choice for all types of epilepsy except absence seizures. The chemical structure of phenytoin is shown in Figure 21.6; as can be seen, it is similar in structure to primidone and other barbiturate-type compounds. It does not, however, tend to produce the same degree of sedation found with the barbiturates. The pharmacokinetic characteristics are shown in Table 21.4. Phenytoin is usually prescribed in doses of 250 to 500 mg/day in adults, and because of its long half-life can be given once per day except in children or when acute side effects associated with peak drug concentrations occur. This dose range will generally produce the desired plasma concentrations of 8 to 20 μg/ml.

Phenytoin is hydroxylated in the liver and then conjugated and excreted in the urine. The major metabolite is a 5-phenyl-5-parahydroxyphenylhydantoin (HPPH). At high plasma concentrations, biotransformation to HPPH becomes saturated, and disproportionately large increases in plasma concentrations may occur with only small increases in dosage. Thus, phenytoin at low concentrations exhibits *first order* kinetics, and this gives way to *zero order* kinetics as serum levels increase.

Phenytoin is a potent inducer of hepatic metabolism; the addition of the drug to patients receiving other compounds such as phenobarbital will result in enhanced metabolism. Competition for metabolic enzymes or direct enzyme inhibition in the liver can reduce metabolism of phenytoin and result in increased concentrations. Drugs such as sulthiame (another anticonvulsant), isoniazid, cimetidine, erythromycin, and chloramphenicol can produce such an effect.

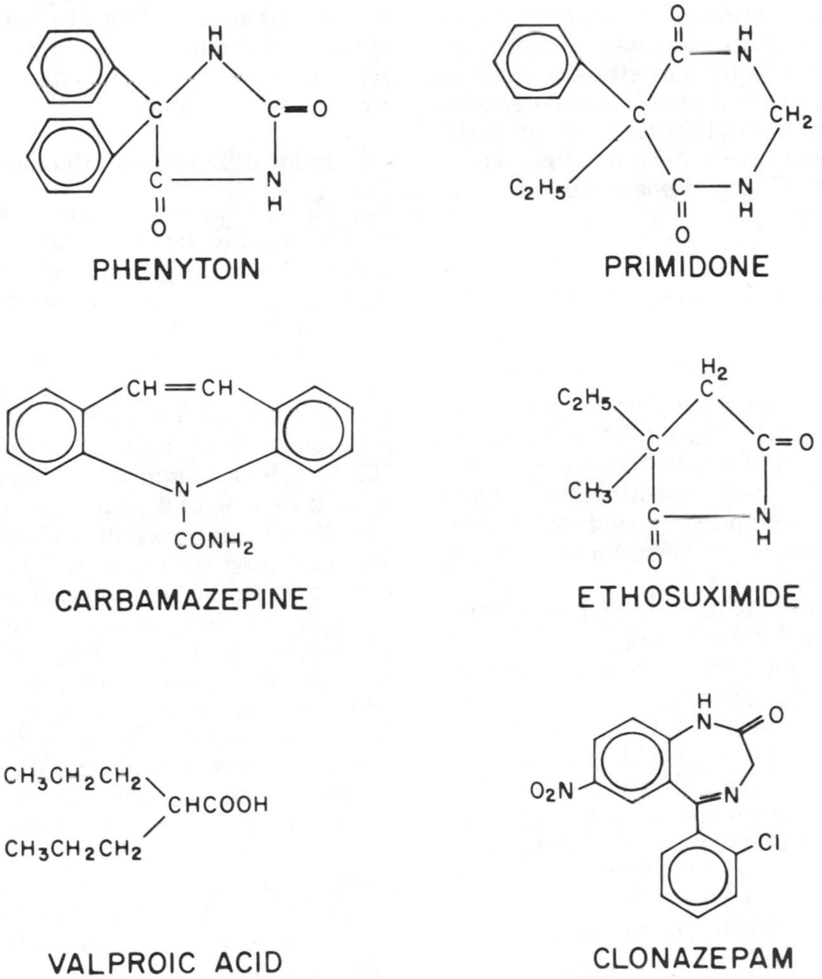

Figure 21.6.   Chemical structures of some important antiepileptic drugs.

Plasma protein binding of phenytoin is high, and therefore small changes in binding produce large changes in the concentration of free drug. Many drugs (such as aspirin, sulfonamides, oral hypoglycemics, clofibrate, warfarin, antidepressants, etc.) compete with phenytoin for plasma protein binding sites and can produce toxicity. Further binding is reduced with protein depletion and renal failure.

Adverse effects include gingival hyperplasia, osteomalacia, gastrointestinal symptoms (nausea, vomiting, diarrhea), lupus-like reactions, and hepatocellular hypersensitivity reactions. Depletion and altered metabolism of folate can cause megaloblastic anemia or peripheral neuropathy; these effects can be prevented by the coadministration of folic acid. Other hematological reactions can occur, such as leukopenia, anemia, and more rarely agranulocytosis and aplastic anemia. Toxicity is manifested as sedation, ataxia, confusion, nystagmus, diplopia, and increased frequency of seizures. Chronic (mild) toxicity can result in reversible impairment of intellectual functioning and memory, as well as the rare occurrence of dyskinesias. Nondepolarizing neuromuscular blockade has been shown to be enhanced by the concomitant administration of a wide variety of anticonvulsant drugs, including phenytoin, phenobarbital, and ethosuximide in laboratory experiments. Patients receiving chronic phenytoin therapy are resistant to metocurine, pancuronium, vecuronium, possibly d-tubocurarine, but not atracurium.

Barbiturates—Phenobarbital

The general pharmacology of the barbiturates is described in Chapter 8. Phenobarbital is commonly prescribed alone or in combination with other anticonvulsants in doses of 100 to 180 mg daily. Because of the long half-life of the compound, an extended period of time is required to achieve steady-state concentrations (Table 21.4).

Adverse effects include rash and osteomalacia (responsive to high-dose vitamin D), and hypoprothrombinemia can occur. Megaloblastic anemia and peripheral neuropathy can result from depletion of folate and respond to replacement. Toxicity causes ataxia, dysarthria, sedation, nystagmus, confusion, and at increasing concentrations respiratory depression and death. Levels above 80 μg/ml may increase seizure frequency. Hyperactivity and irritability can be seen in both therapeutic and toxic concentrations in children.

Deoxybarbiturates—Primidone

The pharmacological properties of primidone are of both the parent compound and those of its active metabolites. It is rapidly transformed to phenylethylmalenamide (PEMA) and more slowly to phenobarbital. Primidone and PEMA have little protein binding and phenobarbital only moderately so, and therefore alterations in availability of protein binding sites are of less importance relative to other anticonvulsants.

Adverse effects such as rash, osteomalacia, leukopenia, thrombocytopenia, systemic lupus erythematosus-like reactions, and gastrointestinal effects have been reported. Megaloblastic anemia and peripheral neuropathy are generally responsive to folate administration. Toxicity includes sedation, ataxia, vertigo, nystagmus, and nausea.

Iminostilbenes—Carbamazepine

Carbamazepine is structurally related to the tricyclic antidepressants (Fig. 21.6) and has been used effectively as an alternative antidepressant and in the prophylaxis of bipolar disorder. It is a useful agent in the treatment of temporal lobe epilepsy and is considered by some to be the first choice for this indication. The average daily adult dose is in the range of 600 to 1200 mg, and it is usually administered in a 3- to 4-times per day schedule. Its pharmacokinetic characteristics are described in Table 21.4 Carbamazepine is metabolized in the liver to yield an active stable epoxide, carbamazepine-10,11-epoxide. This derivative is approximately 50% protein bound in plasma and has a half-life ranging from 5 to 23 hours. In normal volunteers, carbamazepine half-lives range from 20 to 55 hours after a single oral dose. This is significantly reduced (8 to 24 hours) after repeated administration due to "autoinduction" of hepatic enzymes. It has been demonstrated that the time required to reach a plateau for autoinduction in normal volunteers is 20 to 30 days.

Adverse reactions to carbamazepine include rash, lymphadenopathy, and splenomegaly. Vomiting, confusion, and headache may be related to water retention due to the antidiuretic effect of the drug. This may be a particular problem in patients with cardiac disease. A substantial proportion of patients develop a transient leukopenia, and persistent leukopenia can occur. Agranulocytosis and aplastic anemia have been reported and, though rare, are seriously life threatening. These hematological effects have led to the recommendation that complete blood counts be followed regularly. Though it is unclear whether this can predict the more serious hematological events, at no point should the total neutrophil count be allowed to fall below 1000 per ml. Nystagmus, ataxia, and diplopia can occur at levels above 10 $\mu g/ml$, while lethargy, sedation, irritability, respiratory depression, and increased seizure frequency are associated with plasma concentrations above 20 $\mu g/ml$.

Succinimides—Ethosuximide

Ethosuximide is the drug of first choice in the treatment of absence epilepsy. The structural formula is shown in Figure 21.6, and its pharmacokinetic characteristics are outlined in Table 21.4. Ethosuximide is extensively metabolized in the liver with only 12 to 20% of the dose excreted unchanged in the urine. Therefore alterations in hepatic drug-metabolizing enzymes will have significant effects on circulating blood levels. The metabolites of ethosuximide are inactive. Plasma protein binding is negligible and, therefore, this is not an important pharmacokinetic variable.

Adverse effects include urticaria and other rashes, hematological reactions (leukopenia, thrombocytopenia, eosinophilia, aplastic anemia), and systemic lupus erythematosus-like reactions, and diminished intellectual abilities can occur. At higher plasma levels, headache, lethargy, vertigo, euphoria, agitation, confusion, and gastrointestinal effects (nausea and vomiting) have been reported.

Valproic Acid

Valproic acid is a derivative of carboxylic acid (Fig. 21.6) that is particularly useful in the management of childhood absence epilepsy. The pharmacokinetic parameters of this drug are shown in Table 21.4. Valproic acid undergoes extensive hepatic metabolism such that only 1 to 4% of the administered dose is excreted unchanged. In addition, it is highly bound to plasma proteins.

Adverse effects with this compound are relatively uncommon and include gastrointestinal effects (nausea, vomiting, anorexia), rash, alopecia, central nervous system activity (sedation, ataxia, etc.), stimulation of appetite, and rarely, fulminant hepatitis.

Benzodiazepines—Diazepam and Clonazepam

Diazepam is commonly used in the management of status epilepticus, administered intravenously in doses of 5 to 10 mg for adults as required. Plasma concentrations of 600 to 1200 ng/ml are reported to be necessary to suppress seizure discharges. It is discussed in detail in Chapter 8. Table 21.4 describes its pharmacological characteristics. Diazepam steady-state plasma concentrations following dosages of 20 to 40 mg/day for 7 to 10 days are generally in the range of 200 to 600 ng/ml. Chronic oral diazepam is, however, relatively ineffective in the management of epilepsy.

Clonazepam is used for the chronic management of a wide variety of seizure disorders. Unlike other benzodiazepines, this generally occurs at doses that do not produce significant sedation. The chemical structure can be seen in Figure 21.6 and its pharmacokinetic properties in Table 21.4. Clonazepam is almost completely metabolized in the liver and is highly protein bound. Alterations of these pharmacokinetic parameters can result in significant changes in clinical pharmacology. Clonazepam is a difficult drug to manage for the treatment of epilepsy because of a narrow "therapeutic window" of plasma concentrations (see Chapter 1). Monitoring of plasma concentrations is, therefore, important. In addition to chronic administration, it is useful in the treatment of status epilepticus in adults, in doses of 1 to 3 mg by slow intravenous infusion.

Adverse effects of benzodiazepines are relatively uncommon but include sedation, ataxia, and dysarthria. Behavioral disturbances such as irritability and hyperactivity are commonly seen in children, less so in adults. Respiratory and cardiovascular depression is rare and occurs primarily after intravenous administration.

ANALEPTIC DRUGS

Analeptic drugs act by stimulating the chemoreceptors of the carotid body or by direct stimulation of the respiratory center of the medulla. These agents are not recommended for the management of overdosage from sedative-hypnotic drugs, where supportive therapy and mechanical assistance to respiration are superior to the use of analeptics. Doxapram is the drug of choice if an analeptic drug is desired, because of its higher margin of safety. Strychnine and picrotoxin are obsolete. Analeptic drugs can cause tonic-clonic convulsions if given in large enough doses.

Doxapram

Doxapram is a respiratory stimulant which acts on the peripheral carotid chemoreceptors at low doses and, as the dosage is increased, stimulates the central respiratory centers of the medulla. The onset of respiratory stimulation occurs within 20 to 40 seconds of intravenous injection with a peak effect at 1 to 2 minutes. It has a short duration of action of 5 to 12 minutes. Respiratory stimulation is manifest as an increase in tidal volume and slight increase in respiratory rate. The respiratory stimulating effects are accompanied by an increase in arterial blood pressure. Doxapram has been used in the treatment of postoperative surgical patients with chronic pulmonary disease to stimulate deep breathing and also as a temporary measure in the treatment of patients with chronic pulmonary insufficiency with acute hypercapnia. It is not recommended in the treatment of patients with hypertension, coronary artery disease, thyrotoxicosis, or epilepsy. Doxapram may be administered by single intravenous injection in doses in the region of 0.5 to 1.5 mg/kg or by continuous intravenous infusion at a rate of 1 to 3 mg/minute.

BIBLIOGRAPHY

General

Baldessarini RJ: *Chemotherapy in Psychiatry.* Cambridge, MA, Harvard University Press, 1985.

Baldessarini RJ: Drugs and the treatment of psychiatric disorders. In Gilman AG, Goodman LS, Gilman A (eds): *The Pharmacological Basis of Therapeutics,* ed 7. New York, Macmillan, 1985.

Ghoneim MM: Drug interaction in anaesthesia, a review. *Can Anaesth Soc J* 18:353–375, 1971.

Potter WZ: Psychotheraputic drugs and biogenic amines, current concepts and theraputic implications. *Drugs* 28:127–143, 1984.

Risch SC, Groom G, Janowsky DS: The effects of psychotropic drugs on the cardiovascular system. *J Clin Psychiatry* 43:16–31, 1982.

Antipsychotics

Balant-Gorgia AE, Balant L: Antipsychotic drugs, clinical pharmacokinetics of potential candidates for plasma concentration monitoring. *Clin Pharmacokinet* 13:65–90, 1987.

Baldessarini R, Cole J, Davis J, Gardos G, Preskorn S, Simpson G, Tarsy D: *Tardive Dyskinesia.* Washington DC, APA Press, 1980.

Davis JM: Dose equivalence of the antipsychotic drugs. *J Psychiatr Res* 11:65–69, 1974.

Davis JM, Janicak P, Chang S, Klerman K: Recent advances in the pharmacologic treatment of the schizophrenic disorders. In Grinspoon L (ed): *American Psychiatric Association, Annual Review 1982.* Washington, DC, American Psychiatric Association Press, 1982, pp 178–262.

Germesh H, Aizenberg D, Lapidot M, Munitz H: The relationship between malignant hyperthermia and neuroleptic malignant syndrome. *Anesthesiology* 70:171–172, 1989.

Levenson JL: Neuroleptic malignant syndrome. *Am J Psychiatry* 142:1137–1145, 1985.

Lipinski JF, Zubenko J, Cohen BM, Barreira P: Propranolol in the treatment of neuroleptic-induced akathisia. *Am J Psychiatry* 141:412–415, 1984.

Snyder SH: Dopamine receptors, neuroleptics, and schizophrenia. *Am J Psychiatry* 138:460–464, 1981.

Antidepressants

Ballenger J, Post R: Carbamazepine (tegretol) in manic depressive illness: a new treatment. *Am J Psychiatry* 137:782–790, 1980.

Blackwell B: Newer antidepressant drugs. In Meltzer HY (ed): *Psychopharmacology, The Third Generation of Progress.* New York, Raven Press, 1987.

Brotman AW, Falk WE, Gelenberg AJ: Pharmacologic treatment of acute depressive subtypes. In Meltzer HY (ed): *Psychopharmacology, The Third Generation of Progress.* New York, Raven Press, 1987.

Fink M: Convulsive therapy in affective disorders: a decade of understanding and acceptance. In Meltzer HY (ed): *Psychopharmacology, The Third Generation of Progress.* New York, Raven Press, 1987.

Folks DG: Monoamine oxidase inhibitors: reappraisal of dietary considerations. *J Clin Psychopharmacol* 3:249–252, 1983.

Glassman AH, Bigger JT: Cardiovascular effects of therpeutic doses of tricyclic antidepressants: a review. *Arch Gen Psychiatry* 38:815–820, 1981.

Joyce PR, Paykel ES: Predictors of drug response in depression. *Arch Gen Psychiatry* 46:89–99, 1989.

Quitkin F, Rifkin A, Klein DF: Monoamine oxidase inhibitors: a review of antidepressant effectiveness. *Arch Gen Psychiatry* 36:749–760, 1979.

Stack CG, Rogers P, Linter SPK: Monoamine oxidase inhibitors and anaesthesia. *Br J Anaesth* 60:222–227, 1988.

Stern SL, Ruch AJ, Mendels J: Toward a rational pharmacotherapy of depression. *Am J Psychiatry* 137:545–552, 1980.

Drug Treatment of Anxiety and Insomnia

Greenblatt DJ, Shader RI, Abernethy DR: Current status of benzodiazepines. *N Engl J Med* 309:354–358, 1983.

Guentert TW: Time-dependence in benzodiazepine pharmacokinetics, mechanisms, and clinical significance. *Clin Pharmacokinet* 9:203–210, 1984.

Hartmann E: *The Sleeping Pill*. New Haven, CT, Yale University Press, 1978.

Lader M: Antianxiety drugs: clinical pharmacology and therpeutic use. *Drugs* 12:362–373, 1976.

Paton DM: Webster DR: Clinical pharmacokinetics of H$_1$-receptor antagonists (the antihistamines). *Clin Pharmacokinet* 10:477–497, 1985.

Paul S, Skolnick J, Tallman J, Uskin E: *Pharmacology of Benzodiazepines*, New York, Macmillan, 1983.

Richter JJ: Current theories about the mechanisms of benzodiazepines and neuroleptic drugs. *Anesthesiology* 54:66–72, 1981.

Rickels K, Schweizer EE: Current pharmacotherapy of anxiety and panic. In Meltzer HY (ed): *Psychopharmacology, The Third Generation of Progress*. New York, Raven Press, 1987.

Lithium

Dunner DL, Clayton PL: Drug treatment of bipolar disorder. In Meltzer HY (ed): *Psychopharmacol-ogy, The Third Generation of Progress*. New York, Raven Press, 1987.

Havdala HS, Borison RL, Diamond BI: Potential hazards and applications of lithium in anesthesiology. *Anesthesiology* 50:534–537, 1979.

Jephcott G, Kerry RJ: Lithium: an anesthetic risk. *Br J Anaesth* 46:389–390, 1974.

Ramsey TA, Cox M: Lithium and the kidney: a review. *Am J Psychiatry* 139:443–449, 1982.

Small JG, Kellams JJ, Milstein V, *et al*: Complications with electroconvulsive treatment combined with lithium. *Biol Psychiatry* 15:103–112, 1980.

Antiepileptics

Beghi E, Di Mascio R, Tognoni G: Drug treatment of epilepsy, outlines, criticism, and perspectives. *Drugs* 31:249–265, 1986.

Commission on Classification and Terminology of the International League against Epilepsy: Proposal for revised clinical and electroencephalographic classification of epileptic seizures. *Epilepsia* 22:489–501, 1981.

Eadie MJ: Anticonvulsant drugs, an update. *Drugs* 27:328–363, 1984.

Evans DEN: Anaesthesia and the epileptic patient. *Anaesthesia* 30:34–45, 1975.

Morselli PL, Franco-Morselli R: Clinical pharmacokinetics of antiepileptic drugs in adults. *Pharmacol Ther* 10:65–101, 1980.

Ornstein E, Matteo RS, Schwartz AE, Silverberg PA, Young WL, Diaz J: The effect of phenytoin on the magnitude and duration of neuromuscular block following atracrium or vecuronium. *Anesthesiology* 67:191–196, 1987.

22

Drugs and the Coagulation System

ALASTAIR J. J. WOOD

Therapeutic agents which interfere with blood coagulation fall into four classes:

1. **Anticoagulants.** This group includes heparin and the coumarin-indanedione oral anticoagulants.
2. **Thrombolytic** agents such as streptokinase, urokinase and recombinant tissue-type plasminogen activator (rt-PA).
3. **Antiplatelet** drugs. These agents alter the aggregating ability of platelets and have recently received considerable attention.
4. **Defibrinogenating** agents. Agents in this group remove the fibrinogen from circulating blood.

Antithrombotic drugs are used clinically either to prevent (anticoagulant) the formation of blood clots within the circulation or to dissolve a clot (thrombolytic) which has already formed. Sometimes, as in extracorporeal circulation, the necessity for anticoagulation is obvious, and the benefits do not need formal evaluation. In other situations, the benefits are much more subtle and, in some cases, are still the source of considerable controversy.

HEPARIN

Heparin is a highly anionic mucopolysaccharide produced by mast cells of most animal species. It is prepared commercially from bovine lung and porcine and bovine intestine. Because of the heterogeneous composition of heparin in terms of both its origin, length, and composition of the mucopolysaccharide chains, and the absence of a chemical assay, commercial preparations are standardized in terms of the anticoagulant activity and should, therefore, be prescribed in units (one unit is the amount of heparin required to prevent 1.0 ml of sheep blood from clotting for 1 hour following the addition of 0.2 ml of $\frac{1}{100}$ calcium chloride solution). Heparin forms a complex with antithrombin III and potentiates the ability of this natural inhibitor to inhibit the coagulation proteins (principally activated factor X and thrombin). The rate of formation of anti-thrombin III-thrombin complex is accelerated by heparin so that clotting is inhibited. The action of heparin is immediate, and it is effective both in vivo and in vitro. The inhibition of thrombin prevents the conversion of fibrinogen to fibrin and the resultant clot formation, so that the *whole blood clotting time* and *activated partial thromboplastin time* (APTT) are prolonged. These tests can be used to monitor heparin therapy. The dose of heparin should be adjusted to prolong the whole blood clotting time or activated partial thromboplastin time to about 2 times normal (or twice the patient's pretreatment time).

Because of its large molecular weight (approximately 15,000) and polarity, heparin crosses membranes poorly. It is, therefore, not absorbed following oral administration, does not cross the placenta to the fetus in appreciable quantities, and is not excreted in breast milk. The higher molecular weight heparins are thought to interact with platelets and may increase the risk of bleeding. For that reason, low-molecular-weight heparins are currently being investigated.

The lack of a specific chemical assay for heparin means that its pharmacokinetics cannot be described in conventional form. Instead the half-life of its effect has been determined and appears to be dose dependent, ranging from $\frac{1}{2}$ to 3 hours. It is removed from the blood by the reticuloendothelial system and by metabolism by heparinase in the liver. It appears that both the clearance of heparin and heparin requirements are increased in patients with pulmonary embolic disease compared to either normal controls or patients with thrombophlebitis. Although one group found a prolonged heparin half-life in liver disease (Teien *et al.*, 1977), a second group (Simon *et al.*, 1978) found the half-life of heparin to be shortened and the clearance to be increased in patients with liver disease. Renal dysfunction did not appear to affect the kinetics. Heparin elimination is markedly reduced during hypothermia, for example, during cardiopulmonary bypass with hypothermia.

Heparin is usually administered intravenously, either by intermittent bolus or preferably by continuous infusion. When continuous infusion is used, a loading dose of 5,000 to 10,000 units is administered prior to starting the infusion. Patients usually require around 1,000 units/hour or 300 to 600 units/kg/24 hours, but the dose should be individualized by monitoring the whole blood clotting time or activated partial thromboplastin time and adjusting the dose to maintain this at 2 times normal, the first APTT test being performed 6 hours after initiating therapy with the frequency of subsequent tests dictated by the quality of control. The volume of fluid which is coadministered can be kept to a minimum by the use of a slow running infusion pump for heparin administration. Intermittent intravenous therapy can be initiated by a loading dose of 10,000 units followed by 5,000 to 10,000 units every 4 to 6 hours (or a total of 35,000 units/24 hours). The clotting studies should be monitored before the next dose is due and the dose adjusted accordingly. The conventional dose of heparin prior to the institution of cardiopulmonary bypass is 300 to 400 units/kg of body weight and 1000 to 2000 units per 500 ml of clear pump prime. However, many workers use the activated clotting time (ACT) to determine heparin requirements during cardiopulmonary bypass. The normal ACT is 90 to 105 seconds and for cardiopulmonary bypass is increased to 300 seconds by heparin administration.

Low dose subcutaneous heparin has been shown to significantly decrease the incidence of postoperative deep venous thrombosis and pulmonary emboli in patients over the age of 40 undergoing major elective abdominal-thoracic surgery. Five thousand units are administered subcutaneously 2 hours before operation, and the dose is repeated every 12 hours thereafter. It is important to begin therapy prior to surgery, as many of the clots which become clinically apparent postoperatively actually begin during the period of paralyzed immobility during the surgical procedure. No monitoring of anticoagulant effect is required during low-dose heparin therapy. The patients must have normal clotting studies and hematocrit prior to beginning therapy and should not have received any antiplatelet agents such as aspirin for at least 5 days prior to operation. The safety of this regimen is not established when spinal or epidural anesthesia is used, or in operations on the eye or brain. It is, therefore, not recommended under these circumstances. Following general surgical, orthopedic, and urological surgery, a 60 to 70% reduction in the odds of deep vein thrombosis is produced by subcutaneous heparin. The chance of pulmonary embolus occurring appears to be reduced by about 50%. It appears that low-dose heparin can slightly increase the extent of postoperative bleeding. However, the reduction in the incidence of pulmonary embolism results in an overall reduction in mortality and clearly justifies the use of low-dose heparin in patients over 40 to prevent vein thrombosis and its complications in the perioperative period.

Complications and Other Effects of Heparin

The most common complication of heparin therapy is hemorrhage. This can be minimized by careful monitoring of heparin effect using whole blood clotting time or activated partial thromboplastin time, with appropriate dosage adjustment if indicated. Particular care should be taken with women over 60 where a very high incidence of bleeding complications has been reported. Other complications of heparin therapy include alopecia (often delayed), osteoporosis and spontaneous fractures (after very prolonged therapy), hypoaldosteronism, and thrombocytopenia. Heparin also liberates lipoprotein lipase from tissues. This enzyme is responsible for hydrolyzing to fatty acids the triglycerides which circulate in blood either bound to very low density lipoproteins or in chylomicrons. This increase in free fatty acid levels is probably responsible for the reduced binding of a number of drugs in plasma samples when heparin is used during cardiopulmonary bypass and to flush "heparin locks."

Dihydroergotamine—Heparin

Dihydroergotamine, because of its vasoconstrictive effects, may decrease venous stasis during surgery and, hence, help to lessen the risk of deep vein thrombosis. A combination of 5000 units of heparin along with 0.5 mg of dihydroergotamine mesylate has been used as prophylaxis for deep vein thrombosis following surgery. However, the true additional benefit of the combination of dihydroergotamine-heparin over heparin alone is unclear, while it appears that there may be an increased risk of vasospastic adverse effects. For example, bowel necrosis, peripheral ischemia resulting in amputation, and skin and muscle necrosis have been described after the use of the dihydroergotamine-heparin combination.

PROTAMINE

Protamine is, in contrast to heparin, highly basic and combines with heparin to form stable inactive complexes. It is used to counteract the anticoagulant effects of heparin but, because it has anticoagulant activity of its own when administered in excess, the dose of protamine must be carefully titrated against either the amount of heparin *remaining* in the patient (1 mg of protamine to every 100 units of heparin remaining) or by determining by titration the amount of protamine required to overcome the anticoagulant activity of the remaining heparin in a sample of blood. Thus, since the half-life of heparin is short (approximately 90 minutes), protamine reversal is often not required, and heparin is merely discontinued. However, following termination of cardiopulmonary bypass, protamine must be administered to reverse heparin anticoagulation. When used within a very short time of heparin administration, 1.0 mg of protamine to every 100 units of heparin may be given but, after a longer time interval, the prot-

amine dose should be reduced. Various protocols have been used to calculate the exact dose of protamine required; the activated clotting time is frequently used in the operating room to determine the optimal dose of protamine for each patient.

Protamine administration has been shown to produce adverse hemodynamic effects in some patients; these reactions range from mild cardiovascular depression and transient hypotension to catastrophic systemic hypotension and pulmonary hypertension. A fall in systemic vascular resistance occurs in some patients, and many investigators have suggested that mild transient hypotension commonly associated with protamine is due predominantly to vasodilation following too rapid intravenous administration. Little evidence exists to suggest that protamine has negative inotropic effects in the human heart. There are rare reports of true anaphylaxis to protamine, with profound hypotension, decreased systemic vascular resistance, flushing, edema, and bronchospasm.

The etiology of protamine-associated cardiovascular changes is controversial; they may be due to protamine-induced histamine release, while activation of the complement system may also be important. In some of the patients who experience the catastrophic reaction of profound hypotension, pulmonary vasoconstriction, and bronchoconstriction immediately following protamine reversal of heparin, increased concentrations of thromboxane B_2 and C_{5a} anaphylatoxin fragments have been reported. Thromboxane B_2 is the stable metabolite of thromboxane A_2, a well-recognized potent pulmonary vasoconstrictor and bronchoconstrictor. Animal studies suggest that pretreatment with a cyclooxygenase inhibitor has beneficial effects on this adverse hemodynamic response to protamine. An IgE-mediated type I hypersensitivity reaction may also occur following previous exposure to protamine or to protamine-containing insulin preparations, so that antibodies against protamine are produced. Thus, insulin-dependent diabetics may have an increased risk of protamine reactions due to prior sensitization. Patients allergic to fish may also be at increased risk for the development of a hypersensitivity reaction to protamine. Adverse cardiovascular reactions to protamine have now been classified into three distinct types: type I, hypotension related to rapid drug administration; type II, anaphylactoid responses; and type III, catastrophic pulmonary vasoconstriction. The anaphylactoid responses have been further subdivided into three groups: type IIA, true anaphylaxis mediated by antibodies; type IIB, immediate anaphylactoid response not mediated by antibodies but possibly through complement activation; and type IIC, a possible less well-defined delayed anaphylactoid response that appears to have an insidious onset. To avoid hypotension, protamine must be administered slowly intravenously (not more than 50 mg in 10 minutes and at a rate not exceeding 20 mg/min). After cardiopulmonary bypass, protamine should be given slowly and cautiously, especially to patients with poor left ventricular function, who are unable to increase cardiac output in response to a fall in systemic vascular resistance.

ORAL ANTICOAGULANTS

In contrast to heparin, the orally active anticoagulants of the coumarin-indanedione class act only in vivo, having no effect in vitro. Warfarin is the most widely used drug of this class, although others, such as phenindione and dicumarol, are also used on occasion. These drugs act by inhibiting the production in the liver of the vitamin K-dependent clotting factors II, V, VII, IX, and X. Inhibition of their production while their degradation continues unchanged results in a fall in their concentration in blood. As these clotting factors have relatively long half-lives (ranging from 6 hours for factor VII to 60 hours for factor II), it takes some days for the maximal effect of a warfarin dose to be apparent.

The effects of these drugs are usually monitored by some test of the extrinsic coagulation pathway, such as the one stage prothrombin time which is depen-dent on the concentrations of factors II, V, VII, and X (factor IX is not measured by this test). The concentration of factor VII will fall first as it has the shortest half-life, so that the prothrombin time may appear to be prolonged before there has been much decrease in the levels of the other clotting factors. The aim of therapy is to prolong the prothrombin time to an extent sufficient to prevent thrombosis while minimizing the risk of hemorrhage. There is considerable variability between laboratories in the measurement of prothrombin time which is partly due to the use of different sources of thromboplastins. This has given rise to a greater intensity of anticoagulation being used in the United States than in Great Britain with consequent greater risk of hemorrhage. The introduction of a method of standardization and the reporting of prothrombin times in a standardized fashion (international normalized ratio, INR) will allow easier control and comparison between laboratories. The degree of anticoagulation, measured as the ratio of normalized patient to control prothrombin times (INR) required for adequate anticoagulation with minimal risks of bleeding, is shown in Table 22.1.

Pharmacokinetics

Warfarin is rapidly and completely absorbed from the gut. It is highly bound (99%) to plasma albumin and is an example of a low hepatic extraction compound (see Chapter 1), so that its rate of

Table 22.1.
Extent of Anticoagulation for Different Indications

Indication for Anticoagulation	INR*
Prophylaxis of DVT	1.5–2.5
Treatment of DVT or pulmonary embolus	2.0–3.0
Recurrent DVT	2.5–4.0
Arterial thromboembolism, prosthetic cardiac valve	3.0–4.5

*INR, international normalized ratio of patient's prothrombin time to control prothrombin time; DVT, deep venous thrombosis.

removal is dependent on both liver drug-metabolizing ability and the extent of protein binding. Warfarin is administered as the racemic mixture of its two optically active enantiomers. *R*- and *S*-forms of warfarin have different pharmacokinetics and give rise to complicated stereospecific pharmacokinetic interactions (for example, with phenylbutazone, discussed later). *R*-warfarin is eliminated more slowly (half-life, 35 hours), than *S*-warfarin (half-life, 24 hours). On the other hand, *S*-warfarin is about 4 times as potent as *R*-warfarin.

DOSAGE

Therapy is usually begun with a dose of 10 to 15 mg, and the subsequent doses are adjusted to maintain the prothrombin time at the appropriate level (Table 22.1). A loading dose is no longer indicated as this does not significantly increase the rate of onset of effect (which is determined by the rate of disappearance of the clotting factors) and may increase the likelihood of bleeding. Following deep venous thrombosis, 3 months of warfarin therapy appear to be adequate.

ADVERSE EFFECTS

Bleeding is the most common adverse reaction. The risk of major hemorrhage is increased by:

1. Presence of additional disease such as cardiac, renal, or hepatic dysfunction, neoplastic disease, or severe anemia;
2. Prior intravenous heparin in patients over 60 years of age;
3. Prolongation of the prothrombin time above the recommended values;
4. Worsening liver dysfunction during warfarin therapy.

The anticoagulant effects of the oral anticoagulants can be reversed by the administration of vitamin K_1 (phytanadione). However, as the synthesis of new clotting factors is required to reverse warfarin's effect, it may take at least 24 hours before the prothrombin time has returned to normal. If the situation requires more urgent action, fresh frozen plasma or concentrates of the vitamin K-dependent clotting factors may be administered.

For patients scheduled to undergo elective surgery in whom continued anticoagulation is required, the oral anticoagulant can be stopped preoperatively and heparin substituted during the perioperative period, after which oral anticoagulation can be restarted. Pregnant women should not receive warfarin because of the fetal wastage and teratogenic effects produced, and heparin is the preferred anticoagulant in pregnancy (see later in chapter). Because of the risk of hemorrhage resulting in neurological sequelae, spinal and epidural anesthesia should not be performed on patients receiving anticoagulants.

Drug Interactions

Because of its low therapeutic index and the ready identification of its dose-related toxicity (hemorrhage), drug interactions are a serious problem with warfarin administration. These can involve all of the mechanisms discussed in Chapter 4.

ABSORPTION

Cholestyramine decreases warfarin concentrations either by binding warfarin prior to its absorption from the gut or by interfering with the enterohepatic circulation, thereby decreasing the reabsorption of warfarin following biliary excretion.

METABOLISM

Drugs which alter the activity of the microsomal mixed-function oxidase system which is responsible for warfarin elimination in humans will alter plasma warfarin concentration and effect. Enzyme inducers (see Chapters 2 and 4) which increase the rate of metabolism and, hence, result in reduced warfarin effect include the barbiturates, glutethimide and rifampin (Fig. 4.1). Enzyme inhibition will result in increased anticoagulation effect and, if appropriate adjustment of dosage is not made, may cause increased risk of hemorrhage. It has been suggested that chloramphenicol and disulfiram impair the elimination of oral anticoagulants. Cimetidine has been clearly shown to slow warfarin metabolism and result in increased warfarin plasma concentrations.

Phenylbutazone produces an interesting stereoselective interaction with warfarin. It halves the plasma clearance of the more potent S-warfarin, while doubling the clearance of the less potent R-warfarin. The net effect is that the overall clearance of the racemic mixture is unchanged, while the anticoagulant effect is increased.

PROTEIN BINDING

In vitro protein binding interactions have been frequently described with warfarin. However, the clinical significance of many of these reported interactions was not critically evaluated. Our improved understanding (see Chapter 1) of the factors determining drug elimination has clarified thinking on this issue. Warfarin is an example of a low-clearance drug (see Chapter 1) whose clearance is dependent on the free fraction of drug in plasma. Increase in the free fraction will result in a transient increase in the free concentration (and possibly increased effect); however, as the clearance is increased, the total level will fall, restoring the free concentration to pretreatment levels (see Figure 1.21).

EFFECTS OF AGE

Age appears to be an important determinant of warfarin sensitivity (Fig. 22.1). As age advances, the anticoagulant response increases, in spite of the patients receiving lower warfarin doses. These changes are not explained by changes in warfarin kinetics but appear to be due to increased sensitivity to warfarin. At the same warfarin plasma concentrations, greater inhibition of vitamin K-dependent clotting factor synthesis occurs in elderly patients than is produced in the young.

ANTICOAGULATION IN PREGNANCY

Heparin is the preferred anticoagulant in pregnancy because of its poor lipid sol-

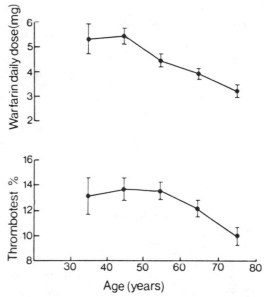

Figure 22.1. Effects of age on warfarin dose requirements and anticoagulant effect (thrombotest). As age advanced, the dose of warfarin administered fell, while the anticoagulant effect increased (reduced thrombotest). (With permission from O'Malley K, Stevenson H, Ward CA, Wood AJJ, Crooks J: Determinants of anticoagulant control in patients receiving warfarin. *Br J Clin Pharmacol* 4:309–314, 1977.)

ubility and, hence, very limited access to the fetus and the reported teratogenic effects of the oral anticoagulants. Warfarin induces a characteristic embryopathy and abnormalities of the central nervous system when given during the first trimester of pregnancy. Because of this risk, oral anticoagulants should not be given to pregnant women and should be used with caution in women of child-bearing potential.

THROMBOLYTIC THERAPY

Thrombolytic agents are listed in Table 22.2 and include *streptokinase, urokinase,* and the new *tissue plasminogen activators* (tPA) or recombianant tPA (rt-PA). The mechanism of action of the thrombolytic agents is to activate plasminogen to the fibrinolytic enzyme plas-

Table 22.2.
Pharmacologic and Clinical Features of Thrombolytic Preparations

	Streptokinase	APSAC*	Urokinase	Recombinant single-chain urokinase	Recombinant-tissue-PA
Half-life (min)	23	90	16	7	5†
Fibrin enhancement	+	+	++	++++	+++
Plasma proteolytic state	++++	++++	+++	++	+
Duration of infusion (min)	60	2–5	5–15	Several hr	Several hr
Thrombus *vs.* hemostatic plug specificity	0	0	0	0	0
Incidence of reperfusion (within 3 hr) (%)	60–70	60–70	60–70	60–70	60–70
Frequency of reocclusion (estimated %)	15	10	10	NK	20
Simultaneous administration of heparin	No	No	No	Yes	Yes
Bleeding complications	++++	++++	++++	++++	++++
Allergic side effects	Yes	Yes	No	No	No
Antigenicity	Yes	Yes	No	NK	NK

Modified with permission from Marder VJ, Sherry S: Thrombolytic therapy: current status. *N Engl J Med* 318:1512–1520, 1988.
†Terminal half-life, 41 to 50 minutes.
*APSAC, anisoylated plasminogen-streptokinase activator complex; NK, not known.

min (Fig. 22.2). In addition to circulating in plasma, plasminogen binds to fibrin during the formation of a clot. It is the activation of this fibrin-bound plasmin to lyse thrombus that is the therapeutic goal of thrombolytic therapy. However, simultaneous activation of the circulating plasma plasminogen results in the breakdown of circulating fibrinogen to fibrinogen degradation products. This so-called lytic state results in hypofibrinogenemia, increased fibrinogen degradation products, and decreased plasma concentrations of the clotting factors V and VIII. This systemic loss of hemostasis coupled with the continuous breakdown of newly formed clots results in increased risk of hemorrhage.

It was hoped that the development of plasminogen activators which are relatively selective for fibrin-bound plasmin (such as rt-PA) would result in a lower incidence of hemorrhagic complications. However, it is not clear that in clinical use the incidence of hemorrhage differs significantly between the various agents.

The risk of bleeding following the use of thrombolytic therapy is substantially increased if the patient has undergone invasive monitoring or cardiac catheterization, and it should be recognized that hemorrhage following thrombolytic therapy is not only due to the production of a systemic hypocoagulable state but is also (perhaps mainly) due to lysis of hemostatic plugs which would normally seal a site of vascular disruption. Even highly fibrin-selective agents will be unable to distinguish between the pathological thrombus responsible for obstruction of, for example, a coronary artery and the hemostatic plug which is maintaining the integrity of the vascular system.

The available agents vary considerably in the ability of fibrin to enhance their plasminogen-activating actions (Table 22.2). It is this enhancement by fibrin that conveys the relative selectivity of rt-PA and the recombinantly produced single-chain urokinase (SCU-PA). Streptokinase and urokinase, on the other hand, show much less enhancement by fibrin (Table 22.2). Conversely, the effects of streptokinase on circulating plasminogen will be greater at therapeutic doses, resulting in greater systemic fibrinolysis.

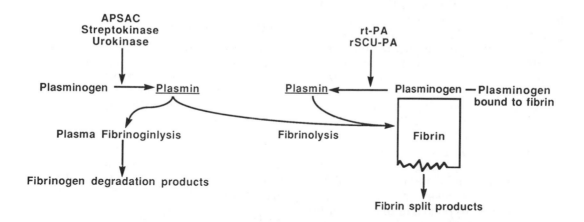

Activation of plasma plasminogen   **Activation of Fibrin bound plasminogen**

APSAC = Anisoylated plasminogen-streptokinase activator
rt-PA = recombinant tissue type plasminogen activator
rSCU-PA = recombinant single chain urokinase-PA

Figure 22.2.   Mechanism of action of plasminogen activators.   APSAC is inactive until it is deacylated in vivo to yield streptokinase. APSAC, streptokinase, and urokinase activate plasminogen in plasma to break down plasma fibrinogen, resulting in systemic fibrinolysis *(left)*. Recombinant SCU-PA and rt-PA have a greater selectivity for plasminogen bound to fibrin *(right)* and have been called "fibrin selective."

A number of thrombolytic agents have been studied. Streptokinase was the first agent to undergo widespread use in humans and is produced by streptococci. Urokinase was initially extracted from human urine but is now made using human renal cell cultures. Single-chain urokinase and rt-PA are produced using recombinant-DNA technology. Two forms of rt-PA were studied. The early studies used rt-PA made by a production technique which yielded the two-chain form, while subsequent studies used the single-chain form (Alteplase). Anisoylated plasminogen streptokinase activator complex (APSAC) is streptokinase which has been acylated at the site responsible for activation of plasmin, rendering it inactive. The complex is, however, still able to bind normally to fibrin where deacylation occurs to yield streptokinase which activates plasmin in the clot to lyse fibrin. On the other hand, acylation prevents the circulating APSAC from interacting with plasma plasminogen, and the small amount of active plasmin produced by the circulating active deacylated APSAC will be rapidly inactivated by plasma antiplasmin.

The source of the available agents determines their antigenicity and, hence, their propensity to produce allergic-type side effects (Table 22.1). Streptokinase and APSAC are products of streptococcal bacteria and, hence, are antigenic. Administration of these products stimulates an antibody response beginning 5 to 6 days after administration. Patients who have previously had streptococcal infections may have developed antibodies to streptokinase which will block its action. The recombinantly produced agents should not be antigenic themselves, but impurities introduced during the production process conceivably could be.

Indications

ACUTE MYOCARDIAL INFARCTION

Acute thrombosis of a coronary artery is the usual precipitating event for myocardial infarction. The subsequent ischemia results in progressive death of myocardium. The goal of thrombolytic therapy is myocardial preservation, not just the reopening of the thrombosed artery. That being the case, therapy needs to be undertaken as early as possible to ensure that the blood supply is restored at a time when the myocardium is still viable. In addition, having restored perfusion to the affected area, the long-term outcome is likely to be affected by the frequency of reocclusion. Thus, sustained antithrombotic effect is required to prevent the stimulus which produced occlusion in the first place from causing reocclusion. The long half-life agents which produce systemic fibrinolysis, such as streptokinase and APSAC, result in a prolonged hypocoagulable state after short-term administration, and therefore, simultaneous administration of heparin is not required to prevent reocclusion. With rt-PA because of both its shorter half-life and lesser systemic effects, heparin is coadministered to prevent reocclusion (Table 22.2).

A number of studies have shown that early intravenous administration of thrombolytic therapy reduces mortality and/or improves cardiac function in patients with myocardial infarction. The earlier in the course of the infarction thrombolytic therapy is administered, the more likely it is to be successful. The mode of administration varies between agents. Those with a long half-life can be given by a single injection either as an intravenous bolus or by a short infusion, whereas the shorter half-life agents such as rt-PA require a prolonged infusion for sustained effect. In addition, because of their greater effect on systemic hemostasis, the less fibrin-selective agents do not require the coadministration of heparin, whereas the fibrin-selective agents require heparin to prevent reocclusion. The risk of hemorrhage is similar with all the available agents.

Following successful thrombolytic therapy and reperfusion, the preexisting narrowing of the coronary artery will still be present, and definitive therapy, either transluminal angioplasty or bypass grafting, may be required. It appears that immediate angioplasty following thrombolytic therapy is neither required nor desirable and may be more dangerous than angioplasty delayed until after the acute event.

PULMONARY EMBOLISM

Administration of thrombolytic therapy to patients with a pulmonary embolism appears to result in more rapid reperfusion than the use of heparin alone. This may result in improved pulmonary perfusion later and perhaps reduce the subsequent development of pulmonary hypertension. However, the long-term benefits of thrombolytic therapy in patients following a pulmonary embolism are unclear.

DEEP VEIN THROMBOSIS

If thrombolytic therapy is administered early enough, lysis of the obstructing thrombi can be produced in a significant number of patients. However, deep vein thrombosis often does not present until the thrombosis has extended up the leg to the thigh, at which time the thrombosis is relatively mature and less susceptible to lysis. Thus, clinical presentation may not occur until too late for effective thrombolysis. The rationale for the treatment of deep vein thrombosis with thrombolytic therapy depends on whether therapy preserves the integrity of the venous valves and prevents the subsequent development of the postphlebitic syndrome. Whether thrombolytic therapy reduces the incidence of postphlebitic syndrome is unclear.

PERIPHERAL ARTERIAL OCCLUSION

Local infusion of thrombolytic agents directly into a thrombosed artery has been used to treat occlusions of peripheral arteries.

AMINOCAPROIC ACID

Aminocaproic acid is an antidote to the fibrolytic agents.

DESMOPRESSIN

Desmopressin (DDAVP; 1-desamino-8-D-arginine vasopressin), a synthetic vasopressin analogue, which does not produce the vasoconstriction seen with vasopressin itself, has been used for the treatment of patients with hemophilia and von Willebrand's disease to treat bleeding episodes and to prevent excessive blood loss when these patients undergo surgery. Administration of DDAVP results in an increase in factor VIII, von Willebrand's factor, and Ristocetin factor levels in blood. These increases seem to be sufficient to prevent bleeding in patients with mild hemophilia and patients with von Willebrand's disease undergoing surgery. The drug can be administered either intravenously or subcutaneously and is usually given intravenously prior to surgery and for a period thereafter.

Desmopressin (0.3 μg/kg of body weight) administered after protamine administration following cardiopulmonary bypass has been shown to reduce perioperative blood loss, probably due to increase in von Willebrand factor and improved platelet function. However, hypotension related to desmopressin administration has been reported following cardiopulmonary bypass. Desmopressin has also been used successfully to reduce blood loss during spinal fusion surgery and insertion of Harrington rods. In uremic patients, desmopressin shortens the bleeding time and may reduce hemorrhage.

Aprotinin is a trypsin inhibitor which inhibits plasmin's fibrinolytic activity and has been shown in some studies to reduce perioperative blood loss.

ANTIPLATELET AGENTS

These are drugs which interfere with platelet function and, therefore, have been evaluated in the prevention of thromboembolic disease. The most extensively studied in this group include aspirin, sulphinpyrazone, and dipyridamole. Aspirin and sulphinpyrazone prevent the synthesis os prostaglandins and protaglandin-like substances (see Chapter 24) from arachidonic acid, resulting in impaired platelet aggregation. Dipyridamole, on the other hand, is a phosphodiesterase inhibitor and there-

fore increases platelet cyclic AMP levels. This effect is probably responsible for dipyridamole's ability to reduce platelet adhesion as well as aggregation.

Antiplatelet drugs have been used in the following conditions:

1. Prosthetic heart valves;
2. Cerebral ischemia;
3. Venous thrombosis;
4. Myocardial ischemia and infarction.

BIBLIOGRAPHY

General

Ginsberg JS, Hirsch J: Optimum use of anticoagulants in pregnancy. *Drugs* 36:505–512, 1988.

Kaplan K: Prophylactic anticoagulation following acute myocardial infarction. *Arch Intern Med* 146:593–597, 1986.

Management of venous thromboembolism. *Lancet* 1:275–277, 1988.

Stow PJ, Burrows FA: Anticoagulants in anaesthesia. *Can J Anaesth* 34:632–649, 1987.

Oral Anticoagulants

Gallus A, Tillett J, Jackaman J, Mills W, Wycherley A: Safety and efficacy of warfarin started early after submassive venous thrombosis or pulmonary embolism. *Lancet* 2:1293–1296, 1986.

Hirsch J: Therapeutic range for the control of oral anticoagulant therapy. *Arch Intern Med* 145:1187–1188, 1985.

Holford NHG: Clinical pharmacokinetics and pharmacodynamics of warfarin: understanding the dose-effect relationship. *Clin Pharmacokinet* 11:483–504, 1986.

Hull R, Hirsh J, Jay R, Carter C, England C, Gent M, Turpie AGG, McLoughlin D, Dodd P, Thomas M, Raskob G, Ockelford P: Different intensities of oral anticoagulant therapy in the treatment of proximal-vein thrombosis. *N Engl J Med* 307:1676–1681, 1982.

Landefeld CS, Cook EF, Flatley M, Weisberg M, Goldman L: Identification and preliminary validation of predictors of major bleeding in hospitalized patients starting anticoagulant therapy. *Am J Med* 82:703–713, 1987.

Levine MN, Raskob G, Hirsh J: Risk of hemorrhage associated with long term anticoagulant therapy. *Drugs* 30:444–460, 1985.

O'Malley K, Stevenson IH, Ward CA, Wood AJJ, Crooks J: Determinants of anticoagulant control in patients receiving warfarin. *Br J Clin Pharmacol* 4:309–314, 1977.

Oral anticoagulant control. *Lancet* 2:488–489, 1987.

Roy D, Marchand E, Gagne P, Chabot M, Cartier R: Usefulness of anticoagulant therapy in the prevention of embolic complications of atrial fibrillation. *Am Heart J* 112:1039–1043, 1986.

Shepherd AMM, Hewick DS, Moreland TA, Stevenson IH: Age as a determinant of sensitivity to warfarin. *Br J Clin Pharmacol* 4:315–320, 1977.

Wessler S, Gitel SN: Warfarin: from bedside to bench. *N Engl J Med* 311:645–652, 1984.

Wilcox CM, Truss CD: Gastrointestinal bleeding in patients receiving long-term anticoagulant therapy. *Am J Med* 84:683–690, 1988.

Heparin

Bjornsson TD, Wolfram KM, Kitchell BB: Heparin kinetics determined by three assay methods. *Clin Pharmacol Ther* 31:104–113, 1982.

Cipolle RJ, Seifert RD, Neilan BA, Zaske DE, Hause E: Heparin kinetics: variables related to disposition and dosage. *Clin Pharmacol Ther* 29:387–393, 1981.

Cohen JA, Frederickson EL, Kaplan JA: Plasma heparin activity and antagonism during cardiopulmonary bypass with hypothermia. *Anesth Analg* 56:564–570, 1977.

Collins R, Scrimgeour A, Yusuf S, Peto R: Reduction in fatal pulmonary embolism and venous thrombosis by perioperative administration of subcutaneous heparin. *N Engl J Med* 318:1162–1173, 1988.

Council on Thrombosis of the American Heart Association. Prevention of venous thromboembolism in surgical patients by low-dose heparin. *Circulation* 55:423–426A, 1977.

Ellison N: Heparin: new information on an old drug. *J Cardiothor Anes* 1:377–378, 1987.

Green D, Lee MY, Ito VY, Cohn T, Press J, Filbrandt PR, VandenBerg WC, Yarkony GM, Meyer PR: Fixed- vs. adjusted-dose heparin in the prophylaxis of thromboembolism in spinal cord injury. *JAMA* 260:1255–1258, 1988.

Hull RD, Rasbob GE, Hirsh, J, Jay RM, Leclerc JR, Geerts WH, Rosenbloom D, Sackett DL, Anderson C, Harrison L, Gent M: Continuous intravenous heparin compared with intermittent subcutaneous heparin in the initial treatment of proximal-vein thrombosis. *N Engl J Med* 315:1109–1114, 1986.

King DJ, Kelton JG: Heparin-associated thrombocytopenia. *Ann Intern Med* 100:535–540, 1984.

Ockelford P: Heparin 1986: indications and effective use. *Drugs* 31:81–92, 1986.

Salzman EW: Low-molecular-weight heparin: is small beautiful? *N Engl J Med* 315:957–959, 1986.

Turpie AGG, Levine NM, Hirsh J, Carter CJ, Jay RM, Powers PJ, Andrew M, Hull RD, Gent M: A randomized controlled trial of a low-molecular-weight heparin (enoxaparin) to prevent deep-vein thrombosis in patients undergoing elective hip surgery. *N Engl J Med* 315:925–929, 1986.

Protamine

Casthely PA, Goodman K, Fyman PN, Abrams LM, Aaron D: Hemodynamic changes after the administration of protamine. *Anesth Analg* 65:78–80, 1986.

Chung F, Miles J: Cardiac arrest following protamine administration. *Can Anaesth Soc J* 31:314–318, 1984.

Colman RW: Humoral mediators of catastrophic reactions associated with protamine neutralization. *Anesthesiology* 66:595–596, 1987.

Conahan TJ, Andrews RW, MacVaugh H: Cardiovascular effects of protamine sulfate in man. *Anesth Analg* 60:33–36, 1981.

Conzen PF, Habazettl H, Guttmann R, Hobbhahn J, Goetz AE, Peter K, Brendel W: Thromboxane medication of pulmonary hemodynamic responses after neutralization of heparin by protamine in pigs. *Anesth Analg* 68:25–31, 1989.

Dutton DA, Hothersall AP, McLaren AD, Taylor KM, Turner MA: Protamine titration after cardiopulmonary bypass. *Anaesthesia* 38:264–268, 1983.

Hines RL, Barash PG: Protamine: does it alter right ventricular function? *Anesth Analg* 65:1271–1274, 1986.

Hobbhahn J, Conzen PF, Zenker B, Goetz AE, Peter K, Brendel W: Beneficial effect of cyclooxygenase inhibition on adverse hemodynamic responses after protamine. *Anesth Analg* 67:253–260, 1988.

Horrow JC: Protamine: a review of its toxicity. *Anesth Analg* 64:348–361, 1985.

Kim YD, Michalik R, Lees DE, Jones M, Hanowell S, Macnamara TE: Protamine induced arterial hypoxaemia: the relationship to hypoxic pulmonary vasoconstriction. *Can Anaesth Soc J* 32:5–11, 1985.

Lowenstein E, Johnston WE, Lappass DG, D'Ambra MN, Schneider RC, Daggett WM, Akins CW, Philbin DM: Catastrophic pulmonary vascoconstriction associated with protamine reversal of heparin. *Anesthesiology* 59:470–473, 1983.

Michaels IAL, Barash PG: Hemodynamic changes during protamine administration. *Anesth Analg* 62:831–835, 1983.

Morel DR, Lowenstein E, Nguyenduy T, Robinson DR, Repine JE, Chenoweth DE, Zapol WM: Acute pulmonary vasoconstricton and thromboxane release during protamine reversal of heparin anticoagulation in awake sleep. *Circ Res* 62:905–915, 1988.

Morel DR, Zapol WM, Thomas SJ, Kitain EM, Robinson DR, Moss J, Chenoweth DE, Lowenstein E: C5a and thromboxane generation associated with pulmonary vaso- and broncho-constriction during protamine reversal of heparin. *Anesthesiology* 66:597–604, 1987.

Shapira N, Schaff HV, Piehler JM, White RD, Sill JC, Pluth JR: Cardiovascular effects of protamine sulfate in man. *J Thorac Cardiovasc Surg* 84:505–514, 1982.

Tan F, Jackman H, Skidgel RA, Zsigmond EK, Erdos EG: Protamine inhibits plasma carboxypeptidase N, the inactivator of anaphylatoxins and kinins. *Anesthesiology* 70:267–275, 1987.

Thrombolytic Therapy

GISSI Coordinating Group: Long-term effects of intravenous thrombolysis in acute myocardial infarction: final report of the GISSI study. *Lancet* 2:871–874, 1987.

Goldhaber SZ, Buring JE, Lipnick RJ, Hennekens CH: Pooled analyses of randomized trials of streptokinase and heparin in phlebographically documented acute deep venous thrombosis. *Am J Med* 76:393–397, 1984.

Ikram S, Lewis S, Bucknal C, Sram I, Thomas N, Vincent R, Chamberlain D: Treatment of acute myocardial infarction with anisoylated plasminogen streptokinase activator complex. *Br Med J* 293:786–789, 1986.

I.S.A.M. Study Group: A prospective trial of intravenous streptokinase in acute myocardial infarction (I.S.A.M.). *N Engl J Med* 314:1465–1471, 1986.

Loscalzo J, Braunwald E, Tissue plasminogen activator. *N Engl J Med* 319:925–931, 1988.

Marder VJ, Sherry S: Thrombolytic therapy: current status; part 1. *N Engl J Med* 318:1512–1520, 1988.

Marder VJ, Sherry S: Thrombolytic therapy: current status; part 2. *N Engl J Med* 318:1585–1595, 1988.

Rao AK, Pratt C, Berke A, Jaffe A, Ockene I, Schreiber TL, Bell WR, Knatterud G, Robertson TL, Terrin ML: Thrombolysis in myocardial infarction (TIMI) trial—phase I: hemorrhagic manifestations and changes in plasma fibrinogen and the fibrinolytic system in patients treated with recombinant tissue plasminogen activator and streptokinase. *J Am Coll Cardiol* 11:1–11, 1988.

Sheehan FH, Braunwald E, Canner P, *et al*: The effect of intravenous thrombolytic therapy on left ventricular function: a report on tissue-type plasminogen activator and streptokinase from the thrombolysis in myocardial infarction (TIMI phase I) trial. *Circulation* 75:817–829, 1987.

TIMI Research Group: Immediate vs. delayed catheterization and angioplasty following thrombolytic therapy for acute myocardial infarction. *JAMA* 260:2849–2858, 1988.

Williams DO, Borer J, Braunwald E, *et al*: Intravenous recombinant tissue-type plasminogen activator in patients with acute myocardial infarction: a report from the NHLBI thrombolysis in myocardial infarction trial. *Circulation* 73:338–346, 1986.

Desmopressin

Can drugs reduce surgical blood loss? *Lancet* 1:155–156, 1988.

Czer LS, Bateman TM, Gray RJ, Raymond M, Stewart ME, Lee S, Goldfinger D, Chaux A, Matloff JM: Treatment of severe platelet dysfunction and hemorrhage after cardiopulmonary bypass: reduction in blood product usage with desmopressin. *J Am Coll Cardiol* 9:1139–1147, 1987.

D'Alauro FS, Johns RA: Hypotension related to desmopressin administration following cardiopulmonary bypass. *Anesthesiology* 69:962–963, 1988.

Harker LA: Bleeding after cardiopulmonary bypass. *N Engl J Med* 314:1446–1448, 1986.

Kobrinsky NL, Letts M, Patel LR, Israels ED, Monson RC, Schwetz N, Cheang MS: 1-Desamino-8-D-arginine vasopressin (desmopressin) decreases operative blood loss in patients having Harrington rod spinal fusion surgery. *Ann Intern Med* 107:446–450, 1987.

Remuzzi G: Bleeding in renal failure. *Lancet* 1:1205–1208, 1988.

Rocha E, Llorens R, Paramo JA, Arcas R, Cuesta B, Trenor AM: Does desmopressin acetate reduce blood loss after surgery in patients on cardiopulmonary bypass? *Circulation* 77:1319–1323, 1988.

Salzman EW, Weinstein MJ, Weintraub RM, Ware JA, Thurer RL, Robertson L, Donovan A, Gaffney T, Bertele V, Troll J, Smith M, Chute LE: Treatment with desmopressin acetate to reduce blood loss after cardiac surgery. *N Engl J Med* 314:1402–1406, 1986.

Sieber PR, Belis JA, Jarowenko MV, Rohner TJ: Desmopressin control of surgical hemorrhage secondary to prolonged bleeding time. *J Urol* 139:1066–1067, 1987.

23

Histamine and Histamine H$_1$- and H$_2$-Receptor Antagonists; 5-Hydroxytryptamine, Kinins, and the Carcinoid Syndrome; Angiotensin and the Renin-Angiotensin System

R. A. BRANCH
MARGARET WOOD

HISTAMINE

Histamine is a naturally occurring amine, which is formed by decarboxylation of the amino acid histidine under the control of the enzyme L-histidine decarboxylase. The chemical structure of histamine is given in Figure 23.1.

PHARMACOLOGICAL EFFECTS

Histamine relaxes the smooth muscle of the arterioles and fine blood vessels

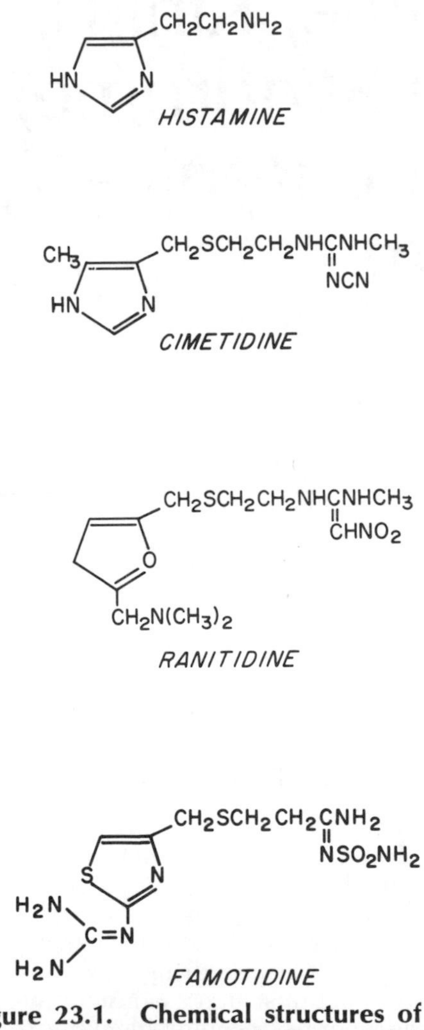

Figure 23.1.   Chemical structures of histamine, cimetidine, ranitidine, and famotidine.   Cimetidine is an imidazole derivative, ranitidine is a substituted furan, and famotidine belongs to the guanidinothiazole group.

leading to a fall in peripheral resistance and arterial blood pressure. Histamine causes capillary dilation throughout the body resulting in the skin of the face and upper part of the body becoming hot and flushed. In addition, capillary permeability to plasma increases and edema may form. When histamine is injected intradermally in humans, a characteristic response (triple response) occurs which comprises (a) a local red response, (b) red flush or flare, and (c) a wheal. The cardiac effects of histamine include increased myocardial contractility and heart rate, and the production of arrhythmias. Histamine generally stimulates extravascular smooth muscle of the gut and bronchi. Histamine has a marked effect on gastric secretion, increasing the acid and pepsin content of gastric juice. Histamine release in the skin can cause pain and itch. The adrenal medulla is stimulated to release epinephrine and norepinephrine; this is usually unimportant in normal subjects but may be sufficient to raise the blood pressure in patients with pheochromocytoma. Administration of histamine has been used as a diagnostic test in this syndrome.

FACTORS AFFECTING HISTAMINE RELEASE

Histamine is one of several vasoactive hormones that are released during anaphylactic or allergic reactions, stress, and injury and by drugs, peptides, snake venoms, and other agents. Drugs that have been implicated in causing histamine release include morphine and muscle relaxants such as d-tubocurarine, atropine, and dextran. Occasionally, the intravenous injection of these drugs may cause bronchospasm and acute circulatory collapse. In addition, the stimulation of the smooth muscle of the gut results in colic, nausea, vomiting, and diarrhea.

HISTAMINE RECEPTORS

Histamine is now known to act in an analogous manner to the neurotransmitters of the adrenergic nervous system, via membrane-located specific receptors, with the individual response being determined by the type of cell being stimulated. There are two populations of receptors for histamine, designated H_1 and H_2, that exhibit specific structural requirements for both binding and pharmacological activity. It has been possible to develop analogs of histamine which can either bind to and stimulate the receptor (agonists) or bind to and prevent histamine gaining access to the receptor (competitive antagonists). The pharmacological effects of histamine such as contraction of the intestine are mediated by stimulation of the H_1-receptors, while the major role of the H_2-receptor is related to acid production by parietal cells in the stomach. H_1-receptors have been found on mast cells, all smooth muscle cells, and in the brain, while H_2-receptors have been found on gastric parietal cells, in vascular smooth muscle, and in the brain where they have been linked to control of prolactin production.

The hypotension due to capillary dilation results from a direct action of histamine on blood vessels and is mediated by both H_1- and H_2-receptors. Histamine increases heart rate, but also slows A-V conduction and, thus, may cause dysrhythmias. The positive chronotropic effects are thought to be due to H_2-receptor stimulation, while slowing of A-V conduction is due to activation of H_1-receptors. Infusion of histamine in normal subjects produces a positive inotropic and positive chronotropic response due to direct stimulation of myocardial H_2-receptors. In summary, therefore, H_2-receptors are mainly responsible for the effects of histamine on gastric secretion and heart rate, while the other effects of histamine are mediated via H_1-receptors. The exception to this rule is that the effect on blood pressure is due to stimulation of H_1- and H_2-receptors and is blocked only by a combination of H_1- and H_2-receptor antagonists. A combination of H_1- and H_2-receptor antagonism has been shown to attenuate the cardiovascular response to morphine administration in patients undergoing cardiac surgery, presumably secondary to the blockade of the effects of morphine-induced histamine release.

In the 1940s, the development of a group of compounds, in which the side chain structure was maintained but the imidazole ring was modified, produced **H₁-receptor antagonists** that blocked the inflammatory, bronchial, and gut smooth muscle activity of histamine. These H_1-receptor blocking agents have no effect on gastric acid production and only a partial effect on the peripheral vasodilation response. In 1972, Black and coworkers developed a group of compounds in which the imidazole ring was left intact but the side chain was modified, resulting in **H₂-receptor antagonists** (Fig. 23.1), which did not affect H_1 responses, but completely inhibited gastric acid production. From this early work, first metiamide (which was withdrawn due to bone marrow toxicity) and later cimetidine were developed for use in humans. More recently, a number of further analogs have been or are being developed as alternatives to cimetidine, for example, ranitidine and famotidine (Fig. 23.1).

A similarity between the adrenergic receptors and the histamine receptors is the concept of selectivity. Histamine and histamine-like agonists stimulate both H_1- and H_2-receptors, with analogs possessing varying selectivity ranging from being predominantly active at the H_1-receptor, equally active at both receptors, or being predominantly active at the H_2-receptor. In contrast, antagonists predominantly inhibit either H_1- or H_2-receptors and leave the other responses intact.

H₁-RECEPTOR ANTAGONISTS

PHARMACOLOGICAL EFFECTS

The pharmacological effects of the H_1-receptor blocking agents can be predicted from a knowledge of the action of histamine on the H_1-receptor. The collective terminology for this group of drugs of "antihistamine" is unsatisfactory because many of these drugs have numerous other actions such as anticholinergic or α-adrenergic receptor blocking properties. However, in general, H_1-receptor antagonists inhibit the increased capillary permeability, flare, and itch responses to histamine and, to some extent, prevent the relaxation of vascular smooth muscle. The residual vasodilation can only be antagonized by the concomitant administration of an H_2-receptor blocking agent. H_1-receptor blocking agents can prevent the effects of histamine on skin and mucous membranes. Although H_1-receptor antagonist drugs can improve bronchoconstriction due to histamine release caused by drugs, they are of little use in the treatment of asthma or allergic bronchoconstriction in humans, presumably because other mediators are also involved. They have no effect on histamine-induced gastric secretion.

PHARMACOKINETICS

The H_1-receptor blocking agents are well absorbed from the gastrointestinal tract and are mainly metabolized in the liver. Diphenhydramine when administered orally achieves peak blood concentrations in about 2 hours and has a plasma terminal half-life of about 3.5 hours.

SIDE EFFECTS

All H_1-receptor blocking agents exert unwanted side effects, which include sedation with a reduction in mental acuity and reflex reaction time, dizziness, fatigue, insomnia, nervousness, diplopia, tremors, gastrointestinal disturbances, and a dry respiratory tract. The combination of ethanol with other psychotropic agents produces additive cerebral effects. Dermatitis and, rarely, agranulocytosis may occur. Newer nonsedating antihistamines (for example, **terfanadine**) are now available. These drugs do not readily penetrate the blood-brain barrier at usual therapeutic doses and, therefore, terfanadine does not cause central nervous system side effects.

THERAPEUTIC USES

H_1-receptor blocking agents have been used in the treatment of allergic diseases such as urticaria and seasonal rhinitis. They are of limited value in the treatment of anaphylaxis and angioedema, and epinephrine is the drug of choice in such life-threatening situations.

PREPARATIONS

Available H_1-receptor blocking agents include diphenhydramine (Benadryl), dimenhydrinate (Dramamine), carbinoxamine (Clistin), tripelennamine (PBZ), chlorpheniramine (Chlortrimeton), brompheniramine (Dimetane), cyclizine (Marezine), and promethazine (Phenergan). The adult oral dose of diphenhydramine is 25 to 50 mg; chlorpheniramine, 2 to 4 mg, and promethazine, 25 to 50 mg. **Terfanadine** (Seldane) is a specific H_1-receptor antagonist which binds to both peripheral and central nervous system H_1-receptors but, because it does not readily cross the blood-brain barrier, does not cause central nervous system effects. It is widely used in the treatment of allergic rhinitis and urticaria. The adult oral dose of terfanadine is 60 mg, twice daily.

H_2-RECEPTOR ANTAGONISTS

The development of H_2-receptor antagonists provides a classical example of the phased development of different generations of drugs. The prototype H_2-receptor antagonist, metiamide, the first administered to humans, was effective but induced bone marrow depression in a minority of subjects. Replacement of the sulfur atom in the side chain with a cyanimino group resulted in cimetidine, a drug which is not toxic to bone marrow. The relatively low incidence of side effects, together with its efficacy in inhibiting gastric acid production, resulted in an exponential growth in the use of cimetidine until it became the most widely administered drug, worldwide. However, with such extensive use, benefits and limitations (such as a short duration of pharmacological action and side effects discussed in the next section) became apparent. This provided the stimulus to develop third generation drugs which inhibit gastric acid production for longer and are less likely to produce some of the side effects seen with cimetidine.

Cimetidine

Cimetidine is an H_2-receptor antagonist that is widely used by anesthesiologists as part of a premedicant regimen to control gastric acid production prior to anesthesia. With its extensive use in a variety of other clinical situations, its potential benefits and limitations are now more clearly appreciated. Cimetidine induces a decrease in gastric acid secretion which is related to the plasma concentration of the drug (Fig. 23.2). At concentrations of about 0.2 μg/ml, there is a minor degree of inhibition of acid production, maximal inhibition occurs with levels of about 0.6 μg/ml, and above this, there is no further therapeutic benefit to be achieved with higher plasma concentrations. As the H₂-receptor is the final common pathway for stimuli for acid secretion, cimetidine inhibits not only overnight basal acid secretion and food-stimulated acid secretion but also acid production due to pentagastrin, histamine, caffeine, and cholinergic agonists. In contrast to its effect on acid production, cimetidine does not influence the lower esophageal pressure, rate of gastric emptying, volume of gastric juice,

production of intrinsic factor, pancreatic function, or intestinal motility.

PHARMACOKINETICS

Oral cimetidine is rapidly absorbed with a bioavailability of approximately 70 to 80%. The drug is optimally given with or directly after meals, when its absorption and duration of action are prolonged. Renal elimination accounts for 80% of total elimination and is impaired linearly with both reduction in renal function and age. Thus, caution must be used in both these groups of patients, and the dosage interval should be lengthened or the dose reduced. The reduced clearance in the elderly allows the dose to be reduced by a half to one-third (see Fig. 1.30). Nonrenal elimination is largely due to metabolism to the sulfoxide by mixed-function oxidase enzymes. In normal subjects, the half-life of cimetidine is 1.5 to 2.5 hours. Total clearance is approximately 10 ml·min⁻¹·kg⁻¹ and the volume of distribution is 1 L·kg⁻¹.

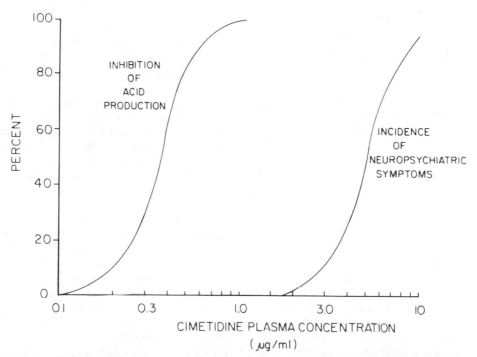

Figure 23.2. Relationship between the plasma concentration of cimetidine and, on the *left*, the percentage of inhibition of gastric acid secretion; on the *right*, the percentage of patients expected to develop neuropsychiatric symptoms.

SUGGESTED DOSAGE AND
ADMINISTRATION

A single oral dose of 300 mg of cimetidine to a normal subject will achieve a
peak plasma concentration of approximately 1.2 μg/ml (i.e., well above maximal inhibition of acid secretion, but
below the toxic range in Fig. 23.2). This
dose will provide almost complete acid
inhibition for a period of 6 to 8 hours
under basal overnight conditions and
after food with normal activity. In elderly
patients and patients with impaired renal
function, the initial peak levels are unchanged, but the duration of action is
prolonged. Furthermore, if repeated
doses are being administered to patients
with reduced renal function, then accumulation possibly to toxic levels is to be
anticipated.

In normal subjects, the generally recommended dose for deuodenal ulcer
therapy is 300 mg orally 4 times daily,
taken with meals (delays absorption and
prolongs action) and with the last dose
taken on retiring to bed.

In acutely ill patients, cimetidine can
be given intravenously. Assuming that
the pharmacokinetic objective is to
achieve a plasma concentration (C_p) of 1
μg/ml, then an initial loading dose of 1
mg/kg should be required.

$$\text{Dose} = V_d \times C_p$$

where V_d, the volume of distrubition, is 1
$L \cdot kg^{-1}$.

In order to maintain a constant level of
1 μg/ml and assuming normal renal function so that cimetidine clearance (Cl) is
10 ml $\cdot$ min$^{-1} \cdot$ kg^{-1}, a constant rate of infusion (I) of 0.6 mg/kg$^{-1} \cdot$ hour^{-1} is
required.

$$I = Cl \times C_p$$

Thus, a 70-kg individual will require approximately 340 mg each 8 hours (Fig.
23.3). If creatinine clearance is reduced,
the same bolus dose should be given, but
the rate of infusion should be decreased
in proportion to the reduction in creatinine clearance. If no dosage reduction occurs, then the normal dosage regimen
would be expected to result in accumulation to toxic levels as indicated by the

dashed lines in Figure 23.3. Cimetidine
(300 mg or 400 mg) may be given orally
on the evening before and on the morning (at least 60 minutes before induction)
of surgery to decrease the acidity of gastric contents prior to the induction of anesthesia. Intravenous administration (200
mg in 50 ml infused over 15 minutes) of
cimetidine has also been demonstrated to
be effective 45 to 60 minutes following
injection.

SIDE EFFECTS

The rapid acceptance of cimetidine
into clinical practice attests to the ease of
use of this drug and its relative lack of
side effects. However, side effects do
occur. The most important, in that it is
preventable, is the dose-related, reversible, neuropsychiatric disturbances of
confusion, slurred speech, hallucinations, delerium, and coma, which commonly occur when plasma concentrations rise above 1.5 μg/ml. These
disturbances have been most often found
in the elderly and in patients with impaired renal function, who have not had
their dosage regimen modified appropriately. A second, adverse reaction of importance to anesthesiologists is its ability
to inhibit the metabolism of other drugs
that are metabolized by the mixed function oxidase enzyme system. Cimetidine
has been shown to inhibit the metabolism of many drugs, including propranolol, metoprolol, lidocaine, diazepam, and
warfarin. Pharmacokinetic drug interactions with cimetidine are due to the
binding of its imidazole group to the
heme portion of cytochrome P-450, and it
is thus an inhibitor of phase I drug metabolism (see page 44). Cimetidine does
not inhibit conjugation mechanisms and
therefore does not affect morphine disposition. Although cimetidine inhibits
the oxidation of diazepam, the glucuronidation of lorazepam and oxazepam is
spared. The effect of cimetidine on anesthetic metabolism has been investigated
in both laboratory studies and humans.
Cimetidine has been shown to inhibit the
oxidative defluorination of methoxyflu-
raine to inorganic fluoride which is responsible for acute polyuria that can be
associated with methoxyflurane; how-

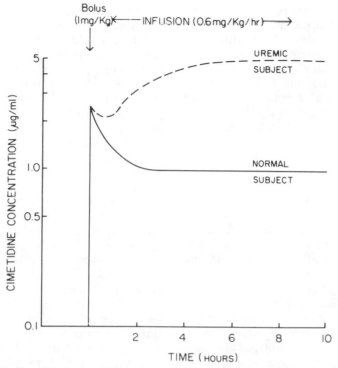

Figure 23.3.   Idealized bolus and infusion of cimetidine to achieve a plasma concentration of 1 µg/ml in a subject with normal renal function (*solid line*) and the same bolus and infusion to a patient with anuria (*dotted line*).

ever, the degree of inhibition is insufficient to allow safe increased use of methoxyflurane. Cimetidine also inhibits the oxidative metabolism of halothane to trifluoroacetic acid and bromide, but does not inhibit the in vivo defluorination of halothane or enflurane under normal conditions. Bradycardia, dangerous arrhythmias, and cardiac arrest have occurred in a small number of patients after oral and particularly after intravenous administration. Cimetidine (200 mg given intravenously over 1 minute) has been shown to reduce blood pressure in intensive care unit patients. It has been suggested that cimetidine, if it is to be given intravenously, should be diluted or injected in an infusion, especially if the patient has severe renal disease. Minor effects have been attributed to an antiandrogen effect, with sperm counts in men being reduced by 40%. This was associated with a reduced pituitary response in releasing luteinizing hormone following administration of gonadotrophin releas-

ing hormone. A small proportion of male patients develop gynecomastia due to elevated serum prolactin levels. A slight rise in serum creatinine almost always occurs and is due to altered renal tubular transport of creatinine rather than a change in glomerular filtration rate. The ability of cimetidine to inhibit renal tubule cation transport can also result in impaired renal elimination of cationic drugs, such as procainamide, producing toxicity by enhanced effect or drug interactions.

THERAPEUTIC USES

Anesthetic Premedication. Aspiration of gastric contents during or after general anesthesia can cause serious lung damage and death. A pH value of less than 2.5 is generally considered the critical level for the development of pulmonary damage. Routine pretreatment with an antacid is established practice in obstetric anesthesia, and, cimetidine, by reducing gastric acid secretion, may be effective for prophylaxis against pulmonary aspiration of acid gastric contents. It has been demonstrated that oral cimetidine, 300 mg, given 90 to 300 minutes preoperatively increased gastric pH above 2.5 in 75% of patients, while in the control patients who did not receive cimetidine only 25% had values over 2.5. When surgical patients were given intravenous cimetidine, 4.5 mg/kg, 45 minutes before induction of anesthesia, 90% had a gastric pH value above 2.5. Cimetidine crosses the blood-brain and placental barrier, apparently without ill effects on the fetus. Although cimetidine decreases bupivacaine clearance when bupivacaine is given intravenously to male volunteers, it has no effect on bupivacaine concentrations during parturition when bupivacaine is given for epidural anesthesia. In conclusion, it appears that cimetidine may play a useful role in the prevention of chemical pneumonitis in both the surgical and obstetric patient.

Duodenal Ulcer. There are now numerous clinical trials indicating the efficacy of cimetidine in the treatment of duodenal ulcer, in providing rapid symptomatic relief, and short-term ulcer healing. However, the long term natural history of duodenal ulcer disease of exacerbations and remissions is not altered so that most patients relapse without continued treatment.

Gastric Ulcer and Gastric Cancer. At the present time, the current general consensus is that cimetidine does provide symptomatic benefit and contributes to ulcer healing in approximately 75% of patients. However, a therapeutic trial without a definitive diagnosis has a risk of overlooking gastric carcinoma, as patients with carcinoma may have their pain relieved.

Acute Esophagitis. Cimetidine causes symptomatic benefit in those patients who have gastric rather than biliary reflux into the esophagus.

Chronic Pancreatitis. Patients with chronic pancreatitis receiving pancreatic supplements have improved fat absorption if cimetidine is administered concurrently. The reduction in acid allows more orally administered pancreatic ex-

tract to pass into the small intestine without being denatured.

Zollinger Ellison Syndrome. There are increasing numbers of case reports of successful management of patients with Zollinger Ellison syndrome, particularly in those patients who have either undergone previous surgery or who are a poor operative risk.

Prophylaxis in the Critically Ill. Cimetidine is now extensively administered to acutely ill patients with the objective of diminishing the incidence of stress ulcers. However, these patients often have impaired renal function so that drug accumulation to toxic levels can easily occur if doses are not modified. Furthermore, these patients often have neurological deficits, and further drug-induced cerebral dysfunction may confuse the clinical picture. It should also be remembered that cimetidine also has the potential to inhibit the metabolism of coadministered drugs (see previous discussion). A further problem is that by increasing gastric pH, the protective effect of gastric acidity in preventing bacteria from entering the body is lost, and it has been suggested that this may be a significant factor in the etiology of systemic infections in patients in intensive care units.

Systemic Mastocytosis and Gastric Carcinoid. Patients with both systemic mastocytosis and gastric carcinoid are subject to episodic release of large amounts of histamine which can cause life-threatening episodes of hypotension. In patients with gastric carcinoid, the effects appear to be due to histamine release alone, as considerable symptomatic benefit can be achieved with a combination of H_1- and H_2-receptor blocking drugs, though it should be remembered that these drugs act by competition, so that if circulating levels of histamine are high, then appropriately high levels of antagonist are required to block a response. In systemic mastocytosis, not all of the effects can be attributed to excess histamine release, as high levels of H_1- and H_2-blockers fail to suppress some of the symptoms. Such patients have been observed to have excess secretion of the prostaglandin, PGD$_2$ (see Chapter 24), and inhibition of its release by a cyclooxygenase inhibitor such as aspirin or indomethacin results in a further improvement in decreasing the frequency and severity of hypotensive episodes.

Newer H$_2$-Receptor Antagonists

The extensive market for H$_2$-receptor antagonists and the appreciation of the limitations of cimetidine have resulted in a search for newer analogs. The major objectives of this search have been to find more potent compounds in the hope that, with a smaller amount of drug being required to achieve the same level of acid inhibition, there will be less non-H$_2$-receptor-mediated adverse reactions or, alternatively, to find a drug whose kinetics permits once or twice daily therapy, rather than 4 times a day administration originally advocated for cimetidine. New H$_2$-receptor antagonists include **ranitidine, famotidine** and **nizatidine**. Table 23.1 indicates that both ranitidine and famotidine appear to have met these objectives without the appearance as yet of any new adverse responses not observed with cimetidine. As both new drugs are available in intravenous and oral formulations, both will be expected to be used widely. Several aspects are worth emphasizing in comparing these three drugs (Table 23.1): (*a*) The therapeutic efficiency of each of these drugs has been equal in all situations investigated. (*b*) By far the greatest experience has been obtained with cimetidine, and the extent of its use has in large part been due to its low incidence of side effects. (*c*) The actual duration of acid inhibition by each of these drugs is almost identical, and the changes in recommendation of prescribing four, two, or one dose a day largely reflect experience over time that indicates that the major therapeutic benefit in peptic ulcer patients is achieved by overnight acid inhibition rather than needing 24-hour inhibition. This can be achieved to an equivalent extent with all three drugs. Thus, the true therapeutic difference between drugs is small. In a situation of therapeutic equivalence, cost can be a rational deciding factor. The one situation of therapeutic nonequivalence is in the severely ill patient requiring prophylactic acid inhibition where renal function may be impaired and there is a need to avoid the neuropsychiatric effects of cimetidine. In this situation, ranitidine has been found to be easy to use, effective, and safe, while evidence with famotidine has not yet been well established.

PHARMACOLOGICAL CONTROL OF GASTRIC ACID PRODUCTION AND VOLUME

The acid aspiration syndrome is a serious complication of general anesthesia,

Table 23.1.
Comparison of H$_2$-Receptor Antagonists

	Cimetidine	Ranitidine	Famotidine
Ability to inhibit acid production	+++	+++	+++
Ability to inhibit pepsin	+++	+++	+++
Relative potency (in comparison to cimetidine)	1	5	32
Neuropsychiatric side effects	+	−	−
Pituitary stimulation	+	−	−
Antiandrogen effect	+	−	−
Inhibition of drug metabolism	++	+	−
Inhibition of cation transport	+	−	−
Frequency recommended for drug administration (doses per day)	4	2	1

and anesthesiologists strive to prevent its occurrence. Mendelson's syndrome (1946) results from the aspiration of stomach contents during childbirth and is most likely to occur if the pH of the gastric contents is below 2.5 and its volume above 25 ml. Thus pharmacological measures are taken to prevent inhalation of acid gastric contents by:

1. Regulation of gastric acid production
2. Regulation of intragastric volume

A variety of anesthetic regimens have been recommended for use in anesthetic practice to raise intragastric pH and reduce the volume of gastric contents at the time of induction of anesthesia. A combination of antacid with an H_2-receptor antagonist is today routine anesthetic practice in many institutions. In many instances, the gastroprokinetic drug metoclopramide may be added to the regimen (see page 89). The combination of metoclopramide and cimetidine is more effective in reducing volume and increasing intragastric pH than either drug alone.

Pharmacologic Regulation of Gastric Acid Secretion

Gastric acid is secreted by parietal cells in the fundus of the stomach. Cells in the fundus are highly resistant to the low gastric pH; thus disease processes aggravated by gastric acid, such as gastric ulcers, duodenal ulcers, esophagitis, and acid inhalation pneumonia, occur at distant sites from the area of production. Gastric acid production is due to an H^+,K^+-ATPase, located on the canalicular membrane of the parietal cell, which acts as a proton pump (Fig. 23.4). The activity of this pump is primarily determined by the intracellular level of cAMP. Numerous hormones, acting via their own specific receptors, can influence cAMP. Of these, the most important are

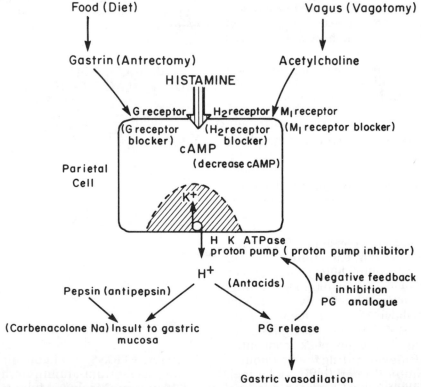

Figure 23.4.   Schematic illustration of the regulation of gastric acid secretion indicating potential sites of intervention.

histamine via the H$_2$-receptor, acetylcholine via the muscarinic (M$_1$) receptor, and gastrin via a gastrin receptor. The H$_2$-receptor appears to have a major role in the integrated response, as the response to gastrin and acetylcholine is trivial in the absence of H$_2$-receptor stimulation and, in addition, a small amount of histamine considerably augments the acid secretion response to both gastrin and acetylcholine. The parasympathetic nervous system via the vagus nerve with acetylcholine as the neurotransmitter causes an early or cephalic increase in gastric acid at the thought of, or at the sight of, food. This early phase is augmented and prolonged by hormonally mediated stimulation due to gastrin release from the gastric antrum following contact of food with the stomach. A consequence of acid release is activation of the prostaglandin system which exerts a negative feedback inhibition on gastric acid production and simultaneously increases gastric blood flow. Figure 23.4 is a schematic illustration of a gastric parietal cell depicting the regulation of gastric acid secretion and indicating potential sites of intervention.

Measures to reduce gastric acidity include:

1. H$_2$-receptor antagonists
2. Antacids
3. Anticholinergics

HISTAMINE H₂-RECEPTOR ANTAGONISTS

Cimetidine, ranitidine, and famotidine are H$_2$-receptor antagonists that inhibit gastric acid secretion and are discussed in previous sections of this chapter. Timing of administration and the rate of gastric emptying are crucial, since these drugs have no effect on acid already present in the stomach. **Cimetidine** (300 mg) given on the evening before and again on the morning of surgery (60 to 90 minutes before induction) is effective in raising gastric pH above 2.5 in the majority of patients. When cimetidine (300 mg) is given intravenously, higher peak concentrations are achieved during the first hour of administration. Cimetidine may be ineffective if the interval between administration and anesthesia is less than 30 minutes or greater than 90 minutes; thus timing of administration is critical.

Ranitidine may also be used to reduce gastric acidity and volume; a dose of 150 mg orally or 50 mg intravenously infused over 15 minutes produces peak blood levels in 60 to 90 minutes and therapeutic concentrations for about 8 hours. Ranitidine does not inhibit the metabolism of other drugs as has been shown for cimetidine, unless very high doses are used, because binding of the furan ring of ranitidine to cytochrome P-450 is less than the interaction between cimetidine's imidazole ring and cytochrome P-450. Thus anesthetic drug interactions may be less likely to occur.

Famotidine is yet another potent selective H$_2$-receptor antagonist that has been used to reduce gastric acidity prior to surgery; the dose is 40 mg orally or 20 mg intravenously. Famotidine does not appear to interfere with hepatic metabolism. Although the duration of action of famotidine is reported to be 10 to 12 hours, for aspiration prophylaxis a bedtime dose and a second dose the morning of surgery are more effective.

ANTACIDS

Application of antacids into the stomach undoubtedly neutralizes gastric acid acutely, raises the pH of gastric contents in the majority of patients, and therefore is effective in such situations as anesthesia and labor. However, clinical trials evaluating the effectiveness of antacids for treating peptic ulcer disease are conflicting, and their efficacy remains questionable. Particulate antacids are not used as frequently by anesthesiologists today because of poor mixing with gastric contents and possible lung damage if pulmonary aspiration of gastric contents should occur. Soluble antacids are thus preferred. It is important to note, in addition, that gastric fluid volume is increased and gastric emptying delayed.

PREPARATIONS. Available antacids include magnesium-aluminum-hydroxide gel (Aludrox, Maalox, Mylanta), aluminum-containing antacids (Amphogel), calcium carbonate (Tums), and sucralfate, a complex of aluminum hydroxide and sulfated sucrose. Sucralfate is an advance on conventional antacids. It is thought to bind to the ulcer base and enhance the integrity of the mucosal barrier. It also binds pepsin and bile salts. It has been shown to be as effective as H_2-blockers in promoting ulcer healing. It is not absorbed, and its only side effect is constipation.

Nonparticulate antacids include sodium citrate, Bicitra, and Polycitra. Particulate antacids do not always raise gastric fluid pH, probably due to inadequate mixing, and if aspiration of gastric contents does occur following particulate antacid ingestion, a pneumonitis may result. In contrast, clear antacids mix well with gastric fluid and are less likely to cause an aspiration syndrome. Sodium citrate, 15 to 30 ml of 0.3 molar solution, given 15 minutes prior to anesthesia induction will raise intragastric pH to above 3 for about 2 to 3 hours. Bicitra contains sodium citrate and citric acid, and Polycitra is a nonparticulate antacid, containing sodium citrate, potassium citrate, and citric acid. It is important to recognize that antacids may increase gastric fluid volume. The effectiveness of antacids in increasing gastric pH depends on many factors, including the volume and pH of gastric contents at the time of administration and the gastric emptying rate. Narcotics reduce gastric motility and, therefore, the effects of antacids are increased if an opiod is also given. The normally low gastric pH provides a barrier to the entry of microbial organisms. By removing that barrier by the administration of H_2-blockers, it is possible that patients such as those in an intensive care unit may be exposed to increased risk of nosocomial infection. It has been suggested that there is less risk with sucralfate.

ANTICHOLINERGIC DRUGS

Anticholinergic drugs used in anesthetic practice are either ineffective or unreliable in raising intragastric pH and, in addition, decrease lower-esophageal sphincter pressure (see later in the chapter); they should be avoided in patients at risk from regurgitation.

Anticholinergic therapy for peptic ulcer disease is sound in theory but, until recently, has not proved effective in practice. Atropine-like drugs, which inhibit both M_1- and M_2-muscarinic receptors, should reduce the vagal stimulus for acid secretion and prolong the action of antacids by delaying emptying of the stomach if given immediately before a meal. In view of the lack of proven efficacy, the potential for side effects, and the introduction of an effective alternative approach with H_2-receptor antagonists, it can be argued that the atropine-like group of anticholinergic drugs no longer has a place in the treatment of uncomplicated peptic ulcer disease or as a therapeutic approach to reducing gastric acid production. More recently, **Pirenzapine,** a specific M_1-receptor antagonist, has been developed which has specific effects on acid secretion but not on the heart and gut. Early clinical studies indicate this drug is as effective as H_2-receptor antagonists in the management of peptic ulcer disease.

Omeprazole, a substituted benzimidazole, is the first generation of a new group of drugs which act directly on the parietal cell proton pump and act as a H^+,K^+-ATPase inhibitor. The drug is eliminated from the body with an elimination half-life of 1 to 2 hours, but its pharmacological half-life is much longer (1 to 2 days) due to its local concentration and persistence at the site of action. It may produce complete inhibition of gastric acid secretion for 48 hours after a single dose and thus would be extremely useful in anesthesia practice. It has been shown to inhibit all forms of acid secretion, even in patients with gastrinomas (Zollinger-Ellison syndrome) which have been resistant to H_2-blockers. In early clinical trials in duodenal ulcer, it has provided almost 100% healing rates. In a single animal species, it has induced gastric carcinoid tumors, but the relevance of this to humans is unknown. Its long-term adverse effects are still unknown.

PROSTAGLANDIN ANALOGS

The majority of agents used in the management of peptic ulcer disease either increase mucosal protection or decrease acid production. The prostaglandin analogs are the only group of drugs that have both mechanisms of action. It has been shown that endogenously produced prostaglandins (predominantly PGE_2) increase mucus production and blood flow to the gastric mucosa, while directly inhibiting gastric acid secretion. It has also been suggested that the therapeutic efficacy of sucralfate, carbonoxolone sodium, and even H_2-receptor antagonists is mediated via local prostanoid release, and that peptic ulcer disease might be considered a prostaglandin deficiency syndrome. Unfortunately, naturally occurring prostaglandins have only a transient action. The pharmaceutical industry has and is developing more stable analogs of the PGE_1 series (rioprostil and misoprostol) or PGE_2 series (**Enprostil,** arbaprostil, and trimoprostil). Misoprostol is used in the prevention of nonsteroidal antiinflammatory induced ulcers.

Pharmacological Regulation of Intragastric Volume

Pharmacological regulation of intragastric volume includes measures taken to increase gastric emptying. The major factors affecting gastric emptying are outlined in Table 23.2. Gastroesophageal reflux is an important risk factor for inhalation of gastric contents and, in general, factors that increase lower-esophageal sphincter (LES) pressure reduce the risk of regurgitation, while those factors that lower LES may increase the risk (Table 23.3). Thus some anesthetic drugs tend to have opposite effects, e.g., atropine and metoclopramide and opioids and metoclopramide.

METOCLOPRAMIDE

Metoclopramide, fully described on page 89, may be used to increase gastric emptying. Metoclopramide, 10 to 20 mg intravenously, given before anesthesia and surgery decreases intragastric volume. However, its effects are abolished by narcotic analgesics.

DOMPERIDONE

Domperidone, a peripheral dopamine antagonist that acts on the chemoreceptor trigger zone (CTZ) and dopamine receptors in the gut, has gastroprokinetic and antiemetic effects that may be useful to the anesthesiologist. It is chemically related to the butyrophenones.

5-HYDROXYTRYPTAMINE (SEROTONIN)

5-Hydroxytryptamine (5-HT) or serotonin is widely distributed in animals and plants.

Table 23.2.
Factors Delaying Gastric Emptying

Pathophysiological	Drugs
Posture	
Food	Opioids
Pregnancy	Anticholinergics
Obesity	Alcohol
Gastrointestinal disease	
Trauma	
Pain	

Table 23.3.
Factors Influencing Lower Esophageal Pressure (LES)

Increase	Decrease
Metoclopramide	Anticholinergics (atropine, hyoscine, glycopyrrolate)
Domperidone	
Cisapride	Thiopental
Succinylcholine	Ganglion blockers
Pancuronium	Sodium nitroprusside
Antacids	Halothane, enflurane
Edrophonium	Opioids
Neostigmine	Pregnancy
Ergometrine	Obesity
	Hiatus hernia

PHARMACOLOGICAL EFFECTS

5-HT rarely causes bronchospasm in humans, except in susceptible individuals such as asthmatics. 5-HT causes direct vasoconstriction resulting in a rise in arterial blood pressure. In addition, 5-HT increases gastrointestinal motility. High doses of 5-HT may cause secretion of catecholamines from the adrenal gland. About 90% of the 5-HT present in humans is found in the enterochromaffin cells of the gastrointestinal tract. The rest is present in platelets and the central nervous system. The major function of 5-HT in humans is as a neurotransmitter for serotonergic neurons within the central nervous system.

5-Hydroxytryptophan is synthesized from tryptophan under the influence of tryptophan hydroxylase (Fig. 23.5). The enzyme, aromatic L-amino acid decarboxylase, then catalyzes the formation of 5-HT (serotonin). 5-HT is degraded to 5-hydroxyindoleacetic acid (5-HIAA), which is excreted in the urine (Fig. 23.5). Large amounts of 5-HIAA are excreted by patients with malignant carcinoid, and the quantitative estimation of 5-HIAA in the urine is used as a diagnostic test for this syndrome. The degradation of 5-HT by the lung is important, 30 to 90% of an administered dose being taken up by pulmonary endothelial cells.

TRYPTOPHAN

       Tryptophan 5-hydroxylase

5-HYDROXYTRYPTOPHAN
    (5-HTP)
       Aromatic L-amino acid
       decarboxylase

5-HYDROXYTRYPTAMINE (SEROTONIN)
    (5-HT)

       Monoamine oxidase

5-HYDROXYINDOLEACETALDEHYDE

       Aldehyde dehydrogenase

5-HYDROXYINDOLEACETIC ACID
    (5-HIAA)

Figure 23.5. Synthesis and breakdown of 5-hydroxytryptamine (serotonin).

KININS

Kallidin (decapeptide) and bradykinin (nonapeptide) are plasma kinins which are cleaved from precursors (kininogens) in the α_2-globulin fraction of the plasma under the control of a group of enzymes known as the kallikreins. Plasma kallikrein forms bradykinin directly from high-molecular-weight (HMW) kininogen. Bradykinin is an extremely potent vasodilator; the fall in total peripheral resistance and arterial blood pressure may elicit a reflex increase in heart rate and cardiac output. The plasma kinins increase capillary permeability and produce edema. In addition, they are involved in pain production. Their mechanism of action may in part be mediated by histamine and prostaglandin release.

CARCINOID SYNDROME

Tumors of enterochromaffin cells (carcinoid tumors) in the gastrointestinal or respiratory tract synthesize and release large amounts of 5-HT (serotonin). It is now recognized that 5-HT alone cannot account for all the symptoms of the syndrome. Other agents elaborated by those tumors include the enzyme kallikrein (which is responsible for the formation of bradykinin in the blood), histamine, prostaglandins, and peptide hormones, such as adrenocorticotropic hormone (ACTH).

The carcinoid syndrome is characterized by episodic cutaneous flushing, telangiectasia, gastrointestinal symptoms (recurrent severe diarrhea and abdominal cramps), cardiac valvular lesions, and bronchoconstriction. The most common clinical feature is cutaneous flushing, which may be provoked by excitement, exertion, the ingestion of alcohol, and the administration of pentagastrin, epinephrine, norepinephrine, and calcium. Many of the stimuli of the carcinoid flush, including epinephrine, calcium, and alcohol, cause gastrin release; somatostatin inhibits both the release and actions of gastrin and has been found to be effective in suppressing pentagastrin-evoked carcinoid flushes. In addition, bradykinin, a potent vasodilator, will stimulate an erythematous reaction in association with tachycardia and hypotension.

TREATMENT

Management of the carcinoid syndrome involves two approaches—pharmacological and surgical. There are five groups of drugs that have been used in an attempt to improve the symptoms of carcinoid syndrome: those with antiserotonin properties; inhibitors of the kallikrein-bradykinin syndrome; corticosteroids; adrenergic receptor blocking agents; and cytotoxic agents.

Diarrhea is largely due to the release of 5-HT, and its antagonist methysergide is of proven value in ameliorating symptoms. However, long-term methysergide may result in retroperitoneal fibrosis. Blockade of serotonin synthesis with the tryptophan hydroxylase inhibitor, p-chlorophenylalanine, may also be helpful.

Patients with gastric carcinoid are subject to episodic release of large amounts of histamine and may benefit from the combined use of an H₁-receptor antagonist (diphenhydramine) and an H₂-receptor antagonist (cimetidine) (see previous discussion). Reports of the use of kallikrein-bradykinin inhibitors have been disappointing, although the kallikrein inhibitor, aprotinin, has been successfully administered during anesthesia to treat a carcinoid crisis, manifest by severe bronchospasm and hypotension. Somatostatin and its long-acting analog have been shown to be useful during such a life-threatening situation. Intravenous somatostatin, a widespread peptide that inhibits the release of many regulatory peptides (growth hormone, insulin, glucagon, gastrin), has been shown to inhibit both spontaneously occurring and pentagastrin-provoked flush in patients with the carcinoid syndrome. It has a very short half-life measured in minutes and is not absorbed orally. Long-acting analogs of somatostatin **(octreotide)** have now been developed and have been used in the long-term management of malignant carcinoid syndromes. The half-life

of octreotide is about 45 minutes after intravenous and 80 minutes after subcutaneous administration. The drug has been shown to be effective as prophylaxis in preoperative management of patients with carcinoid syndrome, and hypotensive episodes associated with surgical manipulation of the carcinoid tumor are also reversed. It has thus become an important mode of therapy in the anesthetic management of these patients. It has also been used in the management of symptoms associated with vasoactive intestinal peptide (VIP)-secreting adenomas. The initial dose of octreotide is 50 μg subcutaneously, but intravenous injection can be used under emergency conditions. The daily dosage of octreotide ranges from 100 to 600 μg per day.

Patients who have tumors arising in ovarian or testicular teratomas or in the bronchus may undergo complete surgical cure; the release of active agents directly into the systemic circulation produces clinical manifestations before metastatic disease occurs. However, as 5-HT and other agents released by tumors that drain into the portal circulation are generally metabolized by the liver, tumors of the ileum and other gastrointestinal sites produce the systemic manifestations of the carcinoid syndrome only after the development of hepatic metastases. In certain instances patients may undergo surgery for palliative resection of hepatic metastases.

ANESTHETIC MANAGEMENT

Anesthesia may be required for the resection of the primary tumor, excision of hepatic metastases, or cardiac valve replacement. Clinical problems arising during anesthesia are thought to be due to the release of 5-HT (serotonin), kallikrein, and histamine. Common intraoperative complications include hypotension, bronchospasm, flushing, hypertension, and tachycardia. Hypotensive episodes should not be treated with β-agonists because, by stimulating the release of vasoactive substances from the tumor, they can exaggerate and prolong the cardiovascular disturbance. Hypotension is best treated with volume expansion and somatostatin and, if hypotension persists or is severe, with methoxamine. Corticosteroids may be beneficial in relieving bronchospasm. Because histamine has also been shown to be involved in the mediation of symptoms in patients with gastric carcinoid syndrome, the combined use of H_1-receptor (diphenhydramine) and H_2-receptor (cimetidine) antagonists may be helpful. As stated previously, a somatostatin infusion would be expected to be beneficial during a life-threatening attack of severe bronchoconstriction, hypotension, and flushing and has now become the treatment of choice.

Premedication with barbiturates, H_1-receptor antagonists, and antiserotonin drugs such as droperidol has been found to be helpful. If there is evidence of excess histamine secretion, cimetidine and diphenhydramine should be given as part of the preanesthetic regimen. Morphine should not be given as part of the premedication because it causes release of 5-HT from the small intestine and may precipitate bronchospasm due to histamine release. Induction with thiopental, followed by intubation facilitated by the muscle relaxant pancuronium, and maintenance of anesthesia with pancuronium, nitrous oxide-oxygen, and fentanyl appear to be a satisfactory regimen. Succinylcholine may cause a rise in intraabdominal pressure which may stimulate the release of hormones from the tumor. Tubocurarine should be avoided, since it may cause hypotension due to ganglionic blockade and, in addition, stimulates histamine release in some patients. Regional anesthesia offers no protection against the carcinoid syndrome.

ANGIOTENSIN AND THE RENIN-ANGIOTENSIN SYSTEM

The pathway of formation of the angiotensins is given in Figure 23.6. The enzyme renin acts on angiotensinogen (plasma substrate), an α-globulin, to give the decapeptide angiotensin I. Angiotensin II, an octapeptide, is formed from angiotensin I by enzymatic cleavage by con-

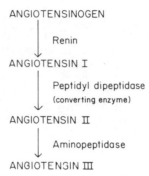

Figure 23.6. The formation of the angiotensins.

verting enzyme, peptidyl dipeptidase. Angiotensin II undergoes hydrolysis by aminopeptidase to yield the heptapeptide, angiotensin III. Angiotensin I has limited pharmacological activity.

Angiotensin II is a potent pressor agent and, in addition, stimulates the synthesis and secretion of aldosterone by the adrenal cortex and potentiates norepinephrine release from nerve terminals. Cardiovascular effects include peripheral vasoconstriction, rise in arterial blood pressure, fall in cardiac output, and reflex slowing of the heart. Angiotensin II is not available commercially in the United States.

FUNCTION OF THE RENIN-ANGIOTENSIN SYSTEM

The renin-angiotensin system is an important homeostatic physiological mechanism for the regulation of water and electrolyte balance. Renin is released from the kidney in response to a reduction in blood volume, fall in renal perfusion pressure, and sodium depletion. Conversely, factors that increase these parameters tend to inhibit its release. The sympathetic outflow is known to stimulate renin release in response to painful stimuli, stress, or emotion via β-adrenergic, stimulation. The role of the renin-angiotensin system in hypertensive states has been the subject of considerable research and has led to the development of antagonists of the renin-angiotensin system that are effective antihypertensive drugs.

ANTAGONISTS OF THE RENIN-ANGIOTENSIN SYSTEM

ANTAGONISTS OF ANGIOTENSIN II

Saralasin is an angiotensin II receptor antagonist. Thus, saralasin causes hypotension in subjects with elevated renin levels and reduces the secretion of aldosterone in sodium-depleted subjects. The use of saralasin as an antihypertensive agent is further discussed in Chapter 15.

INHIBITORS OF PEPTIDYL DIPEPTIDASE

Captopril, enalapril, and lisinopril are potent competitive inhibitors of the enzyme peptidyl dipeptidase, and they may be administered orally in the treatment of hypertension. These drugs are further discussed in Chapter 15.

BIBLIOGRAPHY

Histamine

Editorial: Histamine and antihistamines in anaesthesia and surgery. *Lancet* 2:74–75, 1981.

Editorial: Cardiovascular histamine H₂ receptors. *Lancet* 2:421–422, 1982.

Fahmy NR, Sunder N, Soter NA: Role of histamine in the hemodynamic and plasma catecholamine responses to morphine. *Clin Pharmacol Ther* 33:615–620, 1983.

Haggstrom GD, Hirschowitz BI: Histamine H₁ and H₂ effects on gastric acid and pepsin, heart rate, and blood pressure in humans. *J Pharmacol Exp Ther* 231:120–123, 1984.

Inada E, Philbin DM, Machaj V, Moss J, D'Ambra MN, Rosow CE, Akins CW: Histamine antagonists and d-tubocurarine-induced hypotension in cardiac surgical patients. *Clin Pharmacol Ther* 40:575–580, 1986.

Koga Y, Iwatsuki N, Hashimoto Y: Direct effects of H₂-receptor antagonists on airway smooth muscle and on responses mediated by H₁- and H₂-receptors. *Anesthesiology* 66:181–185, 1987.

Lagunoff D, Martin TW, Read G: Agents that release histamine from mast cells. *Annu Rev Pharmacol Toxicol* 23:331–351, 1983.

Moss J, Rosow CE: Histamine release by narcotics and muscle relaxants in humans. *Anesthesiology* 59:330–339, 1983.

Philbin DM, Moss J, Akins CW, Rosow CE, Kono K, Schneider RC, VerLee TR, Savarese JJ: The use of H₁ and H₂ histamine antagonists with morphine anesthesia: a double-blind study. *Anesthesiology* 55:292–296, 1981.

Rosow CE, Moss J, Philbin DM, Savarese JJ: Histamine release during morphine and fentanyl anesthesia. *Anesthesiology* 56:93–96, 1982.

Thornton JA: Editorial: The problem of histamine in anaesthesia. *Br J Anaesth* 54:1–2, 1982.

Thronton JA, Lorenz W: Histamine and antihistamine in anaesthesia and surgery. *Anaesthesia* 38:373–379, 1983.

H₁-Receptor Antagonists

Brandon ML: Newer non-sedating antihistamines. Will they replace older agents. *Drugs* 30:377–381, 1985.

Clissold SP, Sorkin EM, Goa KL: Loratidine. A preliminary review of its pharmacodynamic properties and therapeutic effect. *Drugs* 37:42–57, 1989.

Paton DM, Webster DR: Clinical pharmacokinetics of H₁-receptor antagonists (the antihistamines). *Clin Pharmacokinet* 10:477–497, 1985.

Pearlman DS: Antihistamines: pharmacology and clinical use. *Drugs* 12:258–273, 1976.

H₂-Receptor Antagonists

Abe K, Shibata M, Demizu A, Hazano S, Sumidawa K, Enomoto H, Mashimo T, Tashiro C, Yoshiya I: Effect of oral and intramuscular famotidine on pH and volume of gastric contents. *Anesth Analg* 68:541–544, 1989.

Abernethy DR, Greenblatt DJ, Eshelman FN, Shader RI: Ranitidine does not impair oxidative or conjugative metabolism: non-interaction with antipyrine, diazepam, and lorazepam. *Clin Pharmacol Ther* 35:189–192, 1984.

Black JW, Duncan WAM, Durant CJ, Ganellin CR, Parsons EM: Definition and antagonism of histamine H-2 receptors. *Nature* 236:385–390, 1972.

Breen KJ, Bury R, Desmond PV, Mashford JL, Morphett B, Westwood B, Shaw RG: Effects of cimetidine and ranitidine on hepatic drug metabolism. *Clin Pharmacol Ther* 31:297–300, 1982.

Burland WL, Duncan WAM, Hesselbo T, Mills JG, Sharpe PC, Haggie SJ, Wyllie JH: Pharmacological evaluation of cimetidine, a new histamine H2-receptor antagonist, in healthy man. *Br J Clin Pharmacol* 2:481–486, 1975.

Collins JD, Pidgen AW: Pharmacokinetics of roxatidine in healthy volunteers. *Drugs* 35:41–47, 1988.

Coombs DW, Hooper D, Colton T: Acid-aspiration prophylaxis by use of preoperative oral administration of cimetidine. *Anesthesiology* 51:352–356, 1979.

Coombs DW, Hooper D, Colton T: Pre-anesthetic cimetidine alteration of gastric fluid volume and pH. *Anesth Analg* 58:183–188, 1979.

Dailey PA, Hughes SC, Rosen MA, Healy K, Cheek DBC, Shnider SM: Effect of cimetidine and ranitidine on lidocaine concentrations during epidural anesthesia for cesarean section. *Anesthesiology* 69:1013–1017, 1988.

Dammann HG, Muller P, Simon B: Parenteral ranitidine: onset and duration of action. *Br J Anaesth* 54:1235–1236, 1982.

Feely J, Wilkinson GR, McAllister CB, Wood AJJ: Increased toxicity and reduced clearance of lidocaine by cimetidine. *Ann Intern Med* 96:592–594, 1982.

Feely J, Wilkinson GR, Wood AJJ: Reduction of liver blood flow and propranolol metabolism by cimetidine. *N Engl J Med* 304:692–695, 1981.

Finkelstein W, Isselbacher KJ: Drug therapy. Cimetidine. *N Engl J Med* 299:922–996, 1978.

Flynn RJ, Moore J, Collier PS, McClean E: Does pretreatment with cimetidine and ranitidine affect the disposition of bupivacaine? *Br J Anaesth* 62:87–91, 1989.

Goudsouzian N, Cote CJ, Liu LMP, Dedrick DF: The dose-response effects of oral cimetidine on gastric pH and volume in children. *Anesthesiology* 55:533–536, 1981.

Greenblatt DJ, Abernethy DR, Morese DS, Harmatz JS, Shader RI: Clinical importance of the interaction of diazepam and cimetidine. *N Engl J Med* 310:1639–1643, 1984.

Greenblatt DJ, Locniskar A, Scavone JM, Blyden GT, Ochs HR, Harmatz JS, Shader RI: Absence of interaction of cimetidine and ranitidine with intravenous and oral midazolam. *Anesth Analg* 65:176–180, 1986.

Guay DRP, Meatherall RC, Chalmers JL, Grahame GR: Cimetidine alters pethidine disposition in man. *Br J Clin Pharmacol* 18:907–914, 1984.

Heining M, Groom J, Luthman J, Aps C: Hypotension following cimetidine administration during cardiopulmonary bypass. *Anaesthesia* 38:260–263, 1983.

Henn RM, Isenbeerg JI, Maxwell V, Sturdevant RA: Inhibition of gastric acid secretion by cimetidine in patients with duodenal ulcer. *N Engl J Med* 293:371–375, 1975.

Howe JP, McGowan WAW, Moore J, McCaughey W, Dundee JW: The placental transfer of cimetidine. *Anaesthesia* 36:371–375, 1981.

Iberti TJ, Paluch TA, Helmer L, Murgolo VA, Benjamin E: The hemodynamic effects of intravenous cimetidine in intensive care unit patients: a double-blind, prospective study. *Anesthesiology* 64:87–89, 1986.

Jacob AI, Lanier D, Canterbury J, Bourgoignie JJ: Reduction by cimetidine of serum parathyroid hormone levels in uremic patients. *N Engl J Med* 302:671–674, 1980.

Jensen JC, Gugler R: Cimetidine interaction with liver microsomes in vitro and in vivo. Involvement of an activated complex with cytochrome P-450. *Biochem Pharmacol* 34:2141–2146, 1985.

Kirch W, Hoensch H, Janisch HD: Interactions and non-interactions with ranitidine. *Clin Pharmacokinet* 9:493–510, 1984.

Klotz U, Arvela P, Rosenkranz B: Famotidine, a new H_2-receptor antagonist, does not affect hepatic elimination of diazepam or tubular secretion of procainamide. *Eur J Clin Pharmacol* 28:671–675, 1985.

Klotz U, Reimann I: Delayed clearance of diazepam due to cimetidine. *N Engl J Med* 302:1012–1014, 1980.

Kuhnert BR, Zuspan KJ, Kuhnert PM, Syracuse CD, Brashear WT, Brown DE: Lack of influence of cimetidine on bupivacaine levels during parturition. *Anesth Analg* 66:986–990, 1986.

Lam AM, Clement JL: Effect of cimetidine premedication on morphine-induced ventilatory depression. *Can Anaesth Soc J* 31:36–43, 1984.

Lineberger AS, Sprague DH, Battaglini JW: Sinus arrest associated with cimetidine. *Anesth Analg* 64:554–556, 1985.

Locniskar A, Greenblatt DJ, Harmatz JS, Zinny MA, Shader RI: Interaction of diazepam with famotidine and cimetidine, two H_2-receptor antagonists. *J Clin Pharmacol* 26:299–303, 1986.

Longstreth GF, Go VLW, Malagelada JR: Cimetidine suppression of nocturnal gastric secretion in active duodenal ulcer. *N Engl J Med* 294:801–804, 1976.

Maile CJD, Francis RN: Pre-operative ranitidine. Effect of a single intravenous dose on pH and volume of gastric aspirate. *Anaesthesia* 38:324–326, 1983.

Manchikanti L, Colliver JA, Grow JB, Dermeyer RG, Hadley CH, Roush JR: Dose-response effects of intravenous ranitidine on gastric pH and volume in outpatients. *Anesthesiology* 65:180–185, 1986.

Manchikanti L, Kraus JW, Edds SP: Cimetidine and related drugs in anesthesia. *Anesth Analg* 61:595–608. 1982.

Martin LF, Staloch DK, Simonowitz DA, Dellinger EP, Max JH: Failure of cimetidine prophylaxis in the critically ill. *Arch Surg* 114:492–496, 1979.

Mojaverian P, Fedder IL, Vlasses PH, Rotmensch HH, Rocci ML, Swanson BN, Ferguson RK: Cimetidine does not alter morphine disposition in man. *Br J Clin Pharmacol* 14:809–813, 1982.

Noble DW, Smith KJ, Dundas CR: Effects of H-2 antagonists on the elimination of bupivacaine. *Br J Anaesth* 59:735–737, 1987.

Osborne DH, Lennon J, Henderson M, Lidgard G, Creel R, Carter DC: Effect of cimetidine on the human lower oesophageal sphincter. *Gut* 18:99–104, 1977.

O'Sullivan GM, Smith M, Morgan B, Brighouse D, Reynolds F: H_2 antagonists and bupivacaine clearance. *Anaesthesia* 43:93–95, 1988.

Patwardhan RV, Yarborough GW, Desmond P, Johnson RF, Schenker S, Speeg KV: Cimetidine spares the glucuronidation of lorazepam and oxazepam. *Gastroenterology* 79:912–916, 1980.

Pounder RE, Williams JG, Russell RCG, Milton-Thompson GJ, Misiewicz JJ: Inhibition of food-stimulated gastric acid secretion by cimetidine. *Gut* 17:161–168, 1976.

Price AH, Brogden RN: Nizatidine. A preliminary review of its pharmacodynamic and pharmacokinetic properties, and its therapeutic use in peptic ulcer disease. *Drugs* 36:521–539, 1988.

Redolfi A, Borgogelli E, Lodola E: Blood level of cimetidine in relation to age. *Eur J Clin Pharmacol* 15:257–261, 1979.

Rendic S, Kajfez F, Ruf HH: Characterization of cimetidine, ranitidine, and related structures interaction with cytochrome P-450. *Drug Metab Dispos* 11:137–142, 1983.

Roberts CJC: Clinical pharmacokinetics of ranitidine. *Clin Pharmacokinet* 9:211–221, 1984.

Sewing KF, Beil W, Hannemann H: Comparative pharmacology of histamine H_2-receptor antagonists. *Drugs* 35:25–29, 1988.

Smith CL, Bardgett DM, Hunter JM: Haemodynamic effects of the IV administration of cimetidine or ranitidine in the critically ill patients. *Br J Anaesth* 59:1397–1402, 1987.

Smith RS, Kendall MJ: Ranitidine versus cimetidine. A comparison of their potential to cause clinically important drug interactions. *Clin Pharmacokinet* 15:44–56, 1988.

Somogyi A, Gugler R: Drug interactions with cimetidine. *Clin Pharmacokinet* 7:23–41, 1982.

Somogyi A, Gugler R: Clinical pharmacokinetics of cimetidine. *Clin Pharmacokinet* 8:463–495, 1983.

Somogyi A, Muirhead M: Pharmacokinetic interactions of cimetidine 1987. *Clin Pharmacokinet* 12:321–366, 1987.

Taylor DC, Cresswell PR, Bartlett DC: The metabolism and elimination of cimetidine, a histamine H$_2$ receptor antagonist in the rat, dog, and man. *Drug Metab Dispos* 6:21–30, 1978.

Tryba M, Wruck G, Thole H, Zenz M: The use of roxatidine acetate in fasting patients prior to induction of anaesthesia as prophylaxis against the acid aspiration syndrome. *Drugs* 35:20–24, 1988.

Tryba M, Zevounou F, Zenz M: Prevention of histamine-induced cardiovascular reactions during the induction of anaesthesia following premedication with H$_1$- and H$_2$-antagonists IM. *Br J Anaesth* 58:478–482, 1986.

Weber L. Hirshman CA: Cimetidine for prophylaxis of aspiration pneumonitis: comparison of intramuscular and oral dosage schedules. *Anesth Analg* 58:426–427, 1979.

Williams JG: H$_2$ receptor antagonists and anaesthesia. *Can Anaesth Soc J* 30:264–269, 1983.

Wood M, Uetrecht J, Phythyon JM, Shay S, Sweetman BJ, Shaheen O, Wood AJJ: The effect of cimetidine on anesthetic metabolism and toxicity. *Anesth Analg* 65:481–488, 1986.

Control of Gastric pH and Volume

Detmer MD, Pandit SK, Cohen PJ: Prophylactic single-dose oral antacid therapy in the preoperative period—comparison of cimetidine and Maalox. *Anesthesiology* 51:270–273, 1979.

Frank M, Evans M, Flynn P, Aun C: Comparison of the prophylactic use of magnesium trisilicate mixture B.P.C., sodium citrate mixture, or cimetidine in obstetrics. *Br J Anaesth* 56:355–362, 1984.

Gallagher EG, White M, Ward S, Cottrell J, Mann SG: Prophylaxis against acid aspiration syndrome. Single oral dose of H$_2$-antagonist on the evening before elective surgery. *Anaesthesia* 43:1011–1014, 1988.

Gibbs CP, Spohr L, Schmidt D: The effectiveness of sodium citrate as an antacid. *Anesthesiology* 57:44–46, 1982.

Gillett GB, Watson JD, Langford RM: Ranitidine and single-dose antacid therapy as prophylaxis against acid aspiration syndrome in obstetric practice. *Anaesthesia* 39:638–644, 1984.

Hodgkinson R, Glassenberg R, Joyce TH, Coombs DW, Ostheimer GW, Gibbs CP: Comparison of cimetidine (Tagamet®) with antacid for safety and effectiveness in reducing gastric acidity before elective cesarean section. *Anesthesiology* 59:86–90, 1983.

Lam AM, Grace DM, Manninen PH, Diamond C: The effects of cimetidine and ranitidine with and without metoclopramide on gastric volume and pH in morbidly obese patients. *Can Anaesth Soc J* 33:773–779, 1986.

Lam AM, Grace DM, Penny FJ, Vezina WC: Prophylactic intravenous cimetidine reduces the risk of acid aspiration in morbidly obese patients. *Anesthesiology* 65:684–687, 1986.

Maliniak K, Vakil AH: pre-anesthetic cimetidine and gastric pH. *Anesth Analg* 58:309–313, 1979.

Manchikanti L, Roush JR: Effect of preanesthetic glycopyrrolate and cimetidine on gastric fluid pH and volume in outpatients. *Anesth Analg* 63:40–46, 1984.

Manchikanti L, Roush JR, Colliver JA: Effect of preanesthetic ranitidine and metoclopramide on gastric contents in morbidly obese patients. *Anesth Analg* 65:195–199, 1986.

Mathews HML, Wilson CM, Thompson EM, Moore J: Combination treatment of ranitidine and sodium bicarbonate prior to obstetric anaesthesia. *Anaesthesia* 41:1202–1206, 1986.

Moir DD: Editorial: cimetidine, antacids, and pulmonary aspiration. *Anesthesiology* 59:81–83, 1983.

Morgan M: Control of intragastric pH and volume. *Br J Anaesth* 56:47–57, 1984.

Morison DH, Dunn GI, Fargas-Babjak AM, Moudgil GC, Smedstad K, Woo J: A double-blind comparison of cimetidine and ranitidine as prophylaxis against gastric aspiration syndrome. *Anesth Analg* 61:988–992, 1982.

Nimmo WS: Effect of anaesthesia on gastric motility and emptying. *Br J Anaesth* 56:29–36, 1984.

O'Sullivan G, Sear JW, Bullingham RES, Carrie LES: The effect of magnesium trisilicate mixture, metoclopramide, and ranitidine on gastric pH, volume, and serum gastrin. *Anaesthesia* 40:246–253, 1985.

Reid SR, Bayliff CD: The comparative efficacy of cimetidine and ranitidine in controlling gastric pH in critically ill patients. *Can Anaesth Soc J* 33:287–293, 1986.

Sutherland AD, Maltby JR, Sale JP, Reid CRG: The effect of preoperative oral fluid and ranitidine on gastric fluid volume and pH. *Can J Anaesth* 34:117–121, 1987.

Carcinoid Syndrome

Ahlman H, Ahlund L, Dahlstrom A, Martner J, Stenqvist O, Tylen U: SMS 201-995 and provocation tests in preparation of patients with carcinoids for surgery or hepatic arterial embolization. *Anesth Analg* 67:1142–1148, 1988.

Bloom SR, Polak JM: Somatostatin. *Br Med J* 295:288–290, 1987.

Dery R: Theoretical and clinical considerations in anesthesia for secreting carcinoid tumors. *Can Anaesth Soc J* 18:245–263, 1971.

Frolich JG, Bloomgarden ZT, Oates JA, McGuigan JE, Rabinowitz D: The carcinoid flush. Provocation by pentagastrin and inhibition by somatostatin. *N Engl J Med* 299:1055–1057, 1978.

Kvols LK, Moertel CG, O'Connell MJ, Schutt AJ, Rubin J, Hahn RG: Treatment of the malignant carcinoid syndrome. Evaluation of a long-acting somatostatin analogue. *N Engl J Med* 315:663–666, 1986.

Marsh HM, Martin JK, Kvols LK, Gracey DR, Warner MA, Warner ME, Moertel CG: Carcinoid crisis during anesthesia: successful treatment with a somatostatin analogue. *Anesthesiology* 66:89–91, 1987.

Mason RA, Steane PA: Carcinoid syndrome: its relevance to the anaesthetist. *Anaesthesia* 31:228–242, 1976.

Nubiola-Calonge P, Badia JM, Sancho J, Gil MJ, Segura M, Sitges-Serra A: Blind evaluation of the effect of octreotide (SMS 201-995), a somatostatin analogue, on small-bowel fistula output. *Lancet* 2:672–673, 1987.

Oates JA: The carcinoid syndrome. *N Engl J Med* 315:702–704, 1986.

Parris WCV, Oates JA, Kambam JR, Shmerling R, Sawyers JF: Pre-treatment with somatostatin in the anaesthetic management of a patient with carcinoid syndrome. *Can J Anaesth* 35:413–416, 1988.

Patel AU, Miller R, Warner RRP: Anesthesia for ligation of the hepatic artery in a patient with carcinoid syndrome. *Anesthesiology* 47:303–305, 1977.

Roberts LJ, Marney SR, Oates JA: Blockade of the flush associated with metastatic gastric carcinoid by combined histamine H_1 and H_2 receptor antagonists. *N Engl J Med* 300:236–238, 1979.

Roy RC, Carter RF, Wright PD: Somatostatin, anaesthesia, and the carcinoid syndrome. *Anaesthesia* 2:627–632, 1987.

Tornebrandt K, Nobin A, Ericsson M, Thomson D: Circulation, respiration, and serotonin levels in carcinoid patients during neurolept anaesthesia. *Anaesthesia* 38:957–967, 1983.

Systemic Mastocytosis

James PD, Krafchik BR, Johnston AE: Cutaneous mastocytosis in children: anaesthetic considerations. *Can J Anaesth* 34:522–524, 1987.

Prostaglandin Analogues

Bright-Asare P, Habte T, Yirgou B, Benjamin J: Prostaglandins, H_2-receptor antagonists, and peptic ulcer disease. *Drugs* 35:1–9, 1988.

Goa KL, Monk JP: Enprostil. A preliminary review of its pharmacodynamic and pharmacokinetic properties, and therapeutic efficacy in the treatment of peptic ulcer disease. *Drugs* 34:539–559, 1987.

Omeprazole

Editorial: Omeprazole. *Lancet* 2:1187–1188, 1987.

Walan A, Bader JP, Classen M, Lamers CBHW, Piper DW, Rutgersson K, Eriksson S: Effect of omeprazole and ranitidine on ulcer healing and relapse rates in patients with benign gastric ulcer. *N Engl J Med* 320:69–75, 1989.

Domperidone

Champion MC: Domperidone: (minireview). *Gen Pharmacol* 19:499–505, 1988.

General

Wolfe MM, Soll AH: The physiology of gastric acid secretion. *N Engl J Med* 319:1707–1715, 1988.

24

Arachidonate Metabolites. Prostaglandins, Prostacyclin, Thromboxane, and Leukotrienes

ALAN R. BRASH

THERAPEUTIC USES
    Therapeutic Abortion
    Congenital Heart Disease
    Alprostadil (PGE$_1$)
    Peptic Ulcer Disease
    Cardiopulmonary Bypass
    Adult Respiratory Distress Syndrome

INTRODUCTION: PROSTAGLANDINS AND OTHER EICOSANOIDS

Essential fatty acids are metabolized through oxygenation pathways to form several biologically active mediators. Arachidonic acid is the most important of the essential fatty acid substrates for these reactions. The prostaglandins were the first group of products to be characterized. Now the list includes, in addition to the "classical" prostaglandins (PGE, PGF, and PGD), the thromboxanes, prostacyclin, slow-reacting substance of anaphylaxis (SRS-A) and other leukotrienes, and simple monohydroperoxy and monohydroxy fatty acids. Because these compounds are all derivatives of polyunsaturated eicosanoic (C_{20}) fatty acids, they are collectively known as *eicosanoids*.

No attempt is made in this chapter to cover all aspects of prostaglandin-related pharmacology. Rather, some common properties of the oxygenated products of essential fatty acid metabolism are described. The account is given in historical perspective; however, it should be noted that general characteristics of the classical prostaglandins, such as their rapid synthesis and metabolism, are equally applicable to the more recently discovered products. The aim is to give the reader a feeling for the biological significance of the eicosanoids and their potential importance in therapeutics.

It is helpful to an understanding of the whole area to have an appreciation of the mechanism of prostaglandin biosynthesis. For this reason, the story of the development of the prostaglandin field is prefaced by a description of this process.

MECHANISM OF PROSTAGLANDIN BIOSYNTHESIS

The classical prostaglandins (PGE, PGF, and PGD), thromboxane A, and prostacyclin are all formed from C_{20} essential fatty acids, such as arachidonic acid, via a common intermediate. Biosynthesis of the intermediate involves an oxygenase enzyme (the fatty acid cyclooxygenase) which catalyzes reaction of two molecules of O_2 with each molecule of the essential fatty acid substrate.

The cyclooxygenase is a more complex example of the simple lipoxygenase enzymes commonly found in plants. A plant lipoxygenase can utilize as substrate any of the essential fatty acids shown in Figure 24.1. Only two double bonds arranged as in linoleic acid are required. One molecule of oxygen (O_2 dissolved in water) is reacted to give a hydroperoxy derivative of the fatty acid as product. The lipoxygenase from soybeans, for example, inserts the O_2 molecule at one end of the two double bonds, whereas the potato lipoxygenase oxygenates the other position (Fig. 24.2A).

The first step in the cyclooxygenase reaction involved in the synthesis of prostaglandins is identical to that catalyzed by the potato lipoxygenase, and it is illustrated as *step 1* in Figure 24.2B. However, in prostaglandin synthesis, the oxygen molecule proceeds to react with another part of the fatty acid. The enzyme swings round the attached oxygen molecule to react it with the third double bond of the substrate (*step 2*). This reaction creates an endoperoxide. For endoperoxide formation to occur, it is necessary to have the third double bond in the substrate (and so prostaglandins cannot be synthesized from linoleic acid). *Step 3* of the cyclooxygenase reaction creates the five-membered carbon ring which is characteristic of the prostaglandins. The cyclooxygenase is now ready to carry out a second lipoxygenase-type reaction using another molecule of oxygen. This time, the enzyme must direct the insertion of O_2 in the opposite position from the first oxygenation. This gives the final product which is now released from the enzyme (*step 4*).

INTRODUCTION TO PROSTAGLANDIN NOMENCLATURE

The product of the cyclooxygenase reaction is known as the prostaglandin endoperoxide, PGG. (When the C-15 OOH group is reduced to OH, the endoperoxide is called PGH.) The endoperoxide is

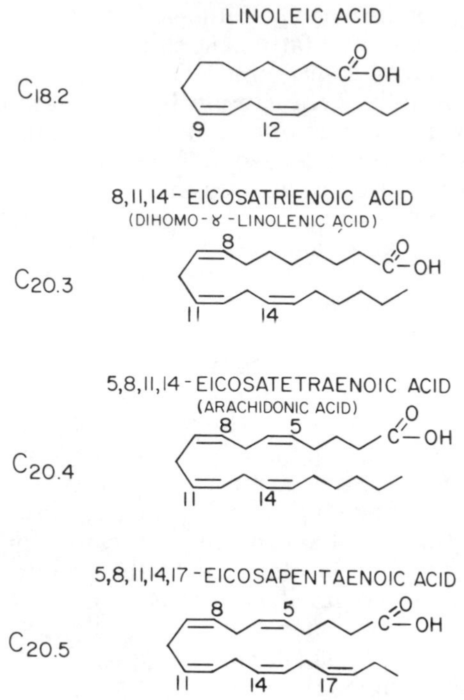

LINOLEIC ACID

$C_{18.2}$

8,11,14 - EICOSATRIENOIC ACID
(DIHOMO - γ -LINOLENIC ACID)

$C_{20.3}$

5,8,11,14 - EICOSATETRAENOIC ACID
(ARACHIDONIC ACID)

$C_{20.4}$

5,8,11,14,17 - EICOSAPENTAENOIC ACID

$C_{20.5}$

Figure 24.1. Essential fatty acid substrates for lipoxygenases. Linoleic acid (18-carbon with two double bonds, $C_{18.2}$) contains the basic structural feature for reaction with a lipoxygenase (the two double bonds arranged as in Fig. 24.2A). The other three essential fatty acids are substrates for lipoxygenases and also for the cyclooxygenase (prostaglandin synthetase). The latter enzyme utilizes the double bonds at 8, 11, and 14 as shown in Figure 24.2B.

attacked by specific enzymes which transform it into either a classical prostaglandin, into prostacyclin (PGI), or into thromboxane A (TxA). The classical compounds differ only in the structure of the cyclopentane ring; TxA is quite distinct in having an oxirane ring (Fig. 24.3).

Whereas the cyclooxygenase is found in almost all animal tissues, the enzymes which catalyze the conversion of the endoperoxide to the prostaglandin, prostacyclin, or thromboxane have a much more specific distribution. Thus, platelets synthesize predominantly thromboxane A_2 from arachidonic acid, the endothelial cells of blood vessels make PGI_2, while $PGF_{2\alpha}$ is a major product in the uterus. The subscript "2" used here refers to the number of double bonds in the side chains of the prostaglandin. It is apparent from the mechanism of prostaglandin biosynthesis that, of the three double bonds required in the substrate, only one remains after biosynthesis is complete. Thus, $C_{20.3}$ essential fatty acid gives rise to "1" series protaglandins; arachidonic acid ($C_{20.4}$) is converted to members of the "2" series (the fourth double bond does not participate in the cyclooxygenase reaction and remains in its original position), and $C_{20.5}$ gives PGE_3, $PGF_{3\alpha}$, etc. The meaning of "α" in $PGF_{2\alpha}$ or $PGF_{3\alpha}$ will be explained later in the chapter.

DEVELOPMENT OF THE PROSTAGLANDIN FIELD

Structure of PGE and PGF

In the 1930s, U. S. von Euler of the Karolinska Institutet in Stockholm showed that a pharmacologically active substance isolated from human seminal fluid was distinct from any previously recognized biological mediator. He found that the new material was an acidic lipid. It would contract or relax various smooth muscle preparations, and it caused a reduction in blood pressure when given intravenously to animals. He coined the term "prostaglandin" because he believed it to come from the prostate. This turned out to be a misnomer, because the

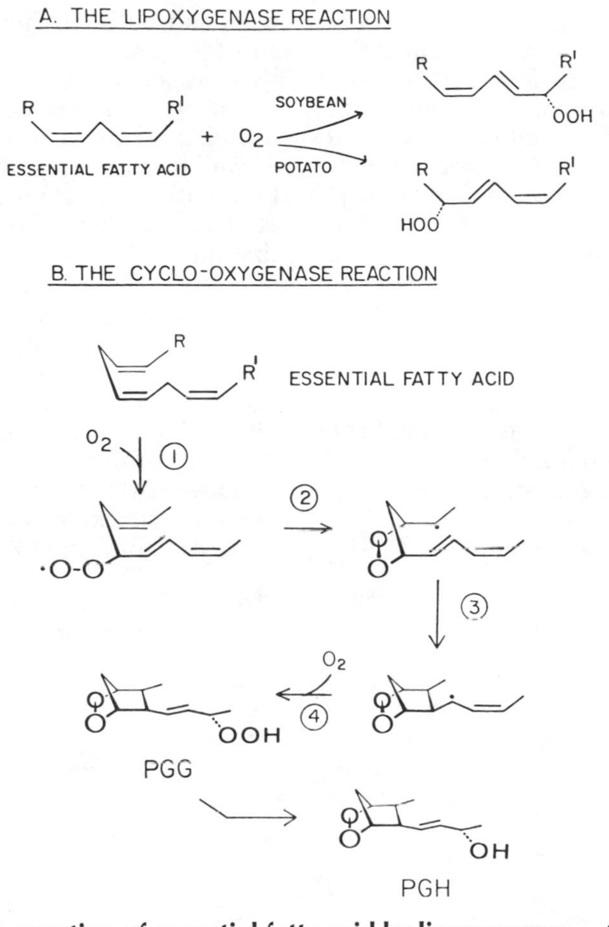

Figure 24.2. A, oxygenation of essential fatty acid by lipoxygenase. Only the important twin double bond unit of the essential fatty acid is shown. The potato lipoxygenase and soybean lipoxygenase form the different fatty acid hydroperoxides as shown. B, oxygenation by the fatty acid cyclooxygenase (prostaglandin synthetase). Step 1, initial lipoxygenase-type oxygenation; step 2, endoperoxide formation; step 3, formation of the 5-membered carbon ring; step 4, second oxygenation to form the product PGG, the endoperoxide intermediate of prostaglandin synthesis. The C-15 OOH group of PGG can be reduced to OH to give the related endoperoxide PGH.

seminal vesicles and not the prostate gland are the major source of prostaglandins in semen.

Von Euler encouraged Sune Bergström to attempt to elucidate the structure of prostaglandin, and this work was begun in earnest in the 1950s. By 1960, Bergström and Sjövall had isolated a few grams of prostaglandin from huge quantities of sheep prostate glands. They were able to separate two components from the extracts; in a mixture of ether and phosphate buffer, one prostaglandin extracted

into the ether phase (PGE), while the more water-soluble component remained in the phosphate buffer (PGF, from *fosfat* in Swedish). The discovery of the chemical structures of PGE and PGF was announced in 1962. Both compounds are 20-carbon fatty acids containing a five-membered carbon ring. The PGE cyclopentane ring has a ketone and hydroxyl substituent, whereas the more water-soluble PGF has two hydroxyl groups (Fig. 24.3). It was soon recognized that prostaglandins with one, two, or three double bonds in the side chain were present in biological extracts—hence, the subscript PGE_1, PGE_2, and PGE_3. It was also noted that treatment of an E prostaglandin with sodium borohydride reduced the C-9 keto group to give two C-9 hydroxy epimers, and invariably the α-isomer (hydroxyl behind the ring) was identical to the PGF isolated from tissues. For this historical reason, the naturally occurring F prostaglandins are always referred to as $PGF_{1\alpha}$, $PGF_{2\alpha}$, and $PGF_{3\alpha}$. In fact, any ring hydroxyl group in a naturally occurring prostaglandin must be of the α configuration, because both oxygen atoms of the endoperoxide are behind the cyclopentane ring (see Figs. 24.2 and 24.3).

Biosynthesis from Essential Fatty Acids

It was not until 1964 that the prostaglandins were shown to be synthesized by oxygenation of C_{20} essential fatty acids. In 1965, Samuelsson reported an experiment which was crucial to our understanding of the biosynthetic process. Incubations of sheep seminal vesicles were performed in an atmosphere of $^{16}O_2$ enriched with the heavy isotope of oxygen ($^{18}O_2$), and the molecular weights of the prostaglandins formed were measured by mass spectrometry. Samuelsson found that the two atoms of oxygen attached to the cyclopentane ring of PGE or PGF both came from the same molecule of O_2. This followed from the observation that either $^{16}O_2$ ($MW = 32$) or $^{18}O_2$ ($MW = 36$) was incorporated on the ring, but never $^{16}O + {}^{18}O$ ($MW = 34$). From this experiment came the hypothesis that an endoperoxide must be formed during prostaglandin biosynthesis. The discovery of PGD in 1968 provided further circumstantial evidence of the existence of an endoperoxide intermediate. Eventually the endoperoxide was isolated and its structure confirmed in the early 1970s.

Activation of Prostaglandin Synthesis: Inhibition of Steroids

During the 1960s, interest in the prostaglandins spread to many other laboratories. PGE and PGF were found in almost all tissues of all animal species examined, and a wide spectrum of bio-

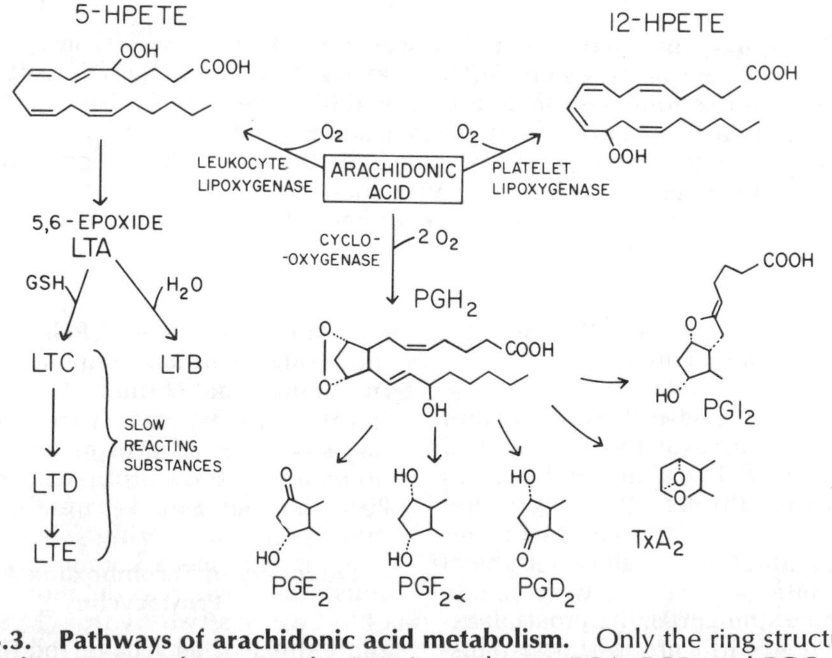

Figure 24.3. Pathways of arachidonic acid metabolism. Only the ring structures of the prostaglandins, TxA_2 and prostacyclin (PGI_2) are shown. PGA, PGB, and PGC are formed from PGE; they are of minor importance and are not shown.

logical activities was characterized. Relatively large amounts of prostaglandins (>1 μg/g of tissue) were found to be synthesized by the lung, kidney, spleen, uterus, and seminal vesicles. It became apparent that prostaglandins are not stored and that release from a tissue can be equated with de novo synthesis. Under normal circumstances, prostaglandin production is almost zero, but synthesis can be activated within seconds of a hormonal or pharmacological stimulation. The liberation of free arachidonic acid from phospholipid stores is the event which initiates prostaglandin biosynthesis, and there is recent evidence that antiinflammatory steroids can block arachidonic acid release from phospholipids, potentially inhibiting all the oxygenation pathways of arachidonate metabolism; however, the relevance of this activity to the mechanism of action of antiinflammatory steroids has yet to be demonstrated.

Any tissue trauma will induce arachidonic acid release and, therefore, activate prostaglandin biosynthesis. For this reason, it is very difficult to measure a true level of prostaglandins in blood or plasma; the disruption of cells and platelets during the sampling procedure is apt to cause biosynthesis and give an artificially high result. In fact, it is clear that biologically active concentrations of prostaglandins do not circulate in blood.

Metabolism

Once the prostaglandins are released into the bloodstream, they are cleared with a very high efficiency as they pass through the lung, kidney, or liver. The prostaglandins are converted on the lower side chain to yield the biologically inactive 15-keto-13.14-dihydro metabolite. More than 90% of an intravenous dose of PGE_2 or $PGF_{2\alpha}$ is metabolized on a single passage through the lungs. The prostaglandins are not hormones in the true sense in that they act at or near their site of synthesis.

By the end of the 1960s, the prostaglandins were viewed as a group of potent biologically active compounds of uncertain function.

Inhibition of Prostaglandin Biosynthesis by Nonsteroidal Antiinflammatory Drugs

Perhaps the most important discovery which helped clarify the role of the prostaglandins was the finding by J. R. Vane and colleagues that aspirin, indomethacin, and other nonsteroidal antiinflammatory drugs are potent inhibitors of cyclooxygenase. The use of this pharmacological tool enabled investigators to test for the involvement of cyclooxygenase products in physiological and pathological processes. This approach was of particular importance for prostaglandin research because effective pharmacological antagonists of the prostaglandins are still not available.

Following Vane's discovery in 1971, it soon became obvious that the prostaglandins are mediators of pain, fever, and inflammation—the very symptoms which nonsteroid antiinflammatory drugs relieve. At this point, it should be noted that the prostaglandins are not often found as the sole mediator of a biological event. Quite commonly, they modulate the activity of other mediators or hormones. For example, the pain caused by an intradermal injection of histamine plus prostaglandin E_2 is considerably more intense than the sum of their individual effects. And PGE_2 will enhance this effect of histamine at a dose which will not by itself cause pain.

The use of cyclooxygenase inhibitors in research has uncovered more subtle actions of aspirin which are due to the inhibition of prostaglandin biosynthesis. For example, the hypercalcemia associated with certain malignancies has been shown to be prostaglandin mediated, and a prostaglandin-dependent component of renin release from the kidney has been identified. In the early 1970s, investigators began to probe for prostaglandin involvement in the well-known inhibition of platelet aggregation caused by aspirin.

Discovery of Thromboxane A₂ and Prostacyclin

The effect of aspirin on platelets was unravelled by Samuelsson and coworker Mats Hamberg. A previously unidentified product synthesized from arachidonic acid via the endoperoxide was shown to be formed during platelet aggregation. This product was unstable (with a chemical half-life of about 30 seconds at 37°C), and it was found to be one of the most proaggregatory substances known. It was named thromboxane A_2 based on its production by the thrombocyte (platelet) and the oxirane ring of TxA and the two double bonds in the side chains (Fig. 24.3). Thromboxane A_2 was also found to be a potent vasoconstrictor and bronchoconstrictor and, indeed, it can also be synthesized by lung tissue. The degradation product of TxA_2 is a chemically stable, but biologically inactive compound called thromboxane B_2 (TxB_2).

It was during a search for tissues which can synthesize TxA_2 that Vane and collaborators discovered yet another previously undetected endoperoxide product. The new compound was formed by the endothelial cells of blood vessels, and it was an extremely potent inhibitor of platelet aggregation. In structure, the compound was a prostaglandin with the upper side chain cyclized to the cyclopentane ring by an internal ether bond (Fig. 24.3). It was named prostacyclin or PGI_2. Prostacyclin is quite unstable in neutral or acidic solutions with a chemical half-life of about 5 minutes at 37°C. It is hydrolyzed to a stable, though biologically inactive compound called 6-keto-$PGF_{1\alpha}$.

Lipoxygenases, SRS-A, and Leukotrienes

When Hamberg and Samuelsson discovered TxA_2, they also detected the formation of a simple hydroperoxy derivative of arachidonic acid in platelets. This was the first time that a lipoxygenase enzyme had been found in animal tissue. (As was mentioned in the section on the Mechanism of Prostaglandin Biosynthesis, lipoxygenase enzymes giving hydroperoxy fatty acid products are quite common in plants.) Since the chemical name of arachidonic acid is eicosatetraenoic acid, the C-12 hydroperoxy derivative formed in platelets is called 12-hydroperoxy-eicosatetraenoic acid (12-HPETE) (Fig. 24.3). The hydroperoxy group is readily reduced to the hydroxy derivative, 12-HETE. The function of the platelet 12-lipoxygenase has yet to be clarified.

In 1976, Samuelsson and coworkers Pierre Borgeat and Mats Hamberg found that leukocytes make the related compound 5-HPETE. The biological relevance of this lipoxygenase pathway was unknown at that time; however, it was later shown that this reaction is the first step in the biosynthesis of slow reacting substance of anaphylaxis (SRS-A). SRS-A was discovered in 1938, but its chemical structure and route of biosynthesis were unknown. It was characterized as a substance which is released in immediate hypersensitivity reactions and which causes a slowly developing contraction of bronchial smooth muscle in vitro. It is thought to be a major mediator of human asthma. 5-HPETE is further converted by leukocytes to an epoxide derivative of arachidonic acid. This intermediate (now called leukotriene A) then reacts with glutathione (the gly–cys–glu tripeptide) to form the first member of a series of C-5 hydroxy, C-6 peptidyl derivatives of arachidonic acid which are slow-reacting substances. The family of compounds formed through this pathway has the double bonds of arachidonic acid conjugated into a triene arrangement which has a characteristic absorbance in the ultraviolet spectrum. Since the compounds are formed in white cells, they were named leukotrienes (Figs. 24.3 and 24.4).

DIETARY ESSENTIAL FATTY ACIDS AND CARDIOVASCULAR DISEASE

In the late 1970s, it was reported that Eskimos have a relatively low incidence of cardiovascular disease, and it was suggested that this correlated with their diet rich in "omega-3" essential fatty acids. Certain fish oils are rich in these polyunsaturated fatty acids. The name "omega-3" comes from the fact that the last double bond in the chain is positioned three carbons from the tail end of the molecule; eicosapentaenoic acid (EPA) (Fig. 24.1) is one of the main omega-3 fatty acids. Because of their

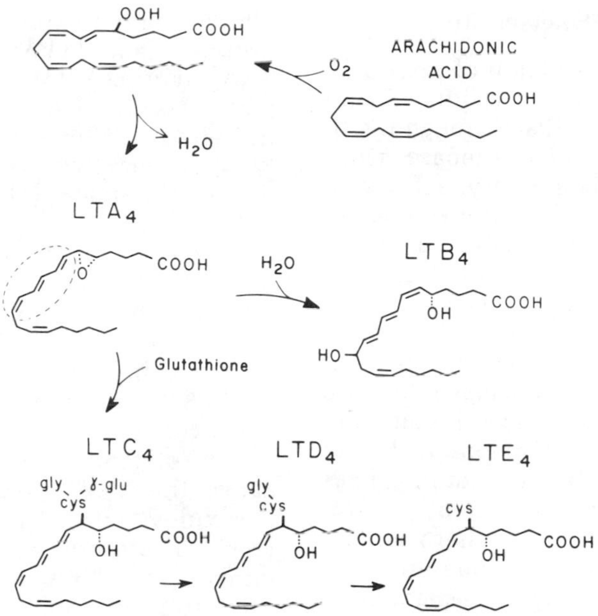

Figure 24.4. Biosynthesis of the leukotrienes. Arachidonic acid is converted to the 5-hydroperoxy compound which is further transformed to the key epoxide intermediate leukotriene A_4. LTA_4 is reacted with water to form LTB_4, a chemotactic leukotriene, or with reduced glutathione to form LTC_4. LTC_4 can be modified by removal of peptide residues to form LTD_4 and LTE_4; all three are constituents of slow reacting substance. The characteristic triene is outlined on the structure of LTA_4.

diet, Eskimos have more EPA (and less arachidonic acid) in their tissue lipids.

The biochemical basis for the claims about Eskimos and fish oils lies in the relative efficiency of conversion of arachidonic acid and EPA to prostaglandins and thromboxanes. It was found that EPA is very poorly converted to thromboxane A_3 in platelets, and moreover, that TxA_3 has relatively weak aggregatory effects compared to TxA_2. On the other hand, EPA is converted quite efficiently to PGI_3, and this is equipotent to PGI_2. Therefore, when EPA substitutes for arachidonic acid, an antiaggregatory effect is anticipated. Indeed, Eskimos were shown to have a prolonged bleeding time, an indication of decreased platelet activation, and possibly explaining their diminished tendency to coronary thrombosis.

Could a fish oil diet be of benefit to others? Although most studies of supplemented omega-3 fatty acids in the Western population have detected platelet-inhibitory effects, very large doses have been used (~50 g/day). These doses have been given for only a few weeks, and the long-term effects are yet to be evaluated. Also, there remains some dispute whether the epidemiological evidence of reduced incidence of cardiovascular disease among Eskimos can be attributed to dietary factors. Current research is focused on further definition of the biochemical and physiological sequelae of the fish oil diet.

PATHOPHYSIOLOGICAL ROLES OF PROSTAGLANDINS AND OTHER EICOSANOIDS

Pain, Fever, and Inflammation

Prostaglandins are important mediators of the inflammatory response. Aspirin and other nonsteroidal antiinflammatory drugs (indomethacin, meclofenamate, ibuprofen, phenylbutazone) act by inhibition of the cyclooxygenase.

Immediate Hypersensitivity

Immunological activation of mast cells and leukocytes results in a burst of arachidonic acid metabolism through the lipoxygenase and cyclooxygenase pathways. The proinflammatory actions of the eicosanoid products are well characterized. Allergic asthmatic bronchospasm is probably mediated in part by a mixture of leukotrienes C, D, and E (formerly known only as SRS-A, slow-reacting substance of anaphylaxis). Both the leukotrienes and the prostaglandins are mediators of local vasodilation and increased vascular permeability. Prostaglandin synthesis by the mast cell is strikingly evidenced in systemic mastocytosis. In this condition, there is sporadic synthesis of large quantities of PGD_2, the major arachidonate metabolite of mast cells. Attacks of flushing and often life-threatening hypotension are the resulting symptoms. The symptoms can be alleviated by the use of aspirin, usually combined with antihistamines.

Control of Platelet Aggregation

In the short time since the discovery of TxA_2 and PGI_2, there has been a great deal of attention focused on their respective roles in the control of platelet aggregation. The activation of platelets is a precipitating factor in acute myocardial infarction and stroke. Inhibition of TxA_2 with aspirin has been shown to be effective in preventing coronary thrombosis. Selective inhibition of thromboxane production in such patients is likely to be of greater benefit because the antiaggregatory effects of the endogenous PGI_2 will now be unopposed. Indeed, aspirin has been found to be effective in the secondary prevention of acute myocardial infarction and stroke.

Although a cyclooxygenase inhibitor should block the production of both TxA_2 and PGI_2, there is evidence that a selective effect on just TxA_2 synthesis in platelets can be obtained with a very low dose of aspirin. The platelet cyclooxygenase is exquisitely sensitive to inhibition by aspirin, and, in addition, aspirin acts as an irreversible inhibitor. Since platelets are unable to synthesize new protein, it should be possible to eliminate TxA_2 synthesis for the life-span of the platelet (several days) with aspirin, while the ability of endothelial cells to make PGI_2 is compromised for only a few hours. Complete inhibition is possible with as little as 40 mg daily. The optimum daily dosage regimen has yet to be defined.

Drugs which inhibit thromboxane synthase (the enzyme in platelets which converts the prostaglandin endoperoxide to TxA_2) also inhibit TxA_2 selectively. However, they have proved disappointing as platelet inhibitors, probably because the TxA_2 precursors (the endoperoxides) can activate the TxA_2 receptor. More promising results are obtained using TxA_2 receptor antagonists; this group of compounds block the actions of both the endoperoxides and of TxA_2, and they are currently being evaluated as therapeutic agents.

Control of Renin Release

Renin secretion by the kidney is regulated by catecholamine and prostaglandin pathways. By this action, renal prostaglandin synthesis has an indirect influence on the regulation of blood pressure and on sodium and water balance. Prostaglandin-mediated renin release is activated by a fall in renal arterial pressure, and it is also sensitive to changes in salt balance in the ascending limb of the loop of Henle. Renal prostaglandins may regulate renal blood flow and glomerular filtration in patients with severe congestive heart failure. In these circumstances, cyclooxygenase inhibitors can precipitate acute deterioration in renal function and worsening heart failure.

Control of Tissue Blood Flow During Anesthesia and Surgery

It is well established that prostaglandin synthesis is activated by interventions such as anesthesia and surgery. When this phenomenon was first encountered, investigators mistakenly attributed functions to the prostaglandins which have subsequently been shown to be of little relevance to the more normal physiological circumstances. Nevertheless, under the altered conditions of anesthesia and manipulation of tissues accompanying surgery, it is certain that arachidonate metabolites are synthesized in relatively large amounts. Under these conditions, they assume an important role in the local control of blood flow in tissues and organs.

Protamine administration to reverse the effects of heparin during cardiac surgery is sometimes associated with profound hypotension, pulmonary hypertension, and severe bronchoconstriction. This syndrome has been shown to be mediated by liberation of TxA_2, a well-recognized vasoconstrictor and bronchoconstrictor. Indomethacin attenuates these changes in the sheep, an animal which is particularly sensitive to the effects of TxA_2.

Seminal Prostaglandins and Infertility

Human seminal fluid is a rich source of prostaglandins. The prostaglandins in seminal fluid are thought to stimulate contraction of the uterus and promote the motility of sperm. Some cases of male infertility are associated with low seminal concentrations of prostaglandins, although there is no evidence that the use of aspirin or other cyclooxygenase inhibitors results in infertility.

Menstruation

The endometrium of the uterus produces prostaglandins in amounts increasing during the luteal phase and reaching a maximum at the time of menstruation. Prostaglandins have been shown to inhibit follicular rupture and ovulation. Excess production of prostaglandins may account for some of the symptoms of dysmenorrhea.

Abortion and Parturition

Prostaglandins, particularly PGF_{2a}, are synthesized by the pregnant uterus. $PGF_{2\alpha}$ production is increased at the onset of labor, and it has been suggested that the initiation and contractions of labor are due to prostaglandins. Conversely, it has been reported that labor can be delayed by the administration of aspirin, which blocks prostaglandin synthesis. Prostaglandins have also been implicated in the process of spontaneous abortion.

THERAPEUTIC USES

The very properties which characterize the eicosanoids as local hormones have limited their application in therapeutics. The endogenous compounds seldom cause systemic effects because biosynthesis is restricted to local areas and systemic metabolism is very fast; but pharmacological doses tend to give unacceptable side effects such as nausea, vomiting, and diarrhea, while lesser amounts are inactive orally or have a short duration of action. Consequently, widespread use of the eicosanoids in clinical medicine is likely to be confined to applications in which local administration is possible.

Therapeutic Abortion

Prostaglandins E and F have been used for many years to induce midtrimester abortion. A vaginal suppository of PGE_2 is now the prefered method, giving a minimum of systemic side effects. At term, a PGE_2 gel is used to promote cervical ripening prior to induction of labor. Postpartum hemorrhage can be controlled using the 15-methyl analog of $PGF_{2\alpha}$; the uterus is stimulated to contract, thus closing down blood flow to the endometrium.

Congenital Heart Disease

Prostaglandin production appears to be important in maintaining the patency of the ductus arteriosus in the fetus, and inhibition of this synthesis is used in treatment of symptomatic patent ductus arteriosus. The cyclooxygenase inhibitor indomethacin is now used routinely for this purpose. Infants with ventricular outflow obstruction and other complex congenital abnormalities may be dependent on the continued patency of the ductus for adequate systemic or pulmonary blood flow. For these patients, closure of the ductus can be disasterous and can be prevented by administration of the E-type prostaglandins, thus maintaining flow through the ductus until surgery can be performed.

Alprostadil

Alprostadil, **prostaglandin E₁,** is available in the United States as 1.0-ml ampules containing 0.5 mg. The drug produces vasodilation, inhibition of platelet aggregation, and stimulation of intestinal and smooth muscle. Alprostadil dilates the ductus arteriosus and increases pulmonary blood flow and therefore oxygenation in neonates with restricted pulmonary blood flow, such as pulmonary atresia and stenosis, tetralogy of Fallot, and tricuspid atresia. Alprostadil is also useful in infants with restricted systemic blood flow with aortic arch obstruction; examples include interruption of the aortic arch and coarctation of the aorta. These infants are often acidotic; alprostadil by improving perfusion to the lower body may also improve the acidosis. When given to neonates for its vasodilatory effects, it is usually infused at an initial rate of 0.1 μg/kg/min, and the rate is subsequently titrated down to the lowest dosage possible to maintain a therapeutic response. Side effects of alprostadil include hypotension, flushing, bradycardia, edema, seizure-like activity, pyrexia, and most important apnea. Apnea has been described in 10 to 12% of neonates with congenital heart defects, and it is therefore essential to monitor neonatal respiratory status and have equipment available for ventilation. Alprostadil has a very short half-life of less than 5 minutes; it is metabolized in the lungs and the metabolites excreted by the kidneys.

Although alprostadil is mainly used in neonates, it has been used by anesthesiologists and internists in adult patients. A prostaglandin E₁ infusion (100 to 150 ng/kg/min) has been used as a hypotensive agent during general anesthesia with halothane. Prostaglandin E₁ has been utilized in the setting of right heart failure and pulmonary hypertension after

mitral valve replacement; high-dose PGE₁ (30 to 150 ng/kg/min) was used to vasodilate the pulmonary circulation, while a left atrial norepinephrine infusion was given simultaneously to maintain systemic blood pressure. This mode of treatment was shown to be of considerable benefit in this situation. The drug has also been used chronically in patients with adult respiratory distress syndrome (ARDS) in moderate doses (30 ng/kg/min) in an attempt to improve both oxygenation and survival. *Epoprosterol* (PGI₂) is available in Europe.

Peptic Ulcer Disease

PGE₂ and PGI₂ suppress gastric acid production, and a synthetic PGE analog has been used for the management of peptic ulcer. The inhibition of endogenous prostaglandin production by anti-inflammatory drugs may be the underlying cause of their tendency to provoke gastric and duodenal ulcers.

Cardiopulmonary Bypass

Infusion of prostacyclin (PGI₂) has been evaluated as an antiplatelet agent to prevent platelet consumption during cardiopulmonary bypass. Also, PGI₂ and its analog PGE₁ have been found effective in preventing thrombotic occlusion during coronary angioplasty. Although the compounds are effective in these applications, there is an extremely narrow therapeutic window, above which the potent hypotensive effects present a hazard which will undoubtedly limit the widespread use of these agents. Ongoing efforts are directed toward the development of analogs which retain antiplatelet actions without the vasodilator properties.

Adult Respiratory Distress Syndrome (ARDS)

In ARDS, an increase in lung TxB₂, the stable metabolite of TxA₂, has been shown to correlate with an increase in pulmonary vascular resistance. In animal models of pulmonary hypertension there is an increase in TxA₂, and cyclooxygenase blockade not only blocks the increase in thromboxane production but also reduces the degree of pulmonary hypertension. Thus, indomethacin, by inhibiting TxA$_2$ synthesis, may be a useful agent in the management of ARDS and has been used in ARDS patients in an attempt to attenuate the early increases in pulmonary artery pressure that occur in this situation. Alternatively, infusions of the vasodilators PGI$_2$ (prostacyclin) and PGE$_1$ have been given to these patients, again to reduce pulmonary hypertension. Prostacyclin (epoprosternol, PGI$_2$) has been given in doses of 5 ng/kg/min to improve oxygen delivery and uptake in critically ill patients in the intensive care unit.

CONCLUSIONS

In view of the problems that beset the administration of the eicosanoids, it is probable that the greatest potential for therapeutic innovations lies in the development of selective inhibitors of the enzymes which catalyze steps in the arachidonic acid cascade. The development of selective antagonists of the actions of the individual prostaglandins also holds promise. In particular, there remain outstanding possibilities for the inhibition and antagonism of the lipoxygenase pathways and their major biosynthetic products, the leukotrienes.

BIBLIOGRAPHY

Aherne T, Price DC, Yee ES, Hsieh WR, Ebert PA: Prevention of ischemia-induced myocardial platelet deposition by exogenous protacyclin. *J Thorac Cardiovasc Surg*, 92:99–104, 1986.

Bihari D, Smithies M, Gimson A, Tinker J: The effects of vasodilation with prostacyclin on oxygen delivery and uptake in critically ill patients. *N Engl J Med* 317:397–403, 1987.

Cairns JA, Gent M, Singer J, et al: Aspirin, Sulfinpyrazone, or both in unstable angina. *N Engl J Med* 313:1369–1375, 1985.

Chelly J, Fabiani JN, Chahine R, Tricot AM, Carpentier A, Passelecq J, Dubost C: Hemodynamic and metabolic effects of prostacyclin after coronary bypass surgery. *Circulation* 66:I45–I49, 1982.

Cotton RB: The relationship of symptomatic patent ductus arteriosus to respiratory distress syndrome in premature newborn infants. *Clin Perinatol* 14:621–633, 1987.

D'Ambra MN, LaRaia PJ, Philbin DM, Watkins WD, Hilgenberg AD, Buckley MJ: Prostaglandin E$_1$: a new therapy for refractory right heart failure and pulmonary hypertension after mitral valve replacement. *J Thorac Cardiovasc Surg* 89:567–572, 1985.

DiSesa VJ, Huval W, Lelcuk S, Jonas R, Maddi R, Lee-Son S, Shemin RJ, Collins JJ, Hechtman HB, Cohn LH: Disadvantages of prostacyclin infusion during cardiopulmonary bypass: a double-blind study of 50 patients having coronary revascularization. *Ann Thorac Surg* 38:514–519, 1984.

Ford-Hutchinson AW, Letts GL: Biological actions of leukotrienes: state of the art lecture. *Hypertension* 8:II44–II49, 1986.

Goa KL, Monk JP: Enprostil: a preliminary review of its pharmacodynamic and pharmacokinetic properties, and therapeutic efficacy in the treatment of peptic ulcer disease. *Drugs* 34:539–559, 1987.

Goto F, Otani E, Kato S, Fujita T: Prostaglandin E$_1$ as a hypotensive drug during general anaesthesia. *Anaesthesia* 37:530–535, 1982.

Higgs GA, Moncada S: Leukotrienes in disease: implications for drug development. *Drugs* 30:1–5, 1985.

Hobbhahn J, Conzen PF, Zenker B, Goetz AE, Peter K, Brendel W: Beneficial effect of cyclooxygenase inhibition on adverse hemodynamic responses after protamine. *Anesth Analg* 67:253–260, 1988.

Holcroft JW, Vassar MJ, Webert CJ: Prostaglandin E$_1$ and survival in patients with the adult respiratory distress syndrome. *Ann Surg* 203:371–378, 1985.

Hudson JC, Wurm WH, O'Donnell TF, Shoenfeld NA, Mackey WC, Callow AD, Su YF, Watkins WD: Hemodynamics and prostacyclin release in the early phases of aortic surgery: comparison of transabdominal and retroperitoneal approaches. *J Vasc Surg* 7:190–198, 1988.

Huttemeier PC, Berry D, Bloch KJ, Watkins WD, Zapol WM: Pulmonary vasoconstriction and profound leukopenia in two sheep experimental models: effects of complement depletion. *Chest* 83:24s–25s, 1983.

Kobinia GS, LaRaia PJ, D'Ambra MN, Fabri BM, Aylesworth CA, Peterson MB, Watkins WD, Buckley MJ: Effect of experimental cardiopulmonary bypass on systemic and transcardiac thromboxane B$_2$ levels. *J Thorac Cardiovasc Surg* 91:852–857, 1986.

Kobinia GS, LaRaia PJ, Peterson MB, D'Ambra MN, Watkins WD, Austen WG, Buckley MJ: Cardiac prostacyclin kinetics during cardiopulmonary bypass. *J Thorac Cardiovasc Surg* 88:965–971, 1984.

Longmore DB, Hoyle PM, Gregory A, Bennett JG, Smith MA, Osivand T, Jones WA: Prostacyclin administration during cardiopulmonary bypass in man. *Lancet* 1:800–804, 1981.

Lowenstein E, Johnston WE, Lappas DG, D'Ambra MN, Schneider RC, Daggett WM, Akins GW, Philbin DM: Catastrophic pulmonary vasoconstriction associated with protamine reversal of heparin. *Anesthesiology* 59:470–473, 1983.

MacKenzie IZ: Prostaglandins: has the initial promise been realised? *Drugs* 25:1–5, 1983.

Mahony L, Carnero V, Brett C, Heymann MA,

Clyman RI: Prophylactic indomethacin therapy for patent ductus arteriosus in very-low-birth-weight infants. *N Engl J Med* 306:506–510, 1982.

McIntyre RW, Flezzani P, Knopes KD, Reves JG, Watkins WD: Pulmonary hypertension and prostaglandins after protamine. *Am J Cardiol* 58:857–858, 1986.

Mitchell JRA: Prostacyclin-powerful, yes: but is it useful? *Br Med J* 287:1824–1826, 1983.

Morel DR, Zapol WM, Thomas SJ, Kitain EM, Robinson DR, Moss J, Chenoweth DE, Lowenstein E: C5a and thromboxane generation associated with pulmonary vaso- and broncho-constriction during protamine reversal of heparin. *Anesthesiology* 66:595–596, 1987.

Nies AS: Prostaglandins and the control of the circulation. *Clin Pharmacol Ther* 39:481–488, 1986.

Reilly CS, Biollaz J, Koshakji RP, Wood AJJ: Enprostil, in contrast to cimetidine, does not inhibit propranolol metabolism. *Clin Pharmacol Ther* 40:37–41, 1986.

Reilly IAG, FitzGerald GA: Aspirin and cardiovascular disease. *Drugs* 35:154–176, 1988.

Schuette AH, Huttemeier PC, Hill RD, Watkins WD, Wonders TR, Kong D, Zapol WM: Regional blood flow and pulmonary thromboxane release after sublethal endotoxin infusion in sheep. *Surgery* 95:444–453, 1984.

Seeling W, Heinrich H, Oettinger W: The eventration syndrome: prostacyclin liberation and hypoxaemia due to eventration of the gut. *Anaesthesist* 35:738–743, 1986.

Swerdlow BN, Mihm FG, Goetzl EJ, Matthay MA: Leukotrienes in pulmonary edema fluid after cardiopulmonary bypass. *Anesth Analg* 65:306–308, 1986.

Ylikorkala O, Saarela E, Viinikka L: Increased prostacyclin and thromboxane production in man during cardiopulmonary bypass. *J Thorac Cardiovasc Surg* 82:245–247, 1981.

APPENDIX 1

Pediatric Dose Schedule

Alprostadil (prostaglandin E₁)	0.05–0.10 µg/kg/min	i.v.
Aminophylline	(see Table 19.3, page 547)	
Atracurium	0.2–0.4 mg/kg	i.v.
Atropine	0.015–0.02 mg/kg	i.m.* or i.v.
Calcium chloride	3.0–10.0 mg/kg	i.v.
Chlorpromazine	0.5 mg/kg	i.m.
Dexamethasone	0.2 mg/kg	i.v. (maximum, 10mg)
Diazepam	0.2–0.4 mg/kg	p.o., i.m.
Diphenhydramine	0.2–0.5 mg/kg	i.v.
Dobutamine	1–10 µg/kg/min	i.v.
Dopamine	1.0–10.0 µg/kg/min	i.v.
Droperidol	0.1–0.15 mg/kg	i.m., i.v.
Edrophonium	0.2 mg/kg	i.v.
Epinephrine†	0.02–0.1 µg/kg/min	i.v.
Epinephrine (cardiac resuscitation)	7–10 µg/kg	i.v.
Fentanyl	0.5–2.0 µg/kg	i.v., i.m.
Furosemide	0.5–1.0 mg/kg	i.v.
Gallamine	1.0–2.0 mg/kg	i.v.
Glycopyrrolate	0.004–0.008 mg/kg	i.m.
Hydrocortisone		
Birth–1 month	25 mg	i.m., i.v.
1 month–12 years	50–100 mg	i.m., i.v.
Hydroxyzine	0.5–1.0 mg/kg	i.m.
Isoproterenol†	0.05–0.1 µg/kg/min	i.v.
Ketamine	2.0 mg/kg	i.v.
Ketamine	4.0–8.0 mg/kg	i.m.
Lidocaine (loading)	0.5–1.0 mg/kg	i.v.
Lidocaine (maintenance)	20–60 µg/kg/min	i.v.
Mannitol	2 g/kg	Slow i.v.
Meperidine	1.0–1.5 mg/kg	i.m.
Methohexital	1.0–2.0 mg/kg	i.v.
Methylprednisolone	5–15 mg/kg	i.v.
Morphine	0.05–0.2 mg/kg	i.m.
Naloxone	0.005–0.01 mg/kg	i.v.
Neostigmine	0.06 mg/kg	i.v.
Pancuronium	0.05–0.1 mg/kg	i.v.
Pentazocine	0.5 mg/kg	i.m.
Pentobarbital	2 mg/kg	i.m.
Phentolamine	0.125 mg/kg	i.v.
Promethazine	0.5 mg/kg	i.m.
Propranolol	0.01–0.02 mg/kg	Slow i.v.
Scopolamine	0.008 mg/kg	i.m.
Secobarbital	2 mg/kg	i.m.
Sodium bicarbonate	0.5–1.0 mEq/kg	i.v.
Sodium nitroprusside	0.5–8.0 µg/kg/min	i.v.
Succinylcholine	1.0–1.5 mg/kg	i.v.
Thiopental	2.0–4.0 mg/kg	i.v.
Tubocurarine	0.3–0.5 mg/kg	i.v.
Vecuronium	0.08–0.10 mg/kg	i.v.

*i.m., intramuscular, i.v., intravenous; 1 mg = 1,000 µg.
†Titrate and increase dose according to clinical response.

APPENDIX 2

Pharmacokinetic Parameters of Some Important Drugs

Drug	Plasma binding (%)	Volume of distribution (L/kg)	Half-life (hr)	Clearance (ml/min/kg)	Urinary excretion (%)	Therapeutic concentration	Toxic concentration
Acebutolol	15–20	1.2	3–6	5	20	Active metabolites	>300 µg/ml
Acetaminophen	25	0.95	2.0	5.0	3.0	10–20 µg/ml	
N-Acetylprocainamide	10	1.4	6.0	3.1	81	12 µg/ml	
Acetylsalicylic acid	49	0.15	0.25	9.3	1.4		
Albuterol			2.7–5.0				
Alfentanil	88–92	0.86	1.6	6.4	<1	200–500 ng/ml	
Alphaxalone	46	0.64	0.17				
Alprenolol	85	3.4	2.0–3.0	15	0.5	30 ng/ml	
Amiodarone	96	66	25 days	1.9	0	0.5–2.5 µg/ml	> 2.5 µg/ml
Amitriptyline	96	8.3	15	6.1		160–240 ng/ml	>1 µg/ml
Amoxicillin	18	0.41	1.0	5.3	52		
Ampicillin	18	0.28	1.3	3.9	90		
Atenolol	<5.0	0.7	6.3	1.3	85	1.3 µg/ml	1.1 µg/ml
Atracurium		0.15	0.33	5.1		0.65 µg/ml	
Atropine	50	2.0–4.0	2.2	16.6	25		
Betamethasone	64	1.4	5.6	2.9	4.8		
Bretylium	0–8	6.0	9.0	10	77		
Bupivacaine	90–97	1.0	3.5	6.7	5.0		
Buprenorphine	96	2.0	3.0–5.0	12.0–18.0	<1		
Butorphanol	80		2.4–3.5		0		
Captopril	30	0.7	2.0	13	45		
Carbamazepine	82	1.4	15–27	0.58–1.3	<1	4–12 µg/ml	>8–10 µg/ml
Carbenicillin	50	0.18	1.0	2.0	82		
Cefazolin	84	0.12	1.8	0.95	80		
Cephalexin	14	0.26	0.90	4.3	96		
Cephalothin	71	0.26	0.57	6.7	52		
Chloramphenicol	53	0.92	2.7	3.6	5.0		
Chlordiazepoxide	96.5	0.30	9.9	0.37	<1.0	>0.7 µg/ml	
Chlorothiazide	94.6	0.20	1.5	4.5	92		
Chlorpromazine	95–98	21	30	8.6	<1.0	30–350 ng/ml	750–1000 ng/ml
Chlorthalidone	75	3.9	44	1.6	65		
Cimetidine	19	2.1	2.1	12	77	1.0 µg/ml	
Clindamycin	93.6	0.66	2.7	3.5	9–14		
Clonazepam	47	3.2	39	0.92	<1.0	5–70 ng/ml	
Clonidine	20	2.1	8.5–12.7	3.1	62	1.0 ng/ml	

Drug							
Codeine	7.0	5.4	3.0–4.0	23	0		
Cromolyn	63–76	0.13	0.6–0.9		0		
Desipramine	92	34	18.0	24	0	>225 ng/ml	>1 µg/ml
Diazepam	96–98	1.1	20–90		<1	>600 ng/ml	
Diazoxide	90–99	0.2	20–35	0.38			
Digitoxin	90–97	0.51	168–192	0.046	33	>10 ng/ml	>35 ng/ml
Digoxin	25–40	5.1–7.4	30–42		72	>0.8 ng/ml	
Diltiazem	78	5.0	3.2	11.0	>4		
Disopyramide	28–68	0.78	7.8	1.3	55	2.8–7.5 µg/ml	
Dobutamine		0.2	0.04				
Dopamine			0.12				
Doxepin		20	17	14	Negligible	30–150 ng/ml	
Droperidol	85–90		2–3				
Edrophonium		1.1	1.8	9.6	45		
Enalapril	50		35	1.5			
Encainide	75	4.0	2.3/11.3	30/3	5/40	Extensive/poor metabolizers of debrisoquine	
Esmolol	56	3.4	0.15	286	0		
Ethosuximide	Negligible	0.72	33	0.26	19	40–120 µg/ml	<100 µg/ml
Etidocaine	94–97	1.9	2.6	17.0			
Etomidate	75	2.3–4.5	1.1–4.5	11.5–25			
Fentanyl	79–86	4.0	3.6	13.0	8	3–20 ng/ml	
Furosemide	95.9	0.11	0.85	2.2	74		
Gallamine	30–70	0.29	2.5	1.6	89–100		
Gentamicin	<10	0.25	2–3		>90		
Guanethidine			43–120				
Haloperidol	92	18–30	13–35		Negligible	3–10 ng/ml	
Heparin	95*	0.06	1.0–2.5	0.28–0.73	<1.0		
Hexobarbital	42–52	1.1	4.4	3.6	12–14		
Hydralazine	87	1.6	2.2–2.6	8–10	95	1 µg/ml	
Hydrochlorothiazide	64	0.83	2.5	4.9			
Hydrocortisone	95	0.3	1.0–2.0				
imipramine	89–94	15	13.0	20	0–1.7	>225 ng/ml	>1 µg/ml
Indomethacin	90	0.26–0.93	2.4–2.6	1.6–2.0	15	0.5–3.0 µg/ml	>6 µg/ml
Isoniazid	Negligible	0.61	1.0–3.0	2.5–7.0	7–30		
Isosorbide dinitrate		1.8	0.5		0		
Kanamycin	0	0.26	2.0	1.4	90		
Ketamine	12	3.0	2.5–3.4	17.0	2.3		
Ketanserin	94	6.2	13	6.0	5	150–1000 ng/ml	

APPENDIX 2 (*Continued*)

Pharmacokinetic Parameters of Some Important Drugs (*Continued*)

Drug	Plasma binding (%)	Volume of distribution (L/kg)	Half-life (hr)	Clearance (ml/min/kg)	Urinary excretion (%)	Therapeutic concentration	Toxic concentration
Labetalol	50	5.6	4.0	20	<5	2.5µg/ml	
Lidocaine	60–75	1.1–1.3	1.6–1.8	9.2–13.5	2.0		>6-10µg/ml
Lithium	0	0.79	22	0.35	95	>0.7mEq/L	>2.0mEq/L
Lorazepam	93	1.3	14	1.1	<1.0		
Lorcainide	85	6.4	7.6	17.5	<2	40–200 ng/ml	
Meperidine	58–64	4.2	3–8	10–18.6	4–22	200–600 ng/ml	
Mepivacaine	75	1.2	1.9	11.0			
Metaproterenol	10		1.5				
Methicillin	28–49	0.43	0.85	6.1	88		
Methohexital	73	1.13	1.6	12.1			
Methyldopa	<20	0.37	1.8	3.1	63		
Metocurine	31.8	0.422–0.460	3.6	1.05–1.4	52		
Metoprolol	12	4.2	3.0–4.0	15	10	25 ng/ml	
Midazolam	94–96	1.1–2.5	1–4	7–9	0		
Morphine	35	3.2	2.9	15.0	6–10	65 ng/ml	
Nadolol	25–30	1.4–3.4	12–24	2.9	70		
Nalbuphine	25–40	2.9	2.0–3.5	15–22	10		
Naloxone		2.0	1.0–2.5	30–38	1		
Neostigmine		1.4	1.3	9.2–16.7	67.0		
Nifedipine	98	1.2	3.4	10	0		
Nitroglycerin (intravenous)	60	2.85	0.01–0.06				
Nortriptyline	94.5	18.0	31.0	7.2	2.0	50–139 ng/ml	
Oxprenolol	80	1.5	1.3–1.5	2.8	2.0–5.0	0.1–0.2 µg/ml	
Pancuronium	6–8	0.24–0.26	1.9–2.4	1.9–2.1	46	30–100 ng/ml	
Pentazocine	60–70	4.9	2.0		2.0–5.0		
Phenobarbital	45	0.6–1.01	50–160	0.093	24	10–25 µg/ml	>30 µg/ml
Phenytoin	87–93	0.51	15–20	Dose dependent	2.0	8–20 µg/ml	>20 µg/ml
Pindolol	46	2.0	2.0–5.0	6.2	40	58 ng/ml	
Prazosin	93	0.60	2.9	3.0	<1.0		
Prednisolone	90–95	0.48	2.1	1.4	Negligible		
Prednisone		0.97	3.6	3.6	Negligible		
Primidone	<20	0.6	4–12	0.21–0.69	42	5–10 µg/ml	>10-15 µg/ml
Procainamide	16	1.9	2.9–3.0	9.8	67	3 µg/ml	9–14 µg/ml
Propofol	98	2.9–14	3–6	24–33	>0.3	3.0 µg/ml	
Propranolol	90	3.0–4.3	4.0–6.0	12.0	<1.0	20 ng/ml	

Drug						
Pryidostigmine	1.1	1.9	8.6	80–90		6 µg/ml
Quinidine	2.7	6.2	4.7	18	2–5 µg/ml	
Ranitidine	1.8	2.0	10	69	100 ng/ml	
Salicylic acid	0.17	6.0–8.0	Dose dependent		150–300 µg/ml	>200 µg/ml
Sotalol	0.7	5.0–13.0	2.3	60		
Sufentanil	1.7	2.7	13,0		≃4.0 ng/ml	
Terazosin	0.9	9.2	1.1	5		
Terbutaline	1.6	3.0–4.0	3.0	55		
Tetracycline	1.3	9.9	1.9	48		
Theophylline	0.50	4–5	0.83–1.16	7–13	10–20 µg/ml	>20 µg/ml
Thiopental	1.96	5–11	3.3		40 µg/ml	
Timolol	1.3–1.7	4.0–5.0	7.6	13–20		
Tocainide	3.0	13.5	2.6	38	6–15 µg/ml	
Tolbutamide	0.15	5.9	0.30	Negligible	80–240 µg/ml	
Triamterene	2.5	2.8	14	3.9		
Triazolam	1	3.0	5	0		
Tubocurarine	0.29–0.3	1.4–1.9	2.2–2.6	38–44	0.6 µg/ml	
Vecuronium	0.24	1.1	5.2	20	92 ng/ml	
Verapamil	4.0	4.8	11.8	<3.0	100 ng/ml	
Warfarin	0.11	37	0.045	Negligible	2.2 µg/ml	

A useful guide to clinical pharmacokinetic data is *Clinical Pharmacokinetics, Drug Data Handbook, 1989,* Adis Press, Ltd., New Zealand, 1989.
*Bound to lipoproteins.

Index

Page numbers in *italics* denote figures; those followed by "t" denote tables.

Antithyroid drugs, 566
Anxiolytics, 583–587
  antihistamines, 586–587
  barbiturates, 587
  benzodiazepines, 583–586
  buspirone, 586
  chloral hydrate, 587
  classification of, 583
  propanediols, 587
Aortic aneurysms, β-blockers for, 422
Apomorphine, chemical structure of, 378
Aprindine, 488
Aprotinin, 607
  for carcinoid syndrome, 625
Arachidonic acid, metabolic pathways of, 636
Arbaprostil, 623
"Artificial pancreas", 557
Asendin. See Amoxapine
Aspirin, antiplatelet effects of, 607
Asthma
  chemical mediators of bronchospasm, 540
  immunoglobulin E in, 539
  treatment of. See also Bronchodilators
    β-agonists, 539–545
    calcium antagonists, 531
    corticosteroids, 549–550
    cromolyn sodium, 549
    ipratropium, 550
    methylxanthines, 545–549
Atarax. See Hydroxyzine
Atenolol
  pharmacodynamics of, 410t
  pharmacokinetics of, 414t, 416, 646t
Ativan. See Lorazepam
Atracurium, 303. See also Neuromuscular blocking
      agents
  administration of, 303
  cardiovascular effects of, 300, 300–301
  chemical structure of, 281
  dose of, 303
  pediatric dose of, 645t
  pharmacokinetics of, 282t–284t, 286–287, 287–
      288, 646t
  in pregnancy, 358–359
Atrial ectopic beats, 465t, 465–466
Atrial fibrillation, 465t, 466–467
  β-blockers for, 422
Atrial flutter, 465t, 466–467
Atrial natriuretic factor, 504–505
Atropine, 112–118
  administration of, 117
  cardiovascular effects of, 115
  CNS effects of, 115
  contraindications to, 117
  dosage of, 117
  effects of, 113
  eye effects of, 116
  gastrointestinal effects of, 115–116
  neostigmine and, 97–98, 98, 116
  other effects of, 116
  pediatric dose of, 645t
  pharmacokinetics of, 116–117, 646t
  poisoning with, 117–118
  for premedication, 124
    of children, 125, 125t
  pyridostigmine and, 100

  respiratory effects of, 115
  structure-activity relationships of, 113–114, 114
Autonomic nervous system, 84, 84, 112, 377
Aventyl. See Nortriptyline
Azathioprine, neuromuscular blocking agents and,
      291
Azumolene, 308

Barbital, chemical structure of, 181t
Barbiturates, 180–193. See also specific drugs
  antiepileptic effect of, 592
  anxiolytic effect of, 587
  chemical structure of, 180, 180, 181t
  classification of, 182
  cumulation and prolonged administration of,
      185–186
  lidocaine and, 473
  methohexital, 192–193
  pharmacokinetics of, 182–185
    distribution, 183–184
    metabolism, 185
    renal excretion, 185
    uptake and redistribution, 184, 185
  structure-activity relationships of, 180–182, 181t
  thiopental, 186–192
BARK, 69–70
Beclomethasone dipropionate, 549–550
Belladonna alkaloids, 113–114
Benadryl. See Diphenhydramine
Benserazide, for Parkinson's disease, 123
Benzodiazepine antagonists, 205–206
Benzodiazepines, 196–206, 583–586, 584t. See
      also specific drugs
  adverse effects of, 593
  antiepileptic effects of, 593
  cardiovascular effects of, 585
  chemical structures of, 196, 196
  CNS effects of, 584–585
  diazepam, 198–201
  lorazepam, 204–205
  mechanism of action of, 196–197, 197
  metabolic pathways of, 585, 585
  midazolam, 201–204
  pharmacokinetics of, 200t, 585–586
  for premedication, 123
    of children, 125t
  receptors for, 197–198
Benztropine, for Parkinson's disease, 122
Beta endorphin, 134
Beta lipotropin, 134
Betamethasone
  pharmacokinetics of, 646t
  pharmacology of, 561t
Bethanechol, 89
Bethanidine, 444–445
  site of action of, 437t
Bier's block, 335
Biguanides, 555–556, 556t
Bipolar disorder, 587
Bradykinin, 624
Bremazocine, 167
Bretylium, 475–477
  administration of, 476
  catecholamine hypersensitivity due to, 476–477
  contraindications to, 476–477
  dose of, 476